Praise for Psychiatric Interviewing, 3rd Edition

ADVANCE PRAISE FOR THE THIRD EDITION

"Readers of this book, whether beginning students or wizened clinicians with decades of experience, will find much that is innovative. . . . . I had the pleasure of running across Shea's interviewing strategy for uncovering suicidal ideation, behaviors, and intent (the Chronological Assessment of Suicide Events – CASE Approach) years ago. . . . . In this book readers will find a remarkably compelling and practical introduction to the effective use of the CASE Approach. Shea's subsequent video demonstrations of the CASE Approach are, in my opinion, unparalleled in the history of mental health training. I have never seen such great teaching videos on eliciting suicidal ideation. They are a treasure, and I believe that many lives will be saved by those lucky enough to view them."

> From the Foreword by Jan Fawcett, M.D.
> Professor of Psychiatry, University of New Mexico
> Recipient of Lifetime Achievement Awards
>   from both the American Association of Suicidology
>   and the American Foundation for Suicide Prevention

"Dr. Shea has done the impossible – written a text that works for bachelors, masters, and doctoral level social workers. Throughout the text, Shea integrates cultural humility, the client perspective, clinical wisdom, and the best that research has to offer. His writing is authoritative yet accessible. The accompanying videos are the most amazing instructional videos I've ever seen – they include mini-lectures, video of an actual client interview, and wondrously realistic role-plays (which invite you into the mind of a master) and speak directly to the content in the text. Instructors will treasure the text because it covers everything that needs to be covered and is presented in a way that inspires the reader to learn the material. I hate to say it, but a medical doctor has written the best social work interviewing text on the market. I hope this text gets adopted in every school of social work."

> Jonathan B Singer, Ph.D., LCSW Associate Professor
> School of Social Work, Loyola University Chicago
> Founder and host, Social Work Podcast

"Insightful, wonderfully practical, and surprisingly comprehensive, Shea's chapter on culturally sensitive interviewing in *Psychiatric Interviewing: the Art of Understanding, 3rd Edition* sets a new bar on effective literature on multiculturalism. Shea not only eloquently delineates important cross-cultural principles for students – while modeling numerous immediately useful questions and strategies – he provides examples of clinician/client dialogue in which the student can actually see the interviewer gracefully transforming awkward cultural disconnects. I've never seen anything quite like it in the clinical literature. Simply superb! PS: Year after year my master level counseling students have raved – and I mean raved – about Shea's textbook, and this Third Edition looks to be even better! I know of no book that better prepares a student for actual clinical practice."

> Dottie R. Morris, Ph.D.
> Chief Officer of Diversity and Multiculturalism, Keene State College
> Former Director of Student Affairs for the Clinical Mental Health Counseling
>   Program at Antioch University New England

"In this highly readable and engaging book, psychiatric nursing students learn the principles and techniques of conducting fluid and individualized assessments. We have been using the second edition of this book for over a decade at our school, and it has been an indispensable resource for both our faculty and our students. This 3rd Edition has been revised and expanded including fascinating new chapters on topics such as wellness, motivational interviewing, cultural diversity and how to collaboratively talk with patients about their medications. Many of the chapters are enriched with engrossing video demonstrations (be sure to watch the video on eliciting suicidal ideation, it brings the practical art of suicide assessment alive). I can't recommend this book enough. It will infuse passion and curiosity in your students. It will be a resource they will return to for learning for years to come."

Palmira Brouwer R.N. BscN, MA (psychology)
Faculty Department of Psychiatric Nursing
Douglas College, B.C. Canada

"Both of the previous editions of Dr. Shea's book have anchored Bryn Mawr's advanced clinical social work practice curriculum for a generation of our master's degree students. This third edition is a masterful integration of text and video instruction. Indeed, it represents a pedagogical leap, in which Dr. Shea brings the beginning and advanced student into the mysteries of the first encounter with his characteristic warmth, compassion, and wisdom that has so enthralled our students over the years. Only now, we can see it, not only in engaging text, but in amazingly effective video instruction and interview demonstrations, that bring to life the clinical encounter. Shea models for students the core interviewing skills, the advanced practice competencies, and the guiding ethical behaviors that are the foundations of all helping professions. With the publication of this book, I personally believe that Dr. Shea has cemented his standing as one of the most influential mental health educators of the 21st Century."

James A. Martin, Ph.D., LICSW
Colonel, U.S. Army (Retired)
Professor of Social Work and Social Research
Bryn Mawr College, Bryn Mawr, PA.

Here is a book I would enthusiastically recommend to all graduate students in psychology on the art of clinical interviewing and to all faculty who teach such courses. Shea's book provides a highly satisfying introduction to the core principles of clinical interviewing but much more. It also, with a refreshingly informal writing style, provides a sophisticated journey into advanced interviewing techniques and strategies as needed in the real world of clinical practice. Even the most experienced clinician will enjoy and learn much from this text. I don't believe I've ever seen an author capture the pain of patients dealing with serious disorders such as major depression, schizophrenia, and bipolar disorder with such sensitivity and compassion, while transforming this understanding into easily learned questions and techniques for use in actual practice. Combine this sensitive and comprehensive approach with Shea's skillful use of advanced technology (over 7 hours of streaming video modules and interviewing demonstrations) and you have a book, whose shelf-life will be measured not in years, but decades."

Lawrence A. Welkowitz, Ph.D.
Co-Editor of *Asperger's Syndrome: Intervening in Clinics, Schools and Communities*
Principle Investigator: Use of iPad Assisted Learning for Autism

Interviewing skills are not only indispensable, they are the rate-limiting factor in providing quality care. In the 3rd Edition of Dr. Shea's classic text, we now have an indispensable book to match the training needs of our psychiatric residents (indeed, of our trainees in any mental health discipline). As a forensic specialist, let me focus on Shea's chapters devoted to exploring suicidal ideation and violent ideation. Using Shea's interviewing principles, especially the Chronological Assessment of Suicide Events (CASE Approach), clinicians will be able to render the best possible care, often exceeding the standard of care. The skills delineated within these chapters should, in my opinion, be taught in all psychiatric residency programs. Every resident should buy and read this entire book before taking his or her first night of call. Every resident. In fact, I recommend reading it twice. I almost forgot to mention, Shea's extraordinary streaming videos will thrust this book to the forefront of web-based learning. Trust me on this point. They're fabulous.

> James L. Knoll, IV, M.D.
> Professor of Psychiatry
> Director of Forensic Psychiatry
> SUNY Upstate Medical University

"While reading the pages of this wonderful book, I kept wishing I could have held this book in my hands when I was a psychiatric resident. Dr. Shea's stand-out chapters on personality dysfunction (from DSM-5 differential diagnosis to the effective application of object relations and self psychology) are suffused with an understanding of the pain experienced by patients with personality disorders, and the confusion and intensity they can stir-up in the interviewer. Using Shea's techniques, clinicians will feel competent at steering through the most turbulent and treacherous of interpersonal eddies in order to connect with and help these patients. Readers of this highly engaging, ground-breaking book, and viewers of its over 7 hours of stunning videos, will be able to become the clinicians their patients deserve, the ones they were meant to be."

> Laura Miller, M.D.
> Professor of Psychiatry, Loyola University Stritch School of Medicine
> Medical Director of Women's Mental Health at Edward Hines Jr. VA Hospital

"This book is a gift – an extraordinary gift – to the field of clinical social work. Its sophisticated yet delightfully readable text and its brilliantly conceived and executed streaming video, combine to create the single most practical and enjoyable clinical textbook that I've ever read. Unlike other books that focus only on *what* needs to be addressed, Dr. Shea teaches the *how* and he does so with unmatched insight, clarifying intensity, a self-effacing humor, a contagious warmth, and a genuine sense of mission. The wealth of comprehensive topics explored, ranging from DSM-5 differential diagnosis to uncovering domestic violence and suicide, sensitively exploring psychotic process, and advanced diversity counseling, make this more than a book or a course – it is a virtual traineeship. It provides social workers and other mental health professional with an opportunity to learn from one of the greatest innovators in the history of clinical interviewing. You'll never have a book that you highlight more. In fact, it's probably simpler to highlight what you don't want to emphasize. You'll save ink."

> Amanda Rowan, Licensed Clinical Social Worker
> Founder, Executive Director, Therapist Development Center

PRAISE FOR PREVIOUS EDITIONS OF PSYCHIATRIC INTERVIEWING: THE ART OF UNDERSTANDING

PRAISE FROM THE REVIEWERS

**10 out of 10 rating on Doody's Score for,
"Is this a worthwhile contribution to the field?"**

"Using a rich palette of information from various fields, including psychoanalysis, behavioral psychology, and sociology, the author writes about the entire interview, and reveals the rich interaction that begins even before the first words are spoken. . . . . It is no surprise that this book has been well received by major psychiatric journals. However, it is always a pleasant surprise to find an engaging book that is both theoretically sound and clinically indispensable."

Doody's Book Reviewer

"This is a book I wish I could have written. . . . . can be read with interest by expert and novice alike."

Clinical Psychology Review
Arthur Weins, Ph.D.

"Rich in information, wisdom, humor, and charm, this book teaches not only interviewing skills but also the attitudes and behaviors that underpin the therapeutic personality and process."

American Journal of Psychiatry

"Provides a well-balanced synthesis of many approaches from various schools of psychiatry, psychology, and counseling. . . . enjoyable and stimulating to read. . . . . written with eloquence and humor."

British Journal of Psychiatry

"Intensely practical, with a riveting chapter on the assessment of risk for suicide and homicide. . . . . Reviewers have a way of telling you that a good book is essential for every psychiatric library. This time it really is true."

Canadian Journal of Psychiatry

PRAISE FROM THE REVIEWERS *(continued)*

Both previous editions chosen for the Brandon/Hill List
as one of the most important psychiatric books
for medical libraries to procure!

"Shea's book, which is now in its second edition, is a valuable counter-weight to the 'one size fits all' approach to interviewing and eliciting data. It is an invaluable book for those training in psychiatry or other mental health professions and indeed for practicing clinicians."

Australian and New Zealand Journal of Psychiatry

"Rich with sensitive observations and practical suggestions and enlivened by frequent examples of diagnostic interviewing."

Transactional Analysis Journal

"A marvelous text on an aspect of psychiatry that often does not receive as much attention as it deserves."

Hospital and Community Psychiatry

PRAISE FROM THE EXPERTS AND FACULTY FOR PREVIOUS EDITIONS

"Year in and year out, one of the most popular, if not most popular, required textbooks for our master level students in counseling. Superbly practical yet filled with a sense of compassion."

Judi Durham, A.P.R.N., M.A., C.S.
Senior Associate Faculty
Antioch University New England

"For mental health professionals this book is a must read. The writing style is fluid, fast paced, and stimulating. I recommend it without hesitation to all nurses and nursing students."

Joan Kyes, M.S.N.
Author of *Psychiatric Concepts in Nursing*

"Practical, sensitive, and comprehensive. . . . . The chapter on handling resistance and awkward questions provides a wealth of practical suggestions for students in mental health from social work to psychiatry."

Carol Anderson, M.S.W., Ph.D.
Author of *Mastering Resistance – A Practical Guide to Family Therapy*

PSYCHIATRIC INTERVIEWING

THIRD EDITION

PSYCHIATRIC INTERVIEWING

THE ART OF UNDERSTANDING

Shawn Christopher Shea MD
Director, Training Institute for Suicide Assessment
and Clinical Interviewing (TISA)
(www.sucideassessment.com)
Private Practice
Keene, New Hampshire, USA

Videography and Post-Production of Integrated Video
by Jeff Kolter
Productions

Artwork for Chapter Facing Pages
by Debra Stevens
and
Meg Maloney

For additional online content visit
http://expertconsult.inkling.com

ELSEVIER   Edinburgh   London   New York   Oxford   Philadelphia   St Louis   Sydney   Toronto   2017

ELSEVIER

ISBN: 978-1-4377-1698-6
E-ISBN: 978-1-4377-3782-0
Inkling ISBN: 978-0-323-32901-9

Dr. Shea retains copyright of chapter opener images.

Notices

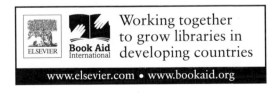

Printed in India
Last digit is the print number: 10

Content Strategist: Charlotta Kryhl
Content Development Specialist: Sharon Nash
Project Manager: Julie Taylor
Design: Miles Hitchen
Illustration Manager: Brett MacNaughton
Marketing Manager: Rachael Pignotti

Dedication

To the memory of my father who showed me the door of creativity,

In fondest memory of my mother who urged me

to open it,

And to Susan, Brenden, and Ryan who were waiting

on the other side.

and

To Juan Mezzich, MD, PhD

my first and most important mentor,

whose unending support and pioneering work

towards Person-Centered Psychiatry and Medicine

will leave a legacy of healing and hope

for untold numbers of people

for many decades to come.

Foreword

It has been my privilege to train and supervise young mental health professionals from many disciplines for over 50 years. I can say that doing so has been one of the great joys of my life. I can also safely say that you are holding in your hands one of the most remarkable books I have had the pleasure to read in all of those years. Enormously practical, elegant in execution and delightfully fun to read, every page holds clinical wisdom.

Shea has an almost uncanny ability to genuinely perceive the complexities of clinical interviewing, while creating frameworks that illuminate, clarify, and simplify those complexities so that young clinicians can actually apply them. And he accomplishes this challenging task with a self-effacing humor and a refreshing sense of compassion that combine to shed a vibrant brilliance on our art. I can think of no better first book for any trainee in mental health, for it is not only, in my opinion, an unsurpassed book about how to interview, it is a book about why we interview. It is a book that captures the wonderment of our work and the soul of our mission.

It is also my opinion, that you are holding in your hands the textbook of tomorrow, today. Shea's graceful integration of over 7.5 hours of streaming video throughout the text provides every psychiatric resident and graduate student the chance to see a truly talented interviewer at work undertaking tasks as complex as exploring sensitive and taboo topics to uncovering suicidal ideation and intent. If this were not enough, the viewer also gets the chance to watch and hear Shea, one of the most dynamic speakers in our field today, discuss these interview excerpts, powerfully consolidating what the student has just read in the text while providing new nuances and insights not even mentioned in the text. It is a stunning wedding of innovative educational theory with today's revolutionary technology. As the student enters their clinical rotations, and ultimately, as they leave their residency and graduate programs to secure their first jobs, they can return to these videos, stream them on their laptops, tablets, and smart phones, wherever they are and whenever they choose. The video illustrations of the book will always be available to them in the palm of their hands.

Readers of this book, whether beginning students or wizened clinicians with decades of experience, will find much that is innovative. Indeed, Shea's innovations, in my opinion, have been pivotal in shaping how interviewing is both done and taught across disciplines. I had the pleasure of running across Shea's interviewing strategy for uncovering suicidal ideation, behaviors, and intent (the Chronological Assessment of Suicide Events – CASE Approach) years ago and promptly invited him to write an article about it in the *Psychiatric Annals*.

As the years have passed, the CASE Approach has become one of the most respected approaches for eliciting suicidal ideation in the world, as reflected by its being chosen as a recommended strategy by the Zero Suicide Initiative and its selection for the Best

Practices Registry from the Suicide Prevention and Resource Center (SPRC). In this book readers will find a remarkably compelling and practical introduction to the effective use of the CASE Approach. Shea's subsequent video demonstrations of the CASE Approach are, in my opinion, unparalleled in the history of mental health training. I have never seen such great teaching videos on eliciting suicidal ideation. They are a treasure, and I believe that many lives will be saved by those lucky enough to view them.

I was pleased to see that Shea's numerous other innovations are equally expertly reviewed and updated in this edition. His internationally respected supervision system for helping trainees to create fluid and naturalistic interviews, known in the clinical interviewing literature as the study of facilics, is beautifully updated in this edition, including an interactive web program. An entire chapter has been dedicated to the topic of "validity techniques," a field of study first delineated by Shea years ago for helping patients to share sensitive and taboo material such as incest, domestic violence, and substance abuse. And, as a bonus, for any clinicians who prescribe medications, there is a chapter on Shea's Medication Interest Model (MIM) as the model is applied to psychiatric medications. If not familiar with the MIM, it is a collaborative model of talking with patients about their medications. In this chapter, the reader will find over 40 specific interviewing techniques that help patients make wise decisions about whether or not medications are a good choice for them and can help clinicians to effectively motivate patient interest in using those medications once chosen. I have been intimately involved in the study and use of medications for decades, and I was fascinated by the principles and techniques delineated in this chapter. I have a feeling that the MIM will someday be as important in the field of improving medication adherence as the CASE Approach has become to uncovering suicidal ideation.

On a final note, Shea is not only a great innovator – he is a wonderful explicator of the ideas and concepts of others. In short, he is a natural born teacher. His eloquent mastery of language and his well-timed wit brings the work of others to life for readers. Two examples will demonstrate my point. Shea has had nothing to do with the development of motivational interviewing (Chapter 22), yet his chapter on motivational interviewing is a remarkably succinct and penetrating introduction to its use. I would recommend it to anyone as a first introduction to the subject. Likewise, Shea's introduction to object relations and self psychology (Chapter 15) is a wonderful monograph on the topic. He brings to life some of the traditionally most difficult concepts in the field of psychodynamic therapy. I feel quite confident that his chapter will delight and fascinate new trainees, who I find have a genuine hunger for learning more about psychodynamic thought. Such students will be hard pressed to find a more practical and compelling introduction to the topic.

In closing, I have always been a believer that every minute counts in this life. I believe that if one values every moment, one essentially stretches life. I close with this thought because I realize that time is at a great premium in our contemporary lives. I just want to reassure any faculty that require this book, and any students that read it, that every minute spent in its pages will be worth it. Every minute will count. And every minute will not only benefit you but all the future patients that your caring will touch.

Jan Fawcett, M.D.

Foreword to the 2nd Edition

This beautiful and immensely useful book is a great gift. It should stand as the best starting clinical text for all mental health professionals, because the ultimate success of our clinical interventions is determined directly by the information we must sensitively garner from the interview. Einstein remarked that in early sciences, examples serve better than concepts; indeed, they form the earliest concepts. Shea introduces the beginning clinician to the work by means of concrete situations and particular examples of actual clinical dialogue. There could be no sounder starting point. Later, I predict, beginning clinicians, and many experienced ones, too, will return to this book the way people return to the books that they find deepest and most evocative, reading a few pages at a time, to be savored and enjoyed, so its wisdom enters their bones.

The book starts where all interviewers start, in the dark, knowing that they must gently feel their way. This is a necessity not only because valid psychological data are extremely difficult to secure but also because our first job is to establish an effective relationship to carry on the work. In other words, Shea takes the interview with deep seriousness, which is the same as taking the relationship seriously and the importance of uncovering valid findings.

On the other hand, in a particularly refreshing light, Shea does not take himself too seriously. He draws our attention to his own mistakes, reflecting on them with a gentle humor, demonstrating directly what can be learned from them. No better model for learning could be demonstrated for the beginning, and often frightened student, allowing the student immediately to feel more at home both with himself or herself and with the author. Moreover, Shea knows that an interview and a relationship can be at cross purposes, so he doesn't want patients to feel that they are "being interviewed," but rather that they are "talking with someone." He states his goal early, "to gather the necessary clinical information efficiently while powerfully engaging the patient."

The focus is on assessment, not ongoing psychotherapy, but there is much here for all psychotherapists. For instance, throughout the book Shea emphasizes the point that a well-crafted initial interview, although it is not psychotherapy, is always therapeutic. He proceeds to demonstrate with practical illustrations, including an entire transcript of one of his own interviews, exactly how to accomplish this complex task.

With "facilics," his innovative set of principles for studying and understanding the methods by which clinicians structure interviews and manage their time, he provides a wonderfully practical method for gracefully navigating the tight time constraints of modern clinical practice. He manages to artfully wed the process of data gathering with compassionate listening. He furthers this integrative task by highlighting the many practical interviewing techniques that other authors have developed from a myriad of disciplines, including analytic, interpersonal, self-psychological, cognitive–behavioral, and existential schools of thought. In short, this is a sophisticated, deeply informed work, the hands-on emphasis of which does not belie a profound understanding.

Too often, clinical discussions have a pretentious, high theoretical cast, whether of putative brain processes or unconscious ones. In our mission to help others, unlike theoretical physicists, it is not our main goal to penetrate the secrets of nature and society. Rather, in clinical care, we are more like engineers whose task is to construct the practical bridges and strong foundations that foster the healing process. We need to get from A to B, from meeting to connecting, from guessing to surmising, from sensing to feeling deeply. Shea breaks down the steps, makes the distinctions, and lets us build our own working methods from the various examples he provides. We are to practice techniques and create new ones, until a wide range of possible actions becomes second nature to us all.

This is where clinical work must begin. We could not be in better hands.

Leston Havens, M.D.

Preface

The purpose of life is to serve and to show compassion and the will to help others. Only then have we ourselves become true human beings.

Albert Schweitzer

It is with great pleasure and excitement that I sit down to write the preface for the 3rd edition of this book. Much has changed in our field since the publication of the 2nd edition 18 years ago – some good, some not so good. My pleasure arises, to a great extent, from the fact that the cornerstone principles of the first two editions – sensitivity and compassion – still resonate in our field today; indeed, in the age of managed care, increasing time pressures, and the advent of the electronic health record, they may play an even more important role as guideposts than ever before. Put more bluntly, many extraneous factors have been introduced into the environment of everyday clinical care that, in my opinion, make it harder to be a sensitive listener today than has been the case in all previous generations.

In this regard, the one over-arching goal of this textbook is to prepare the trainee to function effectively, and with compassion, in the hectic worlds of community mental health centers, inpatient units, emergency rooms, university counseling centers, and private practices. To accomplish this task, today's students require the acquisition of a series of advancing interviewing skills that must be developed sequentially throughout the years of their residency and graduate training (indeed, as an ongoing education throughout the rest of their careers). In these pages I have made my best effort to address these progressive steps in a fashion that makes their acquisition both more pleasant and more effective. I have tried to create a book that, in essence, grows with the trainee through the years of their residency or graduate program and beyond.

Moreover, in an exciting fashion, the field of clinical interviewing has exploded with innovations since the 2nd edition of this book, from the widespread acceptance of motivational interviewing to the numerous advances made with regard to culturally adaptive interviewing and the increased emphasis on wellness interviewing. Towards capturing this excitement, I have tried to keep intact whatever elements of the 2nd edition reader feedback has suggested were most effective, while approaching the topics of each chapter with the same informal writing style that readers seemed to enjoy so much in the previous editions. As they say, don't fix what isn't broken. In addition, as with the 2nd edition, I have given careful attention to presenting the complexities and nuances of each topic with the in-depth sophistication they warrant when training psychiatric residents and graduate students in clinical psychology, psychiatric social work, psychiatric nursing, and counseling.

Concerning the sequential skills that new trainees must master, first and foremost, trainees – no matter what their disciplines – must, in their initial course on clinical interviewing, acquire a set of core interviewing skills of a surprisingly complex nature. More specifically, the trainees must acquire and practice skills ranging from topics as diverse as conveying empathy, nurturing engagement, and sensitively structuring interviews, to effectively uncovering client wellness and strengths, as well as delicately uncovering the truth about sensitive and taboo topics. All of these skills must be learned while simultaneously addressing the interplay between these skills and the complex context of cultural diversity, nonverbal communication, and the interface between the interview and collaborative treatment planning. No small task for an introductory course! Part I of this text – "Clinical Interviewing: the Principles Behind the Art" – was designed to meet this daunting task head-on with individual chapters addressing all of these topics.

And, here is where things get really exciting. As I mentioned earlier, many things have changed since the 2nd edition of this book. A truly great advance has been the ability to stream video through the web. This has revolutionized how we can go about the process of training clinicians in interviewing (as well as psychotherapy). Throughout Part I (as well as Parts II and III) more than 7.5 hours of streaming video have been *integrated directly into the text of the book*. Now readers become viewers. After learning about specific techniques, with the mere click of a link, the reader of the accompanying e-book can view streaming video in which I am not only consolidating and elaborating on what was just read, but I am demonstrating the exact same interviewing techniques with annotated video. Moreover, as Jan Fawcett noted in his Foreword to the 3rd edition: "As the student enters their clinical rotations, and ultimately, as they leave their residency and graduate programs to secure their first jobs, they can return to these videos, stream them on their laptops, tablets, and smart phones wherever they are and whenever they choose. The video illustrations of the book will always be available to them in the palm of their hands."

In Step 2 of their maturation as clinical interviewers, after acquiring their core interviewing skills, the trainee will encounter a new, and particularly challenging set of skills to master. Specifically the graduate student or psychiatric resident must learn how to adapt their newly acquired core interviewing skills for use in the real world of community mental health centers, inpatient units, college counseling centers, private practices, and emergency departments. In these settings, the trainees, during their clinical rotations and internships (and subsequently in their years of employment) will encounter patients suffering from a variety of painful disorders ranging from major depressive disorders, substance use disorders, post-traumatic stress disorder (PTSD), and obsessive–compulsive disorder, to bipolar disorder and schizophrenia.

This requires that a clinical interviewer understand the phenomenology and exquisite pain with which these psychopathological symptoms present themselves to each unique patient (as well as the pain of the family members who love the patient). Moreover, it is not enough to have an introduction to this phenomenology. One must understand, in a particularly sophisticated fashion, the person beneath these symptoms and be able to sensitively explore the experience and meaning of these symptoms, for they are manifested uniquely by each person and the cultural context that shapes that person.

Part II of this textbook – "The Interview and Psychopathology: From Differential Diagnosis to Understanding" – attempts to address these critical concerns. The major diagnostic categories are approached with chapters dedicated not only to sensitively performing a differential diagnosis (in which I provide numerous sample questions and illustrative interview excerpts) but with separate chapters that illustrate various questions and strategies that will take the reader into an even deeper understanding of the pain and symptoms of the person before them. You will note that careful attention is given to cultural and familial factors so that clinicians – who are interviewing a patient who comes from a different culture than the interviewer's culture – will not mistake cultural differences as psychopathology or, on the other side of the coin, miss disorders that are unique to the patient's cultural heritage.

Note that the 3rd edition of this book is specifically designed to allow faculty to literally create the textbook that he or she feels is best suited for the course being taught. Thus some faculty will feel that there is time within their trainees' first course – on core interviewing skills – to assign these chapters on the interface between the clinical interview and psychopathology. Other faculty may decide these chapters are best suited for a separate course on psychopathology. Still others may decide that one or two of the chapters are invaluable in the first course on clinical interviewing so as to ensure that the students immediately understand that their core interviewing skill will be implemented with patients in great pain and with varying disorders.

The third graduated step in the trainee's development of interviewing skills is challenging, indeed, sometimes legitimately intimidating. The student must learn how to sensitively elicit suicidal ideation and intent as well as violent ideation and intent. Many trainees also find the mental status to be confusing and awkward to implement gracefully. These specific tasks are of such importance that separate chapters are dedicated to each of them in Part III of the book – "Mastering Complex Interviewing Tasks Demanded in Everyday Practice."

The expanded chapter on suicide assessment in this 3rd edition includes some of my very favorite pages in the book, which I hope you will enjoy as well. It is an introduction to the interviewing strategy for uncovering suicidal ideation, planning, intent, and actions known in the clinical literature as the Chronological Assessment of Suicide Events (the CASE Approach). It has been one of my greatest satisfactions to see the interest and adoption – both nationally and internationally – of the CASE Approach, which was first delineated in the 2nd edition of the book. In this expanded chapter, I have an opportunity to not only describe the updated version of the CASE Approach (for we are always improving it) but to demonstrate, via streaming video, the interview strategy in its entirety, dissecting its nuanced variations as the clinical risk of suicide presents in varying degrees of severity.

Finally, in a trainee's fourth evolution in clinical interviewing skills, during his or her graduate program or psychiatric residency, the trainee will need to learn advanced skill sets, which are addressed in Part IV, "Advanced Interviewing and Specialized Topics." As noted earlier in this Preface, I have tried to create a book that will grow with the psychiatric resident or graduate student as they progress through their training, while providing a reference that they will pull off the shelf in their subsequent careers as a mental health professional.

The bonus chapters in Part IV are essentially designed as independent monographs regarding each of these topics. I would like to draw the reader's attention to two of these advanced chapters that I think, paradoxically, despite their advanced nature in the sense of requiring a pretty good observing ego to employ their techniques, faculty might find very enticing to include as closing bonus chapters in an introductory course on clinical interviewing. Students really appreciate the usefulness of the topics.

The chapter, "Transforming Anger, Confrontation, and Other Points of Disengagement" covers all of the types of awkward moments that beginning clinicians dread such as patients confronting them on their inexperience, asking personal questions such as, "Do you believe in God?" or "Have you ever had an affair?", or a delusional patient asking, "Do you believe me?" I tried to provide an easily understood framework for handling such questions as well as providing the beginning student with possible answers and illustrative dialogue of clinicians responding gracefully to such moments.

I also think that faculty may find that some of their beginning students will be ready to enjoy the sophisticated introduction to culturally adaptive interviewing to be seen in the chapter, "Culturally Adaptive Interviewing: The Challenging Art of Exploring Culture, Worldview, and Spirituality." I have attempted to create a comprehensive "monograph" that will allow a student – through the reading of a single chapter – to come away with a sound introduction to this fascinating, and critically important, area. I have tried to not only describe what needs to be done during culturally competent interviewing, but I have also tried to give compelling examples of dialogue that demonstrate culturally adaptive interviewing.

Two truly advanced topics, dear to my heart and closely related to each other, also appear as bonus chapters. In this 3rd edition, I finally had a chance to do something that I have wanted to do for years – attempt to provide, in a single chapter, a reasonably sound introduction to the highly innovative work of Miller and Rollnick – Motivational Interviewing (MI). As one would expect in this book, I focus on how the principles of MI can be employed in the initial interview.

It was also a pleasure to be able to introduce to all mental health providers, especially all those who prescribe medications (from psychiatrists to psychiatric nurse clinicians, psychiatric physician assistants, and psychiatric clinical pharmacists) the collaborative and motivational model known as the Medication Interest Model (MIM), which addresses how we can go about the complex process of talking with our patients about the possible use of medications in a truly collaborative fashion. The MIM was first introduced for use in general medicine in my book *Improving Medication Adherence: How to Talk with Patients About Their Medications* as applied to medications being used to treat all disease states from diabetes, hypertension, and congestive heart failure to depression and PTSD. In our bonus chapter in Part IV of this book, I have been able to create a fast-reading monograph on how the collaborative interviewing principles and techniques of the MIM can be specifically applied with patients considering psychiatric medications. I hope this monograph on the psychiatric application of the MIM will help many clinicians to help many patients for many decades to come.

For faculty readers some particularly rich new material has been added in the Appendices. In Appendix IVB the reader will find four popular, unabridged articles from the *Psychiatric Clinics of North America* describing innovative educational strategies and approaches. The articles examine challenges such as designing effective interviewing training programs for psychiatric residents and graduate students and teaching clinical interviewing skills using role-playing from conveying empathy to eliciting suicidal ideation and intent. Separate articles describe, in detail, the real-world application of educational advances such as macrotraining and scripted group role-playing (SGRP).

In addition, over the years I have been repeatedly asked by faculty and interviewing mentors whether there was a readily available resource for quickly teaching both trainees and instructors the schematics to be used in facilic supervision. With the production of this book, readers can now enjoy an easy to use interactive computer module online to do so whenever they choose.

I hope that the reader enjoys this book as much as I enjoyed expanding, revising, and adding video to it. In the final analysis, interviewing should be fun. I think it is important to emphasize that this book does not pretend to show the "correct" way of interviewing, because there is no correct way. Instead, I offer suggestions that will provide the reader with the principles to develop his or her own creative style of interviewing, always flexibly matching the interview to the needs of the patient, not to the dictates of a school of thought.

In closing, this is a book about knowledge – knowledge applied to the art of healing. In the last analysis, as students of this art, it will always remain our great privilege to ensure that the knowledge of our minds is guided by the compassion of our hearts and the wisdom of our souls. As Albert Schweitzer so elegantly stated in our epigram, it is through this art and through our desire to help others that we ultimately find ourselves.

Shawn Christopher Shea, M.D.
July 24, 2016

A Few Stylistic Notes From the Author

Please note that the names of all the patients have been changed. In addition, at times, distinguishing characteristics or facts have been altered to further protect their identity without altering the clinical essence of our interaction.

Also note that, historically, various names have been used to refer to the people we are helping in our therapeutic work including client, patient, consumer, and various other descriptors. To me there are pros and cons to each of these, and I could genuinely make convincing arguments for the use of any of them. I originally began the manuscript by randomly switching such descriptors, but I found that readers then tried to ascribe reasons to why I used each in a particular passage (there were no reasons for I was doing so randomly!).

It became evident that to avoid this type of misunderstanding and for the sake of consistency and ease of reading, I should choose one of them. I chose to use the word "patient" for many readers – at some point in their careers – will be working with people in settings such as hospital units or emergency rooms where, indeed, the term "patient" is viewed as normative. This is not to suggest that the word "patient" is superior or correct, it is merely a way of securing consistency in the text.

With regard to gender identifying words in the text, I also take that topic seriously, for I recognize that language counts. For instance, some experts prefer the word Latino, others the word Latino/a, and still others the word Latina/o (which is my personal preference). I can't pass judgment on any of these descriptors as long as the writers are trying their best to be cognizant of the importance of gender in their writing. I can't assure my readers that we will always agree on my choices, but I can assure the reader that I made my choices with a genuine spirit of addressing gender fairly and in a fashion consistent with the highest current values of our society.

Acknowledgments

I would like to begin by expressing my deep gratitude, once again, to all those who helped with the first and second editions of this book.

With regards to the third edition, many colleagues, clinicians, and patients have coalesced over the years into wonderfully evanescent teams of people whose knowledge, experiences, and bits of self have found themselves into the pages of this book. I can't thank enough all of the clinicians – whom I have had the pleasure to meet during my clinical interviewing workshops – who have shared their interviewing tips with me and, oftentimes, subsequently made contributions to the "Interviewing Tip of the Month" on our website for the Training Institute for Suicide Assessment and Clinical Interviewing (www.sucideassessment.com). Your enthusiasm for clinical interviewing, as well as your clinical wisdom, help to animate the pages of this book.

Regarding my years at Dartmouth spent developing the Dartmouth Interviewing Mentorship Program for the Department of Psychiatry, a special thanks goes to the core members of the so-called "Phantom Gate Club" – Ron Green, MD, Bruce Baker, PhD, Christine Barney, MD, Stephen Cole, PhD and Mark Reed, MD. Your feedback, creative ideas, interviewing expertise, and friendship are reflected throughout the chapters in this third edition.

A special thanks to three wonderful clinicians who provided outstanding input on the chapter entitled, "Culturally Adaptive Interviewing: The Challenging Art of Exploring Culture, Worldview, and Spirituality". Dottie Morris, PhD provided a detailed review of the entire chapter, supplying her insights from her years of work in the field of diversity and multiculturation. I would also like to thank Edward Hamaty, DO for his sensitive review of the section exploring the needs of the LGBT community as well as his cherished friendship since our meeting at Lee Hospital for a summer work program way back in 1970. And thanks to Patsy "PJ" Taucer, M.Ed, a Certified Medical Interpreter, for her hands-on input on the effective role of interpretation. Couldn't have done it without you guys.

With regards to the ongoing development and support of the Chronological Assessment of Suicide Events (CASE Approach) special thanks goes to the never-ending, always appreciated, support of Skip Simpson, JD, as well as his deeply appreciated friendship. Thanks "Skipper". More than anyone, you have taught me the meaning of mission. In addition, both Tom Ellis, PhD and David Jobes, PhD have been staunch advocates of the CASE Approach from its very inception. A very special thanks goes to Donna Amundson, L.C.S.W., whose support, input on training techniques, and unwavering efforts in training clinicians in the CASE Approach has undoubtedly saved many lives. Her selfless efforts are a part of the soul of the CASE Approach and always will be.

Moving on to production support, I want to give much deserved recognition and thanks to the team at Elsevier. In all of my years, this team has been the most talented, professional, and mission-oriented publication team that I have ever encountered. As our "little project" grew and grew, they provided their unequivocal support and patience at every step. I can't thank my editor, Charlotta Kryhl enough. Lotta's encouraging phone-calls with me and her work behind the scenes is the only reason this book appears in its present innovative format and with its many hours of integrated video. Thanks goes to Sharon Nash, content development specialist, who, with skill and savvy, has steadfastly kept us all on track and schedule, no mean accomplishment with regards to myself I might add. Thanks to Julie Taylor and her entire staff for the best production and "look" I have ever had in a book. Finally, Marcela Holmes, my copyeditor. I may be biased, but she's got to be one of the best in the business and has been a joy with whom to work. The book is a much better read for her efforts. Hopefully I'll someday join you all for a round of bitters in a London pub – on me of course.

I would also like to add something about the publisher itself, Elsevier. From the very start they have been believers in the mission of this book. Their genuine belief in its mission was most strikingly reflected in their choosing a remarkably low price for the book – without any hesitation on their part – in an effort to make sure the book would get into the hands of the clinicians who can transform its words into healing and hope. What an extraordinarily refreshing attitude in a world so often consumed by greed and self-interest. Kudos to a great company. Many lives will be changed because of your integrity.

As I come to the production team of our integrated video, I feel a sense of great grati-tude and warmth. Jeff Kolter of Jeff Kolter Productions is a remarkable human being, who put over 500 hours into the project, a large amount of this time for gratis because of his belief in its mission. He is responsible for all videography as well as all post-production and editing. My work with Jeff has been some of the most enjoyable collabo-ration of my life. He brought the didactics and patient interviews to life. And what a gorgeous green screen! Jeff, I'll always remember our times in your studio and dinners at the Co-op. Many thanks to others involved in producing our integrated video includ-ing Xavier Brown and Susan Shea for their creative input, support, and recommendations. A special thanks also goes to both my wonderful role-players and, especially, to my patient for her permission to use the video of her interview with myself.

Another artist warranting much thanks is Debi Stevens. Debi provided the lovely, and sometimes haunting, artwork that forms the facing pages of the many new chapters that appeared in the third edition. Debi, I'll fondly remember our hours at Brewbaker's Café brainstorming and reviewing your remarkable creations.

A thanks goes to the delightful staff of the Susan Colgate Cleveland Library/Learning Center at the Colby-Sawyer College in New London, New Hampshire for their support over the last three years of the project. In particular, I would like to thank Noelle Bassi, Beth Krajewski, Erica Webb, and Kelli Bogan for all of their support as I busily wrote and edited the last half of the book in your beautiful library. You made "the trip" a fun one.

As my acknowledgments draw to a close, I have saved some of the most important for last. I would like to thank Jan Fawcett, MD, for his supportive phone calls and his much appreciated comments and suggestions for the mood disorder chapters in particular. But, most of all, I would like to thank Jan for his truly lovely Foreword. It has been an honor to get to know you better. I believe that anyone who has met you, comes to know that you are not only a gifted clinician and innovator, but a truly good human being. The world is a softer place because you are in it. Many thanks.

Finally, an enormous amount of gratitude to my wife and the Co-Director of the Training Institute for Suicide Assessment and Clinical Interviewing (TISA). Susan, thanks so much for all of your outstanding editorial suggestions on the text as well as the remarkable creative inputs you had on this project. Moreover, for your support over the six years of this project - that required much sacrifice on your part – I will forever be grateful. You are not only the love of my life, you are the keeper of my soul.

Shawn Christopher Shea, MD

Contents

Video Table of Contents

Part I

Clinical Interviewing:
The Principles Behind the Art

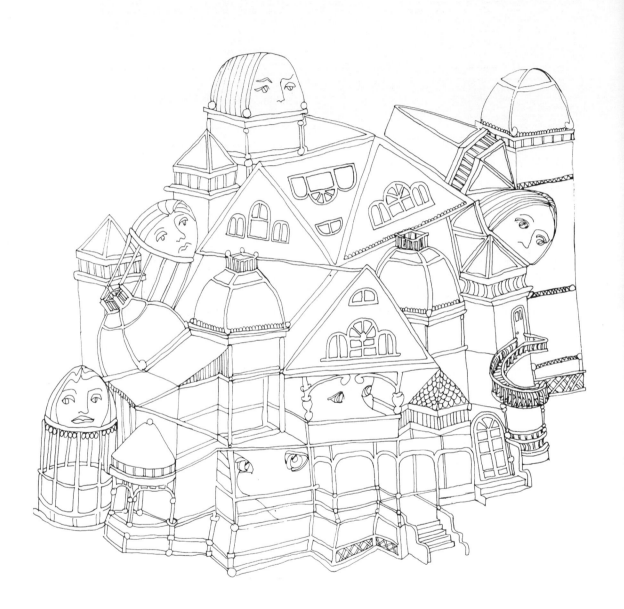

CHAPTER 1

The Delicate Dance: Engagement and Empathy

When a doctor tells me that he adheres strictly to this or that method, I have my doubts about his therapeutic effect. … I treat every patient as individually as possible, because the solution of the problem is always an individual one …

Carl G. Jung
Memories, Dreams, Reflections

In the following pages, we will begin a study of the interviewing process. We will be examining the craft in which one human attempts the formidable task of understanding another human. By way of analogy, this task is not unlike exploring a darkened room in an old Victorian house, holding only a candle as a source of illumination. Occasionally, as one explores the shadows, a brisk wind may snuff the candle out and the room will grow less defined. But with patience, the explorer begins to see more clearly. The outlines of the family portraits and oil lamps become more distinct. In a similar fashion, the subtle characteristics of a patient begin gradually to emerge. This quiet uncovering is a process with which some clinicians appear to familiarize themselves more adeptly than others. It is as if these more perceptive clinicians had somehow known the layout of the room before entering it – and indeed, in some respects, they had.

Their *a priori* knowledge is the topic of this chapter. We will attempt to discern some of the underlying principles that determine whether an initial interview fails or succeeds. As Jung suggests in the epigraph to this chapter, these principles do not harden into rigid rules. Instead they represent flexible guidelines, providing structure to what at first appears structureless.

Perhaps a second analogy may be clarifying at this point. A book on 19th century art by Rosenblum and Janson provides some useful insight.[1] In it, the authors attempt to describe the numerous processes that lead to the creation of a work of art, including environmental influences, political concerns, and the goals and limitations of the artist. With each painting, these historians appear to question themselves vigorously concerning concepts such as color, composition, originality, perspective, and theme. In short, Rosenblum and Janson utilize a specific language of art consisting of concisely defined terms. This language provides them with the tools to conceptualize and communicate their understanding. Since the language is one understood by most artists, the concepts of Rosenblum and Janson can be widely discussed and debated.

The work of the art historian is not at all unlike our own; as clinicians, however, we are concerned with a living art. We can better study the characteristics of this living art once we possess a language with which to conceptualize our interviewing styles. With this language, the principles that seem to provide an experienced clinician with a "map of the Victorian room" naturally evolve. From these principles we will garner a more engaging, flexible, and penetrating style of interviewing.

IN SEARCH OF A DEFINITION

A Bit of Interviewing Examined and the Discovery of a Map

There probably exists no better method for uncovering a definition of interviewing than by analyzing a brief piece of clinical dialogue. Even in a short excerpt, clarifying principles may begin to emerge.

The following dialogue was taken from a videotaped initial interview. Of particular note is the fact that the supervisee was disturbed by a not uncommon problem faced by an interviewer, "the wandering patient." Specifically, the supervisee commented, "I couldn't really even get a picture of her major problem (she had presented complaining of being very depressed), because she took off on every subject that came to her mind." In this excerpt, the interviewer, who had done an excellent job engaging her, uncovering her stresses, and allaying her initial anxieties, for she had never worked with a mental health professional before, was, at this point in the interview, attempting to discover whether she was suffering from the symptoms of a major depressive disorder. He wanted to understand better what symptoms were present and their severity – information that he could subsequently use to collaboratively develop an initial treatment plan with her. The patient, a middle-aged woman, had been describing some problems with her son, who was suffering from an attention-deficit disorder.

Pt.: … He's a behavior problem; maybe a phase he's going through. (Interviewer writes note.) He's exhibiting crying spells, which don't necessarily have a reason. The teacher is trying to interview him to see what exactly is wrong with the child because he's tense and crying, which isn't like him; he's been a happy-go-lucky kid.

Clin.: Is he still kind of hyperactive?

Pt.: Oh yeah … now that we've lowered the medication he's a little bit better, but I was just mad at the doctor; you know, one of them should have explained it to me.

Clin.: I would think that must be very frustrating to you.

Pt.: It was.

Clin.: And how has this affected your mood?

Pt.: Ah … I have a husband who works shifts (interviewer takes note), and he wants to be in charge of everything. I had a job until last February, when I got laid off. I was working more than full time. My husband does not pitch in at all. I was working about 60 hours a week. He wouldn't lift a dish, which really gets to you.

Clin.: Uh-huh; I'm sure.

Pt.:   Especially when you're working Saturdays and Sundays and you start at 6:30 in the morning and don't get home 'til 8:00 at night.

Clin.: What kind of work?

Pt.:   I was working in electronic assembly. I was an X-ray technician for 10 years and then we decided to settle down and have a family. I was working at the hospital up in Terryhill. And, uh, he said, and I can see his point …

At first glance, one can quickly empathize with the interviewer's frustration, for indeed this patient is in no hurry to describe her mood or her depressive symptoms. Instead, when asked directly about her mood, she immediately darts down a side alley into a series of complaints about her husband. She appears to wander from topic to topic. But with a second glance, an interesting observation is apparent concerning the communication pattern between these two co-participants. It is unclear who is wandering more, the patient or the interviewer. It is as if the two had decided to take an evening stroll together, hand in hand.

Specifically, the interviewer had intended to explore for information concerning depression. But when the interviewer asked about mood, the patient chose to move tangentially. At this crucial point, where the patient left the desired topic, the interviewer left with her. Unintentionally the clinician may have immediately rewarded the patient for leaving the desired topic by taking notes. His scribbling may have inadvertently told the patient to continue by suggesting that what the patient was saying was important enough for the clinician to jot down. The interviewer further rewarded the tangentiality of the patient by proffering an empathic statement, "Uh-huh; I'm sure." As if this were not enough, the clinician followed the patient down the alley by asking a question about the new topic (e.g., "What kind of work?").

Thus, both the patient and the clinician had an impact upon each other, their interface defining a dyadic system unconsciously committed to the perpetuation of a tangential interview. If we examined the next 10 minutes of this interview, we would see a continuation of this joint rambling, an unproductive process that resulted in almost no further information regarding the patient's depression and the pain beneath it, material much needed in order to begin collaborative treatment planning and subsequent healing.

This example illustrates the point that interviews define interactional processes, some of which facilitate communication and others of which inhibit communication. These processes are so distinctive that one can name them. For instance, the above process could be named "feeding the wanderer." If one is trying to uncover specific information within a set topic, then the process of feeding the wanderer represents a maladaptive technique. Curiously, if one were attempting to foster an atmosphere conducive to free association, the same technique might be beneficial. In either case, the interviewer can and should be consciously aware of this technique, implementing it when desirable and avoiding it when it would not be efficacious. For example, in Chapter 3 we will discover that the interviewer may have been able, in the above dialogue, to lead this patient effectively into a less digressive mode of speech through the use of sensitively well-timed focusing statements.

As we search for a definition of the interview process, we have already stumbled upon a cornerstone characteristic of all good clinical interviewing. It is not done solely by habit. Good clinical interviewing is the art of choice. The gifted interviewer always tries to match his or her interviewing techniques and strategies to the uniqueness of the patient, the demands of the clinical situation, and the vibrancies of the patient's culture. Allen Ivey, whose books I highly recommend, captured this cornerstone brilliantly with his concept of "intentionality," which is a characteristic both of clinicians, as they engage patients, and patients, as they engage life:

> *Intentionality, along with cultural intentionality, is acting with a sense of capability and deciding from among a range of alternative actions. The intentional individual has more than one action, thought, or behavior to choose from in responding to changing life situations. The culturally intentional individual can generate alternatives in a given situation and approach a problem from multiple vantage points, using a variety of skills and personal qualities, adapting styles to suit different individuals and cultures.[2]*

In this book our task will be, both for beginning and experienced clinicians, to explore a variety of interviewing techniques and strategies that will allow us to creatively choose which of these are most effective for which patients, enabling us to become more and more adept at creating intentional interviews while nurturing intentional interviewees. With this goal in mind, we can now turn our attention to defining exactly what an interview is. This definition would be equally true for an assessment interview by a social worker or a television interview by a talk show host. The general definition reads as follows:

> *An interview represents a verbal and nonverbal dialogue between two participants, whose behaviors affect each other's style of communication, resulting in specific patterns of interaction. In the interview, one participant, who labels himself or herself as the "interviewer," tends to ask questions in attempts to achieve specific goals, while the other participant generally assumes the role of "answering the questions" but undoubtedly has his or her own goals.*

This definition emphasizes the interactional process of the interview. It also allows one to refine the definition depending on the desired goals and the context of the interview. To make this definition more specific to the clinical assessment, one has only to look for the goals particular to the clinical situation.

In a broad sense, these assessment goals are as follows:

1. To establish a sound engagement of the patient in a therapeutic alliance
2. To collect a thorough and valid database
3. To develop an evolving and compassionate understanding of the person being interviewed
4. To develop an assessment from which a tentative diagnosis can be made
5. To collaboratively delineate a set of practical problems to be addressed and therapeutic goals to be set

6. To collaboratively develop an appropriate disposition and tentative treatment plan for achieving these goals
7. To begin the healing process by effecting some decrease of anxiety and pain in the patient
8. To instill hope and ensure that the patient will return for the next appointment

Furthermore, the goals of the initial interview will vary depending on the demands of the assessment situation, including issues such as time constraints and the interviewer's determination of what type of data seems clinically necessary in order to make an appropriate disposition. For instance, a crisis clinician called into an extremely busy emergency department to interview a victim of domestic violence will clearly sculpt a different interview than a therapist performing an initial intake at a community mental health center who, in turn, will create a different initial interview than one undertaken by an analyst asked to spend an hour or two with a well-educated patient requesting psychotherapy for chronic depression. In short, the needs of the clinical situation should determine the style of the interview but can do so only if the clinician remains willing to intentionally and flexibly alter his or her approach.

In any case, the above considerations emphasize one of the frequent challenges facing the initial interviewer, namely to gain a thorough and valid database in a limited amount of time while sensitively engaging the patient. The shorter the time period provided, the more complex the task appears. To return to our Victorian room, it is as if a clinician were being asked to make an inventory of a darkened room in a restricted amount of time while being careful not to disturb the decor too much. No easy task, even for a master of parlor games.

Perhaps this challenge reaches its most formidable peak when an interviewer or consultant is placed in the unenviable role of performing an intake assessment. From his or her assessment, frequently limited to the "50-minute hour" or less time by the numerous time pressures present in a busy clinic, the interviewer must determine the treatment disposition of the patient. We shall now turn our attention to the difficulties inherent in such intake interviews.

The discussion so far has indirectly provided an operational definition of such an assessment interview. From this definition, a map of sorts can be formulated as shown in Figure 1.1. This map, delineating the various goals of the assessment interview, begins with the engagement process, which, in many respects, determines whether the other goals will be successfully achieved. As engagement proceeds, the data-gathering process unfolds, leading to a progressive understanding of the patient. This understanding of the patient as a unique person depends upon the clinician's ability to see the patient's view of the world and recognize the patient's fears, pains, and hopes. As the interview progresses, the clinician begins to formulate a clinical assessment, including a tentative differential diagnosis and a practical list of the patient's concerns and desired goals. From both the assessment of the patient's situation and an understanding of the patient as a person, the clinician and patient can co-formulate a treatment plan suited to the individual needs of the interviewee, while acknowledging the constraints placed on treatment by the limitations of the mental health system itself.

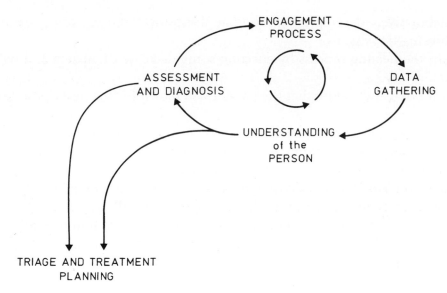

Figure 1.1 Map of the interviewing process.

These processes of engagement, data gathering, understanding, assessment, and treatment planning are, in actuality, longitudinally intertwining processes. The reverse arrows in the center of the map emphasize this fact, highlighting the clinician's need to attend to engagement activities throughout the initial interview.

Person-Centered Interviewing

As we use our map to explore our Victorian room, especially as the shadows darken and we meet areas where the patient is hesitant to share, our efforts must be guided by a compass that can provide a sense of direction in the darkness. What is this compass? It is the realization that our major goal for being in this room is simple, concrete, and unwavering – we are there to help the person who has sought our care.

At first glance this axiom may seem so self-evident as to not need to be stated. But any experienced clinician can relate to the intense time pressures of the work, the weariness engendered by the work, the mountains of paper work attached to the work, the administrative hassles hindering the work, and their own unconscious needs sometimes undermining the work that can make it surprisingly easy to lose this sense of direction.

For decades talented innovators, such as Carl Rogers, have felt this point to be so important that terms have been coined such as "client-centered counseling" (and in the fields of medicine and nursing: "patient-centered medicine") to highlight it. The newest term that has evolved for this concept – "person-centered" – beautifully captures the essence of our mission. It is a term more commonly encountered in European literature.

From the person-centered perspective the clinician views the interviewee as a cascading series of unique moments in time, in which the biology, psychology, intimate relationships, family dynamics, culture, and spirituality of our patient intersect to create the unique person before us. It is an ever-shifting matrix of which we are a part as soon as the patient enters our office. Our goal as clinicians is to understand this uniqueness, help our patients to better understand their strengths and weaknesses, and to learn how to navigate this complex human matrix more effectively.

Throughout the pages of this book we will use a person-centered perspective as our compass. Our interviewing principles, techniques, and strategies will be enriched by our efforts to see the world through the patient's eyes as well as our own, to make sure that we have a collaborative understanding of what the patient views as his or her problems and his or her goals first before sharing some of our own suggestions. It is a perspective that gently reminds us to understand what the person seeking our help wants us to provide before trying to provide it.

In person-centered interviewing the patient is not viewed as the problem but as a unique individual filled with solutions to the many problems that life invariably brings to all of us. There is a humbleness to a person-centered interviewer. It is the wisdom that, even at our best, we do not know all the answers, for we do not even know all the questions. Thus it is intensely important to listen to what our patients have to teach us and the questions that they bring us.

The Next Step

In this book we will focus upon the particularly challenging type of interview described above – the initial assessment – for the principles needed to perform it gracefully can be generalized to most other types of interviews, including emergency department interviews or crisis lines, where a great deal less time may be available. In short, the difficulties presented by the initial assessment interview provide tremendous opportunities for learning skills critical to understanding the core issue of most interviews, the delicate interplay between engagement, data gathering, and time. Many of these same skills will ultimately also be of use in psychotherapy itself.

In Part I of this book we will sequentially explore each of the processes defined by our map with a separate chapter (sometimes multiple chapters). In this chapter we will look at the first way-station on our map, engagement and its relationship to empathy.

Now is an appropriate time to introduce our integrated video program and to view our first video. As described in the Preface, more than 7.5 hours of video instruction are integrated throughout the text. These video modules provide didactic material that consolidates what has been read, adds new material and nuance, and provides video illustrations of the interviewing techniques. Video boxes within the text (as appears immediately below) will alert the reader to the video opportunities as they arise. Note that video modules are accessed via the e-book, for which directions for easy access appear on the inside of the front cover of the book.

VIDEO MODULE 1.1

Title: Introduction to Integrated Video Package

Contents: This short, yet important, video module describes the goals and use of the integrated video package. To utilize the video material most effectively it should be viewed before proceeding with subsequent video modules.

CREATING THE THERAPEUTIC ALLIANCE

First Things First: The Difference Between Engagement and Blending

From the first moment in which they see, hear, smell, and touch each other, the clinician and the patient begin the engagement process. In this complex interplay they reflect their sensory information onto the slippery screen of their memories. From these comparisons, both the clinician and the patient attempt to determine where each will fit into the other's life. Even as simple a gesture as a handshake can lead to lasting impressions. The experienced clinician may note whether he or she encounters the iron fingers of a Hercules bent upon establishing control or the dampened palm of a Charlie Brown expecting imminent rejection.

Ironically, at this same moment, the patient will have begun his or her own "mental status" on the clinician. This process can be seen clearly in the patient who greets the clinician's outstretched hand not with a handshake but with a look of disdain. As the clinician responds to the patient's rejection of a simple social amenity, who can doubt that the patient will be gaining some hints about the psychological workings of the clinician. For example, one interviewer, perhaps with an obsessive need to "do things my way," may further extend his or her hand, testily adding, "Don't you want to shake?" Another clinician, perhaps jaded from overwork, may dryly comment, "Not in the mood for shaking today, are we?"

In either case, the patient has struck a rich vein from which to mine answers to questions such as the following: (1) Will this interviewer get angry with me?, (2) Will this interviewer make me do things I don't want to do?, and (3) Am I safe here? This example hints at the complex and mutual activities affecting the engagement process, during which territorial issues are initially addressed.

Before proceeding, it is important to define two terms, *engagement* and *blending*. Engagement refers to the ongoing development of a sense of safety and respect from which patients feel increasingly free to share their problems, while gaining an increased confidence in the clinician's potential to understand them. Blending represents the behavioral and emotional clues from the interview that suggest that this engagement process is proceeding effectively. Stated differently, engagement defines a set of goals, and the concept of blending provides a method of monitoring the effectiveness of the strategies utilized to achieve those goals.

Not all writers emphasize the distinction between engagement and blending, but I feel it is an important one. Its significance lies in the fact that it does one little good to study engagement techniques if one does not develop a reliable method of measuring the effectiveness of these techniques in the interview itself. The concept of blending provides an avenue for active self-monitoring by the clinician. Problems in blending can alert the interviewer to the need to change interview strategies before serious damage to the clinician–patient alliance has developed.

Using Blending to Gauge the Degree of Engagement

One can assess blending by utilizing three complementary approaches: a subjective method, an objective method, and a patient's self-report. With regard to the subjective technique, an interviewer can learn what sensations he or she experiences when engagement is optimal – in essence, what a good interview feels like. Educators have suggested that once this internal and idiosyncratic feeling stage has been identified, the clinician can use it as a type of thermometer, to determine the intensity of blending at any given moment.[3]

Naturally, this subjective feeling will vary from one interviewer to another. Consequently it may help to examine some of the descriptions clinicians have related concerning this feeling state.

a. "To me good blending feels more like a conversation and a lot less like an interview or interrogation."
b. "I know blending has occurred when suddenly I realize during the interview that I'm actually talking with a person with real pain, not a case with imagined defenses."
c. "When the blending is good, I notice that I feel more relaxed, sometimes even giving off a sigh. Curiously I also feel more interested."

These descriptions suggest the personal uniqueness of the blending process. It is this personal uniqueness that allows the concept of blending to function as such a reliable and sensitive tool for monitoring the degree of engagement. If clinicians can train themselves to intermittently check the progress of blending, they will have discovered a window from which to study the unfolding engagement process. To this extent, the interview becomes less nebulous and more tangible. It evolves into something that can be modified.

This increased tangibility can be furthered by utilizing the second major avenue for monitoring the blending process, an objective look at the behavioral characteristics of the interview itself. The behavioral clues suggested by body language will be discussed in Chapter 8. In this chapter, an examination of the timing and structural characteristics of the verbal exchange will be highlighted.

The issue facing the interviewer involves finding concrete behavioral cues from the verbal exchange that indicate the presence of good blending. Wiens[4] and colleagues have provided some simple but fascinating methods of analyzing the temporal characteristics of speech by studying three major speech variables: duration of utterance (DOU), reaction time latency (RTL), and the percentage of interruptions. The DOU can be roughly equated with the length of time taken up by the interviewee's response following a question. The RTL represents the length of time it takes an interviewee to respond to a question. The percentage of interruptions represents the tendency for the interviewee to cut the clinician off before a question has been finished. One can look at all of these variables in relation to the clinician's speech patterns as well.

With regard to blending, these variables offer a potentially more objective measure of effectiveness, because certain patterns of exchange may suggest weak blending. For instance, a guarded or suspicious patient often produces curt responses to questions (a short DOU), long pauses before answering (long RTL), and occasional cut-offs as the patient corrects the interviewer for inaccuracies in his or her statements. If an interviewer spots such a pattern emerging, it may be a clue to ineffective engagement.

Another example at the opposite end of a continuum concerns the hypomanic, histrionic, or anxious patient who tends to wander. These wandering patients frequently present with a long DOU and a very brief RTL and may also actually cut the interviewer off frequently, a process triggered by the patient's over-eagerness to make their points. Interestingly, the interviewer may find himself or herself reciprocating with cut-offs in a vain effort to get a word in edgewise.

Moreover, with histrionic, hypomanic, or manic patients, the blending is frequently marked by a peculiar superficial quality. With regard to spontaneity of speech, these patients often open-up inappropriately quickly, as opposed to the gradual increase in blending seen with most patients. Consequently, the observed blending possesses a one-sided and shallow quality, aptly called by one student "unipolar blending."

In the above two examples, we have seen that variations in basic patterns of verbal output, such as a DOU and RTL, can provide objective indications of the adequacy of the blending process. One might ask whether this objective technique offers any advantage over the subjective approach described previously. I believe that it does. But one method does not appear more valuable than another; rather each method complements the other. For instance, occasionally clinicians are duped by their subjective sense of blending into missing the psychopathology of patients with histrionic defenses or those experiencing hypomania.

One of the reasons this problem occurs is that the clinician feels at a subjective level that the blending is unusually good. Indeed, the clinician is fascinated by the patient's story. In actuality, the blending is artificially good, representing the unipolar blending just described. In fact, unipolar blending, if recognized by the clinician, could provide the clue that "something is wrong here." The patient's engaging style and subtle dramatics are misleading the clinician. If in this instance the clinician could step back to look at the DOU and RTL, the clinician might recognize the hallmarks of a unipolar blending and consequently evaluate the possible psychopathologic causes of it. In this case, the objective technique sidesteps the confusion created by judging the blending process solely by the subjective method.

The other advantage of paying attention to more concrete parameters such as DOU and RTL is the ability to use these criteria to judge the effectiveness of a specific technique employed by the clinician. If, for example, the clinician attempts to actively engage a patient who seems hesitant to talk, one of the earliest and most easily recognized markers of success will be an increase in DOU. Corresponding changes in the subjective feeling of increased blending may appear only later and may be less easily recognized.

A third method of determining the degree of blending consists of the patient's self-report. Occasionally, a patient will spontaneously tell an interviewer to what degree the interaction is enjoyable. More commonly, the interviewer may inquire, as the interview winds down, "What was it like talking with me today?"

To this question, some patients may pointedly discuss specific concerns, sometimes providing appropriate and constructive criticism. Often, due to a reluctance to appear unappreciative or rude, patients will reply that everything was fine, even if it was not, but their nonverbals may betray their true feelings. A hesitant "yes" surely indicates some discomfort upon the part of the patient, providing us with a rich opportunity to non-defensively uncover their concerns and address them. At such moments of hesitation, the clinician can comment, "You know you look a little hesitant there, is there anything I may have done or said that might have made you uncomfortable?" The answers are sometimes surprising. By non-defensively exploring the patient's concerns, we will have greatly increased the likelihood that there is going to be a second interview.

Other surprises may appear when the self-report contradicts the subjective and objective methods of evaluating blending. For instance, I am reminded of a young man who appeared somewhat disinterested as we spoke. He talked softly and with little animation. As we proceeded, I felt awkward, as if this were going to be a bad mix of personalities. Although both the objective and subjective signs of blending suggested poor engagement, to my surprise, at the end of the interview he reported feeling very at home with me. He stated that he had enjoyed the interview, and he appeared sincere.

His diagnosis was paranoid schizophrenia in remission. It was either a residual blunting of affect from his schizophrenia or perhaps a side effect from an antipsychotic that was creating both an outward and an inward suggestion of poor blending; the engagement was not, in truth, weak. This disparity highlighted the type of miscommunication that this patient could easily convey to other people, an aloofness that was both disarming and misleading. Attention to blending by self-report greatly enhanced my understanding of the manner in which this patient embraces the world and is embraced by the world. It also suggested the possible utility of social skills training or perhaps a medication adjustment.

Thus, the clinician can benefit from learning to judge blending by combining the subjective, objective, and self-report approaches. With these three techniques in mind, the interview becomes at once less mystifying and more gratifying. The gratification arises from the realization that the interviewer can learn to creatively alter the interview process itself.

Once blending has been analyzed, the clinician possesses a concrete idea of the strength of the engagement process with any particular patient at any given moment. Weak engagement may indicate that invalid data is more likely. It may also be a harbinger that the patient may be less interested in the clinician's treatment recommendations or recommendations for follow-up. Moreover, a weak engagement process suggests one of the following three conditions:

1. The interviewer's actions are actively disengaging the patient
2. The interviewee's psychopathologic processes or defenses are interfering with engagement
3. A combination of the above

If the clinician feels that the damaged blending can be attributed to the first condition, then the clinician can attempt to consciously alter his or her style of interaction. For instance, a paranoid patient may be put off by an extroverted style of interviewing. In such an instance, the clinician may decide to tone down their extroversion in an effort to ease the patient's fears.

If the weak blending can be ascribed to the second condition, then the clinician may be alerted to the types of psychopathology that could be blocking the blending, such as with the histrionic process described earlier. Naturally, if the third condition is the issue, increased attention to both style of interaction and psychopathology can be brought into play.

At this point we have reviewed three methods of directly assessing blending that allow us to indirectly assess the engagement process itself. It is valuable to reflect on the map of the interviewing process delineated earlier. On this map, the interviewer begins with the engagement process for a good reason. The engagement process affects all subsequent goals of the interview.

More specifically, poor engagement raises significant doubts about the validity of the database because patients generally do not freely share with people they do not like. Moreover, without effective engagement, one will seldom gain knowledge of the intimate corners of the patient's "room" alluded to in our comparison of an interview with an exploration of a dark Victorian room. Hence, the clinician leaves with only a superficial understanding of the patient's pain. Furthermore, without valid data falling into place, the clinician's assessment and diagnosis are frequently in significant jeopardy. Finally, if the engagement process proceeds poorly, the patient may never return for a second appointment, casting the shadow of irrelevance over the work of the first interview.

Thus one is left with the realization that this somewhat nebulous concept of engagement appears to be the pivotal process on which much of clinical practice turns. Fortunately, this process is not as mercurial as it first appears. The dance of engagement begins with empathy.

CONVEYING EMPATHY: TRAPS, STRATEGIES, AND SOLUTIONS

The Empathy Cycle

Many clinicians assume that empathy is a simple concept. It is not. The large number of research papers devoted to its capture testifies to its elusiveness. Fortunately, over the years insights have been achieved that help to demystify empathy, a quality that all people feel they naturally possess but that in reality may be less ubiquitous than imagined. It seems only appropriate to begin our story with Carl Rogers, who developed the field of client-centered counseling. He conceptualized empathy as the clinician's ability "to perceive the internal frame of reference of another with accuracy, and with the emotional components and meanings which pertain thereto, as if one were the other person, but without ever losing the 'as if' condition."[4] Stated more simply, empathy is the ability to accurately recognize the immediate emotional perspective of another person while maintaining one's own perspective.

As Rogers pointed out, there is an important distinction between empathy and identification, although they can overlap. With empathy, the interviewer quickly recognizes the patient's feelings. Indeed, the interviewer may even begin to automatically "feel" the patient's feelings himself or herself (sadness, anger, etc.) but only briefly. The empathic interviewer has the ability to quickly step back from the process with regard to their own emotional state. The empathic interviewer has no invested acceptance of the patient's feelings as being "correct" or "just like my own would be in such a situation."

In contrast, with identification, the clinician not only recognizes – and briefly shares – the patient's feeling state, the interviewer continues to experience the patient's anger or sadness. Such a misguided clinician fully embraces the patient's feelings as his or her own unconsciously. A clinician who is experiencing identification, in essence, agrees with the patient's feelings and is *personally invested* in accepting these feelings as being both accurate and reasonable.

The importance of this distinction lies in the fact that identification often marks the pathway toward such unrecognized therapeutic gremlins as burnout and unidentified countertransference. The persistent appearance of strong feelings of identification may alert clinicians to the need to begin or return to their own therapy, because such identification can quickly destroy the therapeutic process.

One feels compelled to say a silent prayer for the poor patient with borderline features who meets a clinician that boldly proclaims, "I can feel your pain." Borderline patients have enough problems with identity diffusion without finding "silly putty" coating the edges of their clinician. Thus a simple but important lesson to be learned from the study of empathy is that most patients are not searching for a person who feels as they do; they are searching for someone who is trying to understand what they feel.

G. T. Barrett-Lennard sheds further light on the concept of empathy by recognizing the fact that empathy is effective only if it involves both the interviewee and the interviewer.[5] Thus empathic skill is not limited to the clinician's ability merely to perceive the internal reference of the patient, but also includes the clinician's ability to convey this perception to the patient with an empathic statement or gesture. He calls this shared response the "empathy cycle," a concept providing an excellent framework with which to study the practical application of empathy. Consequently, we will look at each phase of Barrett-Lennard's cycle in detail, using it as our framework for the rest of the chapter.

The empathy cycle consists of the following phases: (1) the patient expresses a feeling, (2) the clinician recognizes this feeling, (3) the clinician conveys recognition of the feeling to the patient, (4) the patient receives this conveyance of recognition, and (5) the patient provides feedback to the clinician that the recognition has been received.[6] With this cycle in mind, the empathic process begins to make significantly more sense. In fact, one can see that a breakdown in empathy can arise at each of these five stages.

First Phase of the Empathy Cycle: Patient Expresses a Feeling

In the first phase of the empathy cycle, in which the patient expresses a specific feeling, a variety of processes can disrupt empathy. For instance, both conscious and unconscious defenses may block the patient from expressing his or her actual emotions. A poignant example of this process is illustrated by the following dialogue, in which a mother of a 7-year-old with marked and permanent developmental problems discusses her son:

> **Clin.:** Tell me a little about John's behavior with other children.
>
> **Pt.:** Oh there is really little wrong there, he's really quite normal, just like the other kids. He doesn't like to play games very much or sports, but then he has a mind of his own, maybe someday he'll be a star golfer or skier.

> **Clin.:** You had mentioned something about his speech earlier.
>
> **Pt.:** Oh, hmm, you must be thinking of his lisp. Well I think we all went through that phase as children. In a few years it'll all work out. You know, I have trouble understanding most little kids when they talk, it's part of being a little person.

One feels the pathos of this situation, in which the mother's defenses of denial and rationalization prevent the expression of core feelings of pain. If the interviewer should attempt to make an empathic statement such as, "It sounds like you're really going through a lot with John," I doubt the response would be positive. In this case the patient's own unconscious defenses have prevented the empathy cycle from spontaneously unfolding.

Second Phase of the Empathy Cycle: Clinician Recognizes the Patient's Feelings

But phase 1 does not have a monopoly on the common breakdowns that prevent the establishment of an empathic contact. In phase 2, the recognition of the patient's feelings, problems may arise if the clinician's perceptual or intuitive skills fall short, perhaps related to his or her own defenses or psychopathologic undertow. In particular, interviewers need to be aware of the impact of their immediate emotional status on their ability to empathize accurately. For example, a clinician who has recently experienced an unsettling session in supervision may have significant trouble attending to a patient's subtle clues of inner pain. At the other extreme, a recently divorced clinician could easily project his own feelings of betrayal onto a patient undergoing a trial separation, when, in fact, the patient is not experiencing such feelings at all. In both situations, the clinician's emotional state prevents an accurate perception of the interviewee's feelings.

In this light, it can be stated that interviewers have only themselves to serve as measuring instruments. The clinician has no microscope or magnetic resonance imaging (MRI) to provide insight. However, like a sophisticated machine, interviewers can unintentionally bias their data. Before beginning an interview, it is often useful to check the bias of the instrument by pausing for a moment of reflection, asking what feelings are present, before proceeding to meet the patient. Such a simple process may alert the clinician to potentially distorting factors such as feeling rushed, angry, sad, or simply weary. Once alerted to their biases, interviewers may hope to stand one step further away from invalid data.

The second phase of the empathy cycle also raises several interesting questions concerning the actual nature of intuition. Margulies and Havens[7,8] have emphasized two frames of mind that appear to be integral aspects of the empathic process. In the first place, the clinician must possess the ability to listen with an attitude of disciplined naiveté, literally attempting to feel the world of the patient without seeking cause and effect, classification, or moral judgment. This receptive listening perspective was masterfully developed by the psychological school of phenomenology, which we shall discuss at greater length later in this book. But the bottom line can be simply stated: The clinician must learn to suspend analytic thought when such thought may be destructive to the engagement process.

The second frame of mind that Margulies discusses concerns the ability of the clinician to imagine the inner experiences of the patient by creatively projecting himself or herself into the patient's world. He likens this ability to the poetic imagination of artists, emphasizing the ability to move actively into the patient's world, or "inscape," as this phenomenon has been called.[9] When the clinician does this well, he or she not only paints a picture of the patient's world, but also enters it.

The ability to listen while suspending analysis and the ability to sensitively project into what another person may be experiencing can be viewed as two skills from which intuition is born. They remain pivotal to effective clinical practice, typically reaching powerful proportions when clinicians achieve a high degree of blending.

Here we stumble upon a fascinating irony, because one of the characteristics of a gifted interviewer is the ability to know not only when to use these intuitive skills but also when not to use them. Phrased slightly differently, a skilled clinician draws from both intuition and analysis. In a matter of a few minutes the skilled interviewer may juxtapose periods of intuitive listening with moments of analytic thought. Indeed, the two processes, in the hands of a seasoned clinician, tend to guide each other. For example, a clinician may intuitively sense a patient's extreme fear of a disintegration of the self. Besides immediately helping the clinician to blend with the patient, this intuitive feeling might prompt the clinician to later explore, in a diagnostic sense, whether the patient may have defenses and behaviors consistent with having a borderline personality or a narcissistic personality.

Similarly, an analytic process can lead a clinician to a higher level of empathy. For instance, a clinician may observe that as the interview proceeds, the patient avoids eye contact and becomes increasingly anxious. This analytic observation may prompt the clinician to be more empathically aware of the patient's feeling of being ill-at-ease. At such moments the clinician may gently ask, "I'm wondering what it has been like for you coming to see a therapist?" Subsequently, an empathic mode of listening may significantly help the patient to relieve his or her sense of guilt or embarrassment. The important point remains that intuition and analysis are complements, not antagonists. Both skills are utilized frequently during the first encounter.

Third Phase of the Empathy Cycle: Clinician Conveys Recognition of the Patient's Feelings

In the third phase of the cycle – the clinician's actual phrasing of the empathic statement – the complexities of human interaction further manifest themselves. It is an arena of considerable complexity in which we will examine some simplifying concepts that can help us to effectively communicate our empathy while navigating the numerous twists and traps in the process.

Strategic Empathy

One such unexpected twist arises from the fact that not all empathic statements work equally effectively with all patients. With many patients appearing for their first appointment, some empathic statements appear to be appropriately engaging, but "nothing special," while other empathic statements appear to be compellingly powerful "grand slams" enhancing the therapeutic alliance. Another perhaps even more puzzling aspect of empathic statements remains their uncanny ability to promptly disengage a small subset of patients, in short, to achieve the exact opposite of their intended use. One is reminded of the varying fashions in which people accept compliments in everyday situations. Some people take compliments well, whereas others take them poorly. Members of the latter group often become decidedly ill-at-ease following a sincere compliment, shrugging it off with "Thank you, but it's really nothing."

One manner of interpreting this peculiar phenomenon consists of viewing the compliment as pushing the recipient towards one of two uncomfortable states: (1) accepting a view of himself or herself that seems inaccurate, or (2) feeling an emotional state (e.g., a pleasant sense of self-worth) that he or she is not currently capable of comfortably experiencing, as may be seen in a person burdened by a chronically punitive superego. So it is with empathic statements, which can backfire when they push people into interpersonal niches they do not wish to occupy. The question is whether or not this situation can be avoided. To a large extent I think it can be.

To understand how to more effectively utilize empathic statements, to more frequently utilize powerfully engaging empathic statements, and to avoid empathic statements that are disengaging, it is critical to return to our compass. From the perspective of person-centered interviewing, it all makes sense, for it is assumed that each patient is unique and each interviewing dyad is also unique. One size does not fit all with regard to empathy. The defenses of the patient will have an immediate impact on how empathic statements are received.

With this acknowledgement, the clinician views empathy as a skill set that is not used in a habitual sense in the same way with every patient who enters the office, but is strategically utilized in a *conscious* fashion depending upon the needs and defenses of the unique patient. Strategic empathy is a classic practical application of Ivey's concept of intentional interviewing. It weds the naturally intuitive skills of the clinician with a sound understanding of the nuances of language, human defenses, cultural proclivities, and dyadic interaction. Two terms are useful for developing a skilled use of strategic empathy: (1) the patient's "interpersonal stance" and (2) "empathic valence."

Interpersonal Stance

One can categorize patients, with some degree of caution, into two types: those who are trusting and those who feel guarded. Most of our patients are reasonably trusting and we will find that the interviewer can effectively use a wide variety of empathic interviewing techniques with such patients with little likelihood of empathic backfiring. It is with the latter patient, the so-called guarded patient, that empathic statements most frequently display the nasty habit of disrupting the engagement process. The guarded quality of these patients may arise from a variety of sources, including high anxiety or fear (perhaps in a patient particularly uneasy about therapy or involuntarily forced to be assessed), an idiosyncratic or situational fear of the clinician (for example, in a patient who has an immediate negative transference to a clinician who physically resembles an abusive parent), a long-standing character trait of suspiciousness (as seen with a paranoid personality), or frankly pre-psychotic or psychotic paranoia.

Empathic statements made to guarded patients, from whatever etiology, frequently decrease the interpersonal distance between these patients and the clinician. This interpersonal intimacy is exactly what guarded patients do not want. At an extreme end, the last thing a truly paranoid patient wants is to be in the room "with someone who can get inside my head." Stripped of their "buffer zones" through the habitual or reflexive use of empathic statements by a well-intentioned clinician, these patients have only one option: to escape through retreat or attack. In short, guarded patients need psychological "distance," a fact too frequently overlooked by interviewers.

So far we have delineated the concept that patients may respond to empathic overtures in different manners secondary to their degree of guardedness. Our understanding can be developed even more fully if we now look at a characteristic of the empathic statement itself – empathic valence – for the valence of the empathic statement often determines what its impact will be in both trusting and guarded patients.

Empathic Valence

Valence refers to the potential "intensity" of an empathic statement, by which we mean the degree to which an empathic statement's impact will tend to be gently or powerfully engaging or gently or powerfully disengaging. Empathic statements with a low valence tend to be only mildly engaging with trusting patients but are much less likely to backfire with guarded patients. Empathic statements with a high valence will tend to be more powerfully engaging (quite powerfully engaging with trusting patients) yet more likely to backfire (often quite disengaging with patients who are guarded or actively paranoid). By recognizing the interpersonal stance of the patient (trusting versus guarded), the clinician can then consciously choose to use empathic statements that have a gentle or powerful valence, hence the concept of strategic empathy. At first glance, this distinction may seem a bit confusing, but with an exploration of its practical application it will clarify quickly.

In this regard, the valence of empathic statements appears to vary along the following two axes: (1) the valence of implied certainty of the interviewee's feelings by the interviewer and (2) the valence of intuited attribution made by the interviewer from statements offered by the interviewee. As one would expect, these axes overlap. However, for purposes of acquiring a more sophisticated understanding, it will be worthwhile to look at them separately, their unique qualities offering the structural foundation from which we can build an ability to effectively use strategic empathy.

Valence of Implied Certainty

To begin our inquiry, let us speculate on the first axis – the valence of implied certainty. Put simply, one considers to what degree the clinician implies that he or she knows exactly what the patient is experiencing. In empathic statements with a low valence of implied certainty, the interviewer expresses considerable uncertainty. In contrast, a clinician using an empathic statement with a high valence regarding certainty will imply a great deal more certitude that what he or she is saying is "on the mark." In the following dialogue, a poetic young man has just suffered the cruelties of an unwanted divorce. This same man had lost his mother to leukemia when he was 13 years old. Following the patient's statement, an example of an empathic statement with a low valence of certainty and one with a high valence will be given.

> **Pt.:** After my wife abruptly left me, it was like a star exploded inward, everything seemed so empty … she seemed like a memory and my life began to fall apart. Very shortly afterwards I began feeling very depressed and very tearful.
>
> **Clin.:** [low valence of certainty] It *sounds like* everything seemed to be collapsing around you.
>
> **Clin.:** [high valence of certainty, said with a gentle tone of voice] Your world had collapsed in so many ways, all of them so very painful. (the patient nods his head in agreement and begins to cry)

As a general rule, empathic statements with a low degree of certainty, which tend to employ words like "It sounds like …" generally can be used effectively to enhance blending with *both* a trusting and a guarded patient.

In the case of a trusting patient, a skilled clinician may strategically choose to use an empathic statement with a higher valence with regard to certainty as shown above. Such a statement may suggest to the patient that he or she is in the presence of a clinician who "really gets it" and is seeing things through their eyes in a phenomenological sense. The well-timed use of an empathic statement with a high degree of valence regarding certainty can be compellingly engaging with a trusting patient.

Sometimes empathic statements with a high valence regarding certainty begin with phrases such as "It is" or "There is." With the above patient, the clinician might have said, "There is so much pain in a divorce of this nature, it's essentially beyond words." These phrases can sometimes be unusually effective for engagement purposes.[9] Such third-person singular impersonal phrases tend to suggest a shared experience to the patient, in the sense that the clinician acknowledges the validity of the patient's experience while simultaneously suggesting one would (or even has) experienced similar emotions. When well timed, these phrases can shore up a faltering alliance.

On the other hand, empathic statements with a high valence of certainty may disengage a guarded patient, as shown in the following:

> **Pt.:** I can't believe how cruel people can be. My ex-boss won't even talk with me, won't even give me a minute of his damn time. It hurts, yes it does. But at this point I've got a million problems and nobody to help me.
>
> **Clin.:** *It is very overwhelming to have so many problems.* [high valence of implied certainty]
>
> **Pt.:** How would you know what it feels like, have you ever been fired?
>
> **Clin.:** No, I can't say I have, but it surely must be a devastating process. [yet another empathic statement with a high valence of certainty]
>
> **Pt.:** To some people perhaps (slight glare from patient).

In this passage, the clinician's attempt at an empathic statement with a high valence of certainty seems to have unsettled the patient, a verbal boomerang of sorts. Perhaps this backfire has its origins in the patient's desire for a private and hence safe world. More explicitly, this patient appears to dislike the process of being told what he is feeling or should be doing, for this world is his world, and trespassers are not encouraged.

This trespass has led to a rather awkward moment, in which the patient challenges the clinician's ability to understand him, which is not exactly the response desired by the interviewer, who suddenly finds himself dodging the cutting edge of an almost paranoid accusation.

One can speculate that if the clinician had used an empathic phrase with a lesser valence of implied certainty such as, "It *sounds like* it could be very overwhelming to have so many problems," instead of the phrase, "*It is very overwhelming to have so many problems*," perhaps the interaction may have been less antagonistic. Perhaps … Nevertheless, as we will see later in this section, even empathic statements with a gentle degree of certainty are often ill advised when the patient is frankly paranoid.

Valence of Intuited Attribution

Now let us turn our attention to the second axis of valence regarding empathy – the degree of intuited attribution. Along this axis, how much the clinician reads into the patient is compared with how much the clinician repeats back exactly what he or she has heard. In empathic statements with a low degree of intuited attribution, the clinician often reflects back the patient's feelings matter-of-factly without much change, trying to communicate that the interviewer understands and is following closely. In contrast, when employing an empathic statement that displays a high valence regarding intuited attribution, the clinician displays the ability to truly enter the patient's inscape as Margulies and Havens described earlier, in order to accurately intuit hidden pain that has not been yet shared. When done with a trusting patient, such statements can be very powerful indeed.

In the following example, the opposing ends of this spectrum will be illustrated. Note that concerning the valence of certainty, both empathic statements show a low degree of certainty (both begin with the words "It sounds like …"). On the other hand, concerning the valence of intuited attribution, they are radically different. This is the poetic patient we saw earlier, who had also lost his mother to leukemia when he was 13 years old:

Pt.: After my wife abruptly left me, it was like a star exploded inward, everything seemed so empty … she seemed like a memory and my life began to fall apart. Very shortly afterwards I began feeling very depressed and very tearful.

Clin.: [low valence of intuited attribution] It sounds as if your whole life *truly* began falling apart.

or

Clin.: [high valence of intuited attribution] It sounds like it was terribly frightening to lose her so suddenly, almost like the loss of your mother so many years ago (the patient pauses for a moment, reflecting on the clinician's intuited association and promptly begins to weep).

In the empathic statement with a low valence of intuited attribution, the clinician essentially employs the same wording as the patient "life began falling apart," but might give a sensitive emphasis by adding a word such as "truly." In this respect, the interviewer has, in an accurate fashion, mirrored back the patient's thoughts. Minimal intuition is displayed here. Consequently, there exists little chance that the statement will be perceived as inaccurate or too invasive by either a trusting or a guarded patient. Moreover, if said in a caring tone, this gentle response can convey concern while demonstrating an attentive listening style. It may represent a rudimentary level of empathy. It does convey caring when done well. Empathic statements that essentially mirror back the exact words of the patient, such as this example, are sometimes simply called *"reflecting statements."* Reflecting statements are useful but have significant limitations, because they do not particularly demonstrate great sensitivity or understanding by the clinician.

In contrast, the second example illustrated above – a nice illustration of an empathic statement with a high valence of intuited attribution – when used with a *patient with a trusting interpersonal stance* may suggest to the patient that he or she is in the presence of a keenly perceptive therapist. For instance, in our example, this sensitivity was suggested by the clinician's use of the term "frightening," a feeling never mentioned by the patient but nevertheless felt to be present by the clinician. When accurate, such empathic connections can be powerful indeed. Moreover, the second part of the clinician's response, suggesting a relationship of the current grief to an earlier mourning for the patient's mother, also represents an intuition made by the clinician. To the trusting patient, such a powerful empathic statement may suggest that he has found a particularly understanding and insightful listener. The use of empathic statements with a high valence regarding intuited attribution often characterize the dialogue of a gifted clinician.

Once again, however, one must ask whether or not an empathic statement with a high valence of intuited attribution can get a clinician into trouble. Not surprisingly, the answer is "yes," especially with guarded patients. By way of example, guardedness is often associated with an inordinate attention to details, demonstrated by an unexpected value on accuracy. This need for *accurate* understanding at all costs is bolstered by the fear that "no one understands what I'm really feeling." With these two processes in mind, one can easily imagine the potential traps awaiting the clinician who unwittingly uses an empathic response with a high valence of intuited attribution with a guarded patient. In this case the patient is veering towards an almost paranoid stance:

> **Pt.:** After my wife abruptly left me, it was like a star exploded inward, everything seemed so empty … she seemed like a memory and my life began to fall apart. Very shortly afterwards I began feeling very depressed and very tearful.
>
> **Clin.:** It sounds terribly frightening to lose her so suddenly, so similar to the pain you felt when your mother died.
>
> **Pt.:** No … no, that's not right at all. My mother did not purposely abandon me. That's simply not true.
>
> **Clin.:** I did not mean that your mother purposely abandoned you, but rather that both people were unexpected losses.
>
> **Pt.:** I suppose … but they were very different. I never was afraid of my mother … they're really *very* different.

Needless to say, this attempt at empathic connection leaves something to be desired. The patient's attention to detail and fear of misunderstanding have obliterated the intended empathic message, leaving the clinician with a frustrating need to mollify a patient who has successfully twisted an empathic statement into an insult of sorts.

Basic Guideposts for Effectively Using Strategic Empathy

At this point, with our understanding of the concepts of interpersonal stance and empathic valence some relatively simple patterns are emerging, which can act as practical guidelines to strategic and effective use of empathy:

1. In general, empathic statements represent extremely valuable methods for strengthening engagement. Consequently, the clinician will usually employ such statements intermittently throughout an interview.
2. The statements themselves vary in their valence from low to high on two axes: their valence regarding implied certainty and their valence regarding intuited attribution.
3. The effectiveness of the empathic statement, as regards its valence, depends upon the interpersonal stance of the patients ranging from trusting to guarded.
4. Low-valence (gentle) empathic statements are generally useful with *both* trusting and guarded patients. Their weakness lies in the fact that they do not convey a particularly sensitive understanding to the patient, although they do demonstrate concern. Their strength lies in the fact that they seldom backfire.
5. With guarded patients it is frequently best to utilize low-valence (gentle) empathic statements. With guarded patients, if one attempts to use a higher valence (powerful) empathic statement, the clinician might find that the patient begins to disengage (often shown by a disavowal of the clinician's empathic comment). At such a point, further high-valence empathic statements are probably best avoided. Indeed, in some instances, all empathic statements may be liable to backfire.
6. On the other hand, with trusting patients, interviewers frequently begin with low-valence empathic statements and progress to high-valenced empathic statements, for such high-valence empathic statements may prove strikingly effective in producing a deepening sense of trust.

VIDEO MODULE 1.2

Title: Effectively Using Empathic Statements

Contents: Contains both expanded didactics and annotated interviewing excerpts.

Three Examples of Using Strategic Empathy to Transform Difficult Moments

1: The Paranoid Spiral

The most extreme form of interpersonal guardedness appears with patients who are actively paranoid and psychotic. There exist few interactions that are more daunting and confusing to the beginning clinician. Unless one has had the misfortune of having a loved one with paranoia, as seen in schizophrenia or some forms of bipolar process, many trainees will have had little or no experience navigating in this interpersonal maelstrom. And the waters are tricky indeed. Fortunately, because of our understanding of strategic empathy, we have some tools for helping both ourselves and our patients to feel more comfortable when paranoid process is active.

Years ago when I was the medical director of a psychiatric emergency room, I would sometimes observe a most striking phenomenon – "the paranoid spiral" – that was common, especially with naturally empathic trainees (who had had little experience with paranoid process up to that date). As mentioned earlier when describing patients with extreme guardedness, paranoid patients have an even more intense need for accuracy in how clinicians describe them and an almost overwhelming need for psychological distance. Even empathic statements with a low valence are often rejected, and empathic statements with a high valence, regarding implied certainty or intuited attribution, are downright anathema to many paranoid patients, because to the patient it feels like the interviewer is trying to "get inside my head." Watch what happens in the following dialogue, which illustrates a paranoid spiral:

Pt.: Things have gotten a little dicey with my husband. I'm not certain what the problem is. He just doesn't communicate the way he used to. He's not warm. We used to show a lot of affection. It's just not good.

Clin.: Sounds like it's gotten pretty tough. [an empathic statement with a low valence of certitude but a relatively high valence of intuition]

Pt.: (said testily) I didn't say "it's gotten tough," I said "It's just not good." (note that the patient has disavowed the clinician's empathic statement, a real red light that paranoia is out and about)

Clin.: Oh (pause) I'm sorry … I think I see what you mean (patient glares). What else have you noticed? (to a naturally engaging clinician, who throughout his or her life has normally engaged very well with people using such empathic statements, this unexpected tenseness with the patient is psychologically jarring – sometimes representing the first time anyone has responded to his or her empathic communications in such an odd way. This psychological jarring was probably the cause of the clinician's somewhat awkward response, "I think I see what you mean.")

Pt.: It's just too weird. It's like he's not the same person. Sort of unpredictable. It's not that I think he is having an affair or anything. But he sure seems to be interested in our pretty next-door neighbor, if you know what I mean. It's pretty upsetting. And I think he might be spying on me.

Clin.: I can see where that would be unsettling to lose trust in someone you have always trusted. [an empathic statement with a high valence of intuition and certitude, which would be quite effective with most people – but this patient is *not* "most people"]

Pt.: It's not unsettling, it's upsetting. (patient glares again) And it has nothing to do with trust.

Clin.: Oh. (pauses) Well, how do you put it all together?

Pt.: Well, finally, we have a good question (pauses). Let's be blunt here, I think my husband has become a strange man. You might call him evil. It's the "divorce game," him trying to drive me nuts so that he can divorce me.

Clin.: How do you mean?

Pt.: For about 3 months he's had them on me. I know they're watching, every night at 6 o'clock. I feel their presence. I think they use telescopes and maybe mind probes to see me, a terrible position to be in.

Clin.:	*That must be* frightening to be constantly watched by others. [high valence of implied certainty]
Pt.:	Just what do you mean by that? How would you know what I'm feeling? (said testily)
Clin.:	Well, in the situation you're describing I think it would be frightening.
Pt.:	Frightening enough to make one lose one's mind?
Clin.:	Well … that's difficult to say, it's not …
Pt.:	It's *what* Dr. Jones? Frightening enough to make one crazy, well I'm not crazy Dr. Jones, no matter what you think, and trust me I'm not defenseless.

In the paranoid spiral, as we are seeing above, the patient may even disavow empathic statements with low valence. The interviewer immediately registers the disengagement, but because they feel less engaged, the interviewer uses, by habit, what they often have used to improve engagement in everyday life and with previous patients – more empathic statements. Naturally, this further disengages the paranoid patient, who wants more distance, not more intimacy, from the interviewer. Because the interviewer acutely feels the progressive uneasiness of the encounter, they often try empathic statements with an even higher valence, for with trusting patients these statements have often been powerfully engaging in the past. Well … "it ain't gonna work here."

I have actually seen such interviews spiral downwards, plummeting into a stony silence, hence the name "paranoid spiral." (This misstep is an easily understandable strategic error for an inexperienced interviewer; in my first year of residency I fell into this trap so many times my supervisors needed a rope to get me out!) In some patients, this reflexive use of empathic statements by the interviewer can stoke considerable hostility, perhaps placing the patient near the edge of violence. In fact, the comment from the above patient, "trust me I'm not defenseless," could be a veiled threat to the clinician, well worth heeding.

Returning to our original definition of an interview, we can see that the paranoid spiral is a beautiful example of the fact that "*an interview represents a verbal and nonverbal dialogue between two participants, whose behaviors affect each other's style of communication, resulting in specific patterns of interaction.*" It is also a beautiful example of the value of one form of intentional interviewing, strategic empathy, for a clinician armed with knowledge regarding strategic empathy does not need to move reflexively. We have choice. Not every patient wants to be on the receiving end of empathy.

Once paranoid process has been spotted, as with the first disavowal of the mixed valence empathic statement seen above ("Sounds like it's gotten pretty tough"), the experienced interviewer can shift gears. Generally speaking, at this point all empathic statements should be avoided, until there is evidence of sound engagement. Once good engagement has been secured, if any empathic statements are going to be employed, one should start with low-valence statements and see the impact on the patient. Any further disengagement suggests empathic statements should probably be avoided for the rest of the interview. For clinicians who routinely use empathic statements throughout their interviews, this process requires true discipline and intentionality. Such discipline will be amply rewarded, for this use of strategic empathy often works remarkably well. The patient experiencing the pangs of paranoia can begin to feel a bit safer because of the intentional shifting away from the use of traditional empathic statements.

Thus far we have seen what *not* to do with paranoid patients. Now let us turn our attention to what interviewing strategies an intentional interviewer might choose to use to avoid the paranoid spiral. If we look closely at the above exchange, we will see that the interviewer is already (albeit, without intentionality) using an interviewing strategy that is often effective with patients coping with the pain of paranoid process. Notice that when the clinician simply showed a genuine interest in how the patient perceived what was happening to him with questions such as, "… how do you put it all together?" and "How do you mean?" the engagement flowed smoothly.

It is critical with a paranoid patient to help them to share as openly as possible, for inside their paranoid delusions the seeds of dangerousness, to both self and others, may be present. The use of an interested, yet non-empathic, conversational manner with paranoid patients may help the clinician to uncover such critical material, while simultaneously helping the patient to feel more comfortable. This interviewing strategy, designed to bring forth the sometimes dangerous secrets hidden within paranoid process, has been called "greasing the wheels" of delusional conversation by David Robinson.[10]

Curiously (yet logically, if one employs what we now know regarding empathic valence), there is one type of empathic statement that might be useful when coupled with Robinson's conversational strategy of greasing the wheels – *reflecting statements*. As we saw earlier, reflecting statements are empathic statements with extremely low valence regarding intuited attribution, for they simply mirror back what the patient has said. With paranoid patients, the clinician might find that the use of absolutely pure reflecting statements (*employing only the exact words of the patient*) works very well. Coupling their use with Robinson's strategy of greasing the wheels, the highly antagonistic exchange seen above might have gone very differently:

> Pt.: Things have gotten a little dicey with my husband. I'm not certain what the problem is. He just doesn't communicate the way he used to. He's not warm. We used to show a lot of affection. It's just not good.
>
> Clin.: What has changed the most in your opinion? (greasing the wheels)
>
> Pt.: It's just too weird. It's like he's not the same person. Sort of unpredictable. It's not that I think he is having an affair or anything. But he sure seems to be interested in our pretty next-door neighbor, if you know what I mean. It's pretty upsetting. And I think he might be spying on me.
>
> Clin.: What have you noticed about him as far as spying behavior? (greasing the wheels)
>
> Pt.: For about 3 months he's had them on me. I know they're watching, every night at 6 o'clock. I feel their presence. I think they use telescopes and maybe mind probes to see me, a terrible position to be in.
>
> Clin.: Sounds like a terrible position to be in (pure reflecting statement). Have you thought what you might need to do about it? (greasing the wheels)
>
> Pt.: Yeah, I just might have to pay a visit to my "pretty next-door neighbor," the little bitch. She's the one who is pushing the spying.
>
> Clin.: When you say pushing the spying (pure reflecting statement), what do you feel needs to be done? (greasing the wheels)

Pt.:   (patient pauses, looks intensely at the interviewer and with a knowing smile says) Maybe a little 22-caliber bullet might catch her attention, if you know what I mean.

What a difference intentional interviewing makes. Language counts. As opposed to our first interviewer, who used empathic statements out of habit, resulting in a striking disengagement, this interviewer has not only skillfully avoided the paranoid spiral, but has uncovered material that might save the life of the neighbor who just happens to be living next door.

On a final unexpected note regarding the paranoid spiral, our understanding of the psychodynamics of the paranoid spiral can help us not only in the engagement process, but also in the diagnostic process. Early in an initial interview, the disavowal of an empathic statement may be the first hint, to an astute clinician, that the patient may be experiencing paranoia. The clinician can then proceed to sensitively search for psychotic process, the discovery of which could have tremendous benefits for the patient, perhaps even saving his or her life (preventing a psychosis-induced suicide or homicide), if appropriate interventions result.

2: Transforming Anger with Defusing Statements

No matter how talented we may become, there are always going to be encounters in which a patient is angry with us. Paradoxically, these moments of confrontation are pregnant with potential for healing and the securing of a more powerful therapeutic alliance. So important is this topic that we will devote an entire chapter to it in Part IV of our book (Chapter 19). At present, though, it is the use of empathic statements as methods for transforming these difficult moments that interests us.

We are going to look at those moments when a patient is specifically mad at us or our institution. As with guarded patients, empathic statements can backfire with angry patients, as we will see in the following exchange with a patient who has been waiting for 20 minutes for a third appointment with an outpatient therapist. The patient has more than his fair share of narcissism:

Pt.:   Where have you been? I've been waiting here for over 20 minutes. What the hell is going on?!

Clin.:   I'm sorry you've been waiting, Mr. Jackson. I know it's not fun to be kept waiting. [empathic statement said sincerely]

Pt.:   Not fun?! You gotta be kidding me. (pause) No, it's *not* fun. How would you like to be kept waiting? You know, I have a job that I had to leave early today just for this appointment.

Clin.:   Mr. Jackson I've already told you I'm sorry, but sometimes I might be late for a very good reason. Today, I got hung up with a patient over at the inpatient unit who needed some extra help and was in crisis. I would do the same thing for you. I will almost always be on time for our appointments, but sometimes these emergencies come up. I'm really sorry. I hope you understand.

Pt.:   Well, I'm really sorry too. (pauses, then continues in a testy voice) I'm really sorry I've got to pay for this type of crap.

This clinician is having another "fun" day at the office. Fortunately there is a style of empathic statement that seldom backfires in these situations. These empathic statements are called *"defusing statements."* I often find that when a patient first makes an angry comment towards me, I often feel flustered and caught off-guard, not entirely certain where to proceed. At such moments, I find that any of the following three defusing statements are often effective:

a. It makes sense to me that you would be upset.
b. No wonder you are so upset.
c. Who wouldn't be upset!

Watch the use of one of these defusing statements with Mr. Jackson and how the defusing statement gives a more powerful genuineness to the clinician's apology:

> **Pt.:** Where have you been? I've been waiting here for over 20 minutes. What the hell is going on?!
>
> **Clin.:** Mr. Jackson, who wouldn't be upset! I'm almost 30 minutes late. I truly apologize. I'm sorry you've been waiting.
>
> **Pt.:** Yeah, well … (said with a mild, but less hostile intensity) you shouldn't keep a patient waiting.
>
> **Clin.:** You're absolutely right. I got hung up with a patient over at the inpatient unit who needed some extra help. Listen, what I'd like to do is give you this session free, for all of your inconvenience. Does that sound okay with you?
>
> **Pt.:** Well (tone of voice softens) well, yeah, sure. You're not gonna make a habit of this are you?
>
> **Clin.:** Of giving you sessions for free? (pauses, then smiles)
>
> **Pt.:** (patient catches the humor) No, of course not. (laughs) Of being late.
>
> **Clin.:** Absolutely not, sometimes emergencies do arise. I'd try to call ahead to my secretary if that happens in the future. Hopefully it won't. Thanks so much for being so patient. (patient shakes his head in a "these things happen" kind of way)
>
> **Pt.:** Don't worry about it.

As this illustration demonstrates, it is hard to keep being angry with someone who agrees with you. The clinician further addresses the situation by using a technique – compensation (offering to do the session for free) – that we will examine in more detail in our chapter on anger transformation, as well as a bit of well-timed humor. But the patient's anger had already been lessened significantly by the adroit use of the defusing statement ("Who wouldn't be upset!") and the sincere apology given immediately upon its use.

Notice also that the first clinician became somewhat defensive and began defending why he was late. In contrast, the second clinician almost presented his appropriate reason for being late as an afterthought, keeping the focus upon agreeing with the patient's perspective, exactly where the focus should be kept after using a defusing statement. Such a stance can seldom do anything but begin to defuse anger as long as it is sincere.

Unlike with guarded and paranoid patients, notice that these defusing statements work well despite having a high valence with regard to implied certainty. In fact, they work precisely *because* they have a high degree of valence regarding implied certainty. It is the power of the clinician strongly agreeing with the patient that transforms the moment. Indeed, each of these three defusing statements has a slightly different valence regarding the degree of certainty, with "It makes sense to me that you would be upset" having the least and "Who wouldn't be upset!" having the most. I have found that the angrier the patient, the higher the valence of the defusing statement that I use. With our new knowledge, we can now use strategic empathy to match the right defusing statement with the right patient. Intentionality, once again, the secret of the art.

3: Shoring Up a Young Empathic Bond with Paraphrasing Statements

Generic Paraphrases. By definition, as the therapeutic alliance is forming during an initial interview, it exhibits a certain fragility. Empathic statements that are paraphrases can be effectively used throughout an interview to help shore up this emerging alliance. Unlike reflecting statements, paraphrases incorporate some of the key words and phrases of the patient, but demonstrate that the clinician has processed the material in his or her own head by the fact that the phrasing is subtly different, perhaps with a slight emphasis or new nuance, but without adding interviewer opinion, reactions, or commentary. This style of empathic statement has been called a "generic paraphrase."[11]

Besides communicating empathy and the fact that the clinician is carefully listening, Ivey points out that paraphrases can sometimes allow a patient, who keeps repeating a story over and over, to move on to the next point. Indeed, sometimes in an initial interview it is important for a patient who has been through a trauma to repeat his or her story, sometimes from slightly differing angles, as a part of working-through the trauma. To such patients, a clinician's sensitive and patient paraphrasing metacommunicates that it is okay to repeat their story. Moreover, the paraphrase conveys that the interviewer has truly heard and respected its telling.[12] Other patients may have deep concerns that "nobody listens to me" or "gets what I mean," so they keep rehashing. An effective paraphrasing statement can let the patient know that he or she has been heard and can now move on.

In their outstanding textbook, Sommers-Flanagan and Sommers-Flanagan give a nice illustration of the power of well-timed paraphrasing to engage an interviewee, even when it is what they call a "simple paraphrase"[13]:

> **Client:**   Yesterday was my day off. I just sat around the house doing nothing. I had some errands to run, but I couldn't seem to make myself get up off the couch and do them.
>
> **Therapist:**   You had trouble getting going on your day off.

They follow with another example as well:

> **Client:**   I do this with every assignment. I wait until the last minute and then whip together the paper. I end up doing all-nighters. I don't think the final product is as good as it could be.

> Therapist: Waiting until the last minute has become a pattern for you and you think it makes it so you don't do as well as you could on your assignments.

Good paraphrases tend be "short and sweet." Also note that like all empathic statements they can vary as to their valence with regard to implied certainty. The paraphrase "You had trouble getting going on your day off" represents a high valence of implied certainty, as does the subsequent paraphrase, "Waiting until the last minute has become a pattern for you and you think it makes it so you don't do as well as you could on your assignments." The latter paraphrase could easily be given a lower valence of certainty, if perhaps the patient seemed a bit wary, by simply rephrasing it as, "It sounds like waiting till the last minute has become a pattern for you and you think it makes it so you don't do as well as you could on your assignments."

Ivey[14] talks about sometimes introducing a paraphrase with a separate phrase alerting the patient that the clinician is trying to make sure that he or she "gets it" – a phrase he calls a "stem." Examples might be: "Demaris, I hear you saying" or "Looks like the situation is …" He also sometimes ends a paraphrase with an added question as to whether the patient thinks the paraphrase was "on the mark," a concept he calls "checking-out accuracy." Illustrations of such check-outs might be as follows: "Am I hearing you correctly?", "Is that close?", and "Have I got it right?"

In an earlier work, as a way of enhancing empathic resonance, Ivey describes the usefulness of matching both stems and check-out questions to the style of communication that the patient uses to express themselves – a concept that Grinder and Bandler, in neurolinguistic programming (NLP), call representational systems.[15] Sommers-Flanagan and Sommers-Flanagan have broadened this approach to include any paraphrase that is based upon matching the patient's sensorial predilection for expressing their personal experiences, a technique they simply call "sensory-based paraphrases."[16] No matter what you want to call it, Ivey succinctly describes this engagement technique with both stems and check-outs below:

> *Visual patients tend to respond best to visual words ("Looks like you're saying you see the situation from this point of view …"); auditory patients respond best to tonal words ("As I hear you, sounds like … does that ring a bell?"); and kinesthetic patients respond to feeling words ("So the situation touches you like … and how does that grab you?). With many patients a mixture of visual, auditory, and kinesthetic words will be even more powerful.[17]*

The Metaphorical Paraphrase. Sommers-Flanagan and Sommers-Flanagan have described a useful empathic statement they call the "metaphorical parphrase."[18] To stressed patients, the world can naturally seem to be a chaotic place, so that their own thoughts are often scattered and not focused clearly upon their problems or their solutions. With a metaphorical paraphrase, the clinician tries to capture the "central message within a patient's communication." When done well, metaphorical paraphrases are not only engaging, but they also may have a therapeutic impact, as the patient's thinking becomes more crystallized by the insightful conciseness of the interviewer's paraphrase. The Sommers-Flanagans nicely capture the essence of a good metaphorical paraphrase as follows:

For instance, often clients come for therapy because of feeling stuck and not making any progress in terms of personal growth or problem resolution. In such a case, a therapist might reflect, "It seems like you're spinning your wheels" or "Dealing with this has been a real uphill battle."[19]

Watch the power of a simple empathic metaphorical paraphrase with a graduate student in sociology who has been struggling to finish her dissertation and is being pressured to wrap things up by her dissertation committee:

Pt.: I just don't feel very motivated right now. And I don't know what is up with me. Maybe I'm just depressed. I really like my topic for my dissertation, but I'm not even fully sure why it is important.

Clin.: That sounds frustrating. [gentle, low-valenced empathic statement]

Pt.: Very much so. (pauses) It's really sort of confusing. I don't really know what I want to do anyway. I'm not really a researcher at heart, but everyone in my class seems dead-set on being an academic and getting grants and stuff. But then what else would I do with a doctorate in sociology?

Clin.: You know, it seems to me that, for you, it feels almost like you're on a treadmill, and you're going nowhere fast. (metaphorical paraphrase)

Pt.: That's exactly it. In fact I *am* on a treadmill of sorts. And I don't have control of the speed of the damn thing, my dissertation committee does.

Clin.: What will happen if the treadmill stops?

Pt.: I'm not sure I follow. What do you mean?

Clin.: Well, if the treadmill stops – you get your dissertation in – you will have to make a decision, won't you, about what you're going to do with your life?

Pt.: Yeah, I suppose. (pauses, reflects for a moment, then sits up more animatedly) Wait a minute, wait a minute. You don't think (pause), you don't think that one of the reasons I am stalling on my dissertation is the fact that, as long as I am stalling, I don't have to make a decision, do you?

Clin.: I don't know, maybe it's one of the things we can look at in therapy.

In an initial interview, we generally use metaphorical paraphrases as a means of enriching the alliance. In this sense the interviewer's empathic comment, "You know, it seems to me that, for you, it feels almost like you're on a treadmill, and you're going nowhere fast" would have accomplished this task very well all by itself. But in this instance, perhaps because the patient clearly liked the metaphor and even spontaneously added to it with "And I don't have control of the damn thing …," the interviewer was able to expand the metaphor into a therapeutic insight.

Frequency, Timing, and Length of Effective Empathic Statements

At this juncture in our discussion of the third phase of the empathy cycle – the actual conveyance of empathy – three further variables determining the effectiveness of empathic statements warrant attention: frequency, timing, and length. With regard to frequency, no magic number exists. I do not think anyone can authoritatively state the number of optimal empathic comments per interview, because this number must surely vary for each paired interviewer and interviewee. On the other hand, I would estimate that well-received clinicians frequently seem to scatter empathic statements throughout their interview, perhaps averaging one statement every 2 to 10 minutes. Moreover, it seems likely that one could either potentially overuse or underuse empathic statements. In the former case, the clinician runs the risk of sounding superficially caring or paternalistic. In the latter case, the interviewer may be perceived to be as inscrutable as the sphinx, hardly an effective tool for ensuring a follow-up appointment.

This discussion of frequency naturally leads into the issue of timing. One underlying principle, perhaps the most important, remains that of using at least two or three, and sometimes significantly more, empathic statements during the first 5 to 10 minutes. Generally speaking, I would suspect that many patients often determine whether they like or dislike the clinician during these initial minutes, and their decision frequently rests upon whether the clinician seems accepting or not. Specifically, patients may fear that the clinician will not understand them or will think they are silly or weak. Few better tools exist in the clinician's repertoire for decisively allaying such fears than an empathic statement. Although an easy maneuver, this technique can set the tone for an entire interview.

Of course, even with the best of intentions, empathic statements can miss their mark, as illustrated below:

> **Pt.:** Well I don't really think it's right for the university to be so upset with me for not paying back the loan. I mean it was 7 years ago and I simply don't have the money. It really hurts me too.
>
> **Clin.:** It sure sounds like a difficult spot to be in, what with all those pressures and financial responsibilities. I bet it seems like you have no place to go, you know, sort of stranded, probably makes you feel like everyone is against you. I bet you feel isolated and lonely, like there is no place to go for financial advice or help, almost like a criminal.
>
> **Pt.:** Uh-huh (painful pause).
>
> **Clin.:** What are you thinking of doing?

In this example, the empathic statement has all the power of a two-page descriptive paragraph in an adventure story. It is far too long. In general, empathic comments display their engagement best when they are concise and unambiguous.

This example also points out one method of determining the effectiveness of any given empathic comment. Put succinctly, effective statements usually result in an increased verbal production by the patient. A decrease in patient speech, as shown earlier, often follows an ineffective comment. Leston Havens describes this process elegantly:

> *A more exacting test of successful empathy is the extent to which our responses stimulate and deepen the other's narrative flow. Does the speaker stop or change subjects? Are the expressions of feeling increased or decreased? One of the moments of greatest clinician drama occurs when a strong empathic flow encounters a memory heretofore forbidden to consciousness or denied.*[20]

There remains one last comment to make before leaving the discussion of the third phase of the cycle. Empathy is probably not primarily conveyed through empathic statements.

Large amounts of empathy appear to be communicated through facial expressions, body language, tone of voice, and other "empathic noises," as Havens calls them.[21] These non-verbal elements will be given the attention they deserve in Chapter 8.

Fourth Phase of the Empathy Cycle: Patient Accurately Perceives the Clinician's Empathic Statement

In the fourth phase of the empathy cycle, in which the patient receives the conveyed empathic statement, problems can also arise. Specifically, the patient's psychopathology may limit his or her ability to perceive empathy or even to understand language itself. Such a situation can occur with delirious patients or severely psychotic patients. In extreme cases, empathic statements can be malignantly transformed into an auditory illusion, perhaps becoming a derogatory statement or threatening insult.

Another situation concerns manic patients who quite simply are sometimes too busy talking to even register an empathic statement. Indeed, at times it is not clear whether they care if the clinician is being empathic or not. With these patients, attempts to empathize may actually be counterproductive, being in some respects contrary to what they most want at that moment, an audience.

Fifth Phase of the Empathy Cycle: Patient Communicates an Appropriate Acceptance of the Clinician's Empathic Statement

In the fifth phase of the empathic cycle, in which the patient provides feedback to the clinician that the empathic statement was received, difficulties may once again surface. As before, the patient's psychopathology may prevent acknowledgment of the clinician's empathic communications. This is perhaps most poignantly demonstrated by the patient ravaged by a severe, regressive depression or a catatonic stupor. Such patients sometimes seem almost hollow, as if our words pass through them unheard and unanswered. But I think it is important not to be misled by this sensation, because these patients may very well be hearing and even responding to empathic statements despite their inability to convey their reception. Clinician statements such as, "I have no real way of knowing what you are feeling, but if you are feeling lonely or sad or want to talk, I will be available, just let me know," can be very important, perhaps even pivotal in providing a new bridge for communication, the first resonation in the empathy cycle.

We should note that how empathy is communicated and how it is received in the empathy cycle can be significantly impacted by the patient's culture as well as the clinician's. We will be looking at the fine points of such diversity issues as they impact on empathy in our chapter on techniques for exploring cultural diversity and spirituality (Chapter 20).

As we wrap up our review of the empathy cycle, we have, it is hoped, moved from a cliché-like understanding of empathy towards a more sophisticated understanding of one of the most practical tools available to the initial interviewer. We have learned how the clinician can use empathic statements in an intentional manner to lay the foundation stones of the therapeutic alliance. The question that now arises is: Are there interviewing techniques and strategies, in addition to the use of empathic statements, that can allow us to deepen the therapeutic alliance? The answer is "yes," and the interviewing techniques that do so are the topic of our next chapter.

REFERENCES

1. Rosenblum R, Janson HW. *19th century art*. New York, NY: Harry N. Abrams; 1984.
2. Ivey AE, Ivey MB, Zalaquett CP. *Intentional interviewing and counseling: facilitating client development in a multicultural society*. 8th ed. Belmont, CA: Brooks/Cole, Cengage Learning; 2014. p. 8.
3. Ward NG, Stein G. Reducing emotional distance: a new method to teaching interviewing skills. *J Med Educ* 1975; **50**(6):605–14.
4. Wiens AN. The assessment interview. In: Weiner I, editor. *Clinical methods in psychology*. New York, NY: John Wiley; 1976.
5. Barrett-Lennard GT. The empathy cycle: refinement of a nuclear concept. *J Couns Psychol* 1981;**28**(2):91–100.
6. Barrett-Lennard GT. 1981. p. 94.
7. Margulies A. Toward empathy: the uses of wonder. *Am J Psychiatry* 1984;**141**(9):1025–33.
8. Margulies A, Havens L. The initial encounter: what to do first. *Am J Psychiatry* 1981;**138**(4):421–8.
9. Margulies A. 1984. p. 1031.
10. Robinson DJ. My favorite tips for exploring difficult topics such as delusions and substance abuse. *Psychiatr Clin North Am* 2007;**30**(2):239–44.
11. Sommers-Flanagan R, Sommers-Flanagan J. *Clinical interviewing*. 2nd ed. New York, NY: John Wiley & Sons, Inc.; 1999. p. 78–80.
12. Ivey AE, Ivey MB, Zalaquett CP. 2014. p. 148.
13. Sommers-Flanagan R, Sommers-Flanagan J. *Clinical interviewing*. 5th ed. Hoboken, NJ: John Wiley & Sons, Inc.; 2014. p. 72.
14. Ivey AE, Ivey MB, Zalaquett CP. 2014. p. 148.
15. Bandler R, Grinder J. *The structure of magic 1: a book about language and therapy*. Palo Alto, CA: Science and Behavior Books; 1975.
16. Sommers-Flanagan R, Sommers-Flanagan J. 2014. p. 75–6.
17. Ivey A, Ivey M. *Intentional interviewing and counseling: facilitating patient development in a multicultural society*. 4th ed. Belmont, CA: Wadsworth Publishing Company; 1998. p. 116.
18. Sommers-Flanagan R, Sommers-Flanagan J. 2014. p. 76.
19. Sommers-Flanagan R, Sommers-Flanagan J. 2014. p. 76.
20. Havens L. Exploration in the uses of language in psychotherapy: simple empathic statements. *Psychiatry* 1978;**41**(4):336–45.
21. Havens L. 1978. p. 338.

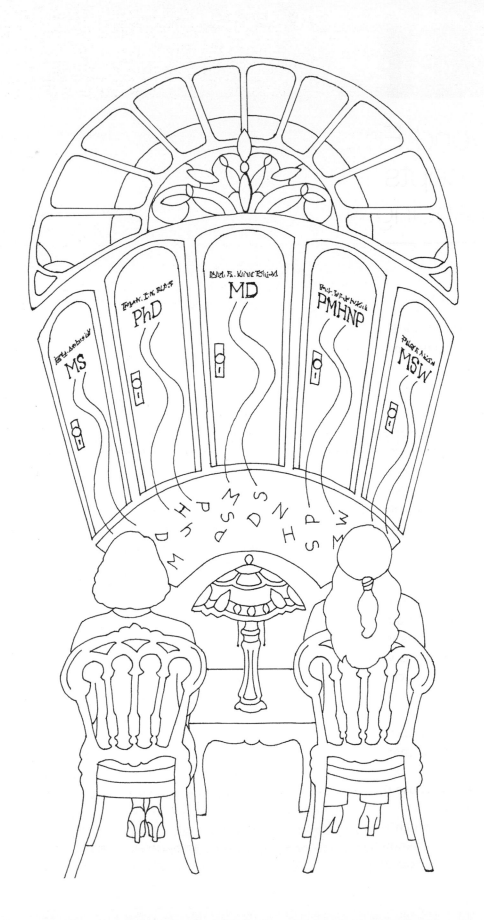

CHAPTER 2

Beyond Empathy: Cornerstone Concepts and Techniques for Enhancing Engagement

The first rule of life is to reveal nothing, to be exceptionally cautious in what you say, in whatever company you may find yourself.

Elizabeth Aston
The Darcy Connection[1]

THE PERSON BEFORE THE LETTERS

Unfortunately many patients when they find themselves in the company of a clinician may adopt the above dictum, especially when exploring sensitive and taboo topics such as suicide, incest, domestic violence, and substance abuse. There are many reasons for their caution. As they approach our office doors, they may notice various letters: M.D., Ph.D., M.S.W., R.N., M.A., but the letters are often relatively unimportant to them. What *is* important to our patients is simple: Who is the person before the letters? Is the person behind the door going to collaborate with them or patronize them? Will they be accepting or critical, warm or cool, trustworthy or irresponsible, capable or incompetent? All good questions. In addition, our task may be made a great deal more difficult because previous encounters with mental health professionals may not have gone so well.

In short, patients want to know who we are, not so much the facts of our personal lives, but our character, our ethics, and our humanness. They also want to know if we know what the hell we are doing – our expertise. In our own personal lives, before we would ever consider sharing intimate details about ourselves, we seek out answers to these questions about the people we are considering as potential friends and confidants, usually requiring many encounters before deciding whether we feel safe "baring our souls." A patient is expected to do this type of sharing within minutes of meeting a total stranger, just because the stranger has some letters after his or her name. It is, at best, an odd situation.

Yet it holds much promise for healing and the relief of suffering, if indeed we can forge a resilient therapeutic alliance. How we address each of the above concerns offers opportunities for deepening the engagement process that goes beyond empathy itself.

These patient concerns are less roadblocks than they are gateways. And the way we address these issues, how our characters and humanness show themselves, is through the interview itself. There are many interviewing principles, techniques, and strategies that provide concrete methods for talented clinicians to intentionally, and surprisingly rapidly, address these issues. This is a chapter about these principles and techniques, and how we can become such clinicians. And it all begins in the waiting room.

INDUCEMENT OF A SAFE RELATIONSHIP

The patient's waiting room period before meeting his or her clinician may pass with an urgent slowness. It is frequently teeming with fears of rejection and with self-recrimination. It is often accompanied by ruminations such as, "Well, it's finally come to this, I'm so weak I need a shrink." As professionals we would like to think patients do not feel this way about us, but we should not deceive ourselves. For most people (including many mental health professionals), it is genuinely upsetting to admit the need for help with psychological problems. The sensitive handling of this anxiety represents one of the centerpiece tasks of the initial interviewer. In fact, if it is not handled well, there may not be a second interview.

In his classic book *The Psychiatric Interview*, Harry Stack Sullivan describes a novel idea he calls "the self-system." This self-system consists of "a vast system of processes, states of alertness, symbols, and signs of warnings, which protects us from a lowering of self-esteem as we meet new people."[2] This self-system, consisting of both conscious and unconscious coping mechanisms, becomes activated in an effort to decrease the anxiety generated by fears of rejection. It is this self-system that rises to a high pitch as a patient absent-mindedly turns the pages of a magazine in the waiting room or plays distractedly with a cell phone.

Three ideas immediately come to mind. First, one of the primary goals of the clinician in the initial interview consists of attempting to decrease the patient's anxiety and hence the need for an extremely active self-system. Second, the activation of the self-system offers the clinician an excellent preview of the patient's defenses against interpersonal anxiety. Thus, the opening 10 minutes of the interview provide an unexpected window into the workings of the patient's mental "guard dogs," both healthy and rabid. And third, in most cases, the clinician's own self-system is also aroused when the clinician meets a new patient. The interplay of these three processes lies at the very heart of the engagement process.

As we have seen, to some extent the conveyance of empathy can significantly decrease the patient's need for an active self-system, but other specific processes can also reassure the interviewee. In the 1950s and 1960s, Carl Rogers developed the concept of "unconditional positive regard," which he defined as follows: "The therapist communicates to his client a deep and genuine caring for him as a person with potentialities, a caring uncontaminated by evaluations of his thoughts, feelings, or behaviors."[3] It is a powerful statement. It is not unlike the suspension of analytic thought seen in the process of intuition.

Placed into the context of the initial interview, as opposed to ongoing therapy, unconditional positive regard translates as a suspension of moral opinion by the interviewer with respect to the interviewee. In short, the patient comes away with the feeling that the clinician is not going to pass judgment on him. In many cases, this safe feeling contrasts starkly with the patient's recent experience (and, at times, lifelong experience) of encountering a long string of raised eyebrows on the faces of friends, family members, and employers. It is up to the interviewer not to follow this parade of frowns.

In this regard, it becomes important for the clinician to work out the potentially disturbing feelings raised by emotionally charged issues such as divorce, religion, sexual orientation, suicide, violence, child abuse, rape, and abortion. No matter what the clinician's view of these activities, in the initial interview, the goal remains to show no judgment to the patient. Instead, the interviewer attempts to convey interest in finding out the significance of these ideas to the patient, recognizing the truth in the very wise statement of Armond Nicholi, Jr., that "whether the patient is young or old, neatly groomed or disheveled, outgoing or withdrawn, articulate, highly integrated or totally disintegrated, of high or low socioeconomic status, the skilled clinician realizes that the patient, as a fellow human being, is considerably more like himself than he is different ..."[4]

Practically, one effective method of spotting potentially disruptive topics for oneself consists of monitoring interviews for topics that one consistently avoids. For instance, one interviewer may discover that he or she seldom knows anything about the religious beliefs of his or her patients, whereas another interviewer never asks about sexuality. Such gaps in data gathering may point to precisely those topics about which the interviewer has strong opinions. It is in these areas that conveying unconditional positive regard may be problematic.

It is not only controversial issues that can disrupt the conveyance of unconditional positive regard. In fact, as clinicians we may unwittingly sound like parents at the most unlikely times. In the following dialogue with a young man suffering from paranoid schizophrenia, this disconcerting process rears its head in a subtle form:

    Clin.:   Tell me more about what you've been doing since your last hospitalization.

    Pt.:   Things are going well. I'm getting along much better at home, and I haven't needed all those drugs the doctor told me to take.

    Clin.:   (pause, clinician looks up from clipboard) So you haven't been taking your medications like you're supposed to.

    Pt.:   No, I just think they fog up my mind.

    Clin.:   We'll need to talk about that a little later.

This clinician's choice of words has created an atmosphere potentially suggestive of a parent's reprimand. Indeed, the interviewer's last statement sounds suspiciously like a threat to go to the principal's office.

As a contrast, in the following dialogue, a different approach yields a different interaction with significantly less activation of the patient's self-system:

    Clin.:   Tell me more about what you've been doing since your last hospitalization.

    Pt.:   Things are going well. I'm getting along much better at home, and I haven't needed all those drugs the doctor told me to take.

    Clin.:   What were some of the medications you were using?

Pt.:	I think it was called Haldol and a little pill … Cogentin or something like that.
Clin.:	Tell me a little bit about what you felt like while you were on these medications.
Pt.:	It was strange. I don't know which one was doing it, but I always felt doped up, like I was in a fog.
Clin.:	That sounds like an unpleasant side effect.
Pt.:	Yes, it was.

This interviewer has successfully conveyed concern without a price tag of obedience. Ironically, later in the interview, I would suspect the latter clinician would be in a more favorable position to persuade the patient to try an antipsychotic again.

This discussion suggests another characteristic – non-defensiveness – that contributes to a feeling of safety for the patient. Patients are very quick to perceive defensiveness in an interviewer. Defensive posturing by the clinician may create in the interviewee the feeling that "I've got to watch what I say here." The following example illustrates a defensive position by the clinician, as a woman describes her anguish concerning her son's problems with schizophrenia:

Moth.:	I just don't know what to do with him. Nothing the doctors do ever helps. It's always the same. I don't think they know what they are doing. They haven't tried megavitamin therapy, and I hear that it sometimes works miracles. I want you to try that treatment.
Clin.:	Well, let's get something straight, these kinds of therapies are simply unproven and maybe unsafe. So we don't use those here.
Moth.:	But some people claim they've been helped.
Clin.:	Don't believe everything you read Mrs. Jones.

Here we see the paternalistic tone that can so readily destroy a patient's trust. The clinician's self-system has been activated, resulting in a defensive, "educational" posture, which only serves to reciprocally activate the patient's own self-system. This interaction might have been avoided with the following approach, beginning with a gentle empathic statement in which the clinician's intuition about the mother's inner world is right on the mark:

Moth.:	… They haven't tried megavitamin therapy, and I hear that it sometimes works miracles. I want you to try that treatment.
Clin.:	It sounds like you've really gone through a lot of frustration, Mrs. Jones. In a little while we'll talk about the pros and cons of different treatments, including megavitamin therapy, but first I want to hear more about your son so that I have a better understanding of exactly what we are dealing with here.
Moth.:	Sure. It's long and complicated. But it all started about 3 years ago …

Our discussion of the principles behind the development of a safe alliance began with the words of Harry Stack Sullivan. Sullivan also provides an important note upon which to close our discussion. One of the contributing factors to the development of an overactive self-system is the not-so-maladaptive fear that strangers may harbor ulterior motives. In short, a patient may fear that he or she is going to be used or even abused.

It is hoped that conscious abuse of a patient is a rarity in our field, but less sinister abuse may enter the picture unconsciously. Clinicians may have ulterior motives of which they have little, if any, awareness. For example, a clinician may depend on a patient for the gratification of the clinician's need to feel liked or important. If the patient feels that the clinician needs something from them, such as respect, caring, or fondness, the relationship is no longer a safe one. Once again, the patient is faced with watching what he or she says, from the fear that professional help will be withdrawn if certain needs are not satisfied.

Sullivan stated this principle elegantly:

> He [the clinician] is an expert having expert knowledge of interpersonal relations, personality problems, and so on; he has no traffic in the satisfactions which may come from interpersonal relations, and he does not pursue prestige or standing in the eyes of his patients, or at the expense of his patients. In accordance with this definition, the psychiatrist is quite obviously uninterested in what the patient might have to offer, temporarily or permanently, as a companion, and quite resistant to any support by the patient for his prestige, importance, and so on. It is only if the psychiatrist is very clearly aware of this taboo, as it were, on trafficking in the ordinary commodities of interpersonal relations, that many suspicious people discover that they can deal with him and can actually communicate to him their problems with other people.[5]

Besides offering a safe relationship, the initial interviewer also actively engages the patient in a positive fashion, utilizing those gestures and words that suggest to the patient that future interaction will be enjoyable and rewarding, as seen in our next topic.

CLINICIAN GENUINENESS

The term "genuineness" has been described by a variety of researchers.[6,7] As was the case with empathy, genuineness appears to be a nebulous term at first glance. Once again, an operative definition provides clarification. One can state that "being genuine" occurs when the following is present:

> The behavioral characteristics of the clinician suggest to the patient that the clinician is feeling at ease both with himself and with the patient. It is frequently marked by three characteristics in the clinician: (1) responsiveness, (2) spontaneity, and (3) consistency.

Perhaps there exists no better arena for examining these characteristics of clinician genuineness than looking at the reactions of a clinician to patient humor. When faced with humor some clinicians display a curious sense of awkwardness, as if humor should not be allowed during an interview. In essence, these clinicians "run-over" the moment of humor. Rather than responding with a smile or a chuckle, they maintain a somber expression.

This rather extreme form of non-responsiveness can produce an immediate increase in patient anxiety, not unlike the discomfort many of us have had the misfortune of experiencing in a social setting, when one of our jokes is followed by an absence of laughter. Ironically, such clinicians may argue that their non-responsiveness represents professionalism, but it seems odd that professional behavior should result in increased patient anxiety during the early stages of an interview. Moreover, this same lack of clinician responsiveness may be uniformly provided in response to a variety of patient affects, including tearfulness, anger, and fear, all in the name of professionalism.

Many patients balk at such pseudo-professionalism, preferring a clinician who interacts with a gentle responsiveness. In the final analysis, the mark of a true professional seems to be his or her lack of a need to feign professionalism. Such clinicians quickly and easily appear at ease with both their body language and their reactivity. They are attentively relaxed. Moreover, they bring to the interview a sense of appropriate spontaneity, the second characteristic of genuine interaction as described in our definition.

This spontaneity does not exist as a license for sharing whatever comes to mind. To the contrary, a skilled clinician consistently assesses the potential impact of all statements, but also possesses the ability to share some spontaneous feelings if they are deemed appropriate for the patient. This spontaneous quality often demonstrates itself in characteristics such as a well-timed sense of humor, a flexible method of structuring the interview, and a non-defensive attitude towards questions voiced by the patient.

As just mentioned, one must be careful about the degree of responsiveness and spontaneity one displays. Both too much and too little can present problems. For instance, a buoyant interviewer can intimidate certain patients, whereas a wooden interviewer may frighten them. In regard to the latter, if the frightened patient feels too uncomfortable with the clinician to share suicidal ideation, then the unresponsive interviewer may truly regret having presented a wooden attitude. The clinician needs to nurture a flexible style. The degree of spontaneity and responsiveness will probably vary from one patient to another and with the clinical setting.

To this point, the myth of "professional blandness" may have evolved from a misinterpretation of the psychoanalytic concept of presenting a neutral screen upon which the patient can project his or her transference. This neutral screen concept does not represent a dictum for unresponsiveness. In the first place, an expressionless presentation hardly represents a neutral stance, as Ryle[8] has commented, for such a bland reaction typically suggests that the non-responder dislikes the other participant. This supposed "neutral stance" is, in actuality, potentially very disengaging. Moreover, rather than providing a blank screen, it seems to bias the patient towards negative transference.

Even if one adhered to this neutral stance theory for therapeutic application, and few talented analysts I have met do so in a strict sense, it does not necessarily follow that the neutral stance is effective for assessment interviewing. Indeed, as we have seen, one of the major goals of the initial interview remains the development of a sound therapeutic alliance, which will, it is hoped, lead to a sincere interest in coming to a second appointment. A wooden interview hardly lends itself to the facilitation of engagement.

It seems timely to examine consistency, the third element commonly characterizing a genuine interaction. Gerard Egan has emphasized the importance of consistency, as demonstrated by the clinician's willingness to explore the patient's world in a shared manner while respecting the patient's present limitations and defenses. More specifically, the clinician avoids discordant actions, such as appearing warmly responsive in part of the interview and coolly distant later; nor does the clinician suddenly become confrontational, as demonstrated by Counselor A in the following example provided by Egan.[9]

> **Patient:** I want to know what you really think of me.
>
> **Counselor A:** I think you're lazy and that you would like things to get better if that could happen by magic.
>
> **Counselor B:** Frankly, I don't find a great deal of value in such direct evaluation, but I think it's good to talk about this directly. Maybe we can take a look at what's happening between you and me.

The response of Counselor B demonstrates a willingness to share exploration, including a foray into the developing interviewer–interviewee relationship.

Together, the traits of appropriate responsiveness, spontaneity, and consistency coalesce to create an appealing milieu for the sharing of problems. When adroitly blended, these three traits of genuineness convey a sense of emotional balance in the clinician, a balance that suggests a possible source of help to the person in need.

In the following dialogue, these traits, as well as a sense of non-defensiveness, are elegantly displayed in a situation in which a therapist could easily have swallowed his or her foot. In this interaction, the clinician, a physician, had determined from the preceding conversation that the patient was pleasant and well integrated but very anxious. Consequently, the interviewer felt that humor could be safely employed.

> **Clin.:** What has it been like coming down to the emergency room today?
>
> **Pt.:** Unsettling, to say the least. I feel very awkward here, sort of like I'm vulnerable. To be honest, I've had some horrible experiences with doctors; I don't like them.
>
> **Clin.:** I see, well, they scare the hell out of me too (smiles, indicating the humor in his comment).
>
> **Pt.:** (chuckle) I thought you were a doctor.
>
> **Clin.:** I am (pause, smiles), that's what's so scary.
>
> **Pt.:** (smiles and laughs)
>
> **Clin.:** Tell me a little more about some of your unpleasant experiences with doctors, because I want to make sure I'm not doing anything that is upsetting you or frightening you. I don't want that to happen.
>
> **Pt.:** Well, that's very nice to hear. My last doctor didn't give a crap about what I said, and he only spoke in huge words.

In this example, the clinician has skillfully transformed a potentially "loaded moment" into a shared resolution through humor. If patients realize that avenues for discussing their needs and complaints are open, they frequently feel less frightened. The presence of pathways for "filing complaints" paradoxically often decreases the need for their use.

This excerpt also illustrates the common finding that experienced interviewers frequently appear to enjoy the process of interviewing itself. Experienced clinicians feel at home in the interviewing process, their own self-systems purring quietly. It is this sense of natural balance in the clinician that remains one of the most powerful of engagement tools. This balance is complemented by the next trait to be discussed, yet another important tool in the engagement process.

CLINICIAN EXPERTISE

In order to explain the concept of clinician expertise most effectively, it may be best temporarily to view the interviewing process solely from the patient's perspective. To the patient, certain questions are of paramount importance. The answer to one of these questions in particular holds unusually powerful significance, perhaps even determining the degree of final interest in whatever treatment recommendations may be made. It is a logical question. It is a natural question. And it can be paraphrased simply as follows: "Can this person help me?"

To ignore the reality that the patient is attempting to answer this question can lead to serious problems in engagement. To begin with, the act of hanging out our shingles as mental health professionals suggests that we have something to offer to patients for which they will exchange money, time, and trust. On a basic level, they are generally expecting to find a good listener, albeit a "paid ear" of sorts. But at a deeper level, they are also expecting something else, something more. They are expecting to find an expert, a term I find mildly threatening, because it comes pre-seasoned with more than a pinch of pride. One feels hesitant to declare oneself an expert in so vast a field as human behavior, feelings, and psychophysiology.

But the term becomes more palatable, and indeed appropriate, if one keeps in mind two of the principles behind it. First, being an expert does *not* mean that one has all the answers or, for that matter, can necessarily provide relief. And second, being an expert *does* suggest that we have been rigorously schooled in an effort to consolidate a body of knowledge found useful in our field. It is the presence of this body of knowledge that may most successfully answer the patient's pressing question, "Can this person help me?"

In this regard, it is also useful to remember that in an anthropological sense, the initial clinician is fulfilling the role of a healer, and whether one is a shaman or a social worker, as a healer one is expected to possess knowledge not commonly available to the patient. From the above discussions, it should be apparent that, at both a personal and a societal level, the clinician's expertise as perceived by the patient is critical to the engagement process.

The next logical question is, "How does one convey expertise effectively during an initial interview?" The answer lies primarily not in what we tell the patient but in what we ask the patient. It is the quality of our questions, not the quantity of our words, that generally convinces a patient that the clinician knows something that might help.

Questions, like empathic statements, can be categorized along a number of continua, including: (1) open-ended versus closed-ended, (2) probing versus non-probing,

(3) fact-finding versus opinion-finding, and (4) structured versus unstructured. Questions along the full range of these continua can be clinically useful, and all can be surprisingly ineffective as well. Their effectiveness or ineffectiveness seems to depend upon their timing as well as their appropriateness for the task facing the interviewer at any specific moment.

In the next two chapters a great deal of time will be spent discussing the flexible use of questions at different phases of the interview. But at this point, I want to focus on an especially useful type of question, a type of question that can unobtrusively yet effectively convey expertise to the patient: the fact-oriented question.

By the term "fact-oriented question," I am referring to questions concerned with the concrete realities of the patient's situation, symptoms, and problems. Questions such as, "Are you having any problem falling asleep?" or "Has your appetite changed?" represent typical examples of fact-oriented questions. Frequently, fact-oriented questions concern diagnostic issues, and they are generally closed-ended in nature.

Some initial interviewers shy away from fact-oriented questions, because they believe that such questions are generally disengaging. In this regard, I agree that they can be disengaging when used at the wrong moments, too frequently, or in checklist fashion. And an interviewer should learn to avoid these pitfalls. But when asked sensitively, fact-oriented questions are powerful engagement tools that also yield large amounts of valuable information for effective treatment planning and triage decisions.

To illustrate the point, let us look at the mid-phase of an initial interview with a woman in her late 20s. Rather than just moving tangentially with the patient, the interviewer begins a more structured effort to tease out the symptoms upsetting this patient in an effort to arrive at a useful diagnosis. Keep in mind that the clinician has used many open-ended questions and empathic statements in the earlier sections of the interview. Indeed she will continue to intermittently utilize both as she explores for the presence of an anxiety disorder by effectively increasing her use of fact-finding questions.

Pt.: I am terribly frightened about going back for my masters, I mean, is it worth it? … When I think about it, I get all uptight.

Clin.: How do you mean?

Pt.: I start to fret and worry. I feel extremely tense and wound up like a crazy alarm clock, ready to explode.

Clin.: Over the course of any given day, say over the last month, how much of your day do you spend worrying like that?

Pt.: Oh, I'd say at least 70%, sometimes almost the whole day.

Clin.: (said gently) Sounds miserable.

Pt.: It really is, and the bad part is, I can't stop it.

Clin.: Sounds like you find it difficult to relax.

Pt.: Oh my God, yes! Even when I come home I feel like I've got to do something, something needs to be done and if I don't do it I'm a bad person. It's strange.

Clin.: People develop a lot of tensions during the day, especially in a job like yours. I'm wondering if you find yourself having muscle aches, trembling sensations, or eye twitches related to your tension.

> **Pt.:** Funny you should ask. You may have noticed, but my left eye twitches when I'm tense, drives me nuts.
>
> **Clin.:** How long has that been going on?
>
> **Pt.:** I've had it … let's see … maybe 5 or 6 years, but ever since deciding on grad school it's been really much worse.
>
> **Clin.:** How do you mean?
>
> **Pt.:** I look like a "mad winker" (patient and clinician chuckle). It really can be embarrassing.
>
> **Clin.:** I'm sure it can be (warmly chuckles again). Tell me, have you noticed any other evidence of tension in your body, other than the twitching?
>
> **Pt.:** I've had a lot of diarrhea lately, I don't know if that's related or not, and I also have been feeling flashes of feeling real hot, makes me think of my mother and menopause, but I've had those kinds of flashes off and on for years.
>
> **Clin.:** With these hot flashes, do you notice any change in your pulse rate or breathing rate?
>
> **Pt.:** No, I can't say I have.
>
> **Clin.:** Have you ever found yourself suddenly having an abrupt episode of being extremely anxious, all at once?
>
> **Pt.:** No … let me think, … not really.
>
> **Clin.:** When you say "not really," what have you experienced?
>
> **Pt.:** About a week ago I really got upset about Bob, but I wasn't really anxious, I was mad.
>
> **Clin.:** What about periods when you suddenly became very frightened, perhaps of dying, without any apparent reason?
>
> **Pt.:** No, that I can clearly say I've never had.
>
> **Clin.:** Any periods when you suddenly found yourself panicing and perhaps short of breath or noticing tingling sensations in your fingers or around your mouth?
>
> **Pt.:** No, I don't get that either.
>
> **Clin.:** What about your concentration?
>
> **Pt.:** Now *that's* shot. I can't concentrate at all. I've particularly noticed that when doing the books at work. Math comes simple to me and usually I fly through that stuff, but over the past 2 months I feel really frazzled. It takes forever.
>
> **Clin.:** Earlier you mentioned the relationship of these feelings to your fears about grad school. What are some of the connections you see?
>
> **Pt.:** Well, in the first place, I don't think I can do it. I mean I'm smart, at least I think I'm reasonably intelligent, but I don't know about the discipline I'd need. I think that worries me most.
>
> **Clin.:** What else worries you?
>
> **Pt.:** What would happen to Bob and me, I mean, when would I see him? I don't know, maybe never …

I have used a rather lengthy example because I want to emphasize the usefulness of sensitively utilized fact-oriented questions. In this excerpt, their gentle structuring, while clearly providing answers to diagnostic questions concerning anxiety disorders, may have also helped to convey a variety of important metacommunications to the patient, such as the following:

1. This interviewer is obviously interested in finding out exactly what symptoms and experiences I have been feeling.
2. This interviewer must have worked with similar problems before because the questions asked hit upon a lot of the feelings and symptoms I have had.
3. This interviewer seems to be thorough and is actively exploring many different issues.

In short, all of these metacommunications serve to increase the patient's confidence in the clinician's expertise and ultimately in the clinician's potential to provide help. Good friends can provide sensitive listening, but only good clinicians can provide both sensitive listening and knowledgeable questioning.

It is also informative to see the frequent peppering of this fact-oriented dialogue with unstructured questions and empathic comments. In fact, it looks as if the interviewer was about to leave structured questioning in order to pursue a region of open-ended inquiries into psychodynamic issues. Once again, the art lies in a flexible attitude – the intentional suiting of the most effective form of questioning to the task at hand.

It is interesting to note that an interviewer who gets stuck on the idea of open-ended questioning throughout most of the initial interview potentially robs himself or herself of the chance to be perceived not only as a good listener but also as a skilled caregiver. In addition, it goes without saying that the clinician limited to an open-ended approach may also come away with an inadequate database for treatment purposes. The use of fact-oriented questions in the previous example has provided a sound exploration of the symptoms of a generalized anxiety disorder, which the patient appears to have. Simultaneously, the exploration of panic disorder symptoms has ruled out that problem. The treatment clearly would have varied for these two disorders. If the questioning around panic episodes had uncovered a panic disorder with an accompanying agoraphobia, specific treatment modalities, such as cognitive behavioral therapy, are available that might provide striking relief.

The above dialogue illustrates the increase in engagement that can be achieved by flexibly mixing fact-finding questions with open-ended questions and empathic statements when exploring diagnostic regions. It is an opportune time to further bring to life such an effective strategy with a video illustration. In this video you will see me helping a patient to share the symptoms of one of the most common presentations you will encounter in everyday clinical practice – a major depressive disorder.

VIDEO MODULE 2.1

Title: Conveying Empathy with Fact-Finding Questions

Contents: Contains both expanded didactics and an annotated interview excerpt illustrating an exploration of depressive symptoms.

When reflecting upon the power of fact-oriented questions to enhance engagement, I am reminded of several of my patients over the years who proved to be suffering from the highly stigmatizing diagnosis of obsessive–compulsive disorder (OCD). OCD has a surprisingly high lifetime prevalence rate of about 2.5%, yet very few outpatient therapists report treating the high number of patients suffering from this disorder that this high prevalence rate would suggest.

The reason is simple. People with OCD are often terribly embarrassed by their symptoms and guilt ridden by the dramatic fall-off in their functioning resulting from their symptoms. I have treated very few people with OCD who have not said things like the following to themselves over the years: "I must be one of the craziest people in the world. There is really something very wrong with me." As a result, the vast majority of people suffering with OCD do not present to us complaining about their OCD symptoms; they present complaining of being depressed or anxious, or having marital problems or problems at work. To uncover OCD symptoms, a clinician often must directly ask about them or forever be unaware of them. Few people feel comfortable meeting a total stranger and saying things like, "It takes me 2 hours to shower each morning because I have to keep repeating my washing because of germs," or "I am plagued by repeated images of knifing my baby even though I know I would never do it. It frightens me so much that I am hesitant to go into the nursery without my husband along."

So strong is the self-recrimination and stigmatization of many people with OCD that studies have shown that they suffer, on average, for about 11 to 14 years before seeking help.[10,11] Sadly, OCD is often a hidden disorder for which many people who could receive help never do.[12,13]

Obviously, all people presenting with depression or anxiety should be screened for OCD, but it is not the importance of screening that interests us here. It is the power of a closed-ended, fact-finding question to enhance engagement that is of interest, as seen in the following illustration, where I have just finished uncovering the depressive symptoms of a patient who had presented complaining, "I've got a really bad depression, and I really need help for it." We are about 20 minutes into the interview:

Pt.: … Yeah, the sleep problems really are rough. Like I told you, I wake up every morning exhausted. I hate getting out of bed. Sometimes I start to sit up to get out of bed and then just lie back down.

Clin.: Sounds really very tough, very painful (said softly).

Pt.: Yeah, it really is. I've been depressed off and on for over 10 years. My marriage has basically been ruined.

Clin.: Hmmm (empathic tone). You know, Mary, some of my patients who are as depressed as you are, tell me that they worry a lot. Now some people worry about stuff that people often worry about, like money or relationships. But I have a fair number of people who worry about stuff that they feel it is very odd to be worrying about. Like some of my depressed patients tell me they are constantly worried they have germs on their hands and wash their hands repeatedly. Others tell me they are worried they have left the stove or an iron on and must repeatedly check it, perhaps spending 10 minutes saying words like "it's off" over and over while looking at the stove or iron. Have you had anything sort of like this happening to you? (closed-ended, fact-finding question)

Pt.: (patient sits up and looks cautiously surprised) Sort of, yeah, sort of.

Clin.: What have you experienced?

Pt.: I'm afraid of germs a lot. (pauses) I mean a real lot. I wash my hands all over the place.

Clin.: Oh, that's very common. I've had patients sitting in that very chair who tell me they wash their hands over 200 times a day (patient looks truly shocked). I've even had patients wash their hands so often they start to damage the skin on the back of their hands.

Pt.: You have? (said with genuine surprise)

Clin.: Oh yeah (nodding head in agreement).

Pt.: I don't wash my hands that much, but I wash my hands a lot, maybe 100 times a day. Sometimes I can't get to work, because I have to keep washing, so I call in sick. It's horrible. It's so weird, and I let everybody down at work.

Clin.: You know what, Mary?

Pt.: What?

Clin.: I think I know what might be going on with you. I think you may have obsessive–compulsive disorder – what we call OCD. I know it feels weird to you, but it's surprisingly common.

Pt.: Other people do these things? I'm not crazy?

Clin.: At this very instant, I would guess several million other people have OCD, and no, you are not crazy. (warmly smiles) In addition they all do exactly what you have done. They are so embarrassed that they tell no one, not even their spouses about their symptoms.

Pt.: Oh my God! (patient bursts into tears) Oh, my God. Can you help me with this?

Clin.: Yeah, I think we can help you. (patient sits back, still crying from relief, wiping away the tears) It is actually a disorder that we have lots of different treatments for.

In 30 years of practice, I am hard pressed to recall any empathic statements that I have made that can match the power of such closed-ended, fact-finding questions to enhance the engagement process as evidenced by the simple, yet sensitive, inquiry into the presence of OCD illustrated above. Their power emanates from their metacommunication of clinician expertise, reassuring the patient that the interviewer has seen "this nightmarish thing" before. In this case, it allowed Mary to share a hugely guilt-producing secret for the very first time, after silently carrying its weight for over 10 years. Simultaneously, such questions also metacommunicate the greatly reassuring fact that many other people have had similar symptoms. Pretty powerful stuff for a single well-timed question.

In a last note concerning clinician expertise, we can see the complementary functions of all the factors discussed so far under the rubric of engagement in both Chapters 1 and 2. Indeed, the ability to blend effectively with a patient is mirrored by the clinician's ability to blend a variety of techniques, such as: (1) the strategic use of empathic statements; (2) the creation of a safe environment; (3) the ability to convey genuineness through spontaneity, responsiveness, and consistency; and (4) the conveyance of a reassuring knowledge base. These four attributes lay the groundwork for quickly establishing an effective therapeutic alliance.

At this point we have nearly completed our exploration of the engagement process, the first way-station in our map of the interview. Yet there remains one more concept that can provide us with a surprisingly robust platform for enhancing engagement – the concept of collaborative interviewing.

COLLABORATIVE INTERVIEWING MODELS: NEW TOOLS FOR ENHANCING ENGAGEMENT

From the very first pages of our book, we have consistently been looking at the interviewing process from a person-centered perspective. In this respect, all of our interviewing techniques can be considered as being "collaborative" in nature, for collaboration is at the heart of effective interviewing, as Carl Rogers demonstrated in his pioneering client-centered approach. In addition though, there has been an exciting development in recent decades of specific therapeutic and interviewing models that emphasize techniques for creating the sensation of "moving with" patients as opposed to "moving against" them. These approaches can collectively be called "collaborative interviewing models." Prominent examples of collaborative approaches include solution-focused therapy,[14-18] motivational interviewing,[19,20] and the medication interest model.[21-23] Jobes has developed innovative collaborative interviewing approaches for helping patients who are being followed for active suicidal ideation to find reasons for living, as well as providing a means for determining patients' ongoing risk.[24]

Collaborative models intentionally enhance engagement by helping patients discover, for themselves, what goals they want to achieve in therapy. In addition, these models further enhance engagement by helping patients choose which methods they want to use to achieve these goals, while finding personally chosen motivators for sticking to these methods until the goals have been achieved. The emphasis is clearly upon collaborative goal setting as a major, if not *the* major, gateway to enhancing engagement. From this perspective, it is believed that collaborative goal setting may be used to forge powerful and sustainable therapeutic alliances, even in situations where empathy does not work particularly well or might even backfire if used.

Cheng points out in an insightful and provocative article that, even in a historical sense, very powerful bonds have occurred among countries based not so much upon empathy, or even respect, but upon common goal setting.[25] He points out that one of the greatest alliances of modern times, the alliance between the Allies in the Second World War, included countries like the United States, Britain, and Russia. It is doubtful that the alliance between the United States and Russia was primarily based upon mutual empathy, trust, and respect; but it most certainly proved to be a powerful alliance, an alliance strong enough to topple the Third Reich. It was an alliance based upon the agreement to have a common goal.

Thus, interpersonal processes, such as jointly arriving upon a set of common goals, working together to achieve these common goals, and sharing in the enjoyment of obtaining them can be powerful tools for nurturing the engagement process. Sometimes, in clinical situations where there may *not* be strong immediate empathy and respect (as with the first meeting with an actively paranoid patient or an angry teenager forced into therapy by his parents), the successful navigation of these collaborative processes may not only forge the core of the initial alliance, but eventually, over time, lead to the development of genuine empathy and respect.

As prototypic person-centered models, collaborative approaches emphasize that the success of many therapeutic alliances is dependent on how well the clinician comes to understand the goals that the patient views as important and the methods the patient wants to use to arrive at these goals. The clinician can then attempt to forge a collaborative and shared understanding both of these goals and the methods for reaching them. It is important to remember that in collaborative interviewing, *we do not necessarily do whatever patients wants us to do, rather we make a sincere effort to help our patients to discover for themselves what it might be best for them to do.*

Cheng points out that decades ago, Borden,[26] with the delineation of his transtheoretical model, helped to lay the foundation for these collaborative approaches when he described a sound therapeutic alliance as having the following three components (note that two of Borden's three "pillars of engagement" are related to collaborative goal setting and treatment planning):

1. Agreement on goals, which are the desired outcomes of the therapeutic process
2. Agreement on tasks, which are the steps that will be undertaken to achieve the goals
3. Bond between patient and therapist, which encompasses Rogerian aspects such as trust, respect, genuineness, unconditional regard, and empathy

It can be seen from Borden's definition that collaborative models fully embrace all of the engagement techniques we have already explored. What they add is merely an emphasis point, but it is an important point – the power of intentionally focusing upon seeing the world first through the patient's eyes, then helping the patient to discover for himself or herself his or her own goals, methods, and motivations for effective change and healing. When done well, such a focus has powerful ramifications for enhancing engagement.

Collaborative approaches, such as motivational interviewing (MI) and the medication interest model (MIM), are so valuable in establishing a powerful alliance in the initial interview that we will devote an entire chapter to each of them in Part IV of our book on advanced interviewing techniques. In the meantime, let us look at two techniques from the psychotherapeutic model known as solution-focused therapy that can be immediately adapted to the initial interview itself.

Solution-Focused Goal Setting

We will begin by looking at an interview that did not go well with a disgruntled teenager who would like to be anywhere but in this clinician's office on this particular day:

Clin.: What's the problem that brings you here today?

Pt.: I don't have a problem. I don't need to be here. My parents need help, not me.

Clin.: Your parents told me that your mood is irritable, you've lost interest in things, and you have trouble with your sleep, appetite, and concentration. Sounds to me like you might have a depression and need treatment for it.

Pt.: I knew this was gonna be a waste of my time. I'm getting out of here![27]

Things aren't going too well here at the ranch, are they? Part of the communication breakdown is that this interview is not person-centered. It is parent-centered. Moreover, the clinician is not waiting to hear directly from the patient what the patient sees as the problem.

In contrast, solution-focused interviewing is goal-directed and attempts to uncover, from the patient himself or herself, exactly what goals they seek. It is important not to assume what the patient wants, but to hear it in the patient's own words. Sometimes there are surprises. Cheng[28] suggests two nice questions for this purpose:

1. "What would make this a helpful visit?"
2. "What would you like to see different from coming here?"

He then offers the following excellent illustration of these techniques at work with the same disgruntled teenager:

Clin.: What's the problem that brings you here today?

Pt.: I don't have a problem. I don't need to be here. My parents need help, not me.

Clin.: Okay – so what would make this a helpful visit?

Pt.: Tell my parents that I don't need to be here; they're the ones who have the problem.

Clin.: Things sound stressful with your parents. What do you wish could be different with your parents?

Pt.: For one, tell them to stop nagging me all the time, they just don't understand how hard it is for me these days.

Clin.: So if we could get things better between you and your parents, would that be helpful? (clinician seeks out healthy goal of improving the relationship between the teenager and parents)

Pt.: Sure, that would make things better.

Clin.: Any other things you wish could be different? (clinician continues to ask about more goals)

When employing solution-focused interviewing techniques for uncovering the patient's goals, notice how the interviewer allows the patient to complain openly, for one can often reframe a complaint as "a goal." This is a process akin to a concept called "rolling with the client's concerns," which we will explore in detail in Chapter 22 on motivational interviewing. The art of engagement here rests in the clinician's gentle, yet persistent, attempt to hear directly from the patient what the patient sees as wrong.

The Miracle Question

Arguably, de Shazer[29] has created one of the most popular of all solution-focused interviewing techniques – the miracle question. Patients often get stuck in the past, convincing themselves that the future cannot be different, a position that undermines problem solving and hope. Such patients often don't see achievable goals, blinded by their own cognitive traps. The initial interviewer can sometimes open these traps, by gently pulling the patient into the "possibilities" of the future with the following question:

"If you woke up in the morning, and a miracle had happened, so that your life was the way you wanted it to be, what are some of the things that would be different?"

There are many ways to phrase the miracle question; I happen to like the one above – for it is direct. Notice that it also asks "what are *some of the things* that would be different" (gently opening the door to multiple goals) as opposed to "how would it be different" (sometimes closes the door to all but one goal).

Cheng[30] provides a beautiful illustration of the miracle question at work:

> Clin.: Imagine that tonight you go to bed, like you normally do. Then, imagine that while you're asleep … [pause] … a miracle happens. Imagine that because of this miracle, your depression [or whatever the patient's problem is] goes away. What will your day be like tomorrow?
>
> Pt.: Well, I guess I would wake up, and rather than sleep in, I'd wake up on time and get ready instead of procrastinating. Then I'd eat breakfast rather than skipping it, and at breakfast, we'd all get along better without fighting. Then I'd go to work, and I'd have more confidence, so I would say "no" to people if they ask me to do too much …

The miracle question has opened up a veritable cornucopia of potential goals for therapy including (1) waking up earlier, (2) decreasing procrastination, (3) eating breakfast on a regular basis, (4) improving discourse at the breakfast table, (5) being more confident, and (6) being able to appropriately set limits on expectations at work.

Now imagine that this was a patient who had been pressured by his wife to enter therapy. Now further imagine that earlier in the interview he had belatedly admitted that he might have "a little bit" of a drinking problem (one of the reasons for not waking up on time) and also had a "tiny" temper problem (breakfast conversation issues). If instead of using the miracle question, the clinician, at the end of the interview, spontaneously suggested that they address both of these obviously important problems, things might not move successfully towards a second interview.

If instead, the clinician, after employing the miracle question, said something like, "Well there are all sorts of things we will be able to focus on in therapy if you'd like, for instance you noted earlier you wished you were drinking less, but let's focus first on some of the things you most want to change like the waking up early and eating breakfast on time. Let's say we could start by working on two of the things you mentioned if a miracle had happened, which two would you be interested in starting with in the therapy?", a second session is much more likely to be in the works.

Ultimately, the number one goal from the clinician's viewpoint in an initial interview is to ensure that there is a second one, for we can't help someone who is not in our office. Paradoxically, as the sessions proceed and the alliance strengthens, this particular patient may discover for himself that it is difficult to get up on time and have civil conversations at breakfast if one drinks heavily. At that point, the patient himself may recognize that the focus needs to shift to recovery issues, and he will be much more self-motivated to do so. The seeds for this subsequent therapeutic breakthrough were directly planted in the initial interview by the clinician's intentional decision to use the miracle question as a means of enhancing engagement.

CONCLUDING STATEMENTS

In our first two chapters we have attempted to develop a practical language through which we can study the engagement process. We began with an operative definition of the interview itself and uncovered a useful map for exploring its nuances. We have subsequently covered a lot of ground, examining key concepts and techniques for securing and enhancing engagement, the first way-station on our map, including blending, strategic empathy, the creation of safety, genuineness, clinician expertise, and collaborative interviewing techniques.

It is hoped our new language offers us a chance to explore effectively our own styles of interviewing, while greatly increasing the opportunity to learn from observing others. This language of the interview has revealed the fact that interviewing is an art and, like the art historians mentioned in Chapter 1, one can discuss this craft precisely and concretely. Indeed, the language we have uncovered, utilizing words such as interpersonal stance, empathic valence, the paranoid spiral, responsiveness, spontaneity and consistency provide us with the details of the map regarding interviewing process. The interior of our Victorian room now appears considerably less foreboding.

We have developed a language with which to begin our study of the interviewing process. But this language is incomplete, for an examination of the complex interplay between clinician and patient, as critical data and history are uncovered, represents a pressing matter as yet unexplored. Other factors have yet to be considered such as the sometimes-daunting tensions existing between the engagement process, time constraints, and the gathering of a useful and thorough database. It is this volatile interaction that creates the dynamic structure of the interview. And it is to an understanding of how to shape this structure that we will now turn our attention.

REFERENCES

1. Aston E. *The Darcy connection*. Austin, TX: Touchstone; 2008.
2. Sullivan HS. *The psychiatric interview*. New York, NY: W.W. Norton; 1970.
3. Egan G. *The skilled helper: a model for systematic helping and interpersonal relating*. Monterey, CA: Brooks/Cole Publishing Company; 1975. p. 97.
4. Nicholi AM Jr. The therapist–patient relationship. In: Nicholi AM Jr, editor. *The Harvard guide to modern psychiatry*. Cambridge, CA: Belknap Press of Harvard University Press; 1978.
5. Sullivan HS. 1970. p. 12.
6. Rogers CR, Traux CB. The therapeutic conditions antecedent to change: a theoretical view. In: Rogers CR, editor. *The therapeutic relationship and its impact*. Madison, WI: University of Wisconsin Press; 1967. p. 97–108.
7. Egan G. 1975. p. 90.
8. Ryle A. *Psychotherapy: a cognitive integration of theory and practice*. New York: Grune & Stratton; 1982. p. 103.
9. Egan G. 1975. p. 93.

10. Pinto A, Mancebo MC, Eisen JL, et al. The Brown longitudinal obsessive compulsive study: clinical features and symptoms of the sample at intake. *J Clin Psychiatry* 2006;**67**:703–11.
11. Cullen B, Samuels JF, Pinto A, et al. Demographic and clinical characteristics associated with treatment status in family members with obsessive–compulsive disorder. *Depress Anxiety* 2008;**25**(3):218–24.
12. Torres AR, Prince MJ, Bebbington PE, et al. Obsessive-compulsive disorder: prevalence, comorbidity, impact, and help-seeking in the British national psychiatric morbidity survey of 2000. *Am J Psychiatry* 2006;**163**(11):1978–85.
13. García-Soriano G, Rufer M, Delsignore A, Weidt S. Factors associated with non-treatment or delayed treatment seeking in OCD sufferers: a review of the literature. *Psychiatry Res* 2014;**220**(1–2):1–10.
14. de Shazer S. *Clues: investigating solutions in brief therapy*. New York, NY: W.W. Norton & Company; 1988.
15. Budman S, Hoyt M, Friedman S. *The first session in brief therapy*. New York, NY: The Guilford Press; 1992.
16. Miller S, Hubble M, Duncan B. *Handbook of solution-focused brief therapy*. San Francisco, CA: Jossey-Bass; 1996.
17. de Jong P, Berg I. *Interviewing for solutions*. New York, NY: Brooke and Cole Publishers; 1998.
18. Guterman JT. *Mastering the art of solution-focused counseling*. Alexandria, VA: American Counseling Association; 2006.
19. Miller W, Rollnick S. *Motivational interviewing: helping people change*. 3rd ed. New York, NY: The Guilford Press; 2013.
20. Rollnick S, Mille WR, Butler CC. *Motivational interviewing in health care: helping patients change behavior (applications of motivational interviewing)*. New York, NY: The Guilford Press; 2007.
21. Shea SC. *Improving medication adherence: how to talk with patients about their medications*. Philadelphia, PA: Lippincott Williams & Wilkins; 2006.
22. Shea SC. The "medication interest model": an integrative clinical interviewing approach for improving medication adherence – part 1 – clinical applications. *Prof Case Manag* 2008;**13**(6):305–17.
23. Shea SC. The "medication interest model": an integrative clinical interviewing approach for improving medication adherence – part 2 – implications for teaching and research. *Prof Case Manag* 2009;**14**(1):6–15.
24. Jobes DA. *Managing suicidal risk: a collaborative approach*. New York, NY: The Guilford Press; 2006.
25. Cheng KS. New approaches for creating the therapeutic alliance: solution-focused interviewing, motivational interviewing, and the medication interest model. *Psychiatr Clin North Am* 2007;**30**(2):156–66.
26. Borden E. The generalizability of the psychoanalytic concept of the working alliance. *Psychother Theory Res Prac* 1979;**16**:252–60.
27. Cheng M. 2007. p. 160.
28. Cheng M. 2007. p. 160.
29. de Shazer S. 1998.
30. Cheng M. 2007. p. 161.

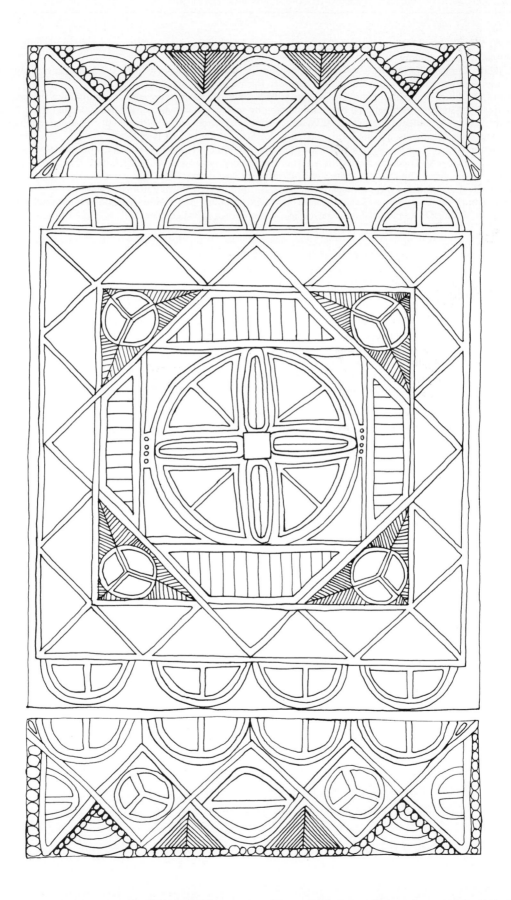

CHAPTER 3

The Dynamic Structure of the Interview: Core Tasks, Strategies, and the Continuum of Open-Endedness

Unceasingly contemplate the generation of all things through change, and accustom thyself to the thought that the nature of the universe delights above all in changing the things that exist and making new ones of the same pattern.

Marcus Aurelius[1]

The clinical interview manifests as a relationship. As with all relationships, it undergoes a continuous process of change. It takes two things that exist, the clinician and the patient, and creates something that did not exist – a therapeutic dyad. This therapeutic dyad, and its accompanying alliance, will change as the needs, agenda, perspectives, and fears of the two participants evolve. This metamorphosis occurs whether either participant wants it to occur or not. The clinician must choose whether to move with these changes gracefully or to struggle against them.

At first glance, these changes can appear almost overwhelming in their complexity, for as noted earlier, daunting tensions exist between the engagement process, time constraints, and the gathering of a useful and thorough database. It is this volatile interaction that creates the dynamic structure of the interview. The complexity becomes significantly more understandable by moving to the next way-station on our map – a study of the art of data gathering (Figure 3.1). By better understanding how the disparate forces of engagement and data gathering shape each other, we will discover that there are principles and "rules" that determine this process. From this understanding we will develop specific strategies and techniques for shaping this unfolding as it occurs, for there is no need for us to be at the mere whim of the universe as it creates this new pattern. Indeed, it is the skilled shaping of this process by the clinician that can maximize the likelihood that the patient's suffering can be most rapidly and effectively relieved.

An interview can be described as having five phases in its macrostructure: (1) the introduction, (2) the opening, (3) the body, (4) the closing, and (5) the termination. Categorizing the stages of the interview in this fashion is somewhat artificial, but this separation temporarily provides an avenue for a more sophisticated study. In reality, these phases merge with one another, a process at least partially determined by the pathways chosen by the clinician. Appreciating that the clinician has a choice in the process creates

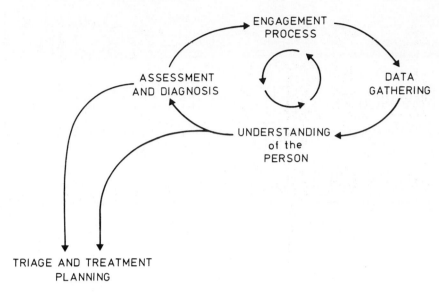

Figure 3.1 Map of the interviewing process.

both a more efficient interview and a more exciting one. As we shall see, the ability to intentionally sculpt the structure of the interview is one of the differences between a good clinician and an outstanding one.

INTRODUCTION: PHASE 1

The introduction begins when the clinician and the patient first see one another. It ends when the clinician feels comfortable enough to begin an inquiry into the reasons why the patient has sought help. When done well, it lasts a minute or two. When done poorly, it hardly occurs at all, or worse yet, the clinician and/or the patient regrets having been a part of it. The introduction represents one of the most important phases of the interview, because patients will frequently have formed their initial impression of the clinician by its end. This initial impression, whether justified or not, may help to determine the remaining course of the interview and perhaps even of therapy itself.

Creating a Safe Environment

The goal of the interviewer during the introduction remains relatively simple: engage the patient by decreasing the patient's anxiety. Employing one of Sullivan's terms mentioned earlier, we can state the goal as follows: the clinician attempts to decrease the patient's need for an overactive self-system. In a similar vein, the goal of the patient is also relatively easy: "to find out what is going on here," because many patients are encountering a mental health professional for the first time.

The patient's need to understand the immediate interview process itself tends to be rather intense, for it is stoked by some of the fears described in Chapter 2. It is worth reviewing these concerns in more detail here, for it is in the introduction phase that we have our first opportunity to address them, before they can create a lasting problem with engagement:

1. Who is this clinician?
2. Is he or she competent?
3. Is this person understanding?
4. What does he or she already know about me?
5. Whose side is this clinician on?
6. How long will this assessment take?
7. Am I going to be hurt?
8. Do I have any control in this matter? (Am I going to be "mind-raped"? as one patient described her initial fear.)

Not all patients are dealing with all these fears, but most patients are probably coping with a good number of them, either consciously or unconsciously. The goal of the clinician and the goal of the patient are really the same at this moment in the interview: in short, to help the patient to feel more at ease. To achieve this more comfortable state of affairs, after some friendly chit-chat the clinician can address some of these questions in the introduction either directly or indirectly. If done sensitively, the patient's initial anxiety should begin to decrease and the interview should begin to gracefully move forward.

There exists no correct method for handling these fears. Consequently, each clinician needs to determine a comfortable style of addressing these issues in his or her own fashion. I shall give two examples. The first example is the work of an inexperienced clinician. The second dialogue demonstrates one method that addresses the issues more smoothly.

[The clinician enters brusquely, shaking the patient's hand very firmly. The clinician does not smile.]

Clin.: Well John, my name is Dr. James, I'll be conducting the interview. I understand you have some problems. Tell me about them.

Pt.: Let me see, I'm not really sure where to begin.

Clin.: Why don't you start at the beginning. I understand you've been acting a little odd.

Pt.: Who told you that?

Clin.: Your wife, but that's neither here nor there, I need to know when it all began.

It is hard not to chuckle at this exchange, for the interviewer has successfully aroused almost all of the anxieties mentioned earlier. Even such word choices as "I'll be conducting the interview" suggest that the patient should expect no control here, although the clinician's overpowering handshake may have already served as a premonition of this fact.

The following dialogue represents a more satisfying solution to the demands of the situation.

[The patient enters the room (or if there is a waiting room the clinician will have greeted the patient there). The clinician smiles warmly and spontaneously. He walks over to the patient at a normal pace and shakes the patient's hand with a gentle firmness.]

Clin.: Hello, my name is Dr. James. I'm one of the senior psychiatrists at the clinic. Why don't we sit over here. By the way, if you like, I can hang your coat up (gestures toward wall).

Pt.: Thank you (patient passes coat and sits down).

Clin.: Did you have any trouble finding a parking space?

Pt.: No, not really. It's not that bad at this time of the day.

Clin.: Good. Sometimes people have some problems with it. ... You ought to see it here when the college kids are coming back – it's a zoo. (clinician pauses, smiles) Don't worry; I'd never schedule us on that day.

Pt.: Good to hear. (patient smiles)

Clin.: Oh, before we get started, would you like some coffee or tea?

Pt.: I don't think so.

Clin.: We got some good chai tea.

Pt.: No, really. Thanks though.

Clin.: Well, why don't we begin by my giving you some idea of what to expect today.

Pt.: That sounds good to me.

Clin.: By the way have you ever seen a therapist before or any type of mental health professional?

Pt.: No. I can't say that I have.

Clin.: Oh, I better be nicer than usual (smiles, patient laughs).

Clin.: First of all, do you like to be called Mr. Fenner or William or Bill?

Pt.: I don't like the name William. "Bill" would be just fine.

Clin.: Good. (pauses) When your wife called to set up your appointment, she passed on some of her concerns. She said you had wanted her to do that.

Pt.: Well, sort of. She said she would, and I told her to go ahead. I didn't know if she had or not.

Clin.: She didn't say a lot, but she did say a few things. And shortly we'll talk about how much you want me to share or not to share with her about our work together as well as how much input you want her to have. I want to make sure that I know directly from you what you're comfortable with, but, for now, let me just summarize my impression from her call. She certainly seems concerned and a little confused about what you've been thinking and feeling recently. She seems to feel that you may be somewhat depressed. What I'd like to do is begin by hearing from you and getting your perspectives on what, if anything, has been going on. We'll talk for about 40, or so, minutes, and then we'll spend about 10 minutes chatting about what might be of value to you and the types of options for work together we might have. How's that sound?

Pt.: That sounds good.

Clin.:   Good, But before we get started, though, this might be a good time to explain more
about confidentiality. I know you haven't been in therapy before, but have you ever
heard the term confidentiality before as far as therapy goes?

Pt.:   Sort of, I think. It's what you were talking about before, about what can or can't be
shared with Sally.

Clin.:   Exactly. Let me fill you in on the details … (interviewer discusses confidentiality, a
process we will address in detail shortly)

[After confidentiality is explained and discussed, the interview might proceed as follows:]

Clin.:   Perhaps we could start with your telling me a little about how you see things at this
point. I know from Sally that she feels you're depressed, but what is more
important is what you think.

Pt.:   It will take me a second to get in gear here … well … let's see … In the first place, I
must admit I've been feeling sort of down, not depressed mind you, but down.
She's right about that.

Clin.:   Uh-huh.

Pt.:   Things have been going poorly at work. My boss left and he was replaced by a, let
me just say, someone more difficult to get along with. The end result has been that
I'm not enjoying my work like I used to.

Clin.:   And where is it you work?

Pt.:   Down at the lumber company.

Clin.:   Go on (said gently).

Pt.:   Well, about 3 weeks ago I did something I've never done in all my 20 years of work
… (pause, clinician waits) I called in sick without actually being sick.

Clin.:   Uh-huh.

Pt.:   It's really unusual for me to do that.

Clin.:   Okay.

In this introduction, which has imperceptibly moved into the opening phase, the clinician has smoothly addressed many of the potential concerns mentioned earlier. In particular, a large element of respect has been conveyed to the patient by the simple gesture
of offering to hang up his coat and by addressing the information his wife communicated
during the appointment call. The clinician also clearly appears to be on no one's side,
emphasizing the desire to hear the patient's opinions, and even stating that the issue of
a problem with the patient has not been determined yet by the comment "and getting
your perspectives on what, *if anything*, has been going on."

Storr[2] points out that the situation may be slightly different if the patient has been
referred by a fellow mental health professional or from an inpatient unit. In these cases,
Storr adds a nice touch, as follows:

Clin.:   I've read your notes and I have some idea of your background and your present
trouble, but I would be grateful if you would go over some of it again. I know that
you have told it all before to various people and that it must be very tedious for
you to repeat it, but I find it difficult to remember details from notes made by other

people. I understand that your present trouble is depression. ... Could we start there? What is your kind of depression really like?[2]

In this example, Storr conveys respect and concern, essentially acknowledging that the patient might find repeating the story again somewhat irksome. The last statement also indicates, from the perspective of person-centered interviewing, the clinician's desire to understand the patient as a unique individual, not just a case. Some clinicians also prefer to end the introduction by asking, "Before we go on, do you have any questions?" Such a question once again conveys a sense of respect, while checking for possible patient concerns.

Going back to our own example of an effective introduction, we find that the clinician has also managed to give a sense of control to the patient with phrases such as, "Perhaps we could start with your telling me a little about how you see things at this point. I know from Sally that she feels you're depressed, but what is more important is what you think."

The clinician also asked the patient how he would like to be addressed. One will encounter many vehemently held opinions both for and against using a patient's first name. I shall not add many pages to this debate, because I think the intensity of the debate has led to overstated arguments on both sides. I, personally, feel that one should not assume a first name basis without asking first. Some patients may find a first name threatening or a "put down," especially if the patient is a young adult or is much older than the clinician. Consequently, when first greeting a patient, I always use his or her last name.

On the other hand, the ability to use the patient's first name can be a powerful asset in engagement. When used sparingly, and with good timing, it can effectively help patients to share difficult material. In a cultural sense, first names are generally used by people who care about us and are privy to our private thoughts. Consequently, I have found it both satisfying and rewarding to simply ask the patient how he or she would like to be addressed. This question accomplishes several tasks:

1. It conveys respect.
2. It gives the patient direct control over an important ego issue. (Some patients do not like to be called by last names and others do not like to be called by first names.)
3. One may learn a significant amount concerning the dynamics of the patient as revealed by the patient's preference.

For instance, very strong opinions voiced by the patient may represent the presence of personality pathology or defensive posturing, thus offering the clinician immediate grist for the mill. A patient developing grandiose thinking as part of a manic episode may adamantly insist on being called "Dr. Jones." At the other extreme, patients with regressive tendencies may sheepishly smile while stating, "Please just call me Jim." With experience one can begin to discern the sense of self-identity implied by the patient's response to this simple question. Indeed, one wonders what psychodynamic issues, if any, may lie beneath ambivalent responses such as, "It doesn't really matter, you can call me Jim,

Jack, or Jimmy." One can see that even in the introduction phase, the data-gathering process has begun.

There are some exceptions to the above guidelines. If the clinician knows beforehand that the patient has a history of paranoia, it may be advisable to use the last name throughout the interview, because such "distance" may be more comfortable for a patient with a paranoid interpersonal stance, as we saw in our exploration of empathic valence. Patients who are much older than the clinician may prefer to be addressed by last name. In the opposite direction, children and adolescents generally should be addressed on a first name basis from the start. In these cases, though, it is often useful to ask the patient which first name to use. For instance, the family may call an adolescent "Sue," yet the adolescent would prefer being called "Susan." Such a simple show of respect can go a long way towards ensuring a powerful engagement.

I should add that with regard to addressing the patient, I have yet to find any problem arising in either the initial interview or subsequent psychotherapy using the above approach. In the end, the reader must decide, from his or her own experience, what feels most comfortable.

In familiarizing the patient with the ensuing interview process, some clinicians go one step further than illustrated above. They specifically describe for the patient what to expect, depending on the goals of the interview, an approach that directly addresses the patient's underlying question of "What is going on here?" After the clinician and patient have introduced themselves, the dialogue may proceed as follows:

> **Clin.:** Perhaps it would be of value to describe what we'll be doing today.
>
> **Pt.:** Sounds good to me.
>
> **Clin.:** Well, first, we'll start by getting a better idea of what some of your concerns are and what types of stresses you're coping with, and also what you're hoping to achieve from today. As we go along I'm sure I'll get a better idea of what you feel the major problems are and what you've already been doing about them. Later in the interview, I'll try to get a little better idea of where you're from and your background by asking some questions about your family, your health, your schooling, and any previous symptoms you might have had. I find that getting an understanding of your background can really help me understand your current problem better. And then, at the end we can brainstorm on ways we might have that could help you to get some relief. The whole appointment will take roughly about 50 minutes. Do you have any questions?
>
> **Pt.:** Not really, no … not really.
>
> **Clin.:** Then let's begin by looking at what brought you here today.
>
> **Pt.:** (sigh) I'll tell you, it's a long story.
>
> **Clin.:** I have big ears (smiles).
>
> **Pt.:** (chuckles) Well, it has to do with some problems with my wife and me. It began about 2 months after our first child, Jenny …

The purpose of a more extended description of the process is twofold. First, it is hoped that the patient's fear of the unknown will be decreased. Second, the description of the process serves as an educational strategy, subtly alerting the patient to the fact that large amounts of data will be covered in 50 minutes. This may allow the clinician to collaboratively structure the ensuing interview more effectively. It also provides one method for smoothly switching gears later with transitions such as, "As I mentioned earlier, I'd like to learn a little more about your family. How many children do you have besides Jenny?" At the end of this interaction, the clinician also demonstrated the use of well-timed humor to break the anxiety of the first meeting.

Before moving on, one final point may be of value. As with all the other aspects of interviewing we have discussed so far, the format of the introduction varies from one patient to another. In some instances in which the patient is extremely psychotic, the patient may quickly cut short the introduction. In such cases, it is wise to follow the patient's lead, because clearly such patients have a need to tell their story quickly. It would be inappropriate to adhere rigidly to the typical format of the introduction with such patients. The format is a guide, not a rule.

Addressing Confidentiality

At some point near the end of the introduction, or as one is transitioning to the opening phase of the interview, it is typical to address confidentiality. It is important to be clear about confidentiality, for it has critical ramifications for building trust. A dialogue might evolve as follows:

Clin.: One thing we should talk about before we get going is the topic of confidentiality. Is that a term you are familiar with?

Pt.: Yeah, sort of.

Clin.: Let me fill you in on what I mean by the term. For the most part, everything you say in here with me never leaves this room. There is total privacy between us, so that you feel comfortable sharing whatever you feel you need to share. Does that make sense?

Pt.: Oh, yeah, I figured that was the case.

Clin.: As with just about anything, there are exceptions to the rule, but these exceptions make good sense. (Note that these exceptions may very a bit from state to state and country to country.) If you share something that indicates to me that you might kill yourself or hurt somebody else, then I might need to talk with somebody else to get more information or to make sure everybody is safe. Naturally, I'd ask your permission to do so, but if you refused – in this rare situation – I would need to break the confidentiality to make sure you or others are truly safe. And, obviously, if there was child abuse or abuse of an elderly person you are taking care of, I actually, by law, have to report that activity to the proper authorities to get you the help you need and to protect any children or elders.

Pt.: Yeah, that makes good sense.

Clin.: Also, other than potentially dangerous situations, if you and I agree that it would be useful for us to talk with somebody else, I would need to get your written approval to do so. So if you wanted me to talk with a family member or friend, you could give me written permission to contact them. I can't just call them up without asking you. If we felt another clinician or a physician, or even a lawyer, would be useful to talk with, I could do so only after you gave me written permission. I take confidentiality very seriously and the bottom line is that, other than exceptions like the above, what you say here is totally private between you and me.

The Sommers-Flanagans make several excellent points about confidentiality.[3] If patients ask further questions about it, then they often are metacommunicating that they might be especially conscious of trust issues, indicating that further open discussion about confidentiality is probably warranted. They also remind us that the confidentiality issues related to written records is important to address with statements such as, "I'll be keeping records of our meetings, but only my office manager and I have access to these files. And the office manager will also keep your records confidential."[3] I also add, "And, of course, in order for you and I to get your insurance company to reimburse us, they may request information about your diagnoses and care."

As electronic health record (EHR) implementation evolves, confidentiality issues will also evolve. Various institutes may handle accessibility to the patient's EHR differently. In a private practice, the confidentiality may be exactly as stated above. In contrast, some hospitals and clinics may allow wider access to records from various clinicians and personnel (for instance every clinician on a given team or all nursing staff may have immediate access to a patient's EHR as well as administrative personnel). Moreover, as confidentiality evolves, we may see some patients allowing records to be proactively transferable to other institutes and clinics. Whatever evolves, it is important for the interviewer to know the exact confidentiality rules within his or her employ, and these rules must be conveyed to the patient explicitly when discussing confidentiality.

If you are in training and will be discussing the case either in individual or group supervision, the Sommers-Flanagans handle this gracefully as follows, "Because I'm a graduate student I have a supervisor who checks my work. Sometimes we discuss my work with a small group of other graduate students. However, in each of these situations, the purpose is to enable me to provide you with the best services possible. Other than the exceptions I mentioned, no information about you will leave this clinic without your permission."[3]

Confidentiality discussions are critical. I seldom encounter problems with them and part of the art is discussing them in a matter of fact tone of voice. But it should be noted that, even when done well, this early introduction of complex and potentially unnerving information, sometimes may disrupt the naturalistic flow of the interview just as it is getting started. Some clinics, hospitals, and emergency rooms alleviate this problem, in a creative fashion, by having a different staff member than the interviewer, such as a well-trained receptionist, review confidentiality issues in detail before the patient sees the clinician. In these situations, the patient has ample time to ask questions and will also sign a written statement of understanding regarding confidentiality.

This process allows the actual interview to unfold very naturally without the need for the discussion of a delicate topic right off the bat. In these instances, I will ask the patient in the introduction if he or she has any questions about confidentiality. And I still review the key points and exceptions of confidentiality with the patient personally, but can now wait to do so during the closing of the interview, where it fits very nicely. Re-addressing confidentiality in the closing phase of the interview also functions to consolidate the patient's understanding of confidentiality for our future sessions. Moreover, for a new patient who has never experienced therapy before, the experience of the therapy hour may have raised new questions about confidentiality by the end of the hour.

OPENING: PHASE 2

With the clinician's first inquiry into the patient's immediate state of affairs, the opening phase heralds a more active phase of data gathering. It ends when the clinician begins to focus his or her questions on specific topics deemed important by the clinician after listening to the patient nondirectively. Whether a 30-minute emergency room interview or a 60-minute initial intake, the opening phase should last about 5 to 7 minutes, because it is the cornerstone of engagement.

Combined with the introductory phase, the opening phase probably represents the most critical time for establishing rapport with the patient. If the end of the introduction marked the formation of the patient's initial impression of the clinician, the end of the opening phase represents the solidification or rejection of that impression. For the most part, patients have determined by the end of the opening whether they basically like or dislike the interviewer. These patient opinions are not irrevocably etched in stone, but it would take a rather large chisel to change them. In many instances when patients abandon therapy after two or three sessions, their disapproval may have been seeded in the opening 7 minutes of the first interview.

The patient has two primary goals during the opening phase: (1) to determine whether it is "okay" to share personal matters with this particular clinician, and (2) to determine which personal matters to share. A third major goal of the patient also surfaces, namely "to tell my story right, so that the clinician understands me." Despite a well-handled introduction, the patient's self-system will usually be activated during this phase, because it is here that conscious self-exposure begins.

With these ideas in mind, one of the complementary goals of the interviewer becomes apparent: The engagement process begun in the introduction must be secured during the opening. The durability and elasticity of this engagement bonding, to a large degree, will determine the depth of probing and the degree of structuring that the patient will tolerate in the subsequent phases of the interview. It is at this time that many of the engagement skills discussed in our first two chapters meet their greatest challenge and yield their highest reward.

The approach to the opening phase generally proceeds along the following lines: Once the clinician has ended his or her introduction, an open-ended technique is used to turn the interview over to the patient on a verbal level. Frequently used openings include the following:

a. "Tell me a little about what brought you here today."
b. "Perhaps you can begin by letting me know what some of your concerns have been recently."
c. "To start with, tell me a little about what has been happening, from your perspective, over the past several weeks or so."
d. "What are some of the stresses you have been coping with recently?"

Such open-ended questions or statements provide the patient with a chance to choose to begin sharing by talking about something with which the patient feels reasonably comfortable. Broadly speaking, the goals are to decrease the patient's self-system while beginning to uncover the patient's viewpoint. Both of these goals are generally met by giving the patient plenty of room to wander during the opening phase.

During this facilitating opening phase, one hopes to begin to see outward signs of good blending, such as the patient's assumption of a more relaxed body posture and a reasonably long duration of utterance (DOU) by the patient following the clinician's questions. This facilitation can be nurtured by the use of phrases such as "Go on," "And then what happened," and frequent short conveyances of the clinician's interest such as "Uh-huh." Generally it appears useful to employ at least several gentle (low valence) empathic statements during the opening phase, because such phrases frequently circumvent the patient's fear of imminent rejection.

The opening phase bears a characteristic that distinguishes it from other phases of the interview. In sharp contrast to the introduction, in the opening phase the clinician speaks very little. Furthermore, there exists a strong emphasis on open-ended questions or open-ended statements in an effort to get the patient talking. Generally speaking, in an uncomplicated opening phase, approximately 60 to 90% or more of the clinician's questions or statements will be open-ended. During an assessment interview, the opening phase will probably represent the least verbally active phase for the clinician, because in the subsequent body of the interview, clinicians tend to increase the frequency of their questions as they attempt to clarify psychological and situational nuances, diagnostic concerns, and triage issues.

With regard to this open-ended emphasis, two frequent problems are encountered: (1) premature structuring of the interview before the patient has begun to relax, and (2) the too frequent use of closed-ended questions. Both of these tendencies remove control of the interview from the patient, a policy that may serve only to heighten the patient's interpersonal anxiety. Perhaps equally important, these activities represent an increased amount of clinician speech, and, at this early stage of the interview, a direct correlation can be drawn between clinician confusion and the amount of time that the clinician spends with his or her mouth open. In short, the opening phase is a time for reflection, not action, unless a specific patient hesitancy needs to be transformed.

Before proceeding, it is worth noting that some clinicians like to employ a bridge between the introduction and the opening. This bridge consists of a brief series of demographic questions that function to provide a cursory background while not intimidating the patient. The clinician may state, "As we get started I'd like to ask a few background questions that can help give me some perspective. For instance, how old are you, Mr. Jones?" Further questions may concern the place of residence, occupation, or a description of the patient's family. Following these questions, the clinician may proceed with the opening as described above. Once again, the emphasis is on effective and rapid engagement. Whether or not to use this approach is an option that becomes a clinician preference. I, myself, tend not to use this approach, for in my experience it ever-so-slightly hinders the natural flow of initiating the conversation.

Active engagement techniques are not the only activities of the clinician during the opening phase. Much of the activity cannot be seen, because it is mental in nature. More specifically, the opening phase represents an intensely productive assessment period for

the clinician. During these initial minutes, the clinician scours the interpersonal coun-
tryside in search of clues that may lead to the most effective engagement techniques for
this particular patient. Simultaneously, the clinician determines the best manner in which
to structure the body of the interview itself. In short, the clinician develops a tentative
game plan, in the sense that a strategy for the interview will be developed, hand-tailored
to the unique needs of the patient.

In the opening phase, the clinician receives a rare opportunity to assess four vital areas:
(1) the patient's conscious view of his or her problems, as well as the patient's conscious
goals for the interview itself (e.g., What does the patient want from the interview?);
(2) the patient's immediate mental state, which can influence the type of interview the
clinician feels would be most clinically appropriate for this particular patient; (3) the
clinician's own conceptualization of the patient's problems, as well as the clinician's view
of the patient's *unconscious* goals for the interview (e.g., What, in reality, does this patient
desire from this interview?); and (4) an evaluation of the interview process itself.

Through an understanding of these four variables, the clinician can begin the delicate
matter of matching the patient's goals with his or her own goals. If common goals are
not collaboratively active, the resultant interview may prove to be relatively unproductive.
It is interesting to note, just as Lazare[4] states that outpatient psychotherapy has a contractual nature; in a sense, each initial interview possesses a contractual element. The
contract can be either implicit or explicit – but it always occurs.

Indeed, as we saw in our section on collaborative interviewing, interviews frequently
break down when the participants cannot agree to shared goals. Many of these communication breakdowns result when the clinician does not recognize the goals of the patient
or, worse yet, knows the goals but does not acknowledge them, resulting in a dysfunctional encounter that is the antithesis of a person-centered interview.

The four analytic tasks of the opening phase are creatively coupled with the intuitive
skills of the clinician. Armed with this interplay between analysis and intuition, the clinician quickly begins an initial "knowing" of the patient. In an attempt to sharpen the
analytic skills of the opening phase, the following acronym, PACE, is useful in reminding
the clinician of the tasks at hand:

Patient's perspectives and conscious goals
Assessment of the patient's immediate mental state
Clinician's perspective of the patient's problems and the patient's unconscious goals
Evaluation of the interview itself

Patient's Perspective and Conscious Agenda

Each patient brings a unique set of perceptions and opinions to the initial interview.
From our person-centered perspective, these views are invaluable for understanding
where to collaboratively move in the interview. Two patient perspectives appear to be
particularly crucial in determining whether contractual agreement will occur: (1) the
patient's concept of what is wrong, and (2) the patient's expectations of the interview

and the interviewer. To uncover these perspectives, I often use the following two questions, or a variation of them, at some point during the opening phase:

1. "In your opinion, what exactly do you think the main problem is at this time?"
2. "What are some of the things that you hope we might be able to accomplish today?"

Many roadblocks to the interview process can arise when the answers to these two questions are not known by the clinician.

On the other hand, sometimes it is the patient's conscious goals that actually get in the way of the interview, as might be seen in malingering or drug seeking. At such moments, it may be even more important that the clinician be able to ferret out what the real agenda of the patient might be. If the interviewer becomes aware of these potentially problematic beliefs or agendas, some roadblocks may be diminished, worked through, or perhaps even nipped in the bud.

To illustrate the usefulness of uncovering a patient's conscious agenda, it may be useful to look at a short piece of dialogue. We will picture a man in his mid-30s, who has scheduled an appointment at the strong urging of his wife. He nervously looks about the office, as if anticipating the appearance of a Grand Inquisitor. He has a small mustache and a nervous nose. Early in the opening phase the following interaction develops:

> **Clin.:** Tell me a little bit about some of the reasons you came here today.
>
> **Pt.:** It is very difficult to say. I don't know what Jane thinks is happening, but I'm not nuts. It's all got something to do with my chemistry, of that I'm sure. Somehow or other I'm a little speeded up.
>
> **Clin.:** In what sense do you feel you're speeded up?
>
> **Pt.:** I'm feeling excitable, ready to rock and roll, very creative, but maybe a little too juiced up. That's why I think it's biologic, not mental. I've been doing some reading about physical fitness and its impact on emotions, and I think I've got some understanding of what the hell is going on here.

The art inherent in the opening phase consists of listening not only to what the patient says his or her goals are, but also to what the patient implies his or her goals might be. A careful examination of this patient's opening dialogue may yield some pertinent information.

His opening comment, "It is very difficult to say," suggests a genuine fear of being misunderstood by the interviewer. This phrase is followed by the statement, "I don't know what Jane thinks is happening, but I'm not nuts." Paradoxically, the patient relates that he does not know what his wife thinks yet he implies that she has labeled him as "nuts." The connection with his fear of being misunderstood seems clearer: one of his goals is to make sure the clinician "gets it" – that he is not crazy; a second goal may be the hope that the clinician will make sure that his wife "gets it." He probably also fears that the clinician will not value his opinions, which he openly shares with the phrase, "It's all got something to do with my chemistry, of that I'm sure."

With this last statement, he offers an explanation for his problem on one level but also provides two more important pieces of information: (1) at some plane of awareness, he recognizes a problem, and (2) he has a need not to view the problem as psychological. With the subsequent phrase, "Somehow or other, I'm a little speeded up," he further describes his perception of the problem.

With the next question, the clinician demonstrates a desire to understand the patient's world by requesting a more phenomenological description of his stated symptom. The patient's reply, once again, confirms his immediate need to conceptualize the problem in physical terms, betraying his fear that the "clinician-inquisitor" will not share this perspective (a second goal has clearly emerged – the need to convince the clinician that the problem is physical not mental). Of course, the patient's insistence on a physical cause may represent an example of a person who "doth protest too much." Even the patient may subconsciously fear a psychological problem.

From this brief dialogue we can see that, in a generic sense, the conscious goal of this patient is to make sure the clinician hears his side of the story and believes it. This generic goal manifests itself as two more specific goals: (1) make the point he is not crazy, and (2) make the point that the problem is physical not mental.

The next question arises: What can be done with this information? First, one can easily imagine what not to do, as would be exemplified by the clinician's proceeding with statements such as, "Perhaps you can start by telling me about some of your stresses with your son, since your wife seems to feel these stresses are at the root of your problem," or "Physiology may play a part here, but first let's look at some of the psychological issues that may be playing a part in your problems." Such blundering inquiries must represent the clinician's hidden masochistic needs, because the clinician is adamantly refusing to explore the patient's world through the patient's eyes. A reciprocal desire by the patient not to accommodate the clinician's goals and recommendations will most likely follow. Two can play at this game.

In contrast, let us look at a possible line of questioning that attempts to move with the patient's needs while ultimately joining both the goals of the patient and of the interviewer:

Pt.: I'm feeling excitable, ready to rock and roll, very creative, but maybe a little too juiced up. That's why I think it's biologic, not mental. I've been doing some reading about physical fitness and its impact on emotions, and I think I've got some understanding of what the hell is going on here.

Clin.: Oh, what kinds of things have you come up with?

Pt.: Well, some people have found that running and jogging can release substances in the brain called endorphins that help people feel good. I'm thinking that maybe that is why I'm speeded up.

Clin.: Hmm, that's interesting. How frequently do you run?

Pt.: About 3 miles every day, sometimes up to 5 miles.

Clin.: It sounds like you must be in pretty good shape. How did you get interested in physical fitness to begin with?

Pt.: I guess you could say it runs in the family, no pun intended (patient and clinician smile). My father was a jock, and my two brothers both went to college on football scholarships.

Clin.: Tell me a little bit about them.

Pt.: Oh, they're both high-powered people, both very successful … (pause), more successful than me, but I do okay. John is a corporate lawyer in Dallas, and Jack is a physician.

As opposed to a denial of the patient's overt goals, this interviewer has implicitly acknowledged them. For example, the clinician picks up on the patient's hint, "… and I think I've got some understanding of what the hell is going on here," by asking, "Oh, what kinds of things have you come up with?" – essentially a variation of our question, "In your opinion, what exactly do you think the main problem is at this time?" The patient is being expressly asked to tell his side of the story.

This particular choice of topics by the interviewer has also reinforced the issue of physiology, which symbolizes an area in which this patient feels safe, a topic in which his self-system is less likely to be activated by discussion. By moving with this patient's needs, the conversation transforms itself gracefully into an exploration of family relations.

This example stands merely as an illustration. Patient needs and perspectives change with each individual. But certain conscious – although not always stated – patient agenda items are fairly common, and the interviewer may want to listen attentively for their presence. The following list includes some of the more common appropriate conscious needs:

1. Somebody to sensitively listen to their story.
2. Somebody to confirm specific beliefs.
3. Somebody to provide, in a generic fashion, relief from their pain.
4. Somebody to provide, in a specific sense, some intervention such as psychotherapy and/or medications.
5. Somebody to "discover secrets," such as suicidal intent or a history of incest, which the patient has been afraid to share previously.
6. Somebody to reassure them that they are "sane," because they fear otherwise.
7. Somebody to uncover that they are "insane," because they are worried that they might be.
8. Somebody to simply "tell me what's happening to me."

As mentioned earlier, there are some goals that may or may not be compatible with the goals of the clinician. In particular, problems arise when the patient's agenda may not originate from a sincere motivation for help, as with the following more manipulative needs:

1. A desire for addictive drugs.
2. A desire to be hospitalized secondary to a need for shelter.

3. A desire to have the clinician help him or her in a legal hassle by proving the patient is "seeing a therapist."
4. A desire to appear mentally ill for legal purposes.
5. A desire to have the clinician confirm that the patient's regular therapist is "all wrong."
6. A desire simply to get a relative "off their back" by "seeing a specialist."
7. A desire for the clinician to tell relatives and friends that there is "nothing wrong."

These latter goals can significantly disrupt the development of a sound therapeutic alliance. If a clinician intuitively becomes suspicious that conscious problematic goals might be present, they can be intentionally sought. If the clinician has not already asked, "What are some of the things that you hope we might be able to accomplish today?" such hidden-agenda items may surprisingly surface with a simple variation of this question said in a gentle and non-accusatory way: "At this point in our talk, it might help both of us to clarify what we want to accomplish in this interview. What specifically would you like me to do for you today?"

Assessment of the Patient's Immediate Mental State

Much can be learned from a single glance if the glance has years of experience behind it. Although the details of the mental status examination will unfold in the body of the interview, during both the introduction and opening phases a simple *passive* noting of the patient's immediate mental state can provide invaluable information. In this "scouting period" of the interview, the clinician searches for mental state clues that may suggest a need for changing the strategy of the interview itself.

These clues are of three major types: (1) clues suggesting possible diagnoses and, hence, suggesting future areas for more extensive diagnostic exploration; (2) clues suggesting significant patient concerns about the interview process itself that need to be addressed; and (3) clues indicating that rather radical changes in the interview format may be needed because severe psychopathology may be present. In Chapter 16 we will look at the mental status in more detail, but for now we will briefly survey these three topics as they pertain to the opening phase.

With regard to diagnostic clues, one of the more interesting findings revolves about the issue of psychosis. If a patient presents with a smoldering psychotic process, it is not unusual for subtle signs to be present during the opening phase. Such subtle signs may include processes such as an infrequent loosening of associations, a slightly inappropriate affect, or an overriding intensity to the patient's feelings and affects. The presence of such clues may suggest that questions dealing with psychosis may yield a rich harvest later in the interview.

In relation to the second area, evidence of patient concerns about the interview process itself, the opening phase is of vital importance. If patient concerns are present and the patient is feeling uncomfortable or angry, it generally becomes necessary to work through these concerns, if possible, before proceeding to the main body of data gathering. Unresolved hesitancies or anger may leave the clinician with an incomplete or erroneous database because invalid data often lie in their wake.

To this end, the clinician keeps an attentive eye out for behavioral evidence suggesting unspoken roadblocks to the development of a therapeutic alliance. As discussed earlier, interpersonal anxiety is to be expected, but unusually high anxiety states may indicate intense fears of rejection, embarrassment, or ridicule. If the clinician suspects the presence of these fears, the following, said gently, may bring them to the surface where they can be dealt with more effectively: "It can be somewhat anxiety provoking to talk with a therapist like myself, especially the first time we are meeting. I'm wondering what, if any, types of things might be concerning you as we are talking here today?" Some interviewers prefer a slightly different wording, which is less assumptive of a problem: "It can be somewhat anxiety provoking to talk with a therapist like myself, especially the first time we are meeting. I'm wondering what you are feeling as we are talking today?"

James Morrison, in his informative book, *The First Interview: A Guide for Clinicians*, takes this one step further in a technique that he refers to as "naming emotions." If a patient appears to be stalled, secondary to such hesitancies, Morrison suggests addressing this process by naming several emotions that could be behind the patient's concerns. His gentle, yet direct, approach is as follows:

> *"I can see that you are having a real problem with that question. Sometimes people have trouble with questions when they feel ashamed. Or sometimes it's anxiety or fear. Are you having any of those feelings now?"*[5]

This technique can open the gate to transform a potentially damaging communication impasse. It should also be kept in mind that patient concerns may be quite direct, as evidenced by purposefully vague answers, an irritated or hostile affect, or no answer at all.

With regard to the third area, the discovery of a need to significantly change the structure of the interview, the issue of disruptive psychopathology rears its head. The question becomes whether a given patient can tolerate a standard initial interview. This question, frequently relevant to the emergency room setting, focuses directly upon the patient's immediate impulse control. A good clinician becomes facile at recognizing the situation in which the best interview may be a short one.

For instance, the clinician may happen upon a patient whose thinking has become laced with delusional ideation. The patient may be furiously pacing about the waiting room, shaking a fist at voices heard only in the private world of a psychotic nightmare. When questioning begins, this type of patient may rapidly escalate towards violence. As such a rapid escalation begins to unfold, the clinician may decide to alter the strategy of the interview drastically, including its length. This type of agitated behavior may also suggest the wisdom of interrupting the interview briefly in order to alert the charge nurse to the possibility of impending violence.

Clinician's Perspective of the Patient's Problems and the Patient's Unconscious Goals

A significant chasm may separate the patient's perspective from the clinician's perspective. For example, a patient may feel that the central problem consists of a vicious harassment devised by the FBI. The clinician may view this patient's problem as the development of a paranoid delusion. In other instances, the clinician and the patient may share similar views concerning the nature of the problem but differ on the issue of its etiology. Fortunately, much of the time, both the clinician and the patient share similar conceptualizations.

It is useful for a clinician to be aware of possible diagnostic issues early in the interview, because this tentative formulation may help determine the basic strategy of the interview itself. By way of illustration, the clinician may be interviewing an elderly man brought by his family because "he can't take care of himself anymore." During the opening phase, the clinician may notice thought disorganization, thought blocking, and a striking memory deficit. Normally, the cognitive mental status examination is brief and generally appears late in the body of the interview. But in this instance, the clinician may decide that a determination should be made of the severity of this patient's cognitive deficit earlier in the interviewing process. Moreover, with this type of patient, the cognitive examination may be lengthened in an effort to explore the degree of cognitive deficit while uncovering the possible presence of a delirium or dementia.

If severe memory deficits are recognized, then little can be gained by a lengthy interview, which would be both tiring and frustrating for the patient suffering with a moderate or severe dementia. Instead, this time may be more profitably spent with members of the patient's family, because they may provide a more reliable history. Once again, the clinician moves flexibly, adjusting to the unique needs of the patient and the clinical situation.

Of equal importance is the determination made by the clinician of the patient's unconscious goals. It is worth emphasizing repeatedly that much of the art of interviewing consists not of analyzing what the patient says but of speculating on what is not said and why it is not said. In a similar vein, patients often "half mention" issues, and the clinician needs to uncover what has been left partially clad. In particular, the issue of unconscious goals remains one of the major tasks of the opening phase.

The unconscious goals include those psychodynamic drives of which the patient may be partially or totally unaware. These needs, frequently arising from core psychological pains, may represent the most telling reasons why the patient has come for help or may also present significant roadblocks to the task of the initial assessment. An example will help to clarify this concept.

In this illustration the patient is a man about 30 years of age. His speech has a pressured quality, as if his words need to escape his mouth. He has been brought by his father, who threatened to commit him after the patient squirted his father with tear gas during a family squabble.

Clin.: Tell me some more about what brought you here today.

Pt.: (patient looks away disdainfully) I'll tell you what brought me here today … No! Before I tell you that, let me reassure you that I'm not crazy! My father's crazy, yeah, crazy, a real nut. … I'm an important person with important business, I don't have time to waste and I don't belong here, my father belongs here, you should see him, let's wrap this thing up here quickly.

Clin.:	Perhaps we could (patient interrupts).
Pt.:	I need a glass of water, you got any?
Clin.:	Yes, I do (clinician brings the patient a cup of water).
Pt.:	Thanks (takes a couple of sips). Look, I need to be out of here by 4 o'clock … the bottom line, the goal line is that there is nothing wrong with me that a little peace and quiet won't help, too many people do all the talking and no one listens. I'm a man whose time is worth big bucks. Here, look at this (patient shows clinician business card).
Clin.:	Let me take a closer look at that (inspects card). I see you are a vice president, no wonder your time is valuable. Perhaps we should start to get to the point.
Pt.:	No kidding, that's a good idea. I think you and I could work this thing out logically. We're both professionals, so professional to professional is the way to work this out. There is a big misunderstanding here. He's got it all wrong, I didn't want to squirt him in the face but he attacked me, he needed a lesson, a whopper, something to put him in his place, always talking, always telling me what to do. That's the way he's always been and I'm sick of it.
Clin.:	Tell me more about the misunderstanding, the way you see it, and take as much time as you need.
Pt.:	The way I see it, no one appreciates me. I just started a mail order business with my fiancée; she is wonderful, she understands. It's a dog-eat-dog world out there and the old man doesn't give a damn, he lives in the age of horse-hoofs, the Stone Age. He thinks the web is something a spider spins.
Clin.:	What are some of the specific stresses you are handling right now?
Pt.:	Financial strain, paying the rent, getting ready for the wedding, this, that, and the other.
Clin.:	Sounds like a lot of bills to pay.
Pt.:	You're darn right. The trouble is my landlord is a jerk. All he thinks about is money and payments. I've been a good tenant, and he has no right to throw me out.
Clin.:	When is he threatening to throw you out?
Pt.:	Two weeks from now, the man's got a lot of nerve. To think I used to say nice things about him.
Clin.:	How have all these pressures affected your sleep?
Pt.:	I don't need much sleep, I get along with very little sleep because I'm energized.
Clin.:	What time do you go to sleep roughly?
Pt.:	Well, that varies. Usually around 12 or 1 o'clock, but recently I've been staying up later to do my work.
Clin.:	And what kinds of things do you do when you stay up?

In this vignette, one can see the subtle maneuverings of the opening phase. The art lies in the interviewer's ability to recognize the unstated needs of the patient, while subsequently attending to some of these same needs. The passage warrants a closer look.

At a conscious level, the patient's agenda includes items such as convincing the clinician that nothing is wrong, convincing the clinician that the patient's father is wrong, and making a quick exit subsequent to an equally quick interview. But it is the unconscious goals that yield the most fertile engagement secrets.

Two of these unstated needs could be described as follows:

1. The need to appear important, possibly related to an underlying fear of inferiority.
2. The need to be in control, perhaps generated by the impending threat of an involuntary commitment, which would represent a total loss of control.

The first unconscious goal, the need for praise, manifests itself early in the dialogue. For instance, the patient immediately raises himself by putting down his father, "the nut," and the interviewer with a disdainful look. These defiant steps, indicative of a frightened ego, are quickly followed by a blunt request for praise, "I'm an important person with important business." Later we hear, "I'm a man whose time is worth big bucks," at which point he proceeds to display his business card.

It is at this moment that the clinician plays a gentle gambit. Specifically, she goes out of her way to provide the much needed praise. The clinician does not merely glance at the offered business card – she calmly admires it. Indeed, it is this quiet admiration that represents the real and immediate business of this interview, for with its presence the engagement process can begin to unfold. This quiet praise is furthered by a simple but elegantly effective acknowledgement of the patient's importance, "I see you are a vice president, no wonder your time is valuable." At last, the patient's self-system receives a chance to relax. Someone has seen his worth. Defenses, such as narcissistic put-downs and accusations, may become less necessary.

Further acknowledgment of the patient's importance resides in the clinician's recognition of the patient's stated time needs, "Perhaps we should start to get to the point." With this apparently appeasing statement, the clinician, in reality, is beginning to structure the interview. In a relatively short time this patient will be providing diagnostic information related to mania instead of demanding a shorter interaction.

The second hidden need, the need for control, begins with a subtle redirecting of the clinician's attention by the patient, "… my father belongs here, you should see him …" and ends with a not so subtle directive, "… let's wrap this thing up here quickly."

The patient continues to control the interview by interrupting the clinician's question by stating a demand, "I need a glass of water …" It is not so hard to imagine that someone close to involuntary commitment would feel threatened, because he is in reality threatened with an imprisonment of sorts. Fortunately, the interviewer recognizes this need and she focuses attention on helping this patient regain some semblance of self-determination.

First, she procures the requested water. Her strategy of releasing control in the service of gaining control is further engendered by the phrase, "Tell me more about the misunderstanding, the way you see it, and *take as much time as you need.*" This conveyance of control is gently bolstered by suggesting that the patient has been appropriately managing at least some aspects of his life as implied by the wording, "What are some of the specific stresses you are handling right now?" How different this phrase must sound compared with a similar content message, "What problems are unsettling you right now?", a phrase that would have ignored the patient's need to feel confident.

This dialogue represents only one of numberless interactions. It is not merely the specific words that are important here. It is the underlying principle of listening for the psychodynamic needs of the patient, even when a major psychiatric illness such as bipolar disorder is active, that warrants emphasis. Uncovering the patient's unconscious goals may yield a more compassionate understanding of his or her pain, an understanding that opens the door to engagement. Because this interviewer has deftly attended to this patient's unconscious needs in the opening phase, she has distinctly decreased the possibility of this patient becoming severely agitated. In the hands of a less skilled interviewer, the mania of this patient could easily be triggered into a violent emergency room incident.

Having completed our examination of the first three tasks of the PACE, it is time to explore the last task of the PACE – the Evaluation of the interview itself. Before doing so, in order to consolidate what we have covered, let's watch an actual interview unfold. We will sit-in during the first 8 or so minutes of an interview with one of my patients. In fact, we will return to the patient that we first met in Chapter 1. This time we will watch the interview consecutively unfold from the introduction through the opening phase and even into the early minutes of the body of the interview. In this sense, it will not only illustrate the real-life dynamics of the introduction and opening, it will give us a preview of how we may transition into the body of the interview itself.

VIDEO MODULE 3.1

Title: Macrostructure of the Interview: The Graceful Unfolding of the Introduction, Opening, and Body of the Interview

Contents: Contains expanded didactics and an annotated interview excerpt.

We are now ready to examine the last task of the PACE acronym – the Evaluation of the interview itself. We will discover that this task serves as a bridge between the opening and the body of the interview, for parts of it may occur in the opening and parts of it in the body. As we shall see, problematic processes – such as shut-down interviews – will generally present and be transformed in the opening phase. Other problematic processes – such as wandering interviews – may provide hints of their presence in the opening phase yet be subsequently transformed by the clinician in the body of the interview itself after more fully manifesting. The successful transformation of all of these hindrances to engagement are made possible by the various techniques I just referred to at the end of our video module and to which we now can turn our attention.

Evaluation of the Interview Itself

Interviews, like the people creating them, tend to develop personalities of a sort. The personality of the interview appears to be determined by the quality and quantity of the communication evolving between the participants. Ideally, a clinician would like to become a co-participant in an interview characterized by a patient who produces relatively large amounts of pertinent and valid information, while easily focusing on issues raised by the clinician. This ideal patient would become increasingly at ease as the interview proceeded, becoming the proverbial open book. Within minutes, an adequate level of engagement would be achieved, the patient and clinician working together towards unified goals.

In reality, ideal interviews are hard to find. Fortunately, good interviews are not. One of the keys to developing consistently productive interviews remains the ability to spot bad interviews before they become painful lessons in frustration. By consciously evaluating the interview process, the clinician opens the door to control and flexibility. Phrased more accurately, once the clinician has determined the personality of the interview, he or she may be better positioned to effectively structure the interview by adaptively altering technique.

To this end, during the opening phase, the clinician needs to attempt a conscious assessment of the progress of the interview. If pleased with its nascent development, then the clinician may continue with similar strategies. If displeased, the clinician may consider new options, yet a further expansion of our abilities to be intentional interviewers.

The interviewer should be on the lookout for a variety of less productive patterns in communication, three of which are the shut-down interview, the wandering interview, and the rehearsed interview. All three of these interview types are common and can lead to serious problems with engagement and data gathering. All three, once spotted, warrant a change in strategy. But before a clinician can spot his or her role in the creation of these problematic interviews, and before we can see how to circumvent them, it is necessary to examine in detail the key component to their transformation – the words that we use when framing our questions.

Degree of Openness Continuum (DOC): Open-Ended Questions, Gentle Commands, Swing Questions, and the Power of Language

In Search of an Answer: What Is an Open-Ended Question?

The concept of an open-ended question appears at first glance to be so self-explanatory that it warrants little discussion. But one could not be more mistaken. In actual practice, the open-ended question is frequently not utilized effectively. Moreover, numerous references to the technique in both research literature (an extensive literature called "response-mode" research exists in which pioneering researchers, such as Clara Hill, have carefully studied how clinicians phrase questions and statements) and interviewing texts tend to disagree with each other about the definition of open-endedness and about which questions are open and which are closed.[6-21]

For instance, how should we classify the following question, "Can you tell me a little bit about your past?" Is it best viewed as open-ended because it certainly opens up an enormous range of possible answers for the patient with minimal limitation by the interviewer. Or should it be viewed as closed-ended, for it can easily be answered with a curt "yes," "no," or "not really," especially by an angry prison inmate forced to see a corrections psychologist by a warden. I could show you outstanding interviewing textbooks that call this question closed-ended and some that view it as a prototypic open-ended question. Puzzling. What exactly is an open-ended question?

Our search for this answer will lead us into one of the most fascinating aspects of clinical interviewing – the realization that every question, as well as every statement that we use, possesses a degree of openness, thus impacting on how easy it is for a patient to talk with us. Moreover, as we saw in Chapter 2, both open and closed questions can be both engaging and useful depending upon the clinical task at that moment of the interview. As we examine this continuum of openness, paradoxes will also appear. For instance, *some statements may be more open-ended than some questions*. In addition, some questions are *simultaneously* open-ended and closed-ended. Understanding these paradoxes is critical for understanding how open or closed our own interviewing style is by habit. With this self-knowledge, we can move away from interviewing by habit to our goal of intentional interviewing.

To make sense of these paradoxes, we will look at a simplifying, yet sophisticated, "supervision language" – the Degree of Openness Continuum (DOC) – for categorizing our own questions and statements. Once mastered, our understanding will allow us to intentionally pick and choose the type of questions or statements that are most likely to transform shut-down, wandering, or rehearsed interviews. From paradox, practicality will be born.

Using the DOC (Table 3.1) we can classify any verbalization we make (whether a question or a statement) into one of nine mutually exclusive types. By definition these nine types of questions and statements fall into one of three broad categories with regard to their degree of open-endedness. These three broad categorizations are: (1) open-ended verbalizations, (2) variable verbalizations, and (3) closed-ended verbalizations. Where specific types of verbalizations fall on the DOC depends upon three characteristics: (1) the degree to which the verbalization tends to produce spontaneous and lengthy responses, (2) the degree to which the verbalization does not limit the patient's answer set, and (3) the degree to which the verbalization, in a generic sense, possesses a tendency to open up moderately shut-down interviewees.

The nine types of clinician verbalizations are as follows. Open-ended verbalizations include open-ended questions and gentle commands. Variable verbalizations include five types: (1) swing questions, (2) qualitative questions, (3) statements of inquiry, (4) empathic statements, and (5) facilitating statements. Finally, closed-ended verbalizations include closed-ended questions and closed-ended statements. Let us take a look at how the system works.

Open-Ended Verbalizations

Keeping in mind that both questions and statements can be classified as open-ended or closed, we immediately encounter our first paradox: some statements are more open-ended than some questions. For example, the statement, "Tell me something about your old high-school girlfriend" is significantly more open-ended than the question, "Did you have a high-school girlfriend?"

By definition, open-ended verbalizations are difficult to answer with one word or a short phrase, even if the interviewee is moderately guarded or resistant, as in a shut-down

Table 3.1 Degree of Openness Continuum (DOC)

VERBALIZATION	EXAMPLE
Open-Ended	
1. Open-ended questions	1. What are your plans for the future? 2. How will you approach your father? 3. What are some of your thoughts about the marriage?
2. Gentle commands	1. Tell me something about your brother. 2. Describe your initial reaction to me. 3. Share with me some of your hopes about the marriage.
Variable	
1. Swing questions	1. Can you describe your feelings? 2. Can you tell me a little about your boss? 3. Can you say anything about the marriage?
2. Qualitative questions	1. How's your appetite? 2. How's your job going? 3. How's your mood been?
3. Statements of inquiry	1. You have never smoked marijuana? 2. You say you were fifth in your class? 3. So you left the marriage after 3 years?
4. Empathic statements	1. It sounds like a troubling time for you. 2. It's difficult to end a marriage after 10 years. 3. It looks like you're feeling very sad.
5. Facilitating statements	1. Uh-huh 2. Go on 3. I see
Closed-Ended	
1. Closed-ended questions	1. Do you think your son will pass? 2. Are you feeling happy, sad, or angry? 3. What medication is he taking?
2. Closed-ended statements	1. Please sit over there. 2. I read the letter Dr. Smith wrote. 3. Anxiety can be helped with behavioral therapies.

interview. It is extremely difficult to respond to open-ended verbalizations with a simple "yes" or "no." Moreover, questions that provide or imply possible answers, or ask for specific facts, items, places, dates, numbers, or names are closed-ended, for they limit the patient's freedom of choice. In contrast, both types of open-ended verbalizations leave the patient significant latitude as to where he or she may want to go with an answer. Broadly speaking, in patients with whom the engagement is high, open-ended verbalizations tend to produce relatively large quantities of speech.

Open-ended verbalizations appear in one of two forms: (1) open-ended questions and (2) what I like to call to call "gentle commands."[22] A classic example of an open-ended question would be as follows, "What would you do if your wife decided to leave you?" (see Table 3.1 for further examples). This question does not guide the patient towards any specific answer, nor can it easily be answered tersely. It invites the patient to share personal experience. Questions that begin with "How" or "What" *and* do not limit the potential answer set by asking for a specific short answer, name, number, time, place, or fact are usually open-ended. Thus the question, "How would you handle your college days differently if you could go back?" is an open-ended question, whereas "How many credits did you take last semester?" is not an open-ended question (even though they both begin with the word "how").

We have already seen one example of a gentle command. They consist of statements such as "Tell me something about your old high-school girlfriend," which direct the patient to speak but do not markedly limit the potential answer. Gentle commands begin with words such as "Tell me ..." or "Describe for me. ..." They are stated with a *gentle* tone of voice while expressing a genuine interest. Such statements, in order to be viewed as a gentle command, as was the case with open-ended questions, *cannot* limit the potential answer set by asking for a specific short answer, name, number, time, place, or fact. Thus, "Tell me what you are finding unpleasant about your new job" is a gentle command. "Tell me who your favorite colleague is at work" is not. A series of gentle commands or a mixture of these statements with open-ended questions frequently increases the blending and spontaneity of even the most shut-down interaction. Generally speaking, gentle commands represent one of the most powerful tools available for helping hesitant patients to share more freely.

Closed-Ended Verbalizations

At the other end of the DOC one encounters closed-ended verbalizations. With closed-ended techniques, it is extremely easy for a moderately shut-down patient to answer with one word, a short phrase, or a simple "yes" or "no." Even in instances in which the engagement is high, these techniques may tend to decrease interviewee response length. Indeed, as we shall see shortly, closed-ended inquiries are frequently useful in focusing wandering patients.

Closed-ended verbalizations come in two types: (1) closed-ended questions and (2) closed-ended statements (see Table 3.1). Closed-ended questions frequently are of a yes/no format such as, "Did you seek therapy at the time of the accident?" or ask for specific details such as, "Which hospital were you at in 1982?" Although frequently hunting for facts, they may also seek out opinions and emotions as seen with, "Do you think your husband is hard working?"

Closed-ended statements do not suggest that any response is expected from the patient and frequently are of an explanatory or educational slant as with, "We will begin by looking at some of your symptoms," or "I spoke with your previous therapist as you suggested."

Variable Verbalizations

Variable verbalizations represent a middle ground with regard to openness, because they tend to vary in the responses they create depending upon the degree of engagement.

When engagement is high, these types of questions often result in the production of large amounts of spontaneous speech. But when engagement is low and the patient is defensive, angry, or embarrassed, the very same questions can be easily answered tersely. And therein lies their danger for the clinician, for these questions and statements are tickets towards monologue when used in a shut-down interview. Consequently, we will examine the five variable verbalizations: swing questions, qualitative questions, statements of inquiry, empathic statements, and facilitating statements, in detail.

Swing questions[23] are characterized by the distinctive fact that the interviewer literally asks the patient whether he or she will answer the question. They often begin with phrases such as, "Can you tell me …", "Can you describe …", and "Would you say something about …" We can now address our earlier question as to how to classify the question, "Can you tell me a little bit about your past?" Here is our second paradox: it seems to be both open and closed simultaneously. But, in actuality, it may be best viewed as laying somewhere in between the two. The impact of such questions literally swings from open to closed depending upon the degree of engagement with the patient. When engagement is high, a patient may merrily chatter away following such a question. But when a patient is hesitant, for whatever reason, these questions can be curtly answered with responses such as, "not really," "don't feel like it," or simply "no." Consequently, as mentioned above, it is generally wise to avoid their use in shut-down interviews.

A second type of variable verbalization is the qualitative question,[24] with which the clinician inquires about the quality of the state of the patient, his symptoms, his relations, or activities. They frequently begin with the words, "How is your …?" Qualitative questions such as, "How's your relationship with your son?" have the potential to produce a significant elaboration if the engagement is high. But, as was the case with swing questions, a shut-down patient could easily answer tersely with a phrase such as, "Just fine." Operationally speaking, if a question begins with the word "how," has a form of the verb "to be" within it, and *theoretically* could be answered by the single word "fine," then it is, by definition, a qualitative question.

The third type of variable verbalization, the statement of inquiry,[25] is represented by a complete sentence followed by a question mark. Unlike closed-ended statements, they are intended to stimulate a response from the patient as seen with, "You were working at the factory right after college?" or "You're viewed as the black sheep in the family?" The tone of voice of the clinician has a lot to do with the transformation of these statements into questions. The clinician's tone of voice can move these statements from a reassuring reflection to a gentle probing to a blunt confrontation. Statements of inquiry tend to perform one of several functions: clarification, summarization, confrontation, or interpretation. As with the two previous variable verbalizations, statements of inquiry can be easily answered tersely or with a "yes" or "no" by shut-down patients, whereas in situations of high engagement these statements may function as springboards for further patient elaboration.

It should also be noted that because statements of inquiry lead with a supposed "statement of fact" by the clinician, they all represent a form of leading question. When it is used to merely reflect back what the patient has said in an engaging fashion, this "leading" quality is minimal. In contrast, when a statement of inquiry raises a new issue and/or communicates a clinician judgment, the leading quality can be striking. State-ments of inquiry that are strongly leading in nature often begin with the word "so," as seen with "So, you were an alcoholic even back in junior high?" If a clinician or supervi-sor wants to find out whether a clinician has a leading style of interviewing, the frequency of statements of inquiry can often provide insight.

Also note that a particularly problematic statement of inquiry, with regard to poor validity, is the "negative statement of inquiry." It includes a negative, such as the word "not," as with, "So, you're *not* feeling suicidal?" Such statements clearly can lead patients to feel that the interviewer expects (or wants) them to answer with a "no." The result is often invalid data – in this case, potentially dangerously invalid data. I see no redeeming value in negative statements of inquiry – with one exception. Some clinicians find that if said with a doubting tone of voice and facial expression on the word "not," they can be utilized to challenge malingering or antisocial patients immediately after they make a patently false statement. But, generally speaking, I suggest eliminating them entirely if you find them as a part of your interviewing style.

The final two types of variable verbalizations, empathic statements and facilitating statements, can be usefully discussed together, because they generally tend to open patients up, although with patients who have a guarded or paranoid interpersonal stance they may backfire, as discussed in Chapter 1. By definition, as described in detail in Chapter 1, empathic statements are attempts to convey to patients that one is gaining an understanding of their feelings and perceptions of the world (see Table 3.1).

Facilitating statements include the wide range of single utterances or short phrases used to signal that the clinician is carefully listening, such as, "Uh-huh" and, "Go on." Although these facilitating phrases tend to urge the patient towards more speech, looked at on an individual basis they are not as powerfully open as a gentle command or an open-ended question. With hostile patients they may even backfire. I recall one instance in the emergency room, when an intoxicated patient began angrily aping both my facili-tating statements and my head nodding, saying, "Yeah, yeah, yeah, you're a shrink all right, yeah, you're a shrink." Several minutes later he attacked a safety officer.

Transforming Shut-Down Interviews

Characteristics of Shut-Down Interviews

Now that we have surveyed the types of questions and statements along the DOC, it is time to see how we can use this knowledge to both recognize and transform common communication gremlins, such as the shut-down interview (Table 3.2). In the shut-down interview, the patient displays a short duration of utterance, a long response time latency, and usually a variety of body language clues indicating that things are not going well. In particular, eye contact is often poor.

I am reminded of a patient that I observed during supervision who sat morosely, her legs propped up on a stool, her own crossed arms representing the main objects of inter-est to her eyes. As if to place appropriate exclamation points in her nonverbal commu-nication, she yawned with impeccable timing. She represented the ideal persona of a shut-down in communication.

Table 3.2 Interview Typologies

INTERVIEW TYPE	CHARACTERISTICS OF PATIENT			CHARACTERISTICS OF INTERVIEWER		
	Duration of Utterance (DOU)	Response Time Latency (RTL)	Natural Body Language such as Eye Contact	Ratio of Open-Ended Questions to Closed-Ended Questions	Focusing Statements	Facilitating Maneuvers, Empathic Statements
Shut-down interview	↓	↑	↓	↓	↑	↓
Wandering interview	↑	↓	↑	↑	↓	↑
Rehearsed interview	↑	↓	↕	↕	↓	↑

KEY: ↑ = increased; ↓ = decreased; ↕ = either increased or decreased.

However, shut-down interviews are not the creation of the patient alone. As emphasized earlier, all interviews represent interaction. In this respect, the action of the patient just described suggests the possibility that the interview will become a shut-down interview. But for this process to unfold fully, the interviewer often must feed it.

This feeding occurs when the interviewer fosters the shut-down pattern by utilizing a low ratio of open-ended to variable/closed-ended verbalizations. In shut-down interviews, both variable and closed-ended techniques generally tend to decrease patient spontaneity and, hence, hinder the engagement process. This tendency becomes further entrenched when the interviewer uses a high proportion of focusing statements and other structuring techniques. It may be even further entrenched if the clinician fails to utilize facilitating nonverbal maneuvers such as head nodding and an encouraging tone of voice.

During shut-down interviews, especially if there is a negative attitude emerging from the patient, it is not uncommon for clinicians to feel frustration, which often manifests itself in a sharpness to their tone of voice and a distinct lack of nonverbal empathic communication. Ironically, such action fosters the further development of the shut-down process itself. Thus, the dyadic nature of the interview surfaces once again.

Unlocking Shut-Down Interviews

Over the course of years of clinical work, variable verbalizations – swing questions, statements of inquiry, and empathic statements – can tend to become habits for interviewers. As an interview becomes more shut-down, habits have a tendency to return, just when they are least useful. As the patient provides short answers and begins to appear more withdrawn, hesitant, or testy, the natural tendency is to ask questions even faster, for the awkwardness of the silence is unnerving. At such points, interviewers tend to rely more upon swing questions, in which the words "Can you say more about …" have an almost apologetic tone or pleading quality. Both low-valence and high-valence empathic statements appear by habit, because the interviewer becomes acutely aware of the poor blending of the interview, and naturally turns towards a technique – empathic statements – that usually improves blending; but not today. Closed-ended questions also seem to appear more frequently, probably because they are easier to formulate than open-ended questions. The unpleasant result may be as follows:

Clin.: How long had you been in prison? (closed question)

Pt.: (looking somewhat disgusted) Two years.

Clin.: Was it a bad experience? (closed question)

Pt.: What do you think? (said sarcastically)

Clin.: Were the guards tough? (closed question)

Pt.: Yeah.

Clin.: Did they get on your nerves? (closed question)

Pt.: Yeah.

Clin.: Did you get time for exercise? (closed question)

Pt.: Sometimes.

Clin.: Pretty bad food, I bet. (empathic statement)

Pt.:	Yeah.
Clin.:	Did you get very lonely there? (closed question)
Pt.:	Yeah. (patient rolls his eyes)
Clin.:	Could you tell me a little about what that felt like? (swing question)
Pt.:	Not much to tell you.
Clin.:	Well, I, uh, was it tough being away from your wife? (closed question)
Pt.:	Sort of.
Clin.:	Would you be able to tell me how she felt about it? (swing question)
Pt.:	Don't really know.
Clin.:	Can you tell me if she still loves you? (swing question)
Pt.:	Don't really know that either.
Clin.:	What do you think? (open-ended question)
Pt.:	I think she might.
Clin.:	How's the communication between you two? (qualitative question)
Pt.:	Just dandy.
Clin.:	How do you mean? (open-ended question)
Pt.:	I mean she still visits, she's got the kids. We're divorced.
Clin.:	Ah, how often does she visit? (closed question)
Pt.:	About twice a year.
Clin.:	When is that? (closed question)
Pt.:	Take a guess … around Christmas and on my birthday.

The only person probably less comfortable than the patient in this room is the interviewer. Indeed, here is a classic shut-down interview moving into a spiral of silence. It illustrates several errors described earlier, including an initial barrage of closed-ended questions. In the latter half, one sees the use of swing questions and an empathic statement, under the mistaken thought that they are open-ended. *The result proves otherwise, for they are variable verbalizations that function as closed-ended with reticent or angry patients.* Then one sees the use of two true open-ended questions, "What do you think?" and "How do you mean?" But two open-ended questions are too few.

The secret to unlocking shut-down interviews lies in using a series of open-ended verbalizations as with a combination of open-ended questions/gentle commands, not just a couple. In addition, the interviewer tries to pick topics that, at a conscious or unconscious level, the patient *wants* to talk about. These are usually topics that have a strong affective charge for the patient or about which the patient has a strong opinion. Following the first couple of open-ended techniques, the patient's responses will probably still be brief. But after six or seven open-ended verbalizations *in a row*, especially if an appealing topic has been broached, many patients will start to yield to the awkwardness of not responding appropriately.

The above exchange also illustrates how easily other variable verbalizations, such as qualitative questions, can be shut down by shut-down patients. In the following example, we will see the course the previous dialogue might have taken if handled differently:

Clin.: How long were you in prison? (closed question)

Pt.:   (looking somewhat disgusted) Two years.

Clin.: Huh … Obviously, most people hate being in prison but some deal with it better than others. What did you do to keep yourself busy? (open-ended question)

Pt.:   Workout in my cell and play cards, workout in my cell and play cards, but it grows old real fast.

Clin.: I really don't know much about what a prison is like; tell me something about it. (gentle command)

Pt.:   Let me put it this way. You wouldn't last a day (patient smiles with a mild disdain, shaking his head from side to side). Yeah, they'd get you real fast.

Clin.: Tell me what it's really like in there. (gentle command)

Pt.:   Well, it's boring, day after day of the same old shit. You're only out of that damn cell for an hour a day. And time goes damn slow. Everything, everything changes for you, man. Eating dinner is something to do; a fucking movie is the highlight of the week. And you become a "con," not a jerk-off.

Clin.: How do you mean, a "con"? (open-ended question)

Pt.:   A "con" is no one's fool. We don't come on to the guards or anyone. You can't survive unless you watch your back. (pauses) There wasn't a minute of the day that I wasn't aware of who was near me. You never know when some asshole is gonna pull a shank on you or something.

Clin.: You know, I gotta plead a little dumb here. I don't exactly know what you mean by a shank. What exactly is it? (open-ended question)

Pt.:   Man (smiling, almost warmly out of pity), you wouldn't last an hour, forget a day. (pauses) A shank's a sharp, a knife. Not a real knife. You make them out of stuff. You know, like you can file down a toothbrush if you have to. It's pretty amazing how creative you can be if you have nothing to do hour after hour for months or years. I've seen some pretty amazing shit made into a shank. One time I saw a guy who …

This clinician is cleverly engaging the patient by utilizing open-ended questions and gentle commands. Notice the rather remarkable increase in spontaneous speech (longer DOU) of the former inmate compared to the first interview. In particular, the clinician has avoided the pitfall of utilizing swing questions and other variable verbalizations, which could function in a closed role, as evidenced in the earlier example. This clinician also wisely went into an area in which the patient felt comfortable and, indeed, could "instruct" the clinician.

The following list reviews the techniques we have discussed for transforming a shut-down interview and also suggests a few more tips:

1. Employ large numbers of combinations of open-ended questions, peppered with some gentle commands, in a series. Too frequently interviewers ask one or two open-ended verbalizations, followed by a close-ended question or a variable verbalization, which can immediately defeat the gains made by the open-ended approach. Often a combination of six or seven open-ended questions or gentle commands *in a row* will be necessary to switch the gears of the interview process towards more open conversation.

2. Even an empathic statement (one of the variable verbalizations) can break up the momentum towards more open patient sharing. Avoid stand-alone empathic statements when trying to unlock a shut-down interview. Instead, if you feel an empathic statement may be of use, couple the empathic statement with an open-ended technique by using it as the lead, a technique known as a "piggy-back" empathic statement (e.g., "That sounds like a really tough divorce, tell me more about what your husband has been doing that is so upsetting.").

3. Follow up any topic that the patient gives the slightest hint that he or she wants to discuss (i.e., any topic on which the patient shows an increasing DOU, even for a brief period of time).

4. Avoid, in general, difficult or sensitive topics such as lethality, drugs and alcohol abuse, and sexual history.

5. Pick topics that gather general background information such as, "Tell me a little bit about the neighborhood you live in?" or "What are the people like where you work?" Or choose topics about which the patient has strong opinions as with, "What are some of the things your boss does that seem unfair?"

6. Avoid the use of swing questions such as, "Can you tell me …?" or "Would you tell me. …?" Such swing questions are easily answered with silence or frowns. Instead, it is frequently best to use gentle commands that often prompt more open sharing. Curiously, if one has a habit of using swing questions, one can easily break the habit. In a shut-down interview, when you find yourself about to use a swing question (e.g., "Can you tell me a little about problems at work?"), drop off the words "Can you" and then proceed with whatever you were about to ask. Notice that you will have immediately transformed your potentially disengaging swing question into an engaging gentle command that begins with the words, "Tell me …"

7. Increase attempts at eye contact, while increasing the reinforcement of verbal output with head nodding, engaging tone of voice and empathic sounds, except with hostile or paranoid patients, with whom a less frequent use of such techniques may be advisable.

8. In initial interviews, avoid long pauses before asking the next question. Long pauses can be effective techniques for eliciting information from reasonably well-engaged patients who stop their flow because of their desire to avoid a topic (as might be encountered in ongoing psychotherapy). On the other hand, long pauses in shut-down patients frequently create further defensiveness and resentment in a first encounter. Effective use of long pauses depends on effective timing and good common sense.

It should also be kept in mind that the above techniques are generally applicable not only in shut-down interviews but also during the opening phase of any interview. In contrast, in interviews with good engagement, patients may spontaneously talk about a variety of painful or sensitive areas fairly early. In even sharper contrast, the first principle outlined above is specific to shut-down interviews. In naturally evolving interviews, open-ended techniques are interwoven with statements of empathy and closed-ended questions, both of which serve to clarify issues and demonstrate the clinician's interest. Thus it is uncommon in naturally unfolding interviews with good initial blending to employ overly long strings of purely open-ended techniques (without using variable verbalizations such as empathic statements), remembering that about 60 to 90% of verbalizations in the opening phase are open-ended.

This list offers some of the guiding principles with which to approach shut-down interviews. Most importantly, a concerted effort should be made to increase patient output before proceeding with information gathering. If these techniques do not work, then a more deep-rooted communication roadblock may have formed. Approaches to resolving such deep-rooted stalemates will be discussed in Chapter 19. Another method of approaching shut-down interviews is to address suspected patient concerns about the interview process or situation itself. This technique is also discussed in Chapter 19.

The most telling point remains that the presence of an evolving shut-down interview, spotted during the opening phase of an initial assessment, indicates a need for an active change in interviewing style before proceeding to the body of the interview, a transformation that we can now accomplish because of our understanding of the DOC. These intentional changes frequently and rapidly result in a more fruitful dialogue, as we saw with the former inmate above.

As with any interview, one must work flexibly and creatively with the individual patient. In some instances of a shut-down interview, the above techniques may actually hinder progress. In particular, some patients whose thinking is grossly disorganized, secondary to either interpersonal anxiety or psychotic process, may respond poorly to open-ended questions or gentle commands. These techniques force these patients to conceptualize at a level at which they may not be capable, further increasing anxiety.

In these instances, very structured and concrete questions may help the patient with organization. In support of this goal, the clinician may employ a higher number of closed-ended questions and statements of inquiry. With experience, one quickly learns which technique works best with which type of patient.

In a similar vein, some adolescents and adults need to "warm up" with a higher ratio of closed-ended questions, because these tend to be less probing and can be more quickly answered. Two other types of questions merit attention. At first glance they seem like classic open-ended techniques – and they are open-ended – but they tend to perplex patients and should, in my opinion, be avoided in shut-down interviews.

The first problematic questions are those that begin with the word "why" such as, "Why did you drop out of school?" As Alfred Benjamin has cogently discussed, questions beginning with "why" frequently sound judgmental and break the feeling of unconditional positive regard, especially if the tone of voice is even mildly harsh.[26] For some patients, hearing the word "why" immediately conjures images of Mom or Dad in "critical mode." Such questions also seem to suggest that there exists one answer to the question, and it may be difficult for the patient to sort through all the confounding factors to produce the single right answer. The fix to phrasing these questions is simple – replace the word "Why" with the words "What were …" Various wordings can be used such as, "What were some of the things going through your mind when you decided that it would be best to leave school?" or "What were the pros and cons of leaving school when you made your decision?"

The second troublesome question that tends to hinder dialogue in a shut-down interview may represent the all-time stereotypical "shrink question," and it reads something like this: "What are you feeling as we talk?" In actuality, it is both uncommon and difficult for most people to be aware of their inner feelings. Thus, in shut-down interviews, this type of question is particularly good at producing looks of consternation on patients' faces. Avoid it. It may be of use in certain communication breakdowns, which we will discuss in a later chapter, or be quite useful later in therapy, or with patients with whom the blending is high. But in shut-down interviews I find little use for it. By the way, children and adolescents, in particular, may find this question puzzling.

Transforming Wandering Interviews

Characteristics of Wandering Interviews

At this point we have spent a large amount of time discussing methods of working through a shut-down interview, because this type of interaction is both common and frustrating. At the other end of the continuum, one may be unfortunate enough to become a participant in a wandering interview, one of the most feared gremlins in a managed care setting or a busy clinic.

We met a mild variant of this entity at the very beginning of the book. As we saw then, in the wandering interview (see Table 3.2) the patient displays a tendency toward tangential thought that can de-rail the interviewer's train of questioning into a frustrating series of unnecessary and unproductive stops. The patient's loquaciousness is often characterized by a mild pressure to speech, resulting in a long DOU, almost tempting the interviewer not to ask questions, because each question creates a new verbal leak. The response time latency (RTL) is short, and eye contact is often good.

A variant of the wandering interview, "the loquacious interview," occurs when the patient demonstrates large amounts of speech but does not stray off the topic. In such interviews, both the patient and the clinician become bogged down in a mass of irrelevant details about the requested topic.

The characteristics described above represent the attributes of a patient that predispose the patient towards the development of a wandering interview. But once again, a true wandering interview remains the joint creation of both the patient and the clinician. Clinicians foster the wandering by using open-ended verbalizations (open-ended questions or gentle commands) and by *not* utilizing focusing statements. In short, as the patient extends his or her hand, the clinician accepts it. And the rambling walk begins.

Frequently clinicians unwittingly further their own demise by employing many facilitating gestures and sounds, which only serve to reward the patient's abundant flow of speech. Note taking can also serve to reward this process, functioning as a metacommunication to the effect of "What you just said is important, keep going." Interviewers can learn to quiet all of these facilitating activities in the service of closing off a runaway interview, but to do so the clinician must first be aware of them.

The patient's contribution to the wandering interview has many etiologies. Such an interpersonal style may accompany histrionic personality structure or indicate the earliest stages of a mania; or this style may represent something much less serious, as seen with a patient who is simply anxious, a very common cause of wandering.

In any case, several principles may be of value in transforming such an interview into a more productive exchange. Generally speaking, one does the opposite of what is used to open-up a shut-down interview. While moving out of the opening phase, begin to help the patient structure his or her answers as follows:

a. Decrease the ratio of open-ended verbalizations and variable verbalizations to closed-ended verbalizations, with only a rare use of open-ended questions or gentle commands and minimal use of any of the variable verbalizations. *Remember that variable verbalizations, especially swing questions and empathic statements, will function as open-ended questions with wandering patients.*

b. Avoid reinforcing the wandering pattern by excessive head nodding or paralanguage cues to "go on." This process was referred to earlier as nonverbally "feeding the wanderer."

c. Begin with a gentle structuring by immediately returning to the topic of the question that led to the tangential sidetrack.

d. If the wandering continues, become progressively more structured with focusing statements such as, "For a moment, let's focus on what your mood was like back then."

e. If the wandering continues, one can further increase the effectiveness of focusing by using statements such as, "This is such an important area I would like us to just focus on it for a few minutes."

f. If the above techniques fail (relatively rare, most patients will have responded nicely to the above techniques), one can more explicitly tell the patient what is needed: "We have a limited amount of time. Consequently, I'm going to focus on some of the very important areas you mentioned in an effort to understand more clearly. It's important for us to focus on one topic at a time so I can get the best possible understanding of what you think is going on."

g. Finally, if all of the techniques above do not work (rare in my experience), one can become very strongly structured: "Because of time, we need to focus directly on the last 2 weeks of your mood. It will be important not to wander on to other topics, because learning specifically about your mood is so important for our understanding. In fact, if *we* wander off, you'll notice that I'll bring *us* back to the last 2 weeks. Is that all right with you? … Let's start with your sleep. Over the past 2 weeks how long has it been taking you to fall asleep?"

h. Another alternative approach if the early and mid-level focusing techniques ("a" through "e" from the above list) fail consists of addressing the interview process itself: "I have noticed that when I ask questions we somehow seem to wander off the subject. What do you think may be going on?"

Generally speaking, unless the patient has some serious underlying psychopathology, such as a manic process, the first several techniques will decrease the wandering process.

In some instances when employing the above techniques, it may also be necessary to literally cut a patient off in mid-sentence. This technique is fairly forceful and consequently should be utilized after less aggressive focusing techniques have failed, although clinicians frequently don't use it early enough. One way to maintain engagement, even when cutting a patient off, is to use a technique we used earlier with shut-down patients – the "piggy-back" empathic statement. Only this time, after leading with the empathic statement, we will follow-up not with an open-ended verbalization but with a closed-ended question that focuses the patient:

Clin.: Exactly how depressed have you been feeling?

Pt.: Well, let's see, in the past several months a lot has been happening to me, you know, what with the move and everything. I was very upset by my mother's nagging and the bills are really mounting, much as they did when I was living with Aunt Louise. Fortunately, I'm not quite as bad off as with Aunt Louise because …

Clin.: (clinician cuts off patient) It really sounds like you've been through a lot. Have you been feeling depressed over the past 2 weeks? (piggy-back empathic state followed by a closed-ended question)

Pt.: Oh, I've been feeling very depressed.

Clin.: Have you cried or felt like crying? (closed-ended question)

Another method of effectively using a cut-off is to include a comment acknowledging the importance of what the patient is saying such as, "So much of what you are saying is important that we need to focus a bit on it to ensure we get the most important points. Has your mood been depressed over the past 2 weeks?" Once again the patient was cut off in mid-stream, but the opening line acknowledges the importance of what the patient is saying while focusing the conversation. If one has appropriately engaged a patient in the introduction and opening phase, I am frequently pleasantly surprised how rarely he or she is disengaged by the effective use of cut-offs deeper into the interview. Patients want us to get the information we need to help them.

To this point, I would like to emphasize that the recognition of a wandering interview occurs during the opening phase, but *the attempt to transform this process actually occurs somewhere in the body of the interview.* This point warrants emphasis because one of the major deterrents to focusing a patient effectively is the attempt to focus too early. Ironically, such premature focusing can leave the patient and the clinician in a duel for control. In such a duel, both participants may go home wounded, because the patient responds by talking even more profusely in an effort to gain control. Or worse, the patient becomes disgruntled and shuts down. The main point remains: engage first, structure second.

A second major factor in successfully focusing a wandering patient is to conscientiously apply the principles regarding the DOC. As stated earlier, the interviewer should be aiming to decrease the ratio of open-ended verbalizations and variable verbalizations to closed-ended verbalizations, with only a rare use (perhaps as the first question when entering a new topic) of open-ended questions or gentle commands, and minimal use of variable verbalizations. It's pretty simple. When directly trying to reverse the wandering style of communication, the interviewer uses essentially *only* closed-ended questions. Remember that *with a wanderer*, all five variable verbalizations essentially function like open-ended questions. Pay particular attention to avoiding swing questions, for their use, in a wandering interview, is opening the gate to a potentially wild gallop into tangential information.

A third major factor in gracefully reining in a wandering interview lies in the effective use of paralanguage and body language during the structuring process. The art is not so much in the choice of words but in the method of presentation. For instance, if said with a concerned tone of voice, a phrase such as, "Let's look again at what your mood was like over the past 2 weeks," will seldom be interpreted as a structuring ploy. On the other hand, the same phrase said harshly, or in frustration, may quickly disengage a timid patient.

Let's examine an interviewer skillfully working with a persistent wanderer. The interviewer recognized the wandering pattern during the opening phase and, consequently, began to structure as the opening phase ended and the body of the interview began. The patient presented saying, "I'm really depressed." We shall pick up the interview at a point where the interviewer is trying to determine both the presence and severity of the patient's depressed symptoms.

Clin.: Tell me what your sleep has been like (gentle command).

Pt.: My sleep, now that's a good question. Nobody in my family has ever been a sound sleeper. I remember my father always talking about his restless nights. Same way with Uncle Harry, although, personally, I think Uncle Harry was a drunk. They say drunks, I shouldn't call him that (patient giggles), have really bad sleep.

Clin.: How has your sleep been over the past 2 weeks? (qualitative question, gently re-focusing the patient back onto the patient's sleep pattern)

Pt.: Pretty bad, more wound up, what with all the worries on my mind. I'm really upset about my decrease in pay. I don't think my boss should have cut my salary. Now there is a guy who needs to see a shrink. I can't believe what he does sometimes. You really ought to see him, a real winner! (note that the patient has "taken off" with this qualitative question, which one would expect to happen if one uses a variable verbalization with a wanderer)

Clin.: It sounds like you've had a lot of worries related to your boss; I'm wondering if it's keeping you up at night. How many hours do you think it takes you to fall asleep? (closed-ended question)

Pt.: Oh, maybe 2 or 3.

Clin.: Once you're asleep, do you stay asleep the whole night or do you tend to wake up occasionally? (closed-ended question)

Pt.: No, no, once I'm out, I'm really out, just like the night after my chem final. I was so tired I literally slept like a log; but fortunately I was alert enough to pack up for home, although I don't know why I should want to go home, why …

Clin.: (cuts off patient) Before we talk about some of the important issues at home, help me to get an even clearer picture of how your sleep has been affected. For instance, over the past 2 weeks have you been awakening earlier than usual for yourself? (closed question)

Pt.: No, I can't say that I have.

Clin.: Do you sleep at all during the day? (closed question)

Pt.: No, once I'm up, I'm really up.

Clin.: How has your energy been recently? (qualitative question)

Pt.: Up and down, mostly down. I guess I'm not as interested in things as I used to be.

Clin.: How do you mean? (open-ended question)

Pt.: Well, I used to be into jazz dance and ballet. On Wednesday nights I did aerobics. My sister, Jane, had gotten me into aerobics, she was always a super athlete. Now there's another example of a big shot. She has been one pain in the ass for years, for instance she …

Clin.: (the open-ended question seemed a reasonable way to clarify the patient's anhedonia, but, sure enough, the patient is "taking off" again – time for another cut-off, but deftly tied into a topic of interest for the patient) What about your own interest in things like dance now – has it increased or decreased? (closed-ended question)

Pt.: Definitely decreased. I'm finding it harder and harder to enjoy all my hobbies. I'm even having a hard time reading.

Clin.: Is your depression making it hard to concentrate when you read? (closed-ended question)

Pt.: Absolutely, it makes it really really hard to read.

In this illustration of some very nice interviewing, the clinician has begun structuring this interview without disengaging the patient. This toning down of a wound-up wanderer was accomplished using a variety of techniques, including focusing statements, closed-ended questions, and even interrupting the patient with cut-off statements when appropriate.

Even when using the initial patient cut-off, the clinician maintained both engagement and blending by conveying the importance of gaining a clear picture of exactly what the patient had been experiencing. Moreover, the clinician also emphasized the importance of what the patient was discussing by implying that the topic would be examined later in the interview. Both of these goals were accomplished with a single elegant phrase, "Before we talk about some of the important issues at home, help me to get an even clearer picture of how your sleep has been affected." Even the use of the words "help me" were part of the process, for they metacommunicated a shared goal and a clinician who was genuinely interested in achieving this goal.

Not surprisingly, working with a wandering patient is one of the most frequent problems for which clinicians request supervision, probably because we are often hesitant to structure, anticipating a rebuff from the patient. This hesitancy prevents us from learning how to structure effectively. In a sense, a wandering interview reminds one of an unchecked nuclear reaction; its ultimate result is a chaotic and sparse understanding of the patient. On the other hand, the ability to effectively, yet sensitively, structure the flow of the interview offers the clinician a method of controlling the reaction, so as to garner the information that can most help the patient and lead to healing.

Later, in the body of the interview, the clinician may find good reasons to unleash the reaction again while exploring the patient's dynamics or feelings. The important point remains that the clinician can intentionally modify the interview process in either direction, depending on what the goals of the interview are at that moment.

To end this discussion of the wandering interview, it is of value to list some of the most common errors that clinicians commit while handling a wandering patient:

1. Continuing to "feed the wanderer" instead of beginning to structure gently as one enters the main body of the interview.
2. Being afraid to focus or interrupt the patient. When done effectively, focusing statements are generally well tolerated by patients.
3. Structuring too early. During the opening phase, one generally lets the patient go wherever the patient wants to go. The interview, at this stage, is highly unstructured. This facilitation period allows one to increase engagement, while letting the clinician assess the various areas of PACE, as mentioned earlier.
4. Focusing too bluntly before trying more subtle approaches. It is best to begin with subtle focusing techniques, increasing the firmness as needed in a graduated fashion.

Transforming Rehearsed Interviews

Characteristics of Rehearsed Interviews

The third type of problematic interview commonly encountered in clinical practice is the "rehearsed interview." It frequently manifests when working with a person coping with a severe and persistent chronic mental illness who "knows the system all too well" or any circumstance in which the patient has been required to tell his or her story many times. In this situation, the patient can relate a story that may even bore the patient himself or herself because it has been told so often. The history seems pat and simple, and therein lies the problem.

Both the patient and the clinician can be lulled into a joint acceptance of half-truths. No person's life history or history of their presenting problems or illness is simple. To get at the appropriate facts, both the patient and the clinician need motivation and involvement. Without these features, the validity and thoroughness of the database may be jeopardized.

A rehearsed interview does not always arise from indifference. Quite the opposite, rehearsed interviews not infrequently grow from a patient's attempt to control the interview. This process may rear its head with patients who are not upfront about their agendas, as seen with malingering, drug seeking, or perhaps during a disability interview for a feigned mental illness. It can also manifest when a patient wants to avoid a given topic, as with a patient trying to hide his or her alcohol dependence from the clinician by focusing on a spouse's personality "issues" instead.

To transform a rehearsed interview, one must first recognize it (see Table 3.2). Such interviews frequently announce themselves with early diagnostic statements by the patient (as with, "I'm a schizophrenic") and/or a quick and unsolicited review of the history of the present illness by the patient (a veteran who rambles off the symptoms of post-traumatic stress disorder as if reading them from the DSM-5). When patients are reeling off lists of malingered symptoms, their monologues frequently result in quite long DOUs and short RTLs. Eye contact varies depending upon the situation. It is generally good, but if the patient is feeling guilt or is uncomfortable with deceit, eye contact may be poor.

Whatever the root causes of a rehearsed interview, a clinician can inadvertently collude with the maladaptive process by focusing poorly or by providing an abundance of facilitating nonverbal activities as seen in the wandering interview. Unfortunately, unlike the process of transforming shut-down or wandering interviews, our knowledge of the DOC provides little advantage, for a rehearsed interview can be fed by the use of open-ended, variable, or closed-ended verbalizations. Any question or statement on the DOC that tracks with the patient can reinforce the direction of the interview.

The following brief vignette conveys a feeling for such an interview:

Clin.: Tell me what brings you here today?

Pt.: Well, I got out of St. Joseph's hospital 2 months ago. After I got out, I moved to a new catchment area, so I need new doctors. I've been feeling a little edgy and need to be on lithium. You see I'm bipolar.

Clin.: I see.

Pt.: Now, I'm not having racing thoughts or problems sleeping, and my energy is just fine. You'll probably be hearing from my sister and don't listen to a word she says. She over-reacts and she doesn't understand this disease. Other than my edginess everything is fine. I'm sleeping just great, no speeded up speech, none of that manic stuff. Oh yeah, don't worry, I'm not spending too much money and I'm not over-sexed or any of that stuff.

The problem here is the validity of this data. All angles are being covered so quickly that one can feel hedged in by the patient's story, almost as if one should not ask any more questions. To break this mechanical storytelling, a variety of methods can be used.

Breaking Through a Rehearsed Interview

One of the methods of transforming a rehearsed interview consists of disrupting the flow of the patient's scripted story by asking for behaviorally specific facts. This type of behavioral questioning serves the dual purpose of forcing the patient to reflect, while also helping the clinician to gain a more effective database.

A second method consists of interrupting the twice-told tale by getting the patient to discuss areas that require new conceptualizations by the patient or bring the patient face to face with affectively charged topics that, at some level, he or she wants to talk about

– a strategy I like to call "affective interjection." These affectively charged topics can lure the patient away from the rehearsed storyline.

For instance, let's return to the above interview. This time we will see the interviewer deftly break the flow of the rehearsed interview by using affective interjection to move the patient into new territory, thus dismantling the patient's attempt to minimize any manic symptoms:

Clin.: Tell me what brings you here today?

Pt.: Well, I got out of St. Joseph's hospital 2 months ago. After I got out, I moved to a new catchment area, so I need new doctors. I've been feeling a little edgy and need to be on lithium. You see I'm bipolar.

Clin.: I see.

Pt.: Now, I'm not having racing thoughts or problems sleeping, and my energy is just fine. You'll probably be hearing from my sister and don't listen to a word she says. She over-reacts and she doesn't understand this disease. Other than my edginess everything is fine. I'm sleeping just great, no speeded up speech, none of that manic stuff. Oh yeah, don't worry, I'm not spending too much money and I'm not over-sexed or any of that stuff.

Clin.: You mentioned your sister several times, tell me a little bit about her.

Pt.: She's sort of a jerk and I'll tell you one thing, I want her to keep her nose out of my affairs.

Clin.: What has she been doing recently that has been so upsetting?

Pt.: She's been mouthing off, getting me in trouble.

Clin.: What sort of ways?

Pt.: She got me into the hospital a month ago, when I didn't want to go. I didn't need to be in there, but she called the cops and the next thing I know, I'm committed. She claims I'm a danger to her children. I would say the greatest danger to her children is their mother.

In this instance, the patient has been led away from his rehearsed story through the gate of affect. With this side trip, important information that may not have been intended for clinician ears has surfaced, namely that the patient was recently committed involuntarily. Perhaps things are not as cut and dried as the patient wanted the clinician to believe.

It is hoped that the above information explains why a large amount of time has been devoted to the opening phase, during which the clinician explores the elements of the acronym PACE. Its importance would be hard to exaggerate, because in it the first hints of understanding are born in the clinician, the alliance with the patient is solidified, and numerous steps will have been taken to set a platform for a productive first encounter and a flowing communication. The clinician is now prepared to enter the patient's world more fully.

If both the introduction and the opening phases have been done effectively, the clinician will generally be asked to enter the patient's world as an invited guest, and there will be no need for a "break in." The question now becomes an issue of finding the most effective method to gather the necessary clinical information efficiently while further enhancing the therapeutic alliance.

BODY OF THE INTERVIEW: PHASE 3

The Gathering of the Database

In this section we will carefully delineate the challenges that we will encounter in this phase of the interview (the nuances of gathering a large database in a sensitive fashion and in a short time period). But we will not yet address the solutions to these challenges, for the interviewing strategies and techniques that provide these solutions are of such critical importance that we will devote the entire next chapter to their study. Our immediate task in this chapter is to better understand both the magnitude of the task and why it tends to create more than its fair share of anxiety in clinicians.

We opened this chapter with the words of Marcus Aurelius, who invited us to accept the simple fact that all is change in the universe, even in a universe as circumscribed as an interviewing dyad. In the first two phases of the interview, the introduction and opening, we saw that, indeed, these phases are less "structures" than they are "constantly changing processes." We have learned a variety of practical strategies and techniques that allow us to intentionally shape these processes to ensure the interview is off to a powerfully reassuring start for the patient. In the body of the interview, we will see that change and flexibility are even more dramatic in nature and that, correspondingly, the skills required to intentionally sculpt these dynamic processes are even more critical.

Let us look at another quotation that will provide us with a guiding principle for understanding the challenges facing us, this one from the T'ai Chi Master Al Chung-liang Huang:

> *Insecurity and uncertainty are everywhere. If you don't let it become part of your flow, you will always be resisting and fighting. If the ground here suddenly shakes and trembles, can you give with it and still maintain your center? … If you can become fluid and open even when you are standing still, then this fluidness and openness makes you able to respond to changes.*[27]

Of course Huang is addressing the insecurity and anxieties encountered in martial art combat and, by extension, into navigating life's everyday hurdles. I have noticed over several decades of training interviewers that such psychological tensions also often arise when exploring the body of the interview. Why is there so much insecurity and uncertainty encountered in this phase of the interview, especially for clinicians in their first several years of training? The answer is simple: *Because it is like nothing they have ever done before in their lives.*

Let me explain. Those of us who have chosen to become mental health professionals, almost by definition, come to the field because we like people and we have generally enjoyed talking and listening to people throughout our lives. Indeed, we naturally come to the field somewhat gifted in listening skills and empathy, or we probably wouldn't be coming to the field in the first place. Thus, the skills we discussed in our first two chapters and were subsequently applied in the introduction and opening phases – empathy and collaborative listening – are not new to us. We use them every time we talk with a friend or a family member. As we saw in these chapters, we can certainly hone these skills and take them to whole new levels of sophistication and competence, but we have already had years of utilizing them in our daily lives.

In contrast, it would be a rare day indeed, when listening to a friend over a steaming café latte in a local café, that we would enter the conversation with an intentional goal of covering, literally, hundreds of pre-determined data points. Moreover, it would be very odd if we entered this conversation having decided in a pre-ordained fashion that this massive database would need to be culled in under the time it would take to finish, let us say, two café lattes apiece. Furthermore, it would be strange indeed if we had decided that we would deliberately "rein our friend in" to topics we deemed to be appropriate if Tommy happened to be a bit too loquacious on this particular evening. Such encounters are the stuff of Monty Python skits. In real life, they would result in a painfully long evening as well as a painfully short list of friends.

The ability to sensitively and intentionally structure a conversation in order to cover a massive pre-determined database is simply not a skill set we bring to our psychiatric residencies and graduate programs from our everyday experiences. Yet this is the exact skill set required to effectively continue the healing process in the body of the interview. And it is complicated. I truly believe it is as complicated as performing surgery, for it is one thing to be empathic when allowing a patient to wander aimlessly. It is entirely a different matter to communicate empathy while gathering the large factual background that one needs in order to most effectively help a patient in pain, as we will be asked to do routinely in a busy community mental health center, hectic private practice, or psychiatric inpatient unit. People are complicated and there is an enormous amount of invaluable information that we can use to collaboratively create the most effective treatment plan for each unique individual from a person-centered perspective.

Just how complex is the task? Let's look at what information we need to gather during the body of the interview in a standard initial intake, as it would be done in a typical community mental health center or inpatient unit. In roughly a 30- to 40-minute time frame (the time available for the body of the interview in a 50-minute intake) the clinician will try to sensitively uncover the following databases:

1. *History of the presenting problem and primary DSM-5 diagnosis:* This database will begin in the opening but will be refined in the body of the interview and there are frequently multiple presenting situational problems and diagnoses.
2. *Interviewee's perspective:* Most of this will be uncovered in the opening, but nuances will usually appear in the body as well.
3. *Screening for other DSM-5 diagnoses:* This includes screening for mood disorders, anxiety disorders, schizophrenia spectrum disorders, eating disorders, substance abuse disorders, personality disorder, etc.
4. *Social history:* This includes educational history, employment history, current living circumstances, and sensitive areas such as incest and domestic violence.
5. *Framework for meaning and spirituality:* This needs to be explored in a fashion that is sensitive to issues of cultural diversity.

6. *Family history.*
7. *Uncovering of suicidal/homicidal ideation, planning, behaviors, and intent.*
8. *Past psychiatric history and treatment.*
9. *Developmental and psychogenetic history.*
10. *Medical history.*
11. *Informal mental status.*
12. *Formal cognitive mental status examination (sometimes optional):* This region is reserved for the more specialized cognitive mental status, in which a clinician examines orientation, attention span, memory functions, and general intellect.

Hmm. This doesn't look easy to do in 30 to 40 minutes. It isn't.

From the above, it is obvious that before we can address the strategies for accomplishing this difficult task in the next chapter, we must first acknowledge that one of the major challenges confronting the intake clinician is that daunting volumes of data often need to be gathered in short periods of time. Stated differently, good clinicians do not merely empathically listen, they actively explore. Patients do not necessarily know which information is relevant for their treatment planning. It is the clinician who must provide the gentle structuring and guidance that will establish a valid foundation for action. Gifted clinicians have the knack for exploring this vast database in such a fashion that patients come away feeling that they have been participating in an engaging conversation with a caring human (which indeed they have) rather than having been interviewed by "some shrink with a clipboard."

The apparent "magic" with which a skilled interviewer accomplishes this task is not really magic. It is a skill. It is a skill based on the knowledge of which questions to ask and when to ask them during the body of the interview, *and a quiet acceptance that one cannot gain all the pertinent information in a single interview.* This craft emerges, as it did with the introduction and opening phases, directly from a study of the dynamic interactions creating the informational flow of the interview.

Conveying Expertise, the Generation of Hope, and the Return Visit

Thus far we have focused upon the immense importance of data gathering in the body of the interview, for it is the resulting information that allows us to develop an effective treatment plan that suits the unique needs of the patient. But something else is happening, something special, in the body of the interview. As an interviewer skillfully weaves together the disparate threads of the patient's story, a second visit is being secured.

As stated in our first chapter, it can be argued that the single most important goal of the initial interview is the securing of a second interview (a return visit). No matter how good the clinical formulation and treatment plan of an initial interview may be, we cannot help a patient who does not return for a second interview. Interestingly, as the body of the interview winds down, it has been my experience that many, if not most, patients have already decided whether or not they are returning.

Let us see why. Naturally, much of the patient's interest in returning has to do with the continued use of our cornerstone engagement skills (such as strategic empathy and genuineness) during the body of the interview. But these engagement skills are far from the whole story, for patients don't come back to see a therapist solely because they feel the therapist is a compassionate and caring person (they may have friends that amply provide them with both of these traits). They come back because they think we can help them. They come back because we have convinced them that we have an expertise that their friends do not have. It is our expertise coupled with our caring that creates the all-important sensation of hope. It is hope that leads to a return visit.

How is expertise communicated? As discussed in Chapter 2, one of the strongest communicators of expertise is the power of our fact-finding questions, for they communicate that we have been there, done that; that we have seen this problem before and we are comfortable helping people with it. Thus, the questions we ask during the body of the interview not only uncover invaluable information, but they also metacommunicate to patients that they are in the presence of someone "who knows what they are doing." It does not matter whether we are a shaman or a therapist, the key to healing is inherently entwined with our ability to create hope through the patient's perception that we possess expertise. A shaman may use the casting of magical stones to communicate their secret knowledge; we do so by the fashion in which we cast our questions.

Fortunately, this magic can be taught, and we will see exactly how to gracefully, and easily, accomplish this task in our next chapter. It is there that we will further develop the fluidness and openness that our T'ai Chi Master Huang described as being critical for success. But before we can do so effectively, it is valuable to view the body of the interview within the context of the entire interview process, for, if handled well, it will gracefully telescope into the closing and termination phases, which also require skilled handling.

CLOSING OF THE INTERVIEW: PHASE 4

As the interview steadily moves towards its closure, certain tensions may arise in the interviewee. From the patient's perspective, the question becomes one of "What have we accomplished here?" or "Was this worth my time and/or money?" A variety of questions may be arising in the patient's mind, either consciously or unconsciously. Not every patient will have all of these concerns, but many patients will be seeking answers to a significant number of them. These include:

1. What is wrong with me?
2. Am I crazy?
3. Did I tell the interviewer what he or she needed to know?
4. Does this interviewer understand my problems?
5. Did this interviewer like me as a person?
6. Do I have a diagnosis?
7. Will I get better?

8. Can I be helped?
9. What are my treatment options?
10. What will happen to me next, and will I see this clinician again?

All of these questions are appropriate and natural. Indeed, the patient, in a sense, has a right to a discussion of these issues with the clinician. The clinician will possess only tentative answers to many of them, and the patient should be made aware of this fact. But even tentative answers may provide a powerfully reassuring experience for the patient. If answered sensitively, the clinician can help decrease the patient's fear of the unknown, including the plaguing question of "What's happening to me?"

Addressing this point, Sullivan has stated that a patient should gain something from the assessment process itself.[28] He emphasizes that patients frequently gain a considerable sense of relief merely by exploring their problems in an orderly fashion with a concerned listener. An orderly inquiry frequently begets a more orderly and calming perspective.

One of the main tasks in the closing is to consolidate the positive feelings and stirrings of hope that have been generated in the first three phases of the interview, while helping the patient to come away with tentative answers to some of the disturbing questions raised above. The types of experiences that, as Sullivan would suggest, a patient can "take away" from an initial intake can be summarized as follows:

a. The patient feels better after the interview.
b. The patient feels comfortable with the interviewer.
c. The patient feels that the interviewer also feels comfortable with the interaction.
d. The patient trusts the clinician.
e. The patient feels that the clinician appears balanced and calm.
f. The patient feels that the clinician appears to be down to earth and accessible.
g. The patient feels that the clinician may be able to help in the future (expertise has been conveyed).

To a significant extent, the presence of such favorable feelings reflects that the interview has achieved one of its greatest goals – the generation of hope. This generation of hope will, at least partially, be determined by the manner in which the clinician has handled the introduction, the opening, and, especially, the body of the interview, as we have already discussed. But it remains the closing phase in which many of these positive feelings can be significantly consolidated and enhanced. Moreover, if the closing is handled poorly, then these positive feelings can be rapidly destroyed.

One of the major methods of enhancing these favorable feelings consists of taking the time to carefully address the questions mentioned earlier. The very fact that the clinician addresses these issues may convey that the clinician can be trusted and seems to understand the patient's needs. Indeed, the clinician's actions represent a direct acknowledgement of the patient's needs at that moment.

One could discuss the issues concerning the closing phase in great detail, but I think it may be of more value to look at a closing phase as it unfolds. This dialogue will represent only one approach to the closing, but it illustrates many of the principles discussed earlier.

In the following illustration, the clinician has been interviewing a middle-aged woman at a local mental health center. The clinician is functioning as an assessment clinician and has decided that the patient is most likely suffering from a major depression. We will pick up the dialogue near the end of the body of the interview. In order to highlight the various aspects of this interview phase, the entire closing phase is included.

Pt.: I don't think any other members of my family ... let me see ... no, I don't think anyone else besides my sister and my uncle have been depressed like this. My mother certainly never went through anything like this, perhaps that's why she doesn't seem to understand.

Clin.: Well, it doesn't seem like too many people in your family have been depressed, but at least two people have. We've covered a lot of ground so far. At this point, we are coming to the close of our interview today. I'd like to spend some time summarizing what we've talked about and discussing some ways of possibly helping you to help yourself. But first, you mentioned that your mother doesn't seem to understand. I'm wondering how you put together what is happening to you?

Pt.: Hmmm ... it all seems so complicated. I think I may have reached a time of life when my bad qualities are catching up with me. Certainly I'm becoming a burden for my husband and I'm not really doing my share.

Clin.: What are some of the reasons that you think it's happening now?

Pt.: Maybe because I deserve it, I don't know. Or maybe because the kids are starting to leave the nest, as they say.

Clin.: Do you think there is anything you might want to add as we close that we haven't covered, that might help us to understand what is going on?

Pt.: No, not really, we've covered an awful lot ... well, one thing though, I didn't mention this because it was so long ago, but in college I had one semester in which I did very poorly in school. Now that I think about it, maybe I was suffering from the same type of thing.

Clin.: What were you feeling back then that makes you feel these experiences were similar?

Pt.: Many of the same things. I couldn't sleep well and I was constantly worried, I was so worried about flunking out I almost did.

Clin.: Did you seek help back then?

Pt.: Are you kidding! My parents didn't think anything was wrong except I was lazy. It never even crossed my mind to get help.

Clin.: Fortunately, you've come for help today and I'm wondering what kinds of ways you thought we might be able to help you?

Pt.: I'm not really certain. Maybe I thought you might have some magic pill that would take all this away (patient smiles and begins a subdued chuckle). I'll tell you one thing though, it was hard to come here.

Clin.: I'll bet it was ... tell me a little about what it was like actually coming here today.

Pt.: Oh, I felt very self-conscious walking in off the street. In fact, I looked around first to see if anybody I knew was around. When the coast was clear, I shot in like a dive-bomber … While I was waiting to see you, I felt very awkward. I didn't know what I was getting into. I almost left.

Clin.: What made you stay?

Pt.: I think I realized I needed help of some sort. I really am at a loss. What do you actually think is happening?

Clin.: First, let me reassure you, most everyone who comes for a first appointment feels much as you have. That's totally normal. It's difficult to share with a stranger. You've done an excellent job of helping me to get a good picture of what you've been experiencing. From what you said I have some ideas of what might be going on. I agree with you that you seem to be dealing with a lot of stresses within your home, including a changing relationship with your children as they leave and a fair amount of tension with your husband.

Pt.: Yes, I really didn't emphasize the problems with Jack but they are there and have been for years. It's not just the kids.

Clin.: I think these issues will be very important for you to try to understand better, so that you can cope with them more effectively. They are complicated. And sometimes some of the pains we feel from the past, like your leaving home at an early age, may also be contributing to the present. Because of this, I think it would benefit you to talk with one of our therapists, perhaps on a weekly basis for a while, to try to sort things out. In addition, I think there is more to the picture as well. You described a variety of symptoms such as an inability to sleep, a loss of energy, decreased enthusiasm, and a loss of sexual drive. All these symptoms suggest that you may be suffering from a depression that has some biological component to it.

Pt.: How do you mean?

Clin.: Over the past 40 or so years, we have made tremendous advances in understanding various forms of depression. It used to be thought that depression was only caused by psychological problems, but now we have discovered that some forms of depression are caused, or in some instances made worse, by chemical imbalances in the brain. No one thinks about how incredibly complicated the brain is. When one realizes how incredibly complicated the brain is, with over one hundred billion brain cells, it is no wonder that sometimes chemical imbalances arise. In any case, the symptoms you have so nicely described today are commonly seen in these forms of depression. Another item pointing that way is the fact that two members of your family seem to have also suffered from a very similar depression, and we have found that the biological forms of depression are frequently seen among family members.

Pt.: What does all this mean?

Clin.: Well, some of these depressive symptoms, perhaps caused, or at least made worse, by your biology, may make it more difficult for you to effectively work on your psychological concerns and interpersonal stresses. They may even be making it harder to cope with your daily chores. Fortunately, we have found a variety of medications that frequently help to get rid of these depressive symptoms. There are no magic pills though, nor are there promises for success, but these antidepressant medications can be very effective with some people. Because your symptoms do suggest that you may also have a biological depression, I'm going to make a referral to our Mood Disorders Clinic. If you are interested in going there, you'll find the therapists are very skilled in both talking therapies and medications. After they get to know you better, they will let you know exactly which psychotherapies, or perhaps medications as well, may help you the most. I am convinced that psychotherapy would be helpful and I think there is a good chance that a medication may help too. Oftentimes we try psychotherapy first and if that doesn't provide enough relief, we add an antidepressant. (pause) I've given you a lot of information, I'm wondering if this is making any sense?

Pt.:   Yes, yeah, I think so at least.

Clin.:   Try to tell me in your own words what I've been explaining to make sure that I'm being clear.

Pt.:   Let me see, you think that I need to talk with somebody about what is going on with my husband and also with my kids taking off for school. You also think there may be something wrong with the chemistry in my brain and that may also be making me feel depressed. And you think some medications may help.

Clin.:   That's right. This means that there may be more than one way to help you feel better. Do you think you'd be interested in seeing our therapist, I think it could really help.

Pt.:   Yes, I think I would like to give it a try, at least. I've read about depression being caused by chemical problems too, I just really never recognized myself as being depressed. And I know I need to talk some of this stuff out, I really do.

Clin.:   I really think you will benefit from therapy, and medications may help too. Depression is complicated. Sometimes depression is hard to recognize. Perhaps back in college your parents didn't recognize it in you, just as you didn't recognize it yourself today.

Pt.:   I never thought of it that way, but I guess it's actually possible.

Clin.:   In any case, as we wrap up here, I'm wondering what this interview has been like for you, was it what you were expecting?

Pt.:   For the most part, yes. I really didn't know exactly what to expect. I really felt we covered a lot of important ground. It seemed very thorough.

Clin.:   Is there anything I could have done differently that might have made you feel more comfortable?

Pt.:   No, no … I felt, I feel very comfortable with you. I do think you could use more magazines out in the lobby though. It really gets uncomfortable sitting out there.

Clin.:   Hmmm … that might be a good idea.

Pt.:   Will I be working with you again at all?

Clin.:   No, as I mentioned earlier, I only work over here in the Assessment Clinic, but I think you'll find the therapists in the Mood Disorders Clinic very knowledgeable and also very nice. Like myself, they will try to gain a broad knowledge of how things have been going for you over the years, in an effort to understand you better.

Pt.:   Good, do I call them or what?

Clin.:   I'll give you a card here (hands card to patient). This has their number on it, and you can call later today for an appointment. This card also has our number on it, if there are any other unexpected problems before your appointment. I think you made a very good decision coming here today. I think they'll be able to help you to help yourself.

Pt.:   Well, thank you. I actually feel a little better.

Clin.:   Good, I have a feeling things are going to go well for you, and I really enjoyed getting to talk with you today. Give us a call if there's a problem.

Pt.:   Thank you very much, I enjoyed talking with you too. (patient exits)

This is a nice example of a straightforward closing phase. The first thing to note is that the closing phase takes time. To have this time available, the clinician must leave appropriate time for the closing to occur. One of the most frequent problems I see in supervision remains the over-extension of the main body of the interview, thus forcing the clinician to rush through the closing phase.

A rushed closing can leave the patient feeling disjointed and uncertain as to what just happened. To the contrary, during this phase, where engagement looms so critical for securing a return visit or following up on our recommendations for referral, the clinician should appear unhurried, concerned, and calm. There is a give-and-take element to the closing phase. The clinician is truly interested in the patient's opinions, and this respect helps the patient to feel a sense of trust and control.

If one looks through this dialogue, most of the questions listed earlier as being pertinent to the closing phase were addressed. The clinician added a nice touch by asking for comments about her own performance. I frequently ask this type of question for several reasons. Sometimes patients provide very good constructive criticism. Second, the metacommunication of the clinician to the patient is reassuring, for the clinician is stating, "I care about how I come across to you and am aware that I sometimes make mistakes and can improve as well." This type of metacommunication can help the patient to feel that he or she will be listened to and not just ordered about.

Before leaving the topic of the closing phase, two areas that are optional components of the closing phase are worthy of note. The first area is of concern for psychiatrists, nurse clinicians, and other potential prescribers who are frequently expected to recommend a medication, if appropriate, at the end of the first session. Introducing a medication is a fine art and it requires time, probably at least 5 to 7 minutes. Not infrequently, in order to do it well, it will take longer. Consequently, the clinician must cut back on the body of the interview by an appropriate amount of time or simply run overtime. I have certainly done both. Sometimes one has the option of introducing the medication at the next session, which can provide a more leisurely approach that also may prove to be more effective.

In any case, it is critical that the discussion of the possible use of medications be done in a sensitive and engaging fashion, optimizing the patient's knowledge, comfort, and interest in the medication. It is unlikely that in the initial interview you will have time to address all of the following topics. But, from following list you can pick and choose several tips that will maximize your ability to collaboratively discuss the possible use of medications and, if applicable, to help the patient match the best medication to his or her unique needs:

a. Ask what his or her previous experiences with medications have been like.
b. Ask if he or she feels particularly sensitive to meds. If the patient states that this is a concern, it is important to listen and convey that this concerns you too. Often such a patient feels better if the physician, nurse clinician, or physician assistant subsequently starts off with a lower than normal dose. This is a powerful metacommunication that the clinician is listening to the patient carefully.
c. Ask if he or she has heard anything about the medication or knows someone who is taking it. If a close friend has had horrible experiences, this might not be the smart

medication to choose. Consider using an equivalent medication. If none are available, addressing the patient's fears directly may alleviate the patient's reluctance to take the med. Not eliciting this information is a way of almost guaranteeing that the med will soon be stopped.

d. Be very open about side effects, and explain common side effects clearly. Any more serious dangers regarding the med should be discussed in a calm and reassuring manner, which accurately reflects any risks.

e. Alert the patient that side effects sometimes occur before benefits, and that if the patient knows what the side effects are, he or she will not be frightened by them. This is one more reason why it is important to explain side effects in detail.

f. Emphasize to the patient that you need his or her help regarding side effects. Only the patient knows what he or she is feeling. Ensure that the patient knows that your goal is not to keep him or her on a medication but to help the patient to find a medication that he or she genuinely wants to be on because it helps.

g. Emphasize that you are the patient's consultant. Ultimately, the patient makes the final decision regarding whether to take a medication or not (this might not be the case in an involuntary commitment), and you are there to help by providing the best possible medical advice.

h. Carefully delineate the benefits of the medication and point out specific areas of relief that you are expecting to see.

i. Emphasize the effectiveness of the medication and describe successes you've had with it and how much better people felt when using it.

There are many other considerations in this area, bridging into the topic of ongoing efforts to increase patient understanding and interest in medications, which are beyond the scope of this chapter but will be highlighted in Chapter 23 on the medication interest model (MIM). However, the above principles provide a starting point.

The second area that sometimes becomes a component of the closing phase of the initial interview is asking permission to contact corroborative informants such as significant others and friends. This is one reason that the topic of confidentiality not infrequently re-emerges for discussion at this time of the interview. In most instances, I find that this is not a problem. If the patient does have concerns about contacting significant others, the wisest course is to explore these concerns in detail. By the way, sometimes the concerns are good ones, and the patient is correct that the person should not be contacted (e.g., the patient is stuck in an abusive relationship and the spouse/partner may be abusive if he or she hears about therapy). Many times the patient's main concerns deal with future confidentiality. Once reassurances are made on this point, most patients will feel comfortable with the contact.

If the patient still seems a little edgy, Morrison has a nice way of phrasing the reasons for contacting a corroborative source:

What you've told me is confidential, and I'll respect that confidence. You have that right. But you also have a right to the best help I can give. For that I need to know more about you. That's why I'd like to talk with your wife. Of course, she'll want to know what's wrong and what we plan to do about it. I think I should tell her, but I'll only tell what you and

I have already agreed upon. I won't tell her anything else we've discussed, unless you give me permission in advance.[29]

Such a reassuring approach often transforms the patient's apprehensions.

Naturally, each closing phase will be different, but the basic principles outlined above offer at least one practical approach. The reader may discover many others. The important thing remains the realization that the closing phase is different from other sections of the interview – its character being formed by the changing needs of the two co-participants.

TERMINATION OF THE INTERVIEW: PHASE 5

The termination phase consists of the actual closing words and gestures of the interviewer and interviewee. As with the introduction, the clinician frequently shakes hands and smiles appropriately. It is not uncommon, if the clinician is functioning as a triage agent and will not be seeing the patient again, to wish the patient good luck with a simple phrase such as, "I hope things go well for you."

The only problems that tend to arise here occur when the clinician feels, for some odd reason, the need to be overly formal and cool. Once again, such pseudo-professionalism runs the risk of creating alienation in the patient. Instead, a quiet warmness seems more appropriate, a warmness generated by two people who have worked together in an attempt to increase understanding.

I would like to add only that if the clinician will be seeing the patient again, perhaps as the patient's therapist, then increased attention to the actions of the patient at termination may be valuable. Indeed, termination functions as a mini-loss to the patient. In responding to such a loss phenomenon, the patient may betray behaviors suggesting dependent feelings and difficulties with separation. These behaviors may offer early clues to more far-reaching psychodynamic processes.

For instance, some patients may dawdle at the door, looking anxiously back at the clinician for one more sign of approval or acceptance. Other patients may suddenly become cooler, as if they resent the ending of their hour. Such a display may be an early sign of narcissistic entitlement or borderline rage. In any case, a sensitive clinician can gain some insight from even a small piece of patient behavior, ranging from a peculiarly soft knock on the door to an unusually rapid series of departing footsteps.

CONCLUSION

In this chapter we have looked at the ever-changing, dynamic structure of the interview with a sophisticated analytical approach. The use of these strategies and techniques may seem awkward at first, but with practice they become a natural and integral part of the clinician's style. A new and more penetrating intuition emerges from the balance, poise, and confidence that characterize an interviewer who understands, not only patients, but the interview process itself. Moreover, patients sense this internal balance and are powerfully attracted to it. As we pointed out in Chapter 1, talented interviewers are neither solely intuitive nor solely analytic. They are both.

With interviewing, one is reminded of a fictional art form described by the writer Herman Hesse in his novel *The Glass Bead Game*. This so-called game was, in reality, the most highly evolved of all art forms. In it, an artist attempts to synthesize two totally opposing views into a unified statement. The more graceful the metamorphosis, the more brilliant the artist. One cannot help but see the parallel between this fictional art form and the craft of clinical interviewing. In this context, the reward is not artistic adulation but increased understanding of the patient and a more powerful sense of caring.

I mention Hesse's game because the following excerpt, depicting the qualities sought for in a glass bead player, illustrates the very essence of a talented and flexible interviewer.

Remember this: One can be a strict logician or grammarian, and at the same time full of imagination and music. One can be a musician or Glass Bead Player and at the same time wholly devoted to rule and order. The kind of person we aim to produce, would at any time be able to exchange his discipline or art for any other. He would infuse the Glass Bead Game with crystalline logic, and grammar with creative imagination. That is how we ought to be. We should be so constituted that we can at any time be placed in a different position without offering resistance or losing our heads.[30]

And so it is with interviewing: flexibility and creativity are born from understanding and discipline.

REFERENCES

1. Schneider MS. *A beginner's guide to constructing the universe: the mathematical archetypes of nature and science.* New York, NY: HarperCollins Publishers; 1994. p. 288.
2. Storr A. *The art of psychotherapy.* New York, NY: Methuen; 1980. p. 9.
3. Sommers-Flanagan R, Sommers-Flanagan J. *Clinical interviewing.* 5th ed. New York, NY: John Wiley & Sons, Inc.; 2013. p. 180–2.
4. Lazare A. *Outpatient psychiatry diagnosis and treatment.* Baltimore, MD: Williams & Wilkins; 1979.
5. Morrison J. *The first interview: a guide for clinicians.* New York, NY: Guilford Press; 1993. p. 176.
6. Campbell AA. Two problems in the use of the open question. *J Abnorm Soc Psychol* 1945;**40**:340–3.
7. Converse JM. Strong arguments and weak evidence: the open/closed questioning controversy of the 1940s. *Public Opin Q* 1984;**48**:267–82.
8. Dohrenwend BS. Some effects of open and closed questions on respondents' answers. *Hum Organ* 1965;**24**:175–84.
9. Elliott R, Hill CE, Stiles WB, et al. Primary therapist response modes: comparison of six rating systems. *J Consult Clin Psychol* 1987;**55**(2):212–23.
10. Friedlander ML. Counseling discourse as a speech event: revision and extension of the Hill counselor verbal response category system. *J Couns Psychol* 1982;**29**:425–9.
11. Hill CE. Development of a counselor verbal response category system. *J Couns Psychol* 1978;**25**:461–8.
12. Lazarsfeld PF. The controversy over detailed interviews – an offer for negotiation. *Public Opin Q* 1944;**8**:38–60.
13. Marquis KH, Marshall J, Oskamp S. Testimony validity as a function of question form, atmosphere, and item difficulty. *J Appl Soc Psychol* 1972;**2**:167–86.
14. Metzner H, Mann F. A limited comparison, of two methods of data collection: the fixed alternative questionnaire and the open-ended interview. *Am Sociol Rev* 1952;**17**:486–91.
15. Naik RD. Responses to open and closed questions: an analysis. *Indian J Soc Work* 1984;**44**:347–351.
16. Rockers DM. *The effects of open and closed inquiry modes used by counselors and physicians in an initial interview on interviewee perceptions and self-disclosure.* Ph.D. dissertation, 1976.
17. Rugg D, Cantril H. The wording of questions. *J Abnorm Soc Psychol* 1942;**37**:469–95.

18. Schuman H. The random probe: a technique for evaluating the validity of closed questions. *Am Sociol Rev* 1966;**21**:218–22.
19. Schuman H, Presser S. The open and closed question. *Am Sociol Rev* 1979;44:692–712.
20. Singleman CK. Evaluating alternative techniques of questioning mentally retarded persons. *Am J Ment Defic* 1982;**86**:511–18.
21. Sigelman CK, Schoenrock CJ, Spanhel CL, et al. Surveying mentally retarded persons: responsiveness and response validity in three samples. *Am J Ment Defic* 1980;**84**:479–86.
22. Shea SC. *Psychiatric interviewing: the art of understanding.* 1st ed. Philadelphia, PA: W.B. Saunders; 1988. p. 77–9.
23. Shea SC. 1988. p. 80.
24. Shea SC. 1988. p. 80.
25. Shea SC. 1988. p. 80–1.
26. Benjamin A. *The helping interview.* 2nd ed. Boston, MA: Houghton Mifflin Company; 1974.
27. Chung-liang Huang A. *Embrace tiger, return to mountain – the essence of t'ai chi.* Moab, UT: Real People Press; 1973. p. 179.
28. Sullivan HS. *The psychiatric interview.* New York, NY: W.W. Norton; 1970. p. 219.
29. Morrison J. 1993. p. 166.
30. Hesse H. *The glass bead game.* New York, NY: Holt, Rinehart and Winston; 1970. p. 68.

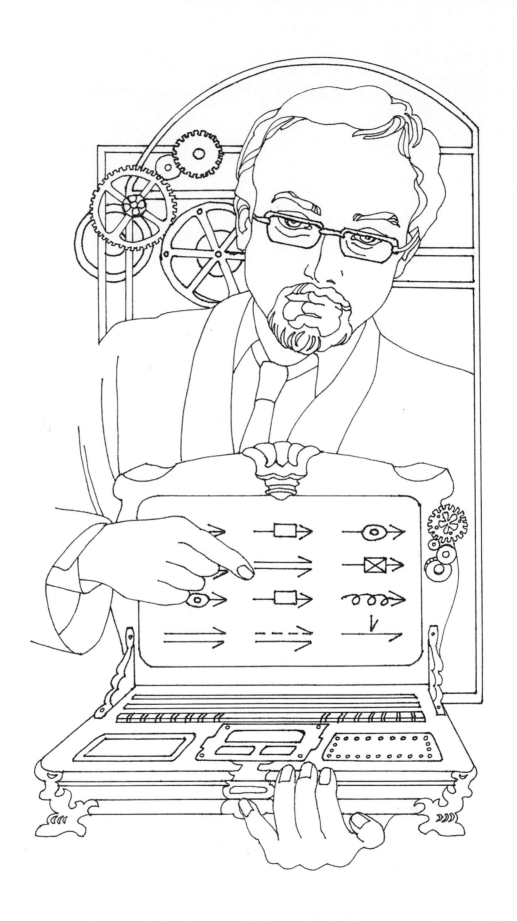

CHAPTER 4

Facilics: The Art of Transforming Interviews into Conversations

It was said that Wang Hsia's brush sometimes waves and sometimes sweeps. The color of his ink is sometimes light and sometimes dark. Following the splotches of the ink he shapes them into mountains, rocks, clouds, and water. His action is so swift as if it were from Heaven. Spontaneously, his hand responds and his mind follows. All at once clouds and mists are completed; wind and rain are painted. Yet, when one looks carefully, one cannot find any marks of demarcation in the ink.

Chung-yuan Chang, discussing Wang Hsia, Chinese master painter
Creativity and Taoism: A Study of Chinese Philosophy, Art & Poetry[1]

SENSITIVELY CREATING CONVERSATIONAL INTERVIEWS

Secrets from Everyday Conversation

We have studied the fashion in which interviews develop discrete phases, which for want of a better term we can call the *macro*structure of the interview. We have also studied what tasks are necessary for each phase, as well as a variety of specific interviewing strategies and techniques for achieving these tasks. What we haven't covered, though, is: How does one effectively, within each of these phases, actually weave together all of these specific tasks, strategies, and techniques?

Within each phase of an interview, every single sentence and question bears a relationship to the immediately preceding and subsequent statement or question. This complex, almost microscopic analysis of the weave of an interview represents a *micro*structure of the interview. Indeed, especially in the body of the interview, how an interviewer achieves the interlacing of this microstructure may very well determine whether the patient perceives the initial encounter as a cold example of "being interviewed" by some guy with a clipboard or a laptop, or as an engaging conversation with a warm and knowledgeable person who genuinely cares about the other person in the room.

In Chapter 1 we observed that an interview in which the engagement and blending is high seems to take on many of the characteristics of an everyday conversation. A natural flow emerges. The two participants appear to move with one another. Common hall-marks of a flowing conversation appear, such as humor and natural body posturing, as the two become "engaged" in conversation.

The engagement process, spontaneously developed during natural conversation, holds within itself some pertinent clues as to how we might create a similar naturalistic flow to a clinical interview itself. Consequently, we will begin our study of the microstructure of the clinical interview by examining the processes involved in an everyday conversation as it might unfold in a local café teeming with people, tablets, and smart phones. It is here, with the sounds of alternative rock and animated chatter bouncing off the walls, that we may stumble upon some unexpected secrets.

To begin with, if one observes two café habitués chatting over some coffee and cheese-cake, one will quickly notice – if one possesses a habit of eavesdropping – that their conversation is not simply a potpourri of unrelated statements. Quite to the contrary, such conversation usually possesses a gentle structure, determined, albeit unconsciously, by its participants. In general, one friend brings up a topic, which both friends animatedly expand. Often the second member of the conversation will ask questions in an effort to more thoroughly understand the first, while also showing an appropriate increase in interest.

Once the topic has been discussed, one of the friends will move the conversation to a new topic. This transition is often prompted by something that has already been dis-cussed. Frequently the new topic is triggered directly by a preceding statement. And so the conversation between the friends moves, swelling and ebbing, as more or less inter-esting topics arise. The basic structure of the conversation consists of succeeding topics connected by transitions.

A smoothly flowing interview possesses many of these same structural elements. One of the keys to generating a natural flow of speech during the body of the interview con-sists of learning to move gracefully from one topic to another while taking cues from the interviewee's statements. The interviewer is aware of which topics are most pertinent for the type of interview being undertaken (initial intake in a community mental health clinic, university counseling center, private practice office, inpatient unit, emergency room, telephone crisis center) and can gently guide the conversation to these topics. Once within a desired topic, the interviewer takes advantage of the natural conversational mode in order to fully expand that topic. When done well, the interviewer has structured the interview imperceptibly. The clinician establishes a powerful engagement with the interviewee while efficiently gathering a strategic database for collaborative treatment planning.

This ability to structure patients naturally while uncovering a dauntingly large data-base is one of the most, if not *the* most, difficult set of skills for clinicians to acquire. As mentioned in Chapter 3, part of the difficulty is the simple fact that the skills needed to sensitively gather a large database in a constricted time limit is simply not a skill set used in everyday life. It is a novel skill set that must be learned.

We have already seen how a carefully delineated supervision language, such as the DOC, can help a trainee to rapidly learn complex interviewing skill sets such as opening up a shut-down interview or effectively structuring a wandering interview. The question is, can we develop a supervision language that can effectively help a trainee to learn how to sensitively structure an initial interview? In addition, a clear and concise supervision language could provide a gateway for self-supervision for the remainder of a clinician's career, for once a clinician possesses a behaviorally concrete and unambiguous language for tagging interviewing patterns and techniques, each interview becomes a potential new learning experience.

In this regard, I certainly hope that I will be learning something new during my very last clinical interview. I am reminded of the wise words of the great internist Sir William Osler, "The hardest conviction to get into the mind of a beginner is that the education upon which he is engaged is not a college course, not a medical course, but a life course, for which the work of a few years is but a preparation."[2] Our goal is to create such a system for our ongoing self-development in the art of transforming interviews into healing conversations.

Of course, the reason that, historically, trainees had to "wing it" through the complexities of sensitively structuring the body of the interview was that a simplifying supervision language, as described above, did not exist for approaching this task until the first edition of this book. Supervision languages existed for talking about a variety of interviewing skills, such as recognizing defense mechanisms and the use of specific types of clinician responses (e.g., open-ended questions and empathic statements), but no language had been developed to understand and describe how interviewers structure and shape interviews as they gather data.

A Solution to the Dilemma

To address this dilemma, at Western Psychiatric Institute and Clinic at the University of Pittsburgh we developed a new field of study and an accompanying supervision language with which to train graduate students across disciplines including clinical psychology, counseling, social work, psychiatry, and psychiatric nursing.[3-5] The system was subsequently refined in the Dartmouth Interviewing Mentorship Program of the Psychiatry Department at the Dartmouth Hitchcock Medical Center, with a heavy emphasis upon direct coaching and the mentoring of trainees longitudinally.[6]

The resulting system, "facilics," is the study of how interviewers structure interviews while gathering data (e.g., what topics they choose to explore, including why and when, how they go about exploring those topics, and how they make transitions from topic to topic), including the manner in which they approach this task while managing tight time constraints. The term "facilics" is derived from the Latin root *facilis*, indicating grace in movement.

The practical application of facilics is composed of two activities: (1) learning how to mindfully be aware of how we are structuring the interview as it proceeds, a process that will form the foundation for our ability to intentionally and sensitively shape the data-gathering process and (2) learning how to apply specific facilic interviewing strategies and techniques that can facilitate the graceful procurement of a unique database. In the following pages, we will learn how to apply both of these activities in a simple and practical fashion. By the end of this chapter, the apparently daunting task of sensitively gathering a powerful database in a short amount of time will appear a good deal less daunting.

INTRODUCTION TO THE PRACTICAL APPLICATION OF FACILICS

Part I: Learning How to Tag the Flow of the Interview – What Topics, When?

Descriptions and Characteristics of Facilic Regions

In the body of the interview, one of the first problems facing the novice interviewer remains the issue of determining what information is important to gather in a full intake assessment. In this regard, the concept of a "region" is the first facilic concept that we need to examine.

A region is defined as any section of an interview, lasting at least several sentences, in which there exists either: (1) a unified attempt to gather data related to a specific topic or (2) a unified focus upon the process of interaction or upon a non-data-gathering task. In this sense, two general categories of regions exist, content regions and process regions.

Content Regions

As with an everyday conversation, an interview tends to revolve around discrete topics. A "content region" is any area of an interview in which the primary focus of the interviewer is the delineation of a specific database. As one would expect, during the exploration of content regions the interviewer continues to carefully attend to patient engagement.

As we saw in the last chapter, in an initial interview ten or more broad regions are often focused upon *in no set sequence*. In order to explore these regions effectively, one must become familiar with their intricacies. (Some broad regions are composed of smaller specific content regions. Thus the broad DSM-5 region of substance use disorders is actually composed of numerous smaller content regions such as cocaine use, opiate use, marijuana use, etc. And the broad content region of social history is composed of smaller content regions such as living conditions, employment history, domestic violence history, etc.) In later sections of this book we will look at methods for sensitively exploring these more specific content regions in detail. At present, it is only important to emphasize that most topics of discussion can be categorized within one of the following broad regions. In order to ensure a common, initial understanding of these critical content regions, let us review them in a little more detail than we did in Chapter 3:

1. *History of the presenting problem and/or stresses:* This region examines the presenting situational and psychological problems of the patient. Often this content region is spontaneously shared by the patient during the opening phase of the interview and is not part of the body of the interview.
2. *Interviewee's perspective:* Most of this material will also be uncovered in the opening, but nuances will usually appear in the body as well. It generally includes an attempt

to understand the interviewee's views on his or her problems/solutions and what type of help the interviewee is hoping to receive. It also touches upon the interviewee's fears, pains, and general expectations for the interview.

3. *History of the presenting illness (HPI):* The HPI delineates the chronological development of the patient's presenting primary DSM-5 psychiatric disorder (if one is present), exploring the types, characteristics, and severity of the patient's symptoms and their duration. This database will sometimes also spontaneously begin during the opening phase of the interview, but it will generally need to be continued and refined in the body of the interview.

4. *Comorbid DSM-5 diagnoses:* Many people have multiple diagnoses, some of which they may even initially try to hide because of stigma, guilt, and/or fear of consequences. Throughout the interview, the clinician will periodically pose various screening questions about common DSM-5 diagnoses. If the patient comments positively to the possible presence of a disorder, then the diagnostic criteria for that disorder will be sensitively explored, an exploration that will subsequently constitute a discrete content region. The uncovering of any of these disorders, if initially hidden, can be of immense importance to helping the patient. Missing comorbid psychiatric disorders can result in significant unnecessary pain or even suicide (for instance obsessive–compulsive disorder [OCD] and substance use disorders are frequently missed disorders, both of which have significant suicide attempt rates).

   Note that the process of intermittently asking single screening questions for the various DSM-5 diagnoses – timed to best fit the natural flow of the patient's conversation – is a clinical task known as the "psychiatric review of symptoms." The questions themselves are not asked in sequence in a specific area of dialogue but are gracefully integrated into the interview conversation. Thus the *individual questions* of the psychiatric review of symptoms do not constitute a facilic content region. But if the clinician follows up a screening question with an exploration of criteria for a specific DSM-5 diagnosis, that diagnostic exploration does, indeed, constitute a content region.

   Your routine diagnostic screening will include questions covering symptoms suggestive of mood disorders (such as major depressive disorder and bipolar disorder), anxiety disorders (such as panic disorder, OCD, generalized anxiety disorder, social phobia, and post-traumatic stress disorder), the schizophrenia spectrum disorders (such as schizophrenia and schizoaffective disorder), substance use disorders, eating disorders, personality disorders, and, as indicated, miscellaneous disorders such as developmental disorders, attention-deficit disorders, gambling and sexual dysfunction.

5. *Social history:* Broadly speaking, the social history includes both interpersonal and environmental information. With regard to interpersonal history, one is interested in interaction with family, friends, employers, and even strangers, both in the past and present. Concerning environmental history, a clinician is interested in factors such as living conditions, neighborhood, economic status, and availability of food and shelter. This region often includes current and past stressors. It is also the area in which ultra-sensitive topics such as incest and domestic violence are often explored.

One may also uncover evidence that the patient is facing cultural biases and/or bigotry related to any number of characteristics including race, ethnic group, religion, sexual orientation, gender identification, presence of a mental illness/physical disability, body habitus, etc. (see Chapter 20 on culturally adaptive interviewing).

6. *Framework for meaning and spirituality:* The patient's unique worldview will be explored in this region, with a keen sensitivity to issues of cultural diversity and spirituality (aspects of this topic will be explored as they arise spontaneously in other content regions as well throughout the interview).

7. *Family history:* This region includes an exploration of psychiatric illnesses in the patient's blood-related family. It commonly includes a survey of entities such as schizophrenia, mood disorders, anxiety disorders, suicide, excessive alcohol or drug use, developmental delays, and seizure disorders.

8. *Uncovering of suicidal/homicidal ideation, planning, behavior, and intent:* This lethality region requires a careful and sensitive expansion by the interviewer and should never be omitted. It will be documented as part of the mental status, although it is actually always woven gracefully into the flow of the interview itself.

9. *Past psychiatric history and treatment:* This region explores previous mental health problems, as well as previous interventions, such as forms of treatment (e.g., psychotherapy, counseling, medication, hospitalizations).

10. *Developmental and psychogenetic history:* This region traces the development of the individual from birth onwards, and it can selectively include a variety of topics (depending upon the proclivities of the clinician and time constraints) such as birth trauma, developmental milestones, toilet training, schooling, and early relationships as viewed through frameworks such as psychodynamic and/or cognitive perspectives. If time constraints do not allow an exploration of this region in the initial interview, clinicians often opt to explore this region in subsequent sessions.

11. *Medical history:* This region includes past and present illnesses as well as a medical review of systems. Current medications and allergies are delineated here. In addition, current physicians, nurse clinicians, physician assistants, and other health care providers/alternative healers are also elicited in this region.

12. *Cognitive mental status:* This region is reserved for a specialized cognitive mental status, in which a clinician examines processes such as orientation, attention span, memory functions, reasoning, and general intellect. It forms a discrete facilic region that is easily identifiable during an interview. It is not always performed in an initial interview in a formal fashion, but it becomes a major point of focus when the clinician is suspicious that the patient is suffering from a delirium, dementia, or other impairment of cognitive and intellectual functioning such as might occur in schizophrenia or adult attention-deficit disorder (see Chapter 16 where a thorough cognitive examination is illustrated in Video Module 16.2).

This brief survey illustrates that, despite the immensity of an initial database, the contents tend to fall into relatively discrete regions. Some of these regions may overlap. In general, however, a given section of an interview tends to focus on a single region, much as a conversation tends to focus on a single topic at a time.

It is also important to openly acknowledge that this database appears to be intimidating in size. Truth be told, it is. It is important to remember that it is rarely possible – perhaps not possible – to cover all of this information in a single initial interview. I'm not sure I have ever done so in 30 years of practice! Nevertheless, it is all valuable information that can, indeed, help the patient when utilized during treatment planning and triage. The art becomes one of learning how to maximize the amount of useful information that can be elicited during the body of the interview while always powerfully and gracefully engaging the patient in a conversational fashion.

With each patient, this solution is a unique one. Clinicians must learn how to prioritize information effectively as the interview proceeds. Facilics provides us with the interviewing approaches and strategies to do so successfully. When a well-trained clinician applies facilic principles, it is rather amazing how much useful information can be sensitively gathered in a mere 50 minutes. It is the patient who benefits greatly from the clinician's application of this hard-won skill set.

For the purpose of illustrating a content region, in the following excerpt, the general region concerning drug and alcohol use is readily apparent:

> **Clin.:** … So right now, have you been drinking at all?
>
> **Pt.:** No.
>
> **Clin.:** You talked about using drugs in the past. I'm wondering what kinds of things you used then and now.
>
> **Pt.:** Right now I'm only using pot. I don't mess around with anything else.
>
> **Clin.:** Are you using it every day?
>
> **Pt.:** Almost every day.
>
> **Clin.:** How many joints might you have in a day?
>
> **Pt.:** Maybe split two; me and Jack might split two.
>
> **Clin.:** Uh-huh.
>
> **Pt.:** Because it really does calm me down. It doesn't make you sick like alcohol can make you sick, or give you a bad head the next day. It just relaxes you. And now that it's legal here, why not take advantage of it.
>
> **Clin.:** Any type of pills you're taking now?
>
> **Pt.:** No.
>
> **Clin.:** Nothing but the marijuana? (patient indicates with a head nod that nothing else is being used currently) What kinds of drugs were you using in the past?
>
> **Pt.:** Well, I never got into any one drug real heavy.
>
> **Clin.:** Uh-huh.
>
> **Pt.:** But I have taken LSD, speed, different goofballs, and stuff … but I never injected any drugs like dope. And I stay away from any shit like K2. I like the real stuff not some crap some idiot made in a laboratory.

Process Regions

In a typical process region the interviewer is less interested in focusing on content and the gathering of a specific database than on the process of the interview itself – what is happening between the clinician and the patient or in the patient's head as the interview is proceeding. (Note that there are also *atypical* process regions, where once again the focus is not on data gathering *per se*, but on a specific interviewer task, such as providing psychoeducation or a specific therapeutic activity such as crisis intervention.) Let us take a look at the three most common "process" regions.

1. Free Facilitation Regions

This region remains one of the foundations of all interviewing. It is the traditional method of nondirective listening. In it, the interviewer invests effort in creating an atmosphere in which it is optimally conducive for the interviewee to feel safe enough to begin sharing problems. The interviewee is able to wander freely to whatever topics chosen while the interviewer maintains a nondirective attitude. The major interventions of the interviewer are usually facilitating head nods, uh-huhs, empathic statements (both low and high in valence), and simple facilitating statements.

These free facilitation regions can appear anywhere in an interview and are often a very useful method of enhancing engagement. As noted in Chapter 3, during the opening phase of the interview the clinician frequently utilizes a series of free facilitation regions. In actuality, the opening phase is a combination of spontaneously appearing content regions intermixed with free facilitation regions. Furthermore, a psychoanalytically focused therapy session may consist almost entirely of free facilitation regions strung together. Naturally, most *content* regions also place a premium upon engagement; but a free facilitation *process* region differs in the goal of its use, which remains the uncovering of information that the patient reveals spontaneously without direction from the interviewer. In content regions, the interviewer is consciously trying to explore a specific topic. In a free facilitation process region, the interviewer is consciously allowing the interviewee to wander wherever he or she wants to wander.

A brief example may help to clarify when a section of an interview can be labeled as a free facilitation region. Note that most of the interviewer's responses are merely facilitating statements, open-ended questions, or gentle commands:

Pt.:	My wife and I are really at odds.
Clin.:	How do you mean?
Pt.:	Oh, we see the world very differently. She is always money conscious and I tend to see the world as, as … (pauses) I don't know, more of a place to play.
Clin.:	Now that does sound like a bit of a difference (clinician gently smiles). How does this play out for you guys?
Pt.:	Badly (patient smiles). We fight all the time, over the silliest things. And let me tell you, these are nasty arguments, nothing physical or anything, but really hurtful. God, they get hurtful.
Clin:	In what sense?
Pt.:	I've called her things I shouldn't say, and that I didn't really mean. And so does she. And then we both miss the point of what life is all about; what's really important. Like we have enough food to eat, we are both healthy, and other important stuff … (pauses).
Clin.:	Go on.

> **Pt.:** Like our kids for God's sake. We have two really wonderful kids. They mean the world to me.
>
> **Clin.:** Tell me about them.
>
> **Pt.:** They are the best. They are so special. They … (patient proceeds to talk about his children in great detail)

A free facilitation region is generally used to improve engagement. It also often helps to lower the defenses of the interviewee so that his or her major concerns will surface. In some instances it can even be utilized to foster the uncovering of subtle psychotic process, for it tends to bring to the surface whatever is lying just below the surface, as will be described in Chapter 11.

2. Transformational Regions

In a transformational region, the interviewer actively attempts to decrease a specific roadblock to communication stemming from unconscious defense mechanisms or conscious feelings of anger or defensiveness in the patient. In previous editions of this book, these were referred to as "resistance regions," but the term "resistance" seems to miss the point that these regions of disagreement are invitations to transforming the relationship in a positive fashion, if handled well.

They are areas rich in information for understanding what makes the patient tick if approached as an area of collaborative discovery by the interviewer instead of an example of patient opposition. Such potential points of disengagement – whether they are expressed by overt patient anger or by aggressive questions asked of the interviewer by the patient – may arise from any number of factors including the interviewee's fears, expectations, or other ramifications of the self-system. Without a resolution of these concerns, the validity of subsequent data and the power of the therapeutic alliance may be greatly reduced. In any case, the defining characteristic remains that in a transformational region, the interviewer consciously is attempting to resolve a communication roadblock as opposed to gathering information as would be seen in a content region.

In the following dialogue, we see an interviewer deftly navigating a potential point of disengagement arising around the clinician's age, for he is 40 years younger than the patient. Clearly the interviewer is focusing upon addressing the patient's hesitancies, not upon gathering a specific database:

> **Pt.:** My boss was really into my work and thinks I may be a little … you know … I don't really think I ought to go on. Do you have a supervisor around?
>
> **Clin.:** You seem concerned about something …
>
> **Pt.:** Well, I'd just feel a little better if I were talking to someone a little older.
>
> **Clin.:** What are some of the ways in which you think an older clinician might be better able to do to help you than a younger clinician? (note the lack of defensiveness by the clinician)
>
> **Pt.:** He'd understand what I've gone through better, that's for damn sure. He'd have a lot more experiences like I have had, seen a lot more of life.
>
> **Clin.:** You know, Mr. Greyson, I wouldn't argue with that for a second. It's true I am younger than you, and, consequently, I haven't experienced the same things. It's an

undeniable fact and an important point that you make. I guess what I'm hoping to be able to do is to help us both gain an understanding, that is as clear as possible, of exactly what you're experiencing and what solutions might be available. My one advantage is that I've worked with many people your age, and they have taught me a lot about the clever ways they have found for dealing with some of the problems you are describing. In essence, they have shared their years of experience with me, just like you've been doing, and they have taught me a lot, just like you're doing. Maybe some of their experiences, not mine, are what might be useful to you. Does that make any sense?

Pt.: I guess so. (said a bit reluctantly, but softened in tone)

Clin.: I'm sort of hoping that you might give me a chance to share some of their ideas, and see how they match up with your own, because you're right, experience does count. I think we could be a good team that way – at least I hope so. (patient nods head in mild agreement) If, by the end of our session today, you still feel uncomfortable, we can talk about perhaps switching to an older clinician, that's not a problem at all. I hope you can give me a chance first though, because I have the feeling that together, we might be able to turn this thing around for you. Is that okay with you? To just see how the rest of the session goes?

Pt.: Yeah, I guess so. (said with a gentle agreement)

Clin.: You could help me by telling me a little more about how people have been pressuring you about your age.

Pt.: It all started with my wife. She left me about 3 years ago, and you guessed it, for a younger man …

Non-defensively navigating potential points of disengagement, such as the one above, is a complex task and not always easy to do. It is of such importance that we will devote an entire chapter to it later in the book (Chapter 19).

3. Psychodynamic Regions

In a psychodynamic region, the interviewer asks questions but is more interested in how and why the patient responds, as opposed to the content of what the patient says. In general, the clinician attempts to answer questions such as: How reflective is the patient? Does the patient have much insight? How does the patient respond to interpretive questions? How good is the patient's observing ego?

Answers to these questions may help determine the suitability of the patient for specific types of time-limited psychotherapy, as well as provide insight into the patient's intellectual development, ego strength, defense mechanisms, self-concept, or genuine readiness to engage in treatments such as substance abuse counseling. To answer questions in a psychodynamic region, the patient must reflect and offer an opinion.

The following excerpt may clarify when a psychodynamic region is occurring:

Pt.: My father always kept a stranglehold on me. He wanted to know my every move. God pity the boy who wanted to take me out. It was like a Gestapo interview for the guy.

Clin.: What kind of impact do you think your father's behavior has had on you?

Pt.: He's made me scared. I'm afraid of him, and who knows, maybe I keep my distance from him because of it … Sort of strange though, 'cause when I was

> a kid I always wanted to be around him. I even would wait for him when he was at work.

Clin.: Go on.

Pt.: Oh, it's sort of silly, but I wondered if he had a toy or something for me ... I remember a small doll he brought home once, with big black eyes. Just a little doll, but important to me.

Clin.: And?

Pt.: Not too much more to say, except that it's sort of sad the way things have turned out between us.

Clin.: What are you feeling as you talk about your father right now? (patient wells up with tears)

Here, content is clearly taking a second place to process. The interviewee's responses suggest a willingness and a certain degree of proficiency at self-exploration. This type of region can occur anywhere in an interview, often appearing frequently between content regions.

Thus far, three types of process regions have been illustrated: (1) the free facilitation region, (2) the transformational region, and (3) the psychodynamic region. As mentioned earlier, other types of process regions exist, including process regions focusing on interviewee ventilation of emotions, psychoeducation, crisis intervention, or phenomenological regions of questioning. These additional process regions often provide windows through which a better understanding of the patient gradually emerges.

Equipped with a facility to move freely among both content regions and process regions, the clinician possesses a powerful flexibility with which to approach any given interviewing task. It is not a matter of learning to interview only in a fairly structured fashion (emphasizing content) or learning to interview in a nondirective style (emphasizing process regions). One needs to master both styles, often delicately interweaving them into a conversational tapestry.

There does not exist a single "correct style" of interweaving these regions or of sequencing them. Instead, one finds styles of exploring such regions and creates unique sequences for each interview of ordering them that may be more or less useful for any given clinical situation or the needs or personality quirks of a specific patient. Too frequently, students learn only one approach, while building an unfounded bias that other styles of interviewing are inferior. No surer method of handicapping one's clinical flexibility can be found.

The Scouting Region: A Unique Combination of Content and Process

Although an understanding of facilics is particularly useful for helping us to navigate the body of the interview, the system allows us to understand the conversational flow of all five phases of the *macro*structure of the interview described in the last chapter. In this regard, the introduction and the opening phase of the interview are included in a unique facilic region called "the scouting region," which lasts roughly 7 minutes or so. We have already explored the importance, goals, and strategies of these two phases of the interview. Here, it is only necessary to emphasize the conversational flow of these two regions, which merge so wonderfully into an interpersonal dance of sorts. In this arabesque, the clinician introduces himself or herself while both parties "scout-out" who this stranger is and what are they about, hence the name of the region.

Both process and content are pivotal players in a well-executed scouting region. There is a premium on free facilitation regions here as the opening phase unfolds, for the patient is essentially allowed to wander wherever the patient wants to wander, through the use of many open-ended questions and gentle commands, with a few empathic statements sprinkled into the mixture. On the other hand, as much as the scouting region emphasizes the use of process, invariably much valuable content-oriented information will be forthcoming, with patients often spontaneously sharing critical aspects of their histories early in the interview. Thus, the scouting region (the combination of the introduction and the opening phases) is a unique type of facilic region: It is both a process region and a content region at once, with an emphasis on attending to the engagement process, while noting whatever pertinent data spontaneously arises.

Part II: Practical Tips for Applying Facilic Principles to the Exploration of Regions

Using Time Effectively

The Core Conundrum: Well-Timed Tracking Versus Poorly Timed Tracking

In the first place, many interviews are made or broken before a word is spoken, because the pre-interview planning frequently determines the success of the subsequent interaction. As discussed above, the clinician needs to ascertain what demands on information gathering are needed by the clinical situation. In an intake interview situation, as would be undertaken at a community mental health center, college counseling center, or psychiatric inpatient unit, most, if not all, of the content regions discussed earlier may need to be addressed, many of them thoroughly. In contrast, an emergency department evaluation of a patient well known to the system may require a significantly different strategy. In this emergency room situation, the clinician may have only 20 to 30 minutes available. Consequently, a conscious decision will need to be made as to which content regions to decrease or eliminate.

One of the most common complaints voiced by supervisees can be summarized as, "I didn't have enough time to gather the information I wanted!" This complaint is often paralleled by harried clinic directors mumbling phrases such as, "My God, how much longer is he going to take with that patient?" Both exclamations represent the end product of a poorly structured interview.

To counteract this problem, an understanding of facilics provides the clinician with a reassuring awareness of "where he or she is at" with regard to the thoroughness of the database during the interview itself. From this heightened awareness, the clinician develops an ability to intentionally control the pace and flow of the interview.

When discussing the opening phase, we examined the problem of the wandering interview, in which a patient with a loquacious manner encounters an interviewer incapable of focusing the flow of the dialogue. The result can be a disappointing experience for both participants. But many times, a patient with a normal verbal output, who could be easily directed, meets an interviewer with poor focusing abilities. Even in this case, the interview may become quite unproductive, because the patient does not know which information is most needed in order to maximize treatment planning. The resultant hodgepodge of dialogue can best be called an "unguided interview."

One may wonder why unguided interviews are so common. The answer is relatively simple and hinges upon the concept called "tracking." Tracking refers to a clinician's ability to sensitively follow up the statements of a patient with questions pertinent to the area discussed. At a more sophisticated level, good tracking also requires the ability to follow up with questions pertinent to the patient's immediate emotional state. This ability to track well is one of the main attributes of a good listener. Indeed, the ability to track well is a prerequisite to becoming a good interviewer.

And here lies the catch – good tracking must be accompanied by an equally good ability to focus the patient sensitively. Many mental health trainees have developed good techniques for tracking through the process of attentively listening to family and friends. However, few have learned from their previous life experiences equally effective methods of focusing. Fortunately, this crucial ability to focus sensitively can be learned.

Generally speaking, in the *body of the interview*, once within a content region, it is frequently best to expand that region relatively fully (usually to completion), because the patient will generally find such expansions to feel natural, for the topics of discussion are essentially related. If the patient spontaneously spins off at a tangent into unrelated topics, it is often best not to track with the patient into the unrelated topic. If one leaves a specific content region prematurely (before garnering the information needed to help the patient), one will have to return to that region (in order to gather the missing information) in the same interview, sometimes several times. Obviously, if the interviewer makes a habit of approaching most content regions in this haphazard manner, it becomes very difficult to monitor what information has been adequately gathered. Consequently, mistakes of omission occur more frequently.

This haphazard approach also tends to indirectly interfere with engagement and the understanding of the person. The amount of thought and concentration required to remember what has been missed and what still needs to be gathered becomes a significant cognitive burden to the interviewer. This unnecessary burden, which often creates anxiety in the interviewer as he or she becomes progressively aware that valuable information is not being addressed and that time is running out, takes away from the conscious attention on engagement and understanding the human being that has sought help. In addition, such a disorganized gathering of information makes the subsequent creation of the finalized electronic health record, typed after the interview is completed, remarkably more difficult and time consuming.

A Basic Paradigm for Successfully Structuring an Initial Interview

Considering the above pitfalls, one can begin to delineate a general approach to the body of the interview that will decrease the frequency of both wandering and unguided interviews, while maximizing both engagement and a comprehensive database. During the scouting region, the clinician should formulate a tentative plan for structuring the interview, utilizing the data gained from PACE (see Chapter 3). From this analysis, an initial content or process region will be chosen as an entrance into the main body of the interview. Frequently, the patient's own spontaneous discussion will have naturally led into a specific content region, such as the history of the presenting problem and/or a diagnostic area, such as the depression region. If so, the clinician should *expand this region fully* and then proceed to the next pertinent region as desired. Wandering patients are gently refocused if they prematurely leave regions.

To the degree that the clinician determines which content regions are pertinent for a particular patient in a particular clinical situation, subsequent regions are successfully entered and expanded as the main body of the interview unfolds. By the end of the first 15 minutes, interviewers will usually have completed the scouting region as well as two to three content expansions, often having gained a surprisingly good idea of the patient's main problems. In the next 15 minutes (the second quarter of the interview), the clinician continues to choose specific content regions and expands them completely in a sensitive fashion, making sure to always attend to the engagement process by effectively employing the techniques described in our first three chapters. Naturally, as deemed necessary, the clinician may pepper the content expansions with process areas such as psychodynamic regions or free facilitation regions. Slowly the patient's story emerges, and with it an increasing sense of understanding. By 30 minutes, it is impressive how much important information an interviewer, who is intentionally structuring an interview, will have garnered.

If structuring has gone well, the third 15 minutes can be utilized for expanding content regions deemed more important than originally expected, as well as for gathering data from the remaining content regions felt to be pertinent for treatment planning and triage. It is in this third 15 minutes that regions such as family history, medical history, social history, and the cognitive mental status (if indicated) are often explored.

During the last 7, or so, minutes, regional explorations might continue, and new questions, generated by the unfolding information, may be asked. But, truth be told, time is tight here and most of the last 5 to 10 minutes is generally not utilized for further data gathering. Instead, the clinician focuses on the important tasks described in the previous chapter that are necessary for a successful closing and termination.

Recognizing and Transforming Two Structuring Gremlins

1. Overly Lengthy Scouting Region: The "Five-Minute Fix"

One of the most common structuring problems, especially earlier in clinical training, is the tendency to let the scouting region go on and on. It is not uncommon to see scouting regions moving deep into the second quarter of the interview, well past the time necessary to ensure initial engagement and the other critical tasks of the opening phase. If the scouting region is overly long, no matter how well structured the rest of the interview, valuable information for helping the patient will inevitably be lost. There is simply not enough time left in a 50-minute hour to garner it. Thus, this is a clinical gremlin that it benefits all to avoid.

Fortunately, the fix is pretty simple, but requires some not-so-easy cognitive discipline by the interviewer. In short, get into the habit of always checking out in your mind when the first 5 minutes of your interview have unfolded. At that point, ask yourself, what have I learned from the PACE, and intentionally decide how you are going to make a graceful transition into the body of the interview. If engagement is weak, one can intentionally address it and, if necessary, *consciously* lengthen the scouting region as needed to ensure engagement. Using the engagement skills delineated in our opening chapters, I think you will find that, with time, you will seldom need to lengthen the scouting region past the typical 7, or so, minutes. Develop the habit, *right from the beginning of your interviewing career*, to note the passing of the first 5 minutes and your scouting regions will seldom run over-time. Your patients will reap the benefits of being both better understood and leaving your office with more effective treatment plans for relieving their pain.

2.   The Dead Zone: Two Errors in One

One of the most frequent structuring problems occurs during the second 15 minutes of the interview. Picture an interviewer, who by 15 minutes has, thus far, skillfully structured. By 7 minutes, after securing a sound engagement, the interviewer has navigated an effective scouting region. By 15 minutes they have proceeded to sensitively and comprehensively explore two or three particularly pertinent, from the patient's perspective, content regions. So far, so good. And now it gets interesting. Literally, *that* is the problem. Both parties are now so well engaged that the patient often begins to animatedly wander off into all sorts of interesting topics or very detailed extrapolations on the topics already adequately explored. Because the conversation is so interesting, the clinician tracks along into material that, although intriguing, does not provide information that can help the patient.

From a facilic perspective, the clinician is utilizing too many free facilitation regions and following too many spontaneous gates instead of focusing upon and completing appropriate content regions. When this process occurs, the clinician often finds that after 30 minutes very little of the needed information for an effective treatment plan, or even a sound triage decision, has been gathered. I have seen this disruptive process unfold so often in supervision, that my trainees and myself coined the term "the dead zone" for the second quarter of the interview. It is often dead to the process of uncovering useful information.

The inadvertent creation of a dead zone in the second quarter of the interview often begets a second error. When the clinician looks at his or her watch at 30 minutes, perceiving that a substantial amount of material needs to be covered, the response to their watch is like a track runner to a starting gun in the 100-yard dash – they're off and running. The clinician will proceed to force a rapid-paced and rigid structure onto the remaining part of the interview in an effort to catch up. Phrases such as "Let me ask just a few other questions here" or "Oh, I forgot to ask this" frequently appear *en masse*, as the scramble for "needed" information takes over. The result may be a patient who begins to perceive that the clinician is more interested in data gathering than in listening.

This vicious cycle of disengagement can be eliminated if, during the second 15 minutes, the interviewer continues to effectively structure (consistently finishing content regions and effectively re-focusing patients who are wandering), so that by the 30-minute mark, the eight to ten content regions that seem most pertinent to a particular patient have been nicely covered. Once again, it is a matter of developing a sense of time awareness and discipline.

But no matter who we are, and I certainly include myself here, it is easy to slip into the creation of a dead zone, because it is enjoyable to keep talking about "interesting stuff" (some of which might be very useful to explore in subsequent psychotherapy but is not particularly useful during the initial intake). Thus, most of us will occasionally find ourselves at 30 minutes at a problematic point. Here is where we can avoid compounding our first error with the second one.

If at 30 minutes one finds the interview to be far behind schedule, simply re-group. Don't try to gather everything you would normally want to gather. Instead, look at what is left, *consciously decide* what you think is most important, and proceed to gather that information effectively (perhaps a suicide assessment has not been done, a substance abuse history, or an exploration of pivotal social history as with incest). Explore this material in an engaging and normal pace. *Purposely* delete an exploration of the material that is less critical for an initial assessment (for instance, you may decide to completely drop the family history, unless you need it to help determine an appropriate medication) and intentionally shorten other content regions. Less important material can be explored in future sessions or by future clinicians if you are functioning as a triage agent. When such a gradual approach is utilized, rigid focusing is seldom required, and the pace of the interview seems appropriately unrushed to the patient.

Remember, it is okay to miss data. In fact, it is not feasible to perfectly collect all of the data we listed under our ten categories in most interviews. As I mentioned earlier, I don't think I ever have! On the other hand, using the principles, strategies, and techniques of this chapter, it is possible to minimize errors of omission while achieving surprisingly comprehensive databases for creating effective treatment plans.

The Eight Golden Rules for Structuring Effectively

As can be seen, the body of the interview represents a delicate organism, whose growth and development warrant careful attention by the interviewer. Perhaps, at this point, a review and occasional expansion upon the basic facilic principles utilized to move gracefully through this area of the interview would be useful:

1. Before beginning the interview, make a tentative determination of which content regions are most appropriate considering time constraints, the needs of the patient, and the goals of the interview.
2. At the 5-minute point, note how well the scouting region is proceeding; make appropriate adjustments and a decision as to how you are going to move into the body of the interview, thus avoiding an overly long scouting phase.
3. Begin gently, but persistently, structuring as soon as you leave the scouting region and during the second 15 minutes.

4. Generally speaking, once within an appropriate content region, it is often useful to expand it thoroughly. If the patient pivots into a new area, it is usually best to gently pull the patient back to the current region until it is completed. The exception to this principle occurs if the patient pivots into a highly charged or sensitive area such as suicidal ideation or incest. If such topics are spontaneously raised by the patient, it is generally best to move into them, for the patient is indicating that he or she is ready to explore what is often a taboo topic. This invitation may disappear quickly if not accepted promptly by the interviewer.

5. Avoid the overuse of free facilitation regions during the body of the interview.

6. During the remaining interview, occasionally (at least every 5 to 10 minutes) monitor the progress of your data gathering and adjust your pace as needed, paying particular attention to where you are with regard to your structuring every 15 minutes of the interview.

7. In the second quarter, be sure to avoid creating a dead zone regarding information gathering. If at 30 minutes you are behind, consciously decide what topics and data to *not* explore, and proceed to naturalistically explore, at a normal pace, whatever regions you have decided are necessary.

8. Leave adequate time in the last quarter for a graceful closing and termination phase.

Thus far, we have focused on the general strategy needed to determine and monitor the regions of dialogue encountered in an interview. Next we will examine the actual process of exploring a given region once it has been entered.

Exploring Content Regions in a Sensitive Fashion

The process of exploring a given content region is referred to as the "expansion" of the region. Different interviewers may approach this expansion in radically different ways.

Speaking broadly, two methods, forming somewhat opposing extremes, can be defined as "stilted expansions" and "blended expansions." In stilted expansions the expansion lacks a feeling of conversational flow. Instead, the interviewee is asked a series of questions that appear somewhat forced, because the interviewer is rigidly attempting to ask specific questions regarding the needed data points of the content region. This type of expansion may cause interviewees to experience the unpleasant feeling that they are "being interviewed," as opposed to talking *with* someone. I suppose one could call this process a "Meet the Press" type of expansion. Rigidly structured interviews sometimes foster this style of expansion such as illustrated below:

> **Pt.:** The pressures at home have really reached a crisis point. I'm not certain where it will all lead; I only know I'm feeling the heat.
>
> **Clin.:** What's your appetite like?
>
> **Pt.:** I guess it's okay …
>
> **Clin.:** What's your sleep like?
>
> **Pt.:** Not too good. I have a hard time falling asleep. My days are such a blur. I never feel balanced, even when I try to fall asleep. I can't concentrate enough to even read.

Clin.:	What about your sexual drive?
Pt.:	What do you mean?
Clin.:	Have you noticed any changes in how interested you are in sex?
Pt.:	Maybe a little.
Clin.:	In what direction?
Pt.:	I guess I'm not as interested in sex as I used to be.
Clin.:	And what about your energy level? How has it been?
Pt.:	Fairly uneven. It's hard to explain, but sometimes I don't feel like doing anything.

This particular interviewer seems doggedly intent on expanding the depression region, specifically the neurovegetative symptoms of depression. This style of expansion exhibits a mechanical quality, as if the interviewer has a list of questions to reel off. Such rigidity characterizes stilted expansions.

As a study in contrasts, in a "blended expansion" the interviewer once again focuses on a specific content region. However, in this expansion the interviewer attempts to blend the questions into the natural flow of the dialogue. Rather than feeling like they are "being interviewed," this type of expansion creates in interviewees a sense of gentle flow, which tends to foster a conversational feel. Moreover, this type of interviewing, by decreasing the anxiety of the patient, may enhance both the quantity and validity of the database as well. Earlier in the book we saw an excellent example of a blended expansion unfolding – when exploring depressive symptoms – illustrated in Video Module 2.1 from Chapter 2.

In the following illustration, a blended expansion unfolds, with the clinician once again exploring the diagnostic region of depression:

Pt.:	The pressures at home have really reached a crisis point. I'm not certain where it will all lead; I only know I'm feeling the heat.
Clin.:	Sounds like you've been going through a lot. (empathic statement) How has it affected the way you feel in general?
Pt.:	I'm depressed. I always feel drained. I'm always tired. Life seems like one giant chore.
Clin.:	What are some of your everyday things that now seem like chores?
Pt.:	Everything! (smiles weakly) Literally, just about everything, even checking my Facebook page. I love Facebook. I've got a zillion friends. I used to check for messages a couple of times a day, and I was always posting something or other. But I just don't care anymore. It just seems like another chore. It's so strange. Everything that was normal in my life is screwed up now.
Clin.:	That sounds tough. (empathic statement) What about your sleep? Has that been affected too?
Pt.:	Absolutely. Perhaps that's the reason I'm drained. I just can't rest. My sleep is horrible.
Clin.:	Tell me about it. (gentle command)
Pt.:	I can't fall asleep. It takes several hours just to get to sleep. I'm wired. I'm wired even in the day. And I'm so agitated I can't concentrate, even enough to read to put me to sleep.
Clin.:	That sounds pretty bad. (another empathic statement, said gently) Once you're asleep, are you able to stay asleep?
Pt.:	Never, I bet I wake up four or five times a night. And about 5:00 A.M. I'm awake, as if someone slapped me.

Clin.: How do you mean? (phenomenological exploration with an open-ended question)

Pt.: It's like an alarm went off, and no matter how hard I try, I can't get back to sleep.

Clin.: What do you do instead?

Pt.: Worry … I'm not kidding … My mind fills with all sorts of worthless junk.

Clin.: What kinds of things do you worry about?

Pt.: I don't know. You name it. I worry that I've let my family down. I worry about our rent. I worry about my mom's health, just everything, and I can't stop it.

Clin.: That sounds really miserable, I bet it really causes you problems with feeling wound up and unrested the rest of the day (empathic statement) … Does it cause any problems with your concentration?

Pt.: Oh yeah. I just simply can't function like I used to. Typing letters, reading, writing notes, all those things take much longer than usual. It really disturbs me. My system seems out of whack.

Clin.: Do you think your appetite has been affected as well?

Pt.: No question. My appetite is way down. Food tastes like paste; really very little taste at all. I've even lost weight.

Clin.: About how much and over how long a time?

Pt.: Oh, about 5 pounds, maybe over a month or two …

In the above dialogue the same region was expanded as in our first illustration (DSM-5 depressive episode), but this time the questioning appeared to flow naturally, generating an increasing flow of information. The interviewer's questions seemed to relate directly to what the interviewee was saying, thus creating a sense that the interviewer was "with" the interviewee. A nice example of good tracking.

This example also illustrates an important point. While expanding content regions, one continuously attends to the engagement process. For instance, early in the above selection the interviewer sensitively utilized a gentle empathic statement, "Sounds like you've been going through a lot." Further empathic statements followed in a timely fashion. And later, open-ended techniques were used, such as the gentle command, "Tell me about it," and the open-ended question, "How do you mean?" The interviewer thus metacommunicated an interest in how the patient phenomenologically experienced the symptom, not just that the patient had the symptom. Such a consistent and effective use of engagement techniques coalesces to create a feeling in patients that the interviewer is moving with them in a relatively unstructured fashion, while, in actuality, the clinician is gently structuring the interview, harvesting an ever-more meaningful field of information.

A further point to consider concerning the expansion of regions is the usefulness of brief excursions out of a region. For instance, while expanding the anxiety disorder region, the patient may mention the use of Valium (diazepam). At this point, the clinician may choose to expand the medication history briefly, after which he or she can return to the anxiety disorder region to complete its expansion. Such short excursions offer yet another flexible option for the clinician. Humor can also be utilized to further the natural feeling of the interview.

The clinician may also choose to utilize split expansions, with a single region expanded at several different locations during the interview. Although useful, these split expansions can lead to serious omissions if the clinician does not keep track of what information has been gathered. But on a limited basis, split expansions further increase the interviewer's adaptability.

The over-riding point remains the clinician's need to develop an active and conscious awareness of the data flow within a content region while simultaneously creating the sensation of the natural flow of conversation. Perhaps a few facilic principles warrant review at this point:

1. An effort should be made to achieve blended expansions as opposed to stilted expansions; such blended expansions move with the patient.
2. As long as one remembers to monitor the completeness of his or her database, then techniques such as split expansions and brief excursions can be useful, but need to be used judiciously.
3. Always attend to engagement during the expansion of content regions, both on a verbal and nonverbal level.

Before ending our discussion of the various methods of expanding regions, one more point warrants attention. Although stilted expansions generally tend to disengage patients, some patients may, ironically, prefer them. By way of illustration, this peculiar preference may surface in the case of a patient suffering from hypochondriacal concerns, associated with the belief that, "Nothing is wrong with my head." Some of these patients may actually prefer the checklist flavor of a stilted expansion because it parallels the feeling generated by a medical review of systems as performed by his or her family practitioner. Hence, the patient feels more at home with an interaction more redolent of a medical examination than of a psychiatric assessment. Once again, the art consists of adapting one's style to the needs of the patient.

At this time, we can move to the third and last major concern of facilics, the transitions utilized between regions. The ability to master these transitions will determine the clinician's ultimate ability to create a smoothly flowing dialogue.

Part III: Facilic Gating – The Fine Art of Making Graceful Transitions

Gates: The Pathways of Conversational Flow

As a conversation or an interview passes from one topic to another, different types of transitions occur. We will refer to the actual statements or questions joining two regions as "gates." Although there exist numerous types of gates, five major forms are most common: (1) the spontaneous gate, (2) the natural gate, (3) the referred gate, (4) the implied gate, and (5) the phantom gate. An understanding of the use of these gates provides interviewers with a simple but elegant method of gracefully maneuvering an interview.

Spontaneous Gates

The spontaneous gate, as its name suggests, unfolds without any effort by the interviewer. Instead, the transition results from a change in topic *unilaterally* initiated by the interviewee. These gates occur when the patient spontaneously moves into a new region (called a "pivot point") and the clinician proceeds to ask a follow-up question in this new region. The patient does the shifting here. The clinician merely follows, sometimes using phrases as simple as "Tell me more about that," or "How do you mean?" In the following example, a spontaneous gate provides an essentially unnoticeable movement from the expansion of depressive symptoms into a new region:

Pt.: The past 2 months have been so horrible. I think it's the worst time of my life. I just can't get away from the feeling.

Clin.: Which feelings are you referring to?

Pt.: The sadness; the heaviness.

Clin.: What else have you noticed when you're feeling sad and heavy?

Pt.: Nothing seems worth doing. It's late November and my yard is covered with leaves. Usually they'd all be gone into neat little piles, like a little farm, but not now …

Clin.: Besides not having energy for chores, do you find you can still enjoy your bridge club or other hobbies?

Pt.: Not really. Things seem so bland. I haven't even gone to bridge club for several months. It is all so different from before. In fact, there were times in the past when I could barely keep still, I was so active. I was a human dynamo. (pivot point)

*Clin.: How do you mean?

Pt.: Oh, I used to be incredibly active, into bridge, tennis, golf, and everything. It was hard to find anyone who could keep up with me.

Clin.: Did you ever move too fast?

Pt.: In what sense?

Clin.: Oh, sometimes one can get so energized that it gets difficult to get things done.

Pt.: Actually, there were a couple of odd times when people kept telling me to "slow down, slow down."

Clin.: Tell me a little about one of those times.

Pt.: About a year ago I got so wound up I hardly slept for almost a week. I'd stay up most of the night cleaning the house, washing the car, and writing furiously. I didn't seem to need sleep.

Clin.: Did you notice if your thoughts seemed speeded up then?

Pt.: Speeded up. I was flying. Everything seemed crystal clear and moved like lightning. It was strange …

In this example, two topics are being discussed sequentially. In the first content region, the interviewee's symptoms of depression are being explored. In the course of this exploration, the interviewee unilaterally brings up a statement that suggests a different diagnostic region (one dealing with mania). The pivot point into a new content region was, "In fact, there were times in the past when I could barely keep still, I was so active. I was a human dynamo."

The interviewer then followed this movement into a region exploring manic symptoms by simply asking, "How do you mean?" (indicated by an asterisk). Once within the diagnostic region of mania, a blended expansion of mania was begun. This movement into a new topic was practically imperceptible.

Spontaneous gates create movement that seems unblemished by effort or apparent structuring. In this sense, a skilled interviewer will frequently make use of such gates whenever transitions into new regions are desirable. But herein lies a potential pitfall mentioned earlier: It is frequently not desirable to leave a region before it is fully expanded. One does not and should not follow every pivot point with a spontaneous gate into a new region.

Indeed, the concept of spontaneous gates and pivot points provides us with a new way of conceptualizing both the wandering interview and the unguided interview. These interviews occur when pivot points are followed by the clinician whenever they appear, resulting in a consistent pattern of incomplete expansions and a subsequently weak database.

Pivot points represent critical moments in which the interviewer can consciously decide whether to stay within an expansion or move with the patient into a new one. If they want to move (the current region is essentially finished), the interviewer simply employs a spontaneous gate to enter the new region with the interviewee. If the current expansion is incomplete, nine times out of ten the clinician will gently pull the patient back into the current topic and fully complete its expansion.

Any clinician who can gain conscious awareness of such pivot points will gain considerable control over the flow of questioning, clipping the wings of an unguided or wandering interview before it can even take flight. In this light, I believe that the ability to *immediately* recognize pivot points, as they occur, is arguably the single greatest secret to effectively structuring interviews.

As alluded to earlier, although relatively rare in the body of the interview, a clinician may decide it is wise to move with a pivot point by making a spontaneous gate, even in the middle of an incomplete expansion. Such times include the following: (1) the patient may have unexpectedly related highly emotionally charged material that needs to be ventilated; (2) the patient may have spontaneously mentioned highly sensitive material that may best be approached immediately, such as suicide, domestic violence, or incest; and (3) specific memories may warrant immediate follow-up, such as screen memories, dreams, or traumatic events.

Of course, during process regions, such as psychodynamic regions or free facilitation regions, the clinician generally follows most spontaneous gates as they appear, utilizing an occasional restraint. The scouting region is also often filled with "internal" spontaneous gates. Along these same lines, during periods of free association, as may appear in therapy itself, spontaneous gates are essentially always followed; indeed, they are nurtured. But no matter what the facilic situation, we return to the all-important realization that clinicians can exercise significant choice (intentional interviewing) as to the pattern any given interview will pursue as long as they recognize pivot points and consciously decide whether or not to follow them.

Natural Gates

A natural gate consists of two parts: the cue statement and the transitional question. A cue statement consists of the very last sentence or two made by the interviewee and it contains content material that can be creatively used as a bridge into a new region by the interviewer. *Note that the content material of the cue statement is still within the content region that is being expanded.* If the interviewer cues off this statement to enter a new region of the clinician's choice, the interviewee will feel that the conversation is flowing from his own speech, as, indeed, it is. Such a transition seems both natural and caring to the interviewee.

The transitional question is the actual question asked by the interviewer that makes a bridge from the cue statement into the new region, *i.e., in contrast to the spontaneous gate, the clinician, not the patient, is moving the conversation into a new region.*

In the following excerpt we will see a transition made from the content region covering depressive symptoms (which the interviewer has been exploring for the last few minutes and currently feels that she has enough information to make the diagnosis) into the drug and alcohol region. This smooth transformation will be made via a natural gate.

> **Clin.:** Have you been able to enjoy your poker games or your shop work?
>
> **Pt.:** No, I just don't feel like doing anything since I've been feeling depressed. It's a really ugly feeling.
>
> **Clin.:** Tell me more about what it feels like.
>
> **Pt.:** Really pretty miserable. Life doesn't seem the same. I'm tired all the time; no sleep.
>
> **Clin.:** How do you mean?
>
> **Pt.:** Over the past several months sleep has almost become a chore. I'm always having trouble getting to sleep, and then I wake up all night. I must wake up five times and it took me 2 hours to fall asleep in the first place.
>
> ***Clin.:** Have you ever used anything like a nightcap to sort of knock yourself out?
>
> **Pt.:** Yeah, sometimes a good belt really relaxes me.
>
> **Clin.:** How much do you need to drink to make yourself sleepy?
>
> **Pt.:** Oh, not too terribly much. Maybe a couple of beers. Sometimes more than a couple of beers.
>
> **Clin.:** Just, in general, how many drinks do you have in a given day?
>
> **Pt.:** Probably … Now, I'm just guessing, but probably a six-pack or two, maybe three (smiles sheepishly). I hold liquor pretty well. I don't get drunk or nothing.
>
> **Clin.:** What other kinds of drugs do you like to take to relax?
>
> **Pt.:** Well, I might smoke a joint here or there.

In this excerpt, the cue statement was, "I must wake up five times and it took me 2 hours to fall asleep in the first place." Note that the patient's cue statement is still within the region of depression. But the clinician, wanting to change content regions, sensed that this statement could be used as a springboard into a new topic. The succeeding transition question (indicated by an asterisk) imperceptibly achieved this desired transition into the drug and alcohol region with the phrase, "Have you ever used anything like a nightcap to sort of knock yourself out?"

Natural gates of this sort are seldom perceived as structuring mechanisms, because the patient generally feels as if he or she brought up the new topic. This type of smooth transition can greatly enhance a conversational feeling in the interview, slowly bringing the patient into a more powerful sense of safety and spontaneity. The interview begins to take on a self-perpetuating momentum, unique to its own nature.

In Figure 4.1, the immense power of the natural gate, as an intentionally utilized tool by an interviewer, is demonstrated. We shall assume that the expansion of the stressor region has been winding down. The interviewer feels it is time to move on to new material. The interviewer decides to cue off of a statement made by the client regarding his stress, which can be utilized by the clinician to enter one of any number of new content regions as illustrated. The flexibility of the natural gate is essentially only limited by the awareness and creativity of the clinician. The ability to intentionally use natural gates is one of the cornerstone skills for creating conversational interviews. Master clinicians use them frequently.

Manufactured "Gates"

One valuable way of using natural gates consists of coupling several of them *in a quick succession* so as to gracefully enter a particularly delicate topic that is difficult to enter without disengagement. In essence, the interviewer manufactures a smooth transition where one might not have been initially available. I like to call these transitions "manufactured gates," although they are not really a new and distinct type of gate; in essence,

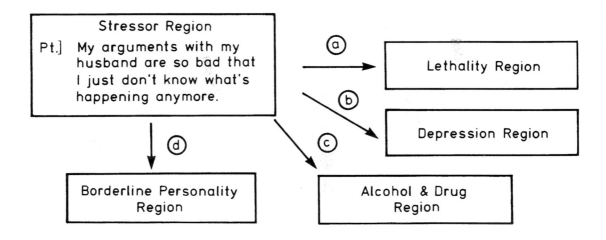

Transition Questions:

a) With all these tensions mounting, have you had any thoughts of wanting to kill yourself?

b) How have all these stresses affected your mood?

c) With all these stresses, have you been drinking at all in an effort to calm yourself?

d). Some people hold all their anger in and others really let it out, maybe even throwing things like glasses or plates. How do you handle your anger?

Figure 4.1 Natural gates utilized as smooth transitions.

this is merely the intentional use of serial natural gates. Let us see this sophisticated strategy put to good use.

Imagine the following situation: About 30 minutes into an initial intake, a counselor at a community mental health center intuitively suspects potentially dangerous domestic violence has been perpetrated by the interviewee. In order to get to this delicate topic, she chooses to manufacture a naturalistic transition. Note that in our illustrative dialogue, the interviewer has been expanding the content region regarding recent stressors with the patient. There doesn't immediately appear to be an apparent way to sensitively move into the topic of domestic violence, but she realizes that if she can position the patient into a conversation about drinking behavior, then the transition could be made much more easily.

The counselor will use her first natural gate ("Does it ever help you to get away from all this stress, and you have a lot of stress, by drinking?") to enter the region of drug and alcohol use, but she is not doing this in order to expand the region of drug and alcohol use (which she will do later in the interview). Rather, she is using it as a stepping stone to an exploration of domestic violence. Look for her timely use of a second natural gate to immediately leave the topic of substance abuse while cleverly raising the new content region of violence:

> **Pt.:** … yeah, money is a real problem. I've got huge credit card debts. And the damn creditors are harassing me constantly. Look, I don't have the money, what do they want me to do – plant a fucking money tree? Times are bad. I don't have a job. The damn repo man took my car. I'm not kidding, they actually hauled it out of my own driveway. I've never really ever been this stressed out. Mind you, I'll get out of it. I always do. But, frankly, I don't know if I'm coming or going.
>
> **Clin.:** Does it ever help you to get away from all this stress, and you have a lot of stress, by drinking?
>
> **Pt.:** You bet. And I deserve a time-out or two. Nothing wrong with a good six-pack or two to lighten the load, if you know what I mean. It usually works too, unless there are just too many assholes bothering me.
>
> **Clin.:** Sometimes when people drink they notice an increased desire to just let off steam, you know, just pick a fight or something, not much, just a little brawl or two to liven things up, a chance to flex the old "beer muscles." Do you know what I mean?
>
> **Pt.:** Oh, yeah. I've been in my share of brawls. (pauses, smiles) Won a few, too.
>
> **Clin.:** Has that ever carried over into other areas when you're drinking? Like when you and your wife are arguing, does it ever get so intense that you feel like hitting her?
>
> **Pt.:** Yeah, sort of (pauses, looks away briefly). Just a few weeks ago I wanted to beat the hell out of her. She can be such a royal pain in the ass.
>
> **Clin.:** Have you ever wanted to hurt her, in an even more serious way?
>
> **Pt.:** (pause) Once in a while I guess I have. And sometimes I still think she deserves it.
>
> **Clin.:** Deserves what?
>
> **Pt.:** (looks away, pauses, then looks the interviewer right in the eye) To be out of the picture. It's crossed my mind, I have to admit it. She's like a fucking albatross around my neck.
>
> **Clin.:** What have you thought of doing?

> **Pt.:** Cracking her upside the head with a hammer or something. I don't know. (pauses) I just don't know anymore. (pauses) I don't think I'd ever do it.

This is a wonderful illustration of skilled interviewing. How does one raise the topic of killing one's spouse in an initial interview while getting at the truth, without harming the alliance or breaking unconditional regard? This appears, at first glance, to be quite a task. It is not exactly easy to ask people if they are potential murderers.

But this counselor makes the difficult seem surprisingly easy. From previous interviews, she knew that the violence region could be frequently entered through a natural gate from the drug and alcohol region, by relating violent thoughts and behaviors unobtrusively to the poor impulse control commonly seen with drinking. Consequently, the clinician steered the conversation into the drug and alcohol region with her first natural gate. She thus manufactured a nice opportunity to immediately setup a second natural gate ("Sometimes when people drink they notice an increased desire to just let off steam, you know, just pick a fight or something …"), through which she subtly entered the region of violence with barely a hint of structuring. She could then gracefully generalize into the topic of domestic violence.

Her skilled interviewing might have just saved the life of this patient's wife and, at the very least, she uncovered a major arena for immediate therapeutic intervention. Many a clinician would not have been able to uncover the murderous thoughts of this patient upon their first meeting. A second meeting might be one meeting too late.

Having secured a sound understanding of how to effectively utilize natural gates – including how they can be used to build manufactured gates – let us explore them in more detail via a video module. Natural gates warrant our further exploration, for, in my opinion, they are one of the most powerful and flexible tools that we have available for creating a conversational feel to our interviews. There exist an almost inexhaustible number of ways to creatively and gracefully transition between topics using natural gates, of which these video illustrations are a tiny sample.

By the way, when using a natural gate to enter a particularly sensitive topic, they are often introduced by using words such as, "Some of my patients who have been experiencing … (at which point the interviewer cues off of the topic of the patient's last sentence)." This added technique is known as a normalization, and we will be discussing it in our next chapter on techniques for improving validity. It metacommunicates to the patient that it is safe to discuss the new topic, for the interviewer has obviously heard it from other people in similar situations. In any case, you will see this validity technique added to our natural gates in several of the video examples. Although normalizations are quite useful when entering a sensitive or taboo topic, they are not a typical – nor a necessary – part of most natural gates.

VIDEO MODULE 4.1

Title: Creating Graceful Transitions Using Natural Gates

Contents: Contains both expanded didactics and annotated interviewing examples. Interview excerpts demonstrate sensitive transitions into difficult topics such as OCD, psychotic process, dementia, violence, and incest.

Referred Gates

A referred gate occurs when the interviewer enters a new region by referring back to an earlier statement made by the interviewee often many minutes earlier. Typical referred gates begin with phrases such as, "Earlier you had said ..." or "I want to hear more about something you mentioned before ..." To the interviewee, a referred gate metacommunicates, "I have been listening very carefully to you; moreover, I want to learn more about something you said to see if I can help." It is a wonderful example of a structuring tool that is simultaneously a powerful engagement technique. Also, it allows the interviewer to enter a fresh region smoothly at almost any place in an interview. It remains extremely useful for re-entering a region that was not fully expanded earlier. Structurally, a referred gate lacks an immediate cue statement, because the cue has been taken from a previous area of the interview.

In the following illustration we will enter the interview at the end of a psychodynamic process region in which the patient's feelings concerning his siblings have been explored. As this process region winds down, the interviewer, by referring to something said much earlier, will enter a content region traditionally viewed to be difficult to gracefully broach – psychotic phenomena – through the use of a referred gate.

Clin.:	What was it like for you when your brother would come home from college?
Pt.:	Sort of odd; a little bit like a trespass. You see, when he was gone I had the room all to myself, even the phone was mine alone. As soon as he came back, boom, the room was his again.
Clin.:	What other feelings did you have?
Pt.:	Some excitement. I really did look up to him, and when he'd come home he'd tell me all about college, frat parties, smoking grass; and it was exciting.
*Clin.:	Earlier you had told me that sometimes when you were alone you'd have scary thoughts. Tell me a little more about those moments.
Pt.:	Okay. It's sort of like this: I might be sitting late at night listening to some music and things seem sort of weird, almost like something bad is going to happen. And then I have thoughts that keep coming at me and they tell me to do things.
Clin.:	Do the thoughts ever get so intense they sound almost like a voice?
Pt.:	They *are* voices. They seem very real. In fact, sometimes I try to cover my ears. I just don't know. I don't know ...

Referred gates, such as the one illustrated above (indicated by asterisk), are unobtrusively powerful tools for structuring. They can be used for entering new regions essentially at will, as well as for re-entering incompletely expanded regions. Moreover, when combined with a creative sensitivity, the clinician can utilize referred gates to enter potentially disengaging regions gracefully as shown above. It is not unusual for 20 to 40% of my gates to be referred in an initial intake.

One of these awkward regions that frequently poses problems for clinicians is the cognitive mental status examination. As mentioned earlier in the chapter, it is often an important aspect of interviewing patients over 50, especially if one is suspicious of the presence of a dementia or delirium, and sometimes is also indicated with younger patients as well. While asking questions about orientation and checking digit spans or serial sevens, clinicians worry that patients will feel insulted by the simplistic nature of the questions. To this end, clinicians may utter phrases such as, "I'm going to ask you some silly questions now, I hope you don't mind," or "Now I have to ask you some routine questions that I have to ask everybody." These phrases are usually accompanied by an apologetic tone of voice or an insecure rustling of the clinician in his or her chair.

The irony of such introductions lies in the fact that rather than dispelling anxiety in the patient, they sometimes create it. The patient can sense that the clinician feels insecure with the subsequent questioning. All that remains for the patient to wonder is why the clinician needs to apologize. What do these *routine* questions mean and why does a professional ask questions if they are silly? In short, the clinician's sudden obsequiousness serves to signal the patient that something odd is afoot.

It is here that one of the many uses of the referred gate becomes apparent. By referring to earlier statements of the patient concerning problems with concentration or thinking, the interviewer can enter the cognitive examination smoothly and without a need to apologize. Quite to the contrary, the interviewer's interest indicates a sincere concern to the patient as well as a display of professional expertise.

By introducing the cognitive exam with a referred gate, the interviewer metacommunicates that these questions are being asked for a specific reason – to clarify collaboratively the degree of cognitive impairment – a point of potential concern to both the clinician and patient. Let us take a look at such an approach in action. The patient is suffering from an agitated major depression and had complained earlier in the interview of problems concentrating:

Pt.: Overall, I know it's all my fault. I should never have retired, it's ruined everything. But life goes on. I only hope I feel better some day.

Clin.: What do you see for yourself in the future?

Pt.: Hopefully, some pretty good stuff. I've always wanted to travel and my wife is interested in doing so as well, so, I think we will probably do a little traveling. And, I also used to paint a little bit, maybe I'll do a little of that too.

Clin.: That sounds sweet. I hope it works out for you.

Pt.: Yeah, me too.

Clin.: You know, a little earlier, you had mentioned that you were concerned about having some problems concentrating and remembering things. I have some questions that would give us both a clearer idea exactly how much your concentration and thinking have been affected by your depression. I think it would be a good idea to check out these concerns in some more detail, does that sound okay?

Pt.: No problem. That's why I'm here, to find out what is going on with me.

Clin.: Some of the questions will be very simple, while some of them may get fairly challenging. Why don't we start with some of the really simple ones first?

Pt.: Sure.

Clin.: What is today's date?

Pt.: I think it's September 21st, 2010.

Clin.: That's correct. What day of the week is it?

> **Pt.:** Wednesday.
>
> **Clin.:** Good. What city is this?
>
> **Pt.:** Pittsburgh.

This interview dyad moved into the cognitive mental status examination with a sense of purpose and no hint of uneasiness on the part of the clinician. Even if the patient does not "pick up" on the referred gate, an easy transition can be made as follows:

> **Clin.:** Earlier you had mentioned how depressed and out of it you sometimes feel at dusk. I am wondering if during this period of the day you notice any problems with concentration or your memory.
>
> **Pt.:** No, I don't think so. No problems with my concentration.
>
> **Clin.:** That's very fortunate, because frequently when people feel depressed, they have problems with concentration or organizing their thoughts. In fact, I would like to ask some questions designed to pick up even subtle problems with concentration or memory, because if we find some subtle problems, it may give us some idea of how we can best help you. Does that sound okay to you?
>
> **Pt.:** Yes. I don't think I've got any problems here, but I guess it's worth taking a look.
>
> **Clin.:** Good, we'll start with some very simple questions and move towards some harder ones. To start with, what is today's date?

We have just seen the usefulness of the referred gate in guiding the discussion into a cognitive examination. In a similar way, referred gates can frequently decrease the awkwardness of entering sensitive regions of discussion such as the drug or sexual history. This effectiveness probably results from the fact that relating the sensitive material to previous statements by the patient decreases the perceived social inappropriateness of the question. This principle may seem a bit abstract at present, but the following illustration will clarify the concept.

In this interview, the patient was an attractive woman of about 30 years of age. She had her blonde hair pulled back in a bun, giving an impression of a young professional. She used her hands to sharply punctuate her words like she was furiously stabbing away at a laptop's keyboard. She described her various plights in a dramatic and telling manner. After 30 minutes, numerous soap opera vignettes had been laid out on the table, including many years of heavy drug abuse in the past, a striking lack of any stable relationships, over 100 sexual encounters, and a current investigation by the FBI of her old friends.

She emphasized her sexual freedom early during the interview stating, "I'm not hung up on having to like the person I have sex with. Sex is something I can easily divorce from my feelings." Later in the interview, as the facts of her life became clearer, I began to wonder if I was talking with someone who might have developed an antisocial personality disorder, slickly camouflaged by an engaging interpersonal style. To this end I wanted to expand the antisocial personality region in more detail.

I wondered if she might be involved in prostitution. Needless to say, asking a person during an initial interview if he or she may be a prostitute can be a delicate matter. In this case, a referred gate provided a smooth entry into this sensitive topic:

Pt.: All of my men have ended up leaving me. None of them want to be fathers. We always fight. I'm bored by it all now.

Clin.: Earlier you had mentioned that you have been able to successfully divorce your sexual feelings from your emotional ones as you've matured. I'm wondering if, because of this ability, you've been able to use your body in a purely practical sense, for instance, did you ever find that desperate financial situations made it necessary to become involved with something like prostitution? (referred gate)

Pt.: Yeah, I've done that too. Back in New York I worked the streets for about 4 or 5 months, not much longer though.

Clin.: What was that like for you?

Pt.: Not really that tough. It's a dirty business though and I'm glad I'm out of it. But it helped when I needed it and believe me I needed the money.

Clin.: Did you ever sell drugs back then to help pay the rent and other needs?

Pt.: No. I never really sold drugs, I would use them like crazy – my life has been a wild one. In fact, someone ought to write a novel about me. I've seen it all, but I never got into pushing drugs.

This referred gate, voiced matter of factly, seemed to flow quite naturally. She did not appear particularly flustered, and the blending remained high. Once again, to the interviewee, referred gates suggest that the clinician has been listening carefully in an effort to piece together the patient's story. One can imagine how differently the above situation may have unfolded if the clinician had abruptly asked without a referred gate, "By the way, are you a prostitute?" This method of transition certainly needs a little more polish. Such abrupt gates are the next topic of discussion.

Phantom Gates

A phantom gate appears to come from nowhere. It lacks a cue statement and also lacks previous referential points, as seen in referred or natural gates. In short, it jolts the spontaneous flow, as the following example will show:

Pt.: I haven't felt the same for months. I'm always down and I'm sick of it.

Clin.: What does it feel like to be down?

Pt.: Very unsettling. I'm like a slab. I don't want to do anything. I don't even have the energy to text message my friends anymore. I'm not kidding! (pauses) The truth is I miss doing things with Jennifer. She was my best friend. Silly as this may sound. I really haven't been the same since she died.

*Clin.: Was your father an alcoholic?

Pt.: No ... (pauses, looks taken aback) I don't think he was. He drank every once in a while.

Clin.: What about your brothers, sisters, or blood relatives? Have any of them had drinking problems?

Pt.: Not that I know of.

Clin.: What about depression? Have any of your relatives been depressed?

This interviewer's sudden leap into the family history region certainly appeared abrupt and ill timed. Obviously, if such phantom gates (indicated by an asterisk) occur frequently throughout the interview, engagement can be seriously hampered. Even in milder forms, they can quickly produce the "Meet the Press" feeling discussed earlier. They often pop up toward the end of interviews, when clinicians suddenly realize several things they forgot to ask, or after the creation of a dead zone in the second quarter of the interview and the clinician ill advisedly tries to cover too much information. If important or critical regions (such as a suicide assessment) have been incompletely expanded or omitted, then referred gates, as opposed to phantom gates, can often return the interviewee to these unanswered questions without substantially interrupting the flow of the interview.

With regard to the possible utility of phantom gates, two instances come to mind. First, when dealing with a wandering interview, phantom gates may be useful in focusing the patient, especially if milder forms of focusing have been unsuccessful. A second use of phantom gates arises during the exploration of certain psychodynamic regions. Specifically, if one wants to catch a patient off-guard in order to observe the patient's spontaneously occurring defenses, then an unexpected phantom gate may be very effective. Phantom gates may also help one break through the communication roadblock caused by a patient bent on manipulating the interviewer or as a method of disrupting a rehearsed interview when used to introduce an affective interjection as described in Chapter 3.

In a less antagonistic sense, phantom gates may also be utilized when attempting to help patients reflect upon themselves through the use of interpretive questions. Interpretive questions may assume more bite if asked at an unexpected moment. These latter uses of phantom gates find minimal applicability during initial interviews, but they are more commonplace during psychotherapy interviews, once the therapeutic alliance has been solidified.

Implied Gates

To complete our summary of transitions used during the body of the interview we can turn our attention to implied gates. These gates are frequently used during chit chat between friends and may have been the predominant gate overheard as we listened in upon the café conversation mentioned earlier.

Implied gates are structurally similar to phantom gates: they do not cue off the patient's immediately preceding statements (as in a natural gate); they do not refer back to earlier statements (as in a referred gate); and the clinician, not the patient (as seen in a spontaneous gate), initiates the movement into the new topic. There is one important difference between an implied gate and a phantom gate: *the implied gate enters a region that is topically similar to the immediately previous region.*

Put slightly differently, in an implied gate, the movement into a new region is characterized by asking a question that seems to be generally related to the region already under expansion. Thus, it is somewhat "implied" that the interviewer is simply expanding a topic already germane to the interviewee. Consequently, implied gates tend to be much less disruptive to flow than phantom gates.

In the following example, movement is made from the content region dealing with immediate stressors into past social history, an area frequently also ripe with stress. The transition (indicated by an asterisk) seems relatively smooth, an effect that is probably secondary to the similarity in content between these two regions.

> **Pt.:** We're living in a fairly nice house now. It has three bedrooms and a couple of acres. Believe me, we need the space with our four kids.
>
> **Clin.:** How are the kids getting along?
>
> **Pt.:** The two oldest, Sharon and Jim, get along pretty well, on different tracks. They stay out of each other's way. But the two little ones – oh my! They live to torture each other … pulling each other's hair, yelling, screaming. It's a zoo.
>
> **Clin.:** I'm wondering if, with all those mouths to feed, money is a problem?
>
> **Pt.:** In some respects, yes; but my husband is a lawyer and is doing well. In fact, if anything, our income has increased recently.
>
> ***Clin.:** Tell me a little bit about what it was like for you when you grew up back in Arkansas.
>
> **Pt.:** First of all, I came from a large family of eight children. So we sometimes, many times, had to do without. I remember all the hand-me-downs and, believe me, I appreciated them. My mother was a loving woman, but beaten down by life. She was tough, but her pain showed through.
>
> **Clin.:** Do you remember a specific time when her pain showed through?
>
> **Pt.:** Oh, yes. I was about 5, I think, and …

As mentioned earlier, unlike a natural gate, an implied gate does not cue directly off the preceding statement. Furthermore, unlike a referred gate, the interviewer does not directly refer back to earlier statements. And, in contrast to the phantom gate, the implied gate seems to fit in fairly naturally with the current flow of the dialogue. Indeed, when the newly entered region appears very similar to the preceding one, an implied gate is practically imperceptible and rivals a natural gate for smoothness of transition.

As the regions connected increase in disparity, the implied gate becomes increasingly more abrupt. Thus, with regard to smoothness, implied gates range on a continuum between natural gates and phantom gates. When the two regions are closely related, implied gates approach the gracefulness of natural gates. On the other hand, if the topics are poorly related, an implied gate may approach the awkwardness of a phantom gate.

Implied gates can frequently be used to enter new regions smoothly. In fact, occasionally, the clinician may simultaneously expand two regions whose contents are similar in nature. For instance, one can easily expand the generalized anxiety disorder region and the major depressive disorder region in a parallel fashion, because anxiety often plays a role in both disorders.

Miscellaneous Gates

There are two miscellaneous gates that are used much less frequently than the five cornerstone gates we have studied. They, too, merit our attention, for they have good uses as well.

Introduced Gate

The first gate is called an "introduced gate." In an introduced gate the interviewer literally tells the interviewee, that a transition is about to be made. One of the few places that I find this type of gate useful is the transition point between the body of the interview and the closing, where it can provide a graceful transition as follows: "Well we have covered a lot of ground so far today. We have about 10 minutes left before we wrap up, and I think it's a great time for me to provide some thoughts on what might be going on and we can brainstorm together on the various options that we have to get you some relief as quickly as possible. As we close, I'm wondering, first, if there is anything that you think we should have talked about that I might have missed?"

Introduced gates are sometimes used to enter a transformative process region, when a slow build-up of interpersonal tension is noted by the clinician and a decision is made to try to dismantle the growing hesitancy. An introduced gate might be utilized as follows: "At this point, let's take a moment to sort of re-group ourselves, if that is okay with you. I might be wrong here, but I've been feeling, for awhile, that there is something I am saying or doing that is bothering you a bit, and I sure don't want that to be happening, because I really want to help. What have you been feeling about where we have been going so far and how we have been doing it?" To which a patient may say something like, "I think you are missing the point here, Doc, I'm not the problem, my wife is the problem. She gets as angry as I do …" If this concern had been left hidden, there probably would be no second appointment, and an introduced gate helped to make the uncovering unobtrusive.

Observed Gate

Our second miscellaneous gate is called an "observed gate." It is used more frequently than an introduced gate and is simple in nature, yet quite helpful. In an observed gate, the clinician makes note of a patient's nonverbal behavior, often to enter a free facilitation region or a psychodynamic region. Observed gates frequently begin with phrases such as, "It looks like you are starting to well-up, what are you feeling?" As with introduced gates, observed gates may also be used to enter a transformative process region as with, "You sound sort of irritated right now, did I say something that offended you or you think is off base?"

THE FINISHING TOUCHES: SUMMARIZING THE PRINCIPLES OF FACILICS

At this juncture, we are nearing the end of our discussion of the various methods by which one can flexibly and sensitively structure the body of the interview. Some of the key facilic principles that can help us to transform a potentially rigid interview into an engaging conversation that gathers a powerfully useful database are as follows:

a. When the patient spontaneously moves into a new region, the clinician always has the choice of whether to follow it or not. These decision moments are called pivot points.

b. If a premium is put upon sensitive, yet efficient, data gathering, as is the case during the body of an initial interview, then it is often best *not* to follow these pivots into new regions. Instead, the clinician can gently pull the patient back into the current content region and continue the expansion of that region until it is completed to the clinician's satisfaction.

c. If a premium is put upon a dynamic understanding of the patient, then these pivots into new regions are frequently completed by the use of simple follow-up questions, creating a spontaneous gate. These wanderings of the patient can provide valuable insights into the patient's psychodynamics. These pivot points are also followed if it appears that the patient has begun spontaneously discussing sensitive areas (such as suicide, incest, or domestic violence) or seems to need to ventilate disturbing emotions.

d. Natural gates, in which the clinician enters a new region by cueing directly off the patient's preceding statement or two, offer another method for creating smooth transitions and should be employed frequently.

e. These natural gates offer a particularly effective means of intentionally structuring an interview while conveying an unstructured conversational feel to the interviewee.

f. Referred gates, in which the clinician refers back to earlier statements by the patient, offer effective methods of re-entering poorly expanded regions or bringing up new regions, and once again provide a graceful tool for sensitive structuring.

g. Referred gates are also useful for tying in sensitive or awkward regions such as the cognitive mental status examination, for the patient feels that this "new topic" appears to relate naturally to the previously referred to dialogue.

h. Implied gates allow one to join topically similar regions and can also provide parallel expansions of related regions (such parallel expansions should be used sparingly for they make it hard to track what information has been gathered and what information needs to be gathered).

i. Phantom gates should be generally avoided unless used for a specific purpose such as a tool for derailing a rehearsed interview when using affective interjection.

Facilics provides a simple language with which to follow the complex structuring techniques of both ourselves and those we supervise. To enhance this system, a supervisor's "shorthand" has been designed in which easily learned symbols are used to represent regions and gates. These facilic schematics allow supervisors to quickly create a permanent record of the supervisee's interview, while providing a concrete and visual springboard for immediate feedback to the student or for subsequent group discussion. The schematic system is easy to learn and to use.

For those supervisors and trainees interested in learning how to use the facilic schematic system for supervision and/or classroom discussion, we have included an ExpertConsult.com short, easy-to-use computerized interactive program in Appendix I. In addition, an article from the Psychiatric Clinics of North America[7] *for faculty and supervisors on how to effectively use the facilic system with trainees is also available in Appendix IV.*

This is also an opportune time to review the annotated, direct transcript of an initial interview that appears in Appendix II. In this interview, taken verbatim from an actual clinical intake of mine, you will get a chance to see the five phases of the interview described in Chapter 3, as they naturalistically unfold. In addition, a variety of the facilic principles we have just examined will be brought to life for you from an interview I performed while working in a community mental health center.

CONCLUDING COMMENTS

Once a clinician understands the principles of facilics, then the body of the interview can be developed and altered almost at the whim of the interviewer. These tricks of the trade can greatly increase engagement with the patient, the effectiveness of the data gathering, and, ultimately, the validity of the database itself.

In short, initiated by the conscious decisions of the interviewer, the clinical dialogue unfolds intentionally and in a person-centered fashion. With each unfolding, the initial hesitancies of the interviewee gradually recede, for the interviewer, instead of opposing these hesitancies, moves with them. Clinicians familiar with the use of natural gates and referred gates, as well as the use of natural expansions as opposed to stilted expansions, can more easily generate interviews that move with the gentle dynamics of an everyday conversation. The patient feels more relaxed, defenses drop, and both the interviewer and the patient are more likely to uncover the information and secrets that lead to healing.

We began this chapter with a quotation concerning a master artist of China, Wang Hsia, who painted in the 8th century C.E. He worked in a different time and in a different medium to the one we have discussed. Yet, he, too, was a student of movement. Like ours, his work was based on a few simple principles, practiced until discipline transformed them into art. Our "painting" is the clinical dialogue we leave behind us. We, too, strive for sensitivity and subtlety. Perhaps, with work, fellow students of interviewing will study one of our future transcripts and find, to their admiration, that "when one looks carefully, one cannot find any marks of demarcation in the ink."

REFERENCES

1. Chung-yuang C. *Creativity and taoism: a study of Chinese philosophy, art, and poetry.* New York, NY: Harper Torchbooks; 1963.
2. Osler W. *Aequanimitas.* 3rd ed. Philadelphia, PA: Blakiston; 1945.
3. Shea SC, Mezzich JE. Contemporary psychiatric interviewing: new directions for training. *Psychiatry* 1988;**51**(4):385–97.
4. Shea SC, Mezzich JE, Bohon S, Zeiders A. A comprehensive and individualized psychiatric interviewing training program. *Acad Psychiatry* 1989;**13**(2):61–72.
5. Shea SC, Barney C. Facilic supervision and schematics: the art of training psychiatric residents and other mental health professionals how to structure clinical interviews sensitively. *Psychiatr Clin North Am* 2007;**30**(2):e51–96.
6. Shea SC, Green R, Barney C, et al. Designing clinical interviewing training courses for psychiatric residents: a primer for interviewing mentors. *Psychiatr Clin North Am* 2007;**30**(2):283–314.
7. Shea SC, Barney C. 2007. p. e51–96.

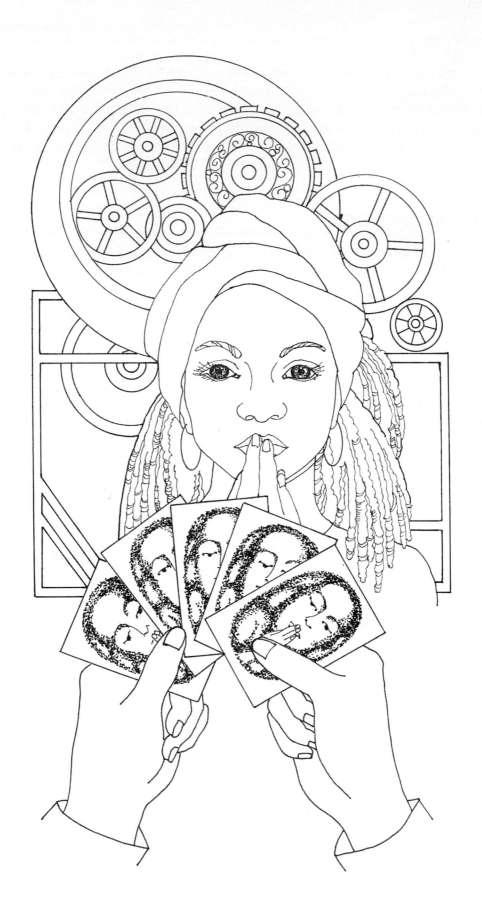

CHAPTER 5

Validity Techniques for Exploring Sensitive Material and Uncovering the Truth

My reality is constantly blurred by the mists of words.

Oscar Wilde, Victorian playwright and dandy[1]

UNDERSTANDING THE CHALLENGE OF EXPLORING SENSITIVE MATERIAL

We have spent the last two chapters exploring the nuances and techniques that can help us to gather a comprehensive database in a sensitive fashion, the second way-station on our map. With these two chapters under our belts, you would think we'd be done with the topic of data gathering. We're not. One critically important caveat to uncovering a useful database has not yet been touched upon – truth. To clarify the issue, let me return to the metaphor with which we opened our study of the clinical interview.

Earlier we had likened the initial interview to a person exploring an old Victorian room with only a candle in hand, the limited light source representing an exterior hindrance to the endeavor at hand. However, a weak light source does not represent the only barrier to the familiarization with the antique furniture scattered about, because the *method* of exploration can provide internal barriers to the effectiveness of gathering an accurate picture of the room. For instance, one explorer may walk about with his hands held only at shoulder level, hence missing all the curios lying upon a well-polished table. A second explorer may underuse her sense of hearing, thus ignoring the presence of a clock tucked away in a quiet niche beside Sarah Bernhardt's portrait. A third explorer may be afraid of dark corners, thus never spotting the elaborately carved chess set hidden away in the shadows. Thus, it is not only a matter of determining what data needs to be gathered, it is also a question of determining how one wants to go about gathering it, for one alters the database by the style with which one elicits it.

For these reasons it is beneficial to explore the issues that determine the validity of the database, issues that are affected not only by the defenses of our patients, but by the defenses and idiosyncratic traits of each clinician's style. On some occasions, it may not be the patient who is standing in the way of accurate information, but rather the clinician.

To understand these limitations and the interviewing techniques that allow us to supersede them, we must first look at what we mean by the term "validity." Statisticians discuss a variety of forms of validity, including content validity, empirical validity, and construct validity. To discuss all three of these concepts is beyond the scope of our study. Instead, we will look at an admittedly simplified concept of validity, which nevertheless sheds considerable light by its clinical application. From our perspectives as everyday clinicians working in hectic everyday environments, validity can be formulated in a no-nonsense fashion as the answer to a simple question, "Are we hearing the truth?"

And this is not to suggest that our patients are lying, for I have found manipulative deceit to be relatively rare with my patients. No. There are a myriad of other factors that prevent us from uncovering the truth including a host of unconscious defense mechanisms (i.e., rationalization, intellectualization, denial, and repression), the vagaries of memory itself, unrecognized miscommunications between clinician and patient, the limitations of all humans to see and know the truth, and genuine fears related to stigmatization as well as realistic concerns of "what will happen to me or my family members, if I tell the truth?"

Indeed, one of the first rude awakenings for any of us that has ever performed a clinical interview is the revelation that we basically function in the dark. We do not know for certain what is going on in our patient's mind. We never will. The delicate arabesques of the mind cannot be easily transferred from one individual brain to the next. Even direct conversation is, at best, a second-generation copy of internal experience, brimming with all of the problems associated with second-generation copies such as information drop-outs and distortions.

Yet our ability to sensitively uncover the troubling secrets of our patients – whether they be thoughts of suicide, histories of incest or domestic violence, substance abuse, an eating disorder, or any act that may create shame or guilt – is at the heart of our ability to relieve their pain. We cannot undertake effective crisis intervention, or begin optimal ongoing therapy, if we do not know what the real crisis, stressors, and diagnoses may be.

Besides the simple fact that we need to know the real problem and its extent in order to maximize our ability to help (with a suicidal patient we cannot get a gun out of a house if we do not know it is there in the first place), there is another reason that uncovering hidden pain is such an important set of skills for an interviewer to master: If we are able to help a patient to share a difficult topic, such as domestic violence, incest, or suicidal thought, which he or she may never have shared with another human being before, we are not only uncovering important information, we are providing a powerful new interpersonal experience.

We will have convincingly demonstrated, directly to the patient, that he or she was able to talk about a stigmatizing topic in detail, and the listener showed both compassion and understanding. Moreover, the listener did not over- or under-react. The reassuring discovery that there are people in this world that one can talk to about topics even as taboo as incest, domestic violence, and suicide may have already set the stage for the immediate first movement towards healing, for once the patient steps out of our office, he or she has a very difficult decision to make: should they return? It is now this patient's first-hand knowledge that "it wasn't so hard to talk with this person about my most frightening secrets" that may prompt them to see us again and to follow up with our immediate treatment recommendations. In these instances, it is the reassuring experience of an unexpected sense of safety, which we created, that has provided the first kindling of hope.

Sometimes the result of helping a patient to share a hidden secret in a safe environment may have an even more dramatic, yet unexpected, effect. It may save the patient's life at a later date. The memory of such a positive interviewing experience with us, even when we may be functioning as a clinician at a telephone crisis center or in an emergency department, may prompt the caller or patient, months later during a particularly desperate night, to reach for a phone and not a gun.

Also of major importance are those situations in which our patients are a danger to others as well as themselves, or perhaps only to others. We have all interacted with an intoxicated patient, who may also be at risk for committing domestic violence (or has recently done so). And on some occasions during a first meeting, as we have already seen, we may become suspicious that our patient is experiencing psychotic process. At such moments, we will need to raise and explore the possibility of psychosis in a fashion that is not disengaging, yet allows us to uncover possibly dangerous psychotic process directed at others, such as command hallucinations or paranoid delusions. It is here that the skills examined in this chapter (and in our chapters on psychosis; see Part II) may help us to prevent tragedies, such as the unpublicized killing of a parent by a teenaged child suffering from a psychotic manic episode to the much publicized slayings at Virginia Tech or an unsuspecting movie theater in a quiet Colorado town.

As if the above reasons were not enough to emphasize the importance of learning how to sensitively raise and explore taboo material, these skills are also useful for revealing those occasions when the patient's intentions may not be in his or her own best interest. For instance, a patient suffering from schizophrenia who wants to return to work too quickly, a decision that might result in a severe relapse and perhaps prevent a return to work for years, may not readily tell the interviewer about the persistence of serious auditory hallucinations. On the other hand, a different patient, not suffering from schizophrenia at all but actively seeking disability, may tell the clinician about a plethora of tormenting yet non-existent voices.

Thus, it is important for the interviewer to be alert for signs that the patient harbors a hidden agenda, such as needing a mental health professional to document that the patient is too ill to appear in court or to provide the patient with addictive drugs. For instance, in an emergency department setting, it is not uncommon for people with imminent court appearances to seem unusually interested in hospital admission, because hospitalization may represent a clever and logical excuse for missing the court date.

The validity techniques we are about to explore have been developed over the past several decades by a variety of interviewing innovators across a variety of disciplines including counseling, psychology, psychiatry, nursing, and social work. Some of these techniques are specifically geared to decrease the likelihood of deception, thus increasing the likelihood of valid information. They can even help a patient with antisocial propensities to share more of the truth about their problematic behaviors such as being a perpetrator of domestic violence or other problems with the law. When utilized effectively, these techniques can elicit sensitive material that one might think would never be revealed during an initial contact. And, indeed, it would not have been revealed had not the patient been provided a safe environment for sharing and the interviewer used skilled interviewing techniques within that environment.

As we begin our study of the validity techniques that address the above issues, we will see that they come in four clusters: (1) techniques for improving generalized recall, (2) strategies for avoiding miscommunication, (3) techniques designed to help us raise a sensitive or taboo topic without disengaging the patient, and (4) techniques for carefully exploring a sensitive area once it has been raised.

VALIDITY TECHNIQUES: KEYS TO ELICITING SENSITIVE MATERIAL

Cluster One: Techniques for Improving Generalized Recall

The Dilemma

It is not only our words that bring on the mists that blur reality, as Oscar Wilde described in our opening epigram. Neurons do. As I have interviewed over the years, it has become increasingly clear to me how unreliable memories actually are, even those reported by patients as, "I remember it like it was yesterday." Neurons are not computer circuits made of microchips; they are biological entities made of goo. This state of affairs contributes to the fact that memories, even when first deposited in long-term biological circuits, are not necessarily exact. Even more striking is the fact that stored memories may be altered by new memories in a completely unconscious fashion.

Let me share two personal, non-clinical, encounters with memory drop-out and distortion that powerfully demonstrate the dilemma. I have had a rare opportunity to study my own memory at work (or rather, not at work, as the case may be), for I have kept a journal intermittently for 35 years.

One day I was perusing a journal entry from a trip to London I undertook when I was a third-year medical student, fortunate to be doing my obstetrics rotation in Nottingham, England, as an exchange student. I had gone to London for about a week and had become good friends with a fellow medical student I met there for the first time. He and I, according to several detailed journal entries, had great adventures hopping around pubs in merry old England and walking about Piccadilly Circus. And here is the catch. Despite having clearly spent days with an individual who was important enough for me to devote pages of journal writing to our shared experiences, I had no memory of him. I could not picture his face, a single conversation, or a single moment of laughter. I don't believe this rather striking example of substantial memory drop-out can be entirely attributed to the pints of bitter (English name for a type of pale beer) I imbibed in our nightly escapades. At least, let's hope not. To the contrary, it illustrates that memory often has a fatigue to it; memory drop-out is a normal, not atypical, aspect of the human brain.

On another day I stumbled upon a journal entry about a big argument I had had with a relative who had inappropriately yelled and sworn at my 5-year-old son. Being the petty person that I try not to be, I recalled this incident for several years and always got angry, especially about his swearing at my son. I remembered it like it was yesterday. Only one problem: He hadn't sworn. I was so mad on the day it had happened that I had written down exactly what he said, in quotations, because I wanted it to be available to show him someday if I needed some interpersonal ammo. Talk about petty! But that's another story altogether. The point for us today is the striking memory distortion that *began within hours*. In this case, my neurological goo created a "fact" that had no basis in fact. Not only a false fact, but it was *the* "fact" that most upset me emotionally about the incident. Strange indeed! I have come to believe that such strange happenings are occurring when our patients are reporting "the facts" much more often than we might be aware.

Anchor Questions

Anchor questions are designed to address the above problems to generalized recall by "stirring" the memory banks of the patient. The goal is to activate important memories that we are trying to uncover by kindling memory circuits that are nearby. Anchor questions come in two main types: time-related and location-related.

Anchor Questions (Focused Upon Time)

Danny Carlat, in his outstanding primer on clinical interviewing, coined the term "anchor question."[2] Carlat pulls on the research of Sudman and Bradburn showing that people tend to remember significant distant events in relation to other memorable events that were happening in their lives, or in their culture, near the moment of the memory being recalled.[3] A person might be better able to tell us when something happened, not with a question such as, "When did you first begin drinking?" but with a question such as, "Did you begin drinking before or after you started high school?"

Carlat suggests that a variety of events can be used to help people pinpoint the timing of recalled events more effectively including: personal events (graduations, accidents, buying a house, moving to a new city, starting a new job), major cultural events (the assassination of President Kennedy, landing on the moon, the O. J. Simpson trial, 9–11), or cultural markers (holidays like Christmas or New Year's Eve, the turn of the century). Let's see the technique at work with a trauma victim, where memories are often hidden in mists. We will picture a woman in her mid-20s who has been dating the same man since high school. They have had their troubles off and on for years. According to her, he has become physically abusive recently:

> **Pt.:** Don't get me wrong, things haven't always been bad, or I wouldn't be with him still.
>
> **Clin.:** It sounds like you have had many good times in the past. I don't doubt that. Obviously, the recent violence is very disturbing to all involved. If you can, try to give me a better idea of when he actually started to become violent?
>
> **Pt.:** Oh, that's pretty recent.
>
> **Clin.:** By pretty recent, how do you mean?
>
> **Pt.:** About a year ago. (pauses) Yeah, I think that's about right.

Clin.: I remember you told me that you moved here to New Hampshire about 2 years ago. Had he ever hit or slapped you before you came to New Hampshire? (anchor question focused on time)

Pt.: Hmm. Well (pauses) … yes, yes he did. I remember he slapped me once pretty bad back in our apartment in Pittsburgh. We used to call it "The Nest." We loved that little place, but yeah, he did slap me there, now that I think about it.

Clin.: How about before that, say back when you were in graduate school? (anchor question focused on time)

Pt.: We weren't living together then.

Clin.: Oh, I know that. Can you remember though if, perhaps on a date or if he stayed over or something, did he ever hit you or slap you back then?

Pt.: My God. (looks up, with a puzzled and surprised expression) You know, he did. I sort of put it out of my mind. One day, after we came back from a party one of my friends in graduate school had given, he got really mad at me, saying I was flirting with another grad student. I wasn't, by the way. But he got really mad.

Clin.: And what happened?

Pt.: He slapped me. Right across my face. It really hurt.

Clin.: Tell me a little more about what happened that night.

Notice the clinician slowly walking the patient back in time with the use of serial time-related anchor questions, a strategy that sometimes yields surprising results both for the interviewer and the patient. In this instance, the gentle uncovering of memories has initiated the therapeutic process. Insight has begun, even during the first interview.

Anchor Questions (Focused on Location)

Here is a technique frequently used by cognitive–behavioral therapists that I have found very useful in the initial interview. It is a form of anchor question, but the goal is slightly different than with the time-focused anchor question of Carlat. It, too, jogs the patient's memory, but not about a date. Instead, it is used if the patient is about to describe a specific event that occurred – a dissociated event, a panic attack, a suicide attempt, an act of domestic violence – that one fears may be distorted or repressed. The goal is to maximize the validity of the reporting by ensuring that the patient is picturing a specific memory and not just a blurred collection of similar memories. If the patient can re-visit a specific memory bank, the hope is that as they "re-live" the specific memory, more and more details of the memory will spring back.

To accomplish this task, the interviewer asks several questions in a row about the details of where the patient was when the experience occurred. Once locked into a specific memory bank in this manner, the subsequent details often begin to tumble out in a more valid fashion. Naturally, with dissociated memories or violent memories, one only uses these techniques if one feels it is important to uncover certain details and one feels the patient can safely, in a psychological sense, re-visit these memories at that moment.

Suppose a patient has come to you complaining of generalized anxiety, but as you hear more of the story, you become suspicious that they are having panic attacks. In the following dialogue, watch how the interviewer locks the patient into a specific potential panic attack.

> **Pt.:** I guess I've always just been sort of wired, but it sure has gotten out of hand.
>
> **Clin.:** When you say "out of hand" does the anxiety ever come on, really suddenly, out of nowhere, and it is really intense, sort of overwhelming?
>
> **Pt.:** That doesn't happen a lot, but it's what has been happening more and more.
>
> **Clin.:** I want you to picture the very worst episode like that. (pauses) Can you picture when that was?
>
> **Pt.:** Oh yeah, absolutely, it was pretty bad.
>
> **Clin.:** Where were you when it happened? (anchor question focused on location)
>
> **Pt.:** I was out driving with my son.
>
> **Clin.:** What road were you on? (anchor question focused on location)
>
> **Pt.:** I had just picked my son up from school. I was just outside of Concord. (the interviewer has now tapped a specific memory bank, the patient is picturing a real event unfolding in real time)
>
> **Clin.:** And what happened?
>
> **Pt.:** Well, it was really weird. I can't really explain why it happened, but all of a sudden I got really worried that something bad, real bad, was going to happen. I started breathing really really fast, and I couldn't stop. It was scary. I actually pulled the car over and …

Tagging Questions

Carlat also describes a nice technique for cuing a patient's memory about a concrete topic from a list that the patient is having trouble recalling even though the topic is not a sensitive one.[4] For instance, a patient may have trouble remembering a specific medication he or she has been on, a type of psychotherapy that has been used, or the name of a therapist.

If one asked a patient, "What medication were you on back in Pennsylvania?" and the patient answered, "You know, I don't really remember what it was called, I know it was for depression." Then one could use a tagging question. The clinician does this by simply offering a list of medications from which the patient then tags the correct answer, "Do you remember if it was called Prozac, Zoloft, Celexa, Effexor?" To which the patient might respond, "Oh yeah, that's it. It was called Celexa. It worked really well for me, but was kind of expensive."

Exaggeration

Before leaving the techniques related to improving generalized recall, there is a creative technique for helping to reduce shame if we begin to see it arise as we explore sensitive material. Sometimes, despite our best efforts to convey Rogerian unconditional positive regard, it is obvious that an overly conscientious patient is suddenly feeling an inordinate amount of shame about a "bad" behavior that he or she has just revealed. Although the behavior may seem fairly insignificant, the interviewer should never forget that the accompanying shame in the patient may be far from insignificant. If this is not addressed, such painful moments experienced in the initial interview may drive the patient away from the entire process of therapy. At such times, Othmer and Othmer sometimes employ a validity technique that they call "exaggeration."[5]

Exaggeration is a technique for immediately decreasing a patient's inordinate shame, so as to increase the likelihood that he or she will continue to share sensitive material, while simultaneously securing engagement. In this sense, the technique of exaggeration is not only a validity technique, it is an effective engagement technique.

Exaggeration works by helping the patient understand that when his or her "shameful activity" is put into perspective with other types of human "wrongdoings," the patient's activity is not of great magnitude, highlighting the fact that you, as an interviewer, are far from aghast at the patient's revelation. Effective "exaggeration" requires a well-timed sense of humor by the clinician, employed in an already well-secured therapeutic alliance. When done well, as demonstrated below, it can release a marked amount of interpersonal tension that otherwise could have resulted in disengagement.

In this vignette, the patient is a conservatively dressed woman with her hair tied into a meticulous bun. She is a successful department store manager with a portable "time-clock" for a superego. She strives for perfection and expects it of herself. She has unfortunately developed a nagging generalized anxiety disorder, for which she has reluctantly sought treatment, despite the admonitions of her superego that "strong people do not go to therapists." In her social history she shares what for her is a major sin of the past, stealing a candy bar from a drugstore when she was 10 years old. And even worse, she got away with it. Up to this point, the interviewer has established a nice rapport with her, but she senses the surprising intensity of the patient's shame:

Clin.: In the past, have you ever had any problems with the law or arrests?

Pt.: I was never arrested (pauses, eyes briefly turn to the floor). But I did steal something once. I know it was a wrong thing to do.

Clin.: Oh, what did you steal?

Pt.: I stole a candy bar when I was about 10. I feel badly about it. I know it wasn't right to do (patient appears clearly uncomfortable with herself and hastens to add) – I haven't stolen anything since.

Clin.: So let me get this straight. At 10 years old you entered a store, pulled out a knife, stole $200 worth of clothing, pocketed $500 of jewelry, and, as you left, kicked the store owner's half-blind cat (clinician smiles).

Pt.: (Absolutely aghast) Oh my gosh no! (she suddenly catches on to the humor and smiles for the first time in 20 minutes) Of course not (sheepishly smiling). I guess it wasn't that bad after all.

Clin.: Not bad (said with a feigned sternness). Why, you stole a Milky Way bar, didn't you! One of the big ones too, I bet. My gosh, I have a mind to call the cops right now, but the statute of limitations has probably expired.

Pt.: (laughing and smiling) Okay, okay, I get the point. I take things too seriously sometimes (continues to chuckle).

Clin.:   (with a normal tone of voice) You know, Jane, let me go out on a limb here. I bet you tend to get down on yourself pretty hard.

Pt.:   Well, I guess you could say that (smiling).

Clin.:   Maybe that is something we can take a look at in the therapy. It may be one of the reasons that you are so anxious. Does that sound like a good idea to you?

Pt.:   Yes. I think that would be a very good thing to do. Although I'm a little bit afraid to do it.

In most cases, "exaggeration" is utilized by employing much shorter phrases. When it is done well, as with this delightful bit of interviewing, it can effectively transform some difficult moments.

Cluster Two: Validity Techniques for Avoiding Miscommunication

Defining Technical Terms

Some terms we use, such as diagnostic terms or terms for complex symptoms, are clearly potentially confusing. Terms such as bipolar disorder, psychosis, and paranoia are inherently technical. Naturally we would always explain them. But, sometimes, a term is frequently used by both professionals and the lay public (depression, addiction) and not always in the same way. It's easy to slip these words into a conversation and not realize that they are being misinterpreted. It is here that Carlat has yet another nice interviewing strategy – simply put, define the technical term even though it doesn't sound that technical. Carlat provides such a nice example of this technique that I'll just let him share it himself[6]:

Clin.:   How old were you when you first remember feeling depressed?

Pt.:   Hard to say. It feels like I have always been depressed.

Clin.:   Just to clarify, I'm not talking about the kind of sadness that we all experience from time to time. I'm trying to understand when you first felt what we call a clinical depression, and by that I mean that you were so down that it seriously affected your functioning, so that, for example, it might have interfered with your sleep, your appetite, your ability to concentrate, your ability to work. When do you remember first experiencing something that severe?

Pt.:   Oh, that just started a month ago. I've never been depressed like this before. Ever.

It's possible that this patient is suffering from a long-term dysthymic disorder in addition to her more recent major depression. The clinician's interviewing skills have prevented the mistake of viewing her as suffering from many years of a major depression, which could have led to some missteps in treatment recommendations.

Clarifying Norms

I have found over the years that it is not just technical terms that can lead to miscommunication between interviewer and patient. A common problem arises when exploring sensitive or taboo topics in which the culture, in general, or the patient's family, in particular, has taken a traditionally enabling stance. I have seen many clinicians ask patients questions such as, "Have you ever been sexually abused by someone" and receive a convincing "no" when, in reality, there has been substantial abuse. This problem is not about stigma. In fact, it is the opposite problem.

This phenomenon arises because the patient grew up in a family where psychological, physical, and/or sexually abusive behavior was the norm, and the patient has no idea (although they often have vague misgivings about the behaviors) that what was done was inappropriate. Thus, the patient above was not minimizing; he or she literally does not know that he or she was abused. I think you will not infrequently encounter this type of miscommunication when enquiring about sexual abuse, physical abuse, verbal abuse, and drinking behaviors (many families accept alcoholic behavior as normal). Be on the lookout for it.

When raising these topics in an initial interview, I often find it useful to use a strategy I call "clarifying norms" early on. I will use sexual abuse as an example:

Clin.: You mentioned that your dad was a heavy drinker and hit you a lot. Sometimes when drinking and violence are around, there can also be sexual abuse. Did your dad ever sexually abuse you that you can remember?

Pt.: Oh no, nothing like that, not that I remember (said with conviction). I mean if he tried something like that, I wouldn't have let him.

Clin.: Of course, problems like that can occur in different ways. At any point, as you were growing up, did your dad try to do things like touching you in your private areas, fondling you or doing things like asking you to watch him undress or did he watch you undress or shower? (clarifying norms) Although these can be hard to talk about, try to remember if he did any of those types of things with you?

Pt.: Well, sort of. I mean, he used to watch me shower all the time (pauses) – he still asks me to do it when I go home sometimes (the patient is 17 years old), but I don't let him anymore.

Clin.: When he used to do that, what exactly did he do?

Pt.: He sort of snuck in the bathroom while I was showering and just asked me to pull back the curtains.

Clin.: When he did that, did he keep his clothes on, or did he take them off?

Pt.: No, he usually pulled his pants down.

Clin.: When he did stuff like that, did he touch himself, you know, masturbate.

Pt.: (patient looks sheepish) Yeah, now that's the part of it I didn't like. Maybe he shouldn't have done that.

Clin.: Did your mom know about this?

Pt.: Nope. (pauses) He told me he would hurt me bad if I ever told my mom. (pauses) You know, I think my dad might have had sex with my little sister.

Here is some really nice interviewing in which important material is being uncovered. The little sister is 12, and she is still at home. The validity technique of clarifying norms has pulled vital information to the forefront with minimal disengagement. If the clinician had accepted the first "no" of the patient and not clarified the norms, possibly none of this information would have emerged.

Cluster Three: Validity Techniques for Raising a Sensitive or Taboo Topic

Normalization

In this technique, first delineated in the clinical literature in the 2nd edition of this book, the interviewer phrases the question so that the patient realizes that he or she is not the only person who has ever experienced the behaviors or problems under scrutiny.[7] We saw normalization demonstrated with some of the natural gates that we viewed in Video Module 4.1 in our previous chapter. This technique can be very useful in raising essentially any sensitive or taboo area. It is particularly useful with a patient who seems to be guilt ridden or filled with social anxiety that they are odd or doing something bad.

It is a simple technique in which we begin the question by stating or implying that we have heard this behavior from others, metacommunicating that the patient is far from alone in having experienced these feelings or behaviors. Normalizations often begin with words such as, "Sometimes people who have …"

Let's look at a couple of examples to see how it works:

a. "Some of my patients who are really worried about their weight, have told me that they will do things to make sure that they don't gain weight like force themselves to vomit after a meal. Have you ever found yourself doing something like that?"
b. "Sometimes when people get really angry they say things they later regret. Has that ever happened to you?"
c. "It's not unusual when there has been a lot of drinking in a family, like you told me your dad was doing when you were growing up, for there to be some violence. Did your dad ever hit you or your mom or brothers and sisters?"

Normalization is also one of my favorite ways to raise the topic of suicide as with:

"Sometimes when people are as depressed as you have been, they find themselves having thoughts of killing themselves. Have you been having any thoughts like that?"

Numerous variations of normalization can be used to raise the topic of suicide, depending upon the painful circumstances of the patient:

"Sometimes when people have lost their spouse, and I know how much Anne meant to you, they find themselves having thoughts of killing themselves. Have you had any thoughts like that?"
"Sometimes when people are in as much pain as you are describing, they find themselves having thoughts of killing themselves. Have you had any thoughts like that?"

Said with a gentle tone of voice, normalizations often allow a patient to share suicidal thought more openly.

Let us take a look at a similar, but slightly different, validity technique, also very useful for raising the topic of suicide, as well as many other sensitive areas.

Shame Attenuation

There are two types of shame attenuation, also first described in an earlier edition of this book.[8] In the first type, the interviewer cues off of the pain or the situational stress of the patient to enter a sensitive topic, such as suicide. In the second type, the interviewer cues off of the patient's own defense mechanisms (typically rationalizations) to uncover material that the culture views as "bad," such as criminal behavior or substance abuse. Let's take a look at the first type of shame attenuation and how it can offer us yet another graceful bridge into suicidal ideation and other sensitive topics.

Shame Attenuation Used to Bridge From Pain or Situational Stress

With the first type of shame attenuation, the patient's *own pain or situational stress* is used as the gateway to sensitive topics such as suicide or psychotic process (note that there is no mention of any other people in the following question, as we would have seen with a normalization). In practice, the first type of shame attenuation, when bridging off of pain, looks like this:

"With all of your pain, have you been having any thoughts of killing yourself?"

If bridging off of the patient's stress, this first type of shame attenuation looks something like this:

"With everything you've been going through, have you been having any thoughts of killing yourself?"

Very simple, and perhaps a tad less wordy than most normalizations. And, when said with a gentle tone of voice, very effective. One of the things I really like about this first type of shame attenuation when used to raise the topic of suicide (or any other sensitive topic) is how easy it is to use, and it can be used with just about any patient, no matter what the patient's circumstances, for psychological pain and personalized stress are ubiquitous. It is one of my favorite ways to raise the topic of suicide.

By using shame attenuation as a bridge from pain, an interviewer can sensitively raise many other difficult topics. For instance, raising the topic of psychosis is often viewed as difficult to do in an engaging fashion, and rightly so. It is safe to assume that not many patients like the idea that their interviewer suspects they are psychotic. But, with the use of shame attenuation, even this daunting challenge to engagement is surprisingly easy. I have found the following question effective at this task: "With all of the pain you have been having, are your thoughts ever so intense that they sound almost like a voice to you?"

It's a wonderfully phrased question for it arises naturally from the patient's immediately preceding self-report of pain and also leaves a "face-saving out" for the patient with the words, "*almost* like a voice." Thus, he or she does not have to admit to hearing voices immediately and can say something like, "Well, sort of, but I don't think they are voices." With further questioning, we can sort out whether or not we feel voices may be present. If present, we can follow up by hunting for command hallucinations (voices that are telling the patient to do something) such as commands to kill themselves or harm another.

As we saw demonstrated in our chapter on facilics, both normalizations and shame attenuations are often utilized with natural gates. Their use with natural gates is particularly popular for transitioning from a non-sensitive topic into a sensitive or taboo topic.

Shame Attenuation Used to Uncover Aggressive, Unethical, and Antisocial Behaviors

Let us, for a moment, take a look at our second type of shame attenuation. It can be highly effective at entering a topic such as substance abuse or violence by cuing off the patient's own rationalizations and defense mechanisms for doing the behavior. Unlike our first type of shame attenuation (in which we cued off of the patient's legitimate pain or reality-based stress), in the second type of shame attenuation we will cue off of a patient's *distorted* view of reality caused by *common everyday* defense mechanisms. Not infrequently, what a patient states as the problem (e.g., "my boss is an asshole") is not necessarily the real problem (or the only problem). The patient's behaviors may be the main problem, as with alcoholism.

The challenge with trying to uncover behaviors viewed as bad by the culture (such as antisocial behaviors) is the fact that if the patient answers positively to our question, he or she may feel they are admitting that "I'm a bad person" or will get into trouble. The natural result is a feeling of shame and/or guilt, which can clearly act as a deterrent to open expression on the part of the patient and can also damage engagement. The word "attenuate," which simply means "lessen," was used for this validity technique because this technique is very effective at lessening the patient's shame or guilt by phrasing the question using the lens of the patient's own rationalizations. The basic premise of this form of shame attenuation is that if we can figure out the patient's rationalizations for why he or she is doing something and then ask the question from the perspective of the patient's own rationalizations, perhaps the patient may be more likely to answer openly.

To effectively use this second type of shame attenuation, the interviewer must be able to do two things: (1) intuit how the patient has rationalized their own behaviors so that they seem okay to do and (2) ask the question while viewing the situation through the eyes of the patient and using the patient's rationalizations. A shame attenuation can either be a statement made before a question (that places the context of the question from the patient's perspective) or can be part of the question itself. This technique is a little harder to understand until we see it used.

For example, picture a patient who relates feeling depressed and angry at the world. As you move deeper into the interview, you begin to intuit that the patient is a big-time drinker with essentially no insight into his or her drinking problem.

If a clinician chose to ask, "Do you think you have a drinking problem?" many such patients would answer with a rather shocked "no." In addition, the question itself might disengage the patient. But in the following example we will see a different approach – the application of shame attenuation – that results not only in more valid information but causes no disengagement at all:

> **Pt.:** I guess some of my best times are with my friends. I really would rather be with my male friends than with my wife and some of her losers. Talk about boring, they invented the word.
>
> **Clin.:** Are these the same guys who are your drinking buddies?
>
> **Pt.:** Yep. They're the ones.
>
> **Clin.:** Well where do you guys like to go for a brew?
>
> **Pt.:** All over the place. We'll tie one on anyplace anytime.
>
> **Clin.:** You know, when you are out with your buddies like that, do you have a problem holding your liquor or are you pretty good at holding your liquor? (shame attenuation)
>
> **Pt.:** Oh, I don't have any problems holding my liquor. I'm not the best mind you, but I can hold my own.
>
> **Clin.:** How much can you put-down in a single night?
>
> **Pt.:** Oh a six-pack, twelve-pack, no problem (said with a cheerful sense of pride).
>
> **Clin.:** How often in a given week do you drink a six-pack or twelve-pack, in all seriousness.
>
> **Pt.:** In all seriousness … I'd say two or three nights a week. Well, make that two nights. It's usually only on weekend nights that I really go after it. By the way, I held down a case one night (pauses) well I sort of held it down (smiles sheepishly).

In this example the interviewer has phrased the question in such a way ("… when you are out with your buddies like that, do you have a problem holding your liquor or are you pretty good at holding your liquor?") that if the patient answers with a positive to the last part of the phrase ("Oh, I don't have any problems holding my liquor. I'm not the best mind you, but I can hold my own"), then he or she is actually stroking his or her own ego as opposed to admitting a flaw. In fact, to admit that "I have problems holding my liquor" represents the answer more likely to produce shame.

This exchange is both more comfortable for the patient while also more likely to yield valid data than a direct question such as, "Do you think you might have a drinking problem?" or "Do you think you are an alcoholic?" Of course, one must also make sure that the patient is not purely bragging. This can usually be accomplished by subsequently delineating the actual drinking history via specific questions aimed at eliciting behavioral specifics, as this interviewer was just beginning to do.

This technique is so valuable that we ought to see it in a different context. In this instance the clinician is suspicious that the patient has had problems with irresponsibility and angry exchanges on the job with his bosses. However, the patient is somewhat cagey around this topic. The clinician has also accurately intuited that this particular patient does not see himself as the problem. In his view, the bosses are the problem.

Consequently, the technique of shame attenuation is used to create a safer environment for the patient to share things as he sees them "going down" at the office.

Clin.: What have your jobs been like?

Pt.: Oh, nothing special, I've always gotten along okay.

Clin.: Ever have any problems on the job?

Pt.: Nah, none worth mentioning.

Clin.: How about with bosses, have you had any bosses who really seemed like they needed to be "big shots," you know, the kind that just like to get on somebody's case? (shame attenuation)

Pt.: Now that you mention it, more than I care to think about.

Clin.: What do you do, when a boss gets off on a power trip like that? (another shame attenuation)

Pt.: Oh, I let them know where I stand, nobody is going to just push me around.

Clin.: Well, what might you do if the boss seemed out of line?

Pt.: I'd tell him to get off my back, that's what I'd do.

Clin.: How do they usually react?

Pt.: Most of them back off.

Clin.: Any of them ever get mad and fire you?

Pt.: A couple have, but I didn't want to work for them anyway.

Clin.: How many times have you been fired, would you say five times, ten times?

Pt.: Hmm … maybe around five times, somewhere around there.

What a difference skilled interviewing makes. We went from a patient reporting, when asked whether there were any problems on the job, "Nah, none worth mentioning," to an open admission of being fired several times, without even a blip in the engagement process.

Shame attenuation can also be useful in uncovering domestic violence as well. Patients who have anger control problems, even when they might feel they need help, can find it very hard to share acts of domestic violence. Shame attenuation can ease their anxieties and lead gracefully into a more useful exploration of abuse issues with questions such as:

"It sounds like you are super stressed. Do you feel the stress has ever pushed you to do something you really regretted, such as striking your wife or your child, something that is just not like you?"

An important point to remember with regard to the technique of shame attenuation is that the clinician must be careful not to side with the patient or condone the described behavior. Such over-identification gives a false impression to the patient and also conveys an inaccurate moral judgment.

With shame attenuation the clinician does not validate the behavior but metacommunicates that from their clinical experience, they understand how people can fall into such a behavior. In the spirit of Rogerian unconditional regard, the clinician attempts to suspend judgment while voicing the question in such a manner that the patient may respond from the perspective of how he or she sees it. Thus, although a patient with an antisocial personality frequently sees other people as the troublemakers, the clinician neither agrees nor disagrees with this stance. Moreover, the phrasing of the question allows the person with the antisocial structure to express the world as it is seen through his or her own eyes.

Induction to Bragging

In their outstanding text, *The Clinical Interview Using DSM-IV*,[9] Ekkehard and Sieglinde Othmer demonstrate a technique that they call "induction to bragging," which takes shame attenuation one step further. As with shame attenuation, they believe that it is quite effective with people displaying an antisocial character structure. In its simplest form, the clinician attaches a positive adjective to a behavior with a negative association, as with the following question, "Were you a good fighter?" In this simple form it is no different than shame attenuation. But when the clinician actually passes on a compliment to the patient in a statement preceding the question, then "induction to bragging" represents a new and distinct validity technique.

In this use of induction to bragging, the clinician begins with a complimentary statement, which makes it easier for the patient to "almost brag" about a behavior that is somewhat less than exemplary. Othmer and Othmer give as an example, "You seem to be sly like a fox …," a description that a person, shall we say, prone to deceit might find a bit more to his or her liking than "You're a deceitful son of a bitch, aren't you?" – not that a clinician would say the latter, although many of us have thought it. After giving the above compliment, the clinician can then proceed to inquire about deceitful behavior in a more productive fashion, fueled by the patient's desire to live up to the compliment.

Let's see how induction to bragging can help a patient to share self-incriminating information:

> **Clin.:** What other types of things did you and your buddies do back in high school?
>
> **Pt.:** Oh, we hung out together. I'm not saying we were a gang or something, but we were somebody you don't mess around with.
>
> **Clin.:** Well, you are obviously very big and clearly work out regularly, I bet you don't take any shit from anybody? (induction to bragging) How many fights have you actually been in?
>
> **Pt.:** Oh, a lot. I could really hold my own.
>
> **Clin.:** Did you ever use a knife on anybody?
>
> **Pt.:** Don't need to. I got these (patient holds fists up and smiles). I used a tire chain on some guy once.

Unlike Othmer and Othmer, I like to limit the use of the term "induction to bragging" to those situations in which the clinician literally compliments the patient in a prefatory statement, so as to clearly distinguish it from shame attenuation. For example, when using *shame attenuation* a clinician might inquire about whether the patient may deserve some praise ("What do you do, do you tend to take their shit or are you the kind of guy who likes to let the boss know where you stand?"). In contrast, with *induction to bragging* there is a direct, clear-cut complement ("Well, you are obviously very big and clearly work out regularly, I bet you don't take any shit from anybody.").

It is not necessary, or typical, to use "swear words" with patients, such as the word "shit" in the example above. But occasionally it may be useful. In this case, the patient had first used the word earlier in the interview, thus the interviewer chose to mirror the patient's own phrasing, a process that potentially enhanced the power of the induction to bragging. If uncomfortable with such a word, the clinician can opt to not use it, for there are many alternative phrasings. Interviewers must use what feels natural to them.

Cluster Four: Validity Techniques for Exploring a Sensitive Topic Once It Has Been Raised

Behavioral Incident

To begin our exploration of this cluster, we will look at a validity technique known as "the behavioral incident," which was developed by Pascal and Jenkins and presented in an eminently useful fashion by Pascal in his book, *The Practical Art of Diagnostic Interviewing*.[10] The basic concept can be delineated as follows.

When a clinician is particularly concerned about gaining accurate information, it is often best to ask the patient to describe specific historical details as opposed to asking the patient his or her opinions about these details. Once a patient is asked to give an opinion, the validity of the data becomes more suspect, because the clinician does not know how accurate the patient's perceptions may be.

All kinds of factors may predispose a patient to provide distorted information when asked for his or her opinion, including unconscious defense mechanisms, fears of stigmatization, fears of the consequences of telling the truth, a need to appear important, a need to minimize bad behaviors, conscious manipulation or malingering, inaccurate perceptions caused by lack of maturity or intellectual dysfunction, a communication misunderstanding of what the interviewer is asking, and peer pressure to distort the truth or protect somebody.

For instance, if the clinician wants to determine whether a patient dates frequently, an interviewee may respond to a patient-opinion question such as "Do you date fairly regularly?" with a simple "yes," because he or she may be embarrassed to relate a sparse dating pattern. To sidestep this problem, the clinician could specifically ask about the frequency of dates over the past several years and ultimately the past several months. If the clinician finds only several dates spanning the past 12 months, then the clinician will have discovered a lack of dating activity without necessarily embarrassing the patient. As Pascal states, in general it is best for clinicians to make their own judgment based on the details of the story itself, for it seems unwise to assume that patients can objectively describe matters that have strong subjective implications.

Pascal calls the discrete historical behaviors elicited "behavioral incidents." I like to also utilize the term "behavioral incident" to refer to the actual interviewing technique itself. In this sense, there are two types of behavioral incidents. In the first style (fact-finding behavioral incidents), the clinician asks for a specific and concrete bit of behavioral information or a train of thought, such as "Did you load the gun?" or "What thoughts were going through your mind at that moment?" In the second type (sequencing behavioral incidents), the clinician simply asks the patient to "chronologically" unfold the story with questions such as, "What happened next?" or "Right after your friend accused you of lying, what was the very next thing you said to him?" Below are some other examples of behavioral incidents:

1. "When you say you 'threw a fit,' what exactly what did you do?" (fact-finding behavioral incident)
2. "Did you put the razor blade up to your wrist?" (fact-finding behavioral incident)
3. "How long did you leave it there?" (fact-finding behavioral incident)
4. "What did your boyfriend say right after he hit you?" (sequencing behavioral incident)
5. "Tell me the next thing that went through your mind?" (sequencing behavioral incident)

Pascal believes that interviewers frequently collect invalid data because they do not ask specifically for such concrete information. It is an extremely useful principle, worthy of illustration.

Let us assume that an interviewer is interested in accurately determining the amount of open affection shared between a woman and her husband. We will look at two hypothetical dialogues with the same woman but with different interviewers. In the first excerpt, the interviewer asks primarily for the patient's opinions, a process that yields invalid data. In the second excerpt, the sensitive use of behavioral incidents provides a different story.

Interviewer 1

    Pt.: Basically I've been very busy, what with the kids and my mother getting sick.

    Clin.: Do you feel happy with your husband's support? (patient-opinion question)

    Pt.: Yes … yes he's been fairly good about it all.

    Clin.: Is he very affectionate? (patient-opinion question)

    Pt.: (pause) Uh-huh, affectionate enough.

    Clin.: Have there been any financial strains?

    Pt.: No, not really. Although the past several months have been a little tight, what with decreased benefits and a new school year starting.

Interviewer 2

    Pt.: Basically I've been very busy, what with the kids and my mother getting sick.

    Clin.: What kinds of things does your husband do to support you? (fact-finding behavioral incident)

    Pt.: Well, he's been a little less demanding, he doesn't get upset if the dirty dishes stack up a little longer or a shirt is a little wrinkled.

Clin.:   When he comes home from work, what is his typical routine? (fact-finding behavioral incident)

Pt.:   That's pretty simple. He'll walk in the door, I usually don't see him come in and he goes straight back to his room to change clothes.

Clin.:   And then? (sequencing behavioral incident)

Pt.:   Well, let's see, I usually knock on the door and let him know dinner will be ready.

Clin.:   Do you go in and talk with him then? (fact-finding behavioral incident)

Pt.:   No, I go straight back. Oh, I usually peek in and say hello, but I have to get back to the stove.

Clin.:   During the course of the night, is he the type of man who likes to hug, or does he prefer to keep a little more to himself? (patient-opinion question)

Pt.:   Well, let me see, he really doesn't hug a lot. No I can't say he does.

Clin.:   Do you remember the last time he hugged you? (fact-finding behavioral incident)

Pt.:   I honestly can't remember (patient's affect is becoming more sad).

Clin.:   You look a little sad. How long has it been since he last hugged you? (fact-finding behavioral incident)

Pt.:   (patient looks at interviewer and pauses with a little sigh) I think the last time he hugged me was about 6 months ago near Christmas. I remember because I was so pleased by it. It's rare for him to touch me like that anymore. (pause) It didn't used to be this way … (breaks into tears).

Clearly, the second interviewer seems to have uncovered a different and more valid story than the first one. Through the gentle use of behavioral incidents, the second clinician has gathered evidence that problems exist in the marriage, a situation the first interviewer missed.

I have found Pascal's concept of the intentional use of behavioral incidents to be one of the most powerful interviewing techniques I have ever learned. It is elegant in its simplicity, powerful in its execution. There is one tough clinical situation where I have found the application of a series of behavioral incidents into a flexible interviewing strategy to be invaluable. Specifically, when one is faced with the task of uncovering a highly sensitive or painful incident, such as a suicide attempt or an act of domestic violence, the serial use of behavioral incidents is remarkably effective at "getting the facts." Here, invalid data (a patient downplaying the seriousness of his or her suicidal intent) is a mistake that can prove to be fatal.

I like to call this strategy "making a verbal video," a term that is very popular with trainees because it so vividly captures the core of the strategy. In cognitive–behavioral therapies the process is often called a "chain analysis."

When making a verbal video, the interviewer interweaves a series of fact-finding and sequencing behavioral incidents that prompts the patient to create a verbal "walk-through" of what happened. If done well, the clinician should be able to see exactly what happened in his or her own mind, allowing him or her to better evaluate the extent of action taken towards suicide by the patient or the degree of violence involved in the act of domestic violence. If the patient suddenly skips ahead, creating a gap in the verbal video (we call these "Nixon Gaps"), the interviewer simply rewinds the video by asking the patient to go back to where the gap began and prompts the story to re-start from there with more behavioral incidents. Let's see this serial use of behavioral incidents at work.

Helping a Patient to Describe an Episode of Intimate Partner Violence (IPV)

We are interviewing a young woman in an emergency department late at night. She has come in following an incident of domestic violence. We have engaged her well, effectively tending to the array of emotional needs of a survivor of recent violence. We are at the point in our interview in which it is critical to determine the extent of the violence, for we need to determine whether the patient can safely return home or whether she needs to stay with a friend or go to a shelter due to a high risk of further violence.

But here's the rub. It can be very hard for any person, no matter how strong they may be, to share the extent of IPV for many reasons: defense mechanisms may be masking the extent of the violence, fears of ramifications for the perpetrator may be present, ambivalent feelings for the perpetrator may be present, feelings of humiliation and shame may be active, it can be painful to describe the incident, the perpetrator may have warned of more violence if "our secret" is shared. It is an ideal situation in which to utilize a verbal video composed of behavioral incidents:

Pt.: … I never expected it to get to this point. I'm not even certain what I want to do. Should I stay with him, should I leave him? I just don't know, I just don't know.

Clin.: Just how bad was it tonight?

Pt.: Not that bad (sighs). I mean he better not do it again, but he's been worse.

Clin.: Anne, if you can help me to get a better feel for exactly what happened tonight, I might be better able to help. You said he was yelling at you and he had been drinking heavily, is that right?

Pt.: Yeah, that's right.

Clin.: And then you told me he hit you. How did it go from yelling to hitting?

Pt.: He was screaming about my not holding up my end of things financially. And I mean screaming.

Clin.: Where were you in the house? (fact-finding behavioral incident, note it is also an anchor question focused on location, to enhance recall)

Pt.: Oh, we were in the kitchen. He likes to drink in the kitchen.

Clin.: What happened next? (sequencing behavioral incident)

Pt.: He said, excuse the language, "Get the fuck out of here!" (shakes her head from side to side with a weak smile of disbelief). I told him I'm not getting the fuck out of here because I live here, in fact it's my house.

Clin.: And then what happened? (sequencing behavioral incident)

Pt.: He screamed, "you little bitch" and he hit me. (looks down and tears well up)

Clin.: It sounds very frightening to me. (gentle empathic statement, clinician hands patient a box of Kleenex)

Pt.: Thanks.

Clin.: Did he hit you with his fist? (fact-finding behavioral incident)

Pt.: Yeah, it really really hurt?

Clin.: Where did he hit you? (fact-finding behavioral incident)

Pt.:	Right here (points to her temple).
Clin.:	Did it knock you to the ground? (fact-finding behavioral incident)
Pt.:	Yeah (note that such a blow can be dangerous and, from a factual perspective, it's not really consistent with her previous description of the violence being "Not that bad.")
Clin.:	Then what happened? (sequencing behavioral incident)
Pt.:	I don't know, it just took its course and he left. (here we have a "Nixon Gap")
Clin.:	Go back for a moment to right after he hit you. What exactly happened next? (clinician returned to where the gap began and re-started the verbal video with a sequencing behavioral incident)
Pt.:	He started screaming again.
Clin.:	And then? (sequencing behavioral incident)
Pt.:	He picked up a knife and said, "I ought to shut you up but good." I told him, look I'll leave, if that's what you want. It was sort of scary. And then he said something like, "Fuck you, I'm leaving." And he left.
Clin.:	What did he do with the knife? (fact-finding behavioral incident)
Pt.:	Oh, he had already thrown that down.
Clin.:	What was the last thing he said? (fact-finding behavioral incident)
Pt.:	(sighs) He said, I'd better watch myself or I'd be really sorry.
Clin.:	Where'd he go? (fact-finding behavioral incident)
Pt.:	I don't have any idea.
Clin.:	I assume he has a key? (fact finding behavioral incident)
Pt.:	Oh, yeah, he's got a key alright.
Clin.:	You know, he sounds like he could still be pretty dangerous, for all we know he is drinking as we speak and I don't think that sounds too good.
Pt.:	Yeah, you're probably right, (pauses) but what can I do?

This interviewer has earned her pay tonight. She might also have just saved this patient from making a very dangerous decision. The facts uncovered through her skilled creation of a verbal video certainly suggest that it would not be wise for the patient to return home on this particular evening, and the patient has discovered, through her own words, the seriousness of the situation.

Also note that the interviewer, near the end of the verbal video, specifically asked what the parting words of the perpetrator of violence were ("What was the last thing he said?"). If the patient does not spontaneously share the last words of the perpetrator, I recommend using a direct question to uncover the information as this interviewer illustrated. Sometimes, as the perpetrator exits, he or she will share a specific threat such as, "I'm gonna get you bad, I'm going kill you real good, real soon." With this question, one sometimes uncovers material clearly indicating immediate or near danger for the patient, suggesting the need for a safe haven.

Limitations of Behavioral Incidents

Before we wrap up on the behavioral incident, there remain a few points worth mentioning. First, this form of questioning can be time consuming, and in initial assessments the clinician will need to utilize verbal videos judiciously in areas in which he or she deems validity to be of particular importance.

Second, the great utility of the behavioral incident does not mean that patient-opinion questions are not useful. Quite to the contrary; as we have seen earlier, as person-centered interviewers, we find the patient's perspective to be of paramount importance. Interviewing techniques are generally neither good nor bad. Interviewing techniques are merely more, or less, useful for specific tasks.

Patient-opinion questions are invaluable for understanding the patient's perspectives, needs, opinions, and goals. We have also seen how they allow us to naturalistically observe the patient's defenses and they provide the foundation for collaborative problem solving. They are just not particularly good for getting at the facts. In contrast, behavioral incidents are poor at all of the above tasks. But when it comes to uncovering the truth, put your money on Pascal's behavioral incident.

Gentle Assumption

With this technique, the clinician, using a gentle tone of voice and non-accusatory wording, assumes that a suspected behavior is occurring. This gentle assumption meta-communicates the reassuring message to the patient that the clinician has already encountered the behavior in other patients.

The technique was first developed by sex researchers, Pomeroy, Flax, and Wheeler,[11] who discovered that questions such as, "How frequently do you find yourself masturbating?" were much more likely to yield valid answers than, "Do you masturbate?" If the clinician is concerned that the patient may be "put-off" by the assumption, it can be softened by adding the phrase "if at all" as with, "How often do you find yourself masturbating, if at all?" I have found very few patients to be bothered by the use of gentle assumptions, if previous engagement has gone well and the tone of voice used with the gentle assumption is non-judgmental.

The definition of a gentle assumption can be clarified by contrasting this technique with questions that are not examples of gentle assumption. Any question that asks whether or not a patient has engaged in a given behavior (e.g., often beginning with words such as "Have you ever …") is by definition not a gentle assumption. For example, when utilizing a gentle assumption to uncover other street drug abuse, after having explored the patient's use of marijuana, the clinician would not ask, "Have you ever tried any other street drugs?" Instead, the clinician would matter-of-factly inquire, "What other street drugs have you ever tried?" Only the latter type of question demonstrates the technique of gentle assumption.

Some prototypic examples of gentle assumptions are:

1. "What other ways have you thought of killing yourself?"
2. "What other problems with the law have you had?"
3. "What other types of problems have you been having with your courses this semester?"
4. "In the past month, how many doses of your medication do you think you may have missed?"

No one knows exactly why gentle assumptions work, but they do. Perhaps, as mentioned earlier, they metacommunicate that the clinician is familiar with the area and has seen other people with similar behaviors, indirectly allowing the patient to feel less odd or deviant. They may also indicate that, at some level, the clinician may be expecting to hear a positive answer and it is okay to provide one.

It is important to note that gentle assumptions are powerful examples of leading questions (a defense attorney on *Law and Order* would be on his feet objecting with each and every one of them). They must be used with care.

More specifically, gentle assumptions should not be used with patients who feel compelled to please the interviewer (e.g., a patient with a histrionic or markedly dependent personality disorder) or who might feel intimidated by the interviewer (e.g., a child or patient with limited intelligence). In such cases, gentle assumptions can lead to a patient reporting something that is not true, for they feel they are "supposed" to have had the experience or behavior in question. In my opinion, gentle assumptions are inappropriate with children when exploring potential abuse issues: in such cases, gentle assumptions can lead to the production of false memories of abuse.

Denial of the Specific

Originally delineated in the first edition of this book,[12] "denial of the specific" has evolved into a technique that can be best conceptualized as a process whereby the clinician asks about specific items from a theoretical "list," such as a list of potentially abused street drugs or a list of potential suicide methods. Strategically, clinicians tend to use denial of the specific directly after a patient has responded with a not-very-believable "no" to a gentle assumption. Sometimes it can ferret out the deceit. At other times it works by simply jogging the memory of a patient who is not being deceitful, but has literally forgotten something on the list.

For example, if a patient said "none" after being asked, "What other ways have you thought of killing yourself?" and the clinician suspected deceit, the clinician might ask, "Have you been having any thoughts of hanging yourself?" If the patient admits to such thoughts, the extent of planning and action taken on hanging would be explored by creating a verbal video with behavioral incidents. If the patient answers negatively, the interviewer proceeds to the next method of which the interviewer is suspicious the patient may be withholding, as with "Have you been having any thoughts of shooting yourself?", and so on, until the interviewer is done with the list. *Remember, denials of the specific are only used if the interviewer is suspicious that information is being withheld.*

As we shall see in Chapter 17 on suicide assessment, patients who are in great pain and at imminent risk of suicide may be hesitant to share their "method of choice" for suicide. With such patients, denials of the specific can be useful at helping them to share this potentially life-saving information.

One of the powers of denial of the specific is the fact it is generally more difficult to shade the truth in response to a specific question as opposed to a generality. Each separate question also allows the clinician to scan carefully for nonverbal evidence of deceit. In the following example, after using a gentle assumption that results in a negative answer from the patient, the clinician will use a series of denials of the specific to tease out the truth:

Clin.: What other street drugs have you tried in the past?

Pt.: Oh … Not much, really.

Clin.: How about coke? (denial of the specific)

Pt.: No, no, not really, it's too expensive.

Clin.: How about if someone gives it to you?

Pt.: (patient smiles) Hey, I'm no fool. Sure, I'll run in the snow if it's falling.

Clin.: Would you say 5, 10, 15 times a week?

Pt.: Nah, maybe three, four times a month.

Clin.: How about when you were younger, has there ever been a time when you used more coke?

Pt.: Oh sure, when I was in the first couple of years of college, I was probably snorting a couple of lines a day.

Clin.: Have you ever tried speed, even once or twice? (denial of the specific)

Pt.: Now that's a drug that I can take or leave. (note that if he can "take it or leave it," it suggests he has indeed tried it, a fact that leads the interviewer to use a gentle assumption)

Clin.: What's it like for you? (gentle assumption)

Pt.: I just don't like it that much. I don't like coming down off it, crashing is no fun.

Clin.: Even though you don't like it very much, how many times have you used it in the last month?

Pt.: The last month, let's see, hmm, maybe two or three times.

Clin.: Was there ever a time in the past where you speeded for days at a time?

Pt.: Sure, when I was in college I might speed for 2, 3 weeks at a time. Hey, I was a Hunter S. Thompson. I was on the road to Vegas (patient chuckles), sort of wish I was there now.

Clin.: Have you ever used some type of downer like Valium or Xanax? (denial of the specific)

Pt.: Well … some … not a lot. When I was speeding I'd sometimes use some shit like that if I needed to come down. But nothing in years.

Clin.: How about marijuana, have you ever used marijuana? (denial of the specific)

Pt.: Yeah, now that's something I've used a little more of. (pauses) And now that it's legal, I plan to use a lot more of the stuff (patient smiles).

The clinician's persistence is paying off. It is not infrequent for patients initially to deny or downplay the use of a drug. But if asked specifically about past use, a patient may then admit to heavier usage. Thus it is often a good idea with a drug history to probe both for the recent past and the distant past.

It is important to frame each denial of the specific as a separate question, pausing between each inquiry and waiting for the patient's denial or admission before asking the next question. The clinician should avoid combining the inquiries into a single question, such as, "Have you thought of shooting yourself, overdosing, hanging yourself, or jumping off of a bridge or building?" A series of items combined in this way is called a "cannon question." Such cannon questions frequently lead to invalid information because patients only hear parts of them or choose to respond to only one item in the string – often the last one. In addition, with each use of a single denial of the specific, the interviewer has an opportunity to observe nonverbal indicators of lying or minimization. Cannon questions undermine this process, for the patient only has to lie once.

Catch-All Question

One of my favorite features on our website for the Training Institute for Suicide Assessment and Clinical Interviewing (www.suicideassessment.com) is our interviewing "Tip of the Month."[13] In this feature, which has well over 150 interviewing tips archived, visitors to our website or participants from my workshops submit interviewing tips that they have found to be particularly useful in their everyday work. Over the years, I've learned an immense amount from these tips and one of my favorites was submitted by Sarah Davila.[14] Her tip, like denial of the specific, helps an interviewer to finish a list. In fact, it is often used after a string of denials of the specific if the clinician is suspicious that an odd outlier may have been missed. Davila's tip was focused upon uncovering unusual methods of suicide. I've broadened its use to other topics and we now call it the "catch-all question." Let's see it at work, first with suicide.

With patients in which one remains suspicious that an important or rather unusual method of suicide has been withheld, the interviewer asks, "We've talked about a lot of different ways that you've been thinking of killing yourself today, is there any method you've thought of, even briefly, that we haven't talked about?" The answers are sometimes surprising. This question can also prompt the patient to share that he or she has done a web search on suicide, offering further glimpses of the patient's intent.

The catch-all question is useful in many situations other than suicide assessment; here are some prototypic examples:

1. "We've talked about a lot of things that your son is doing at school or at home that are upsetting to you; are there any that we haven't talked about yet?"
2. "Are there any other bad experiences you had over in Iraq, perhaps even with fellow soldiers, that we haven't talked about?" (may uncover sexual assault)
3. "We've talked about a lot of things that your wife is upset about with you; are there any we haven't talked about yet?"
4. "Is there any street drug, or perhaps a prescription drug, that you have used to get high that we haven't talked about yet today?"

Symptom Amplification

This technique, also originally delineated in the first edition of this book,[15] is based upon the fact that patients sometimes downplay the frequency or degree to which they have indulged in disturbing behaviors, such as the amount that they drink or the frequency with which they gamble. Symptom amplification allows a clinician to bypass these distorting mechanisms without disengaging the patient, a disengagement that might have occurred if the interviewer had directly challenged the patient's minimization. In fact, with the use of symptom amplification, the clinician allows the patient to naturalistically use minimization as a defense.

This task is accomplished by setting the upper limits of the quantity in question at such a high level that, when the patient downplays the amount, the clinician is still aware that there is a significant problem. For a question to be viewed as symptom amplification, the clinician must suggest an actual number in the question. *This technique is only used if one is suspicious the patient is going to minimize.*

For instance, a clinician suspicious that he or she is in the presence of a heavy drinker can, once the topic of drinking has been raised, ask about the extent of the drinking behavior as follows, "How much liquor can you hold in a single night, a pint, a fifth?" When the patient responds, "Oh no, not a fifth, I don't know, maybe a pint," the clinician is still alerted that there is a problem, despite the patient's minimizations. To be effective, when using a symptom amplification, it is important to start with a high number and go even higher.

Here are some other examples of symptom amplification:

1. "How many physical fights have you had in your whole life, 30, 40, 50?"
2. "How many times have you tripped on acid in your whole life, 25, 50, 100 times or more?"
3. "How many times have you actually struck your wife, 20, 40, 60 times?"
4. "On your very worst days, when you are thinking the most about suicide, how many hours do you spend thinking about it, 8 hours, 12 hours, 15 hours?"

There is one important caveat to the use of symptom amplification. The clinician must be sure that he or she does not set the upper limit at such a high number that it seems absurd or creates the impression that clinician is unfamiliar with the topic at hand. Perhaps the funniest example of this error that I've had the fortune (or misfortune) to encounter was when a trainee asked a street-wizened junkie the following question, "When you've used peyote buttons, how many have you used at a time, 100, 200?" Besides providing an extremely hearty chuckle for the junkie, who immediately began imagining the single most nauseated human being in recorded history, it also provided the clinician with a mildly uncomfortable moment when the patient queried, after containing his glee, "You don't know much about peyote, do you Doc?"

Validity Technique Combinations

Sometimes the effectiveness of validity techniques can be enhanced by combining them into doublets. For instance, one could link normalization with gentle assumption as with, "Some of my patients tell me it is easy to forget their medications, especially when taking them several times a day (normalization); in the past month how many doses of your medication do you think you may have missed, just roughly (gentle assumption)?"[16] In this case, the normalization has "softened" the subsequent gentle assumption.

In the following dialogue with a late-adolescent who presented to our emergency department requesting admission because, "I'm really suicidal and crazy," we will see that it can be very effective to insert one validity technique directly *inside* another one. One of my favorite applications of this strategy involves inserting a shame attenuation inside a gentle assumption or behavioral incident, as illustrated by this direct transcript from my original interview with this adolescent:

Clin.: What about, how frequently have bosses, you know, taken you aside, and complained to you, *or harped to you*, about your work, saying that you're not doing a good job or what they want?

Pt.: I had one boss, and that's after the accident, I worked at the deli on Murray Avenue, I was kinda new there so he couldn't really harp on me, you know, every day he would tell me you're doing this really slow …

With this patient, I inserted a shame attenuation ("or harped to you") directly into the middle of a gentle assumption, for I felt the patient frequently viewed bosses and other authority figures as problematic. By tapping his bias, I thought I might enhance the power of my gentle assumption to uncover the truth. Very shortly, in our next video module, which is based upon this patient, we will see this specific clinical exchange brought to life, and I believe you will see the naturalistic conversational flow that can be generated using doublets.

Clinicians may sometimes find it advantageous to create triplets, as I could easily have done with above: "… how frequently have bosses, you know, taken you aside, and complained to you, *or harped to you*, about your work, saying that you're not doing a good job or what they want, *10 times, 20 times, 30 times*?" (adding a symptom amplification). In this instance we see the coupling of three validity techniques: gentle assumption, shame attenuation, and symptom amplification.

At this point, let me clarify something that, left unaddressed, is sometimes confusing. All of the techniques we have been discussing are specific and cleanly distinct from one another. One will not confuse a shame attenuation with a symptom amplification. This clarity (and lack of overlap) is one of the reasons they are easy to use and easy to teach. But there is one exception.

Almost all of the techniques, in some variant or another, can be simultaneously viewed as being an example of a behavioral incident, for they are often requesting concrete facts, thus fitting the definition of a "fact-finding behavioral incident." For instance, the gentle assumption above ("… how frequently have bosses, you know, taken you aside, and complained to you, … about your work, saying that you're not doing a good job or what they want?") is simultaneously a behavioral incident. Indeed, some validity techniques are always simultaneously a behavioral incident, as is the case with symptom amplification in which case the interviewer is always requesting a number.

In supervision, we explain this overlap area with trainees and relate that if a technique is both a behavioral incident and another more specific validity technique, we will tag it with the name of the more specific technique, for it illustrates better the use and power of the technique. Once explained, we find that trainees have no problems with this definitional overlap.

Now is an opportune time to watch a variety of our validity techniques being utilized clinically. In the following video module, we will be meeting a rendition of the late-adolescent patient introduced above. We will discover that telling the truth is not exactly second nature to him. His presentation will prove to be an ideal setting to put our validity techniques to the test.

VIDEO MODULE 5.1

Title: Validity Techniques: Effective Use

Contents: Contains both expanded didactics and various annotated interview excerpts demonstrating techniques such as shame attenuation, the behavioral incident, gentle assumption, denial of the specific, symptom amplification, induction to bragging, and examples of effective doublets.

Important note to the reader: *After viewing Video Module 5.1 you can proceed directly with the text below regarding techniques for uncovering malingering OR you may view Video Modules 5.2 and 5.3, which are OPTIONAL modules that can be used to consolidate your understanding of the material from Video Module 5.1.*

VIDEO MODULE 5.2

Title: Validity Techniques Illustrated: Complete Interview with Ben without Didactics and without Labels for Interviewing Techniques

Contents: The interview excerpts from Video Module 5.1 appear here as they naturally occurred (without any didactic material inserted), providing a chance to better experience the actual flow of the interview. The labeling of the specific interview techniques as they appeared at the bottom of the video in Video Module 5.1 have also been removed. Thus this module can be used by the reader (individually) or by faculty (within the classroom) to function as a springboard for discussion, consolidate understanding, or as an opportunity to test one's ability to correctly identify the validity techniques as they appear sequentially during the interview.

VIDEO MODULE 5.3

Title: Validity Techniques Illustrated: Complete Interview with Ben without Didactics but *with* Labels for Interviewing Techniques

Contents: This module is identical to Video Module 5.2 except for the return of the labels for the individual validity techniques. With the identifying labels returned as each validity technique is demonstrated, this format provides an ideal method to once again consolidate an understanding of the validity techniques as well as the chance "to check the answers" if one used Video Module 5.2 as an opportunity to test one's abilities to identify the validity techniques.

Miscellaneous Tips for Specific Situations Where Validity Is a Concern

Malingering

Although most of our patients are doing their best to share the truth, some patients are malingering. The reasons for such deceit can vary from easily understood (a patient providing false symptoms to get into a hospital because of homelessness) to more problematic reasons (seeking drugs, attempting to procure inappropriate disability monies, seeking hospitalizations to avoid court appearances). Several diagnoses are easier to fake, such as post-traumatic stress disorder (PTSD) and depression, for the symptoms are subjective. Others, such as psychotic process, are chosen if the patient feels a very serious or dangerous picture needs to be presented to gain the desired goal (such as admission to a hospital or as a prequel for an insanity defense).

One of the clinician's best assets for spotting malingering is a detailed knowledge of what symptoms are present in what diagnoses, how these symptoms appear when really present, and what the pain is like that people feel when these real symptoms are present. Through this person-centered knowledge, we can carefully weigh what the potential malingerer is describing with what patients coping with the real thing actually experience. Taking this a step further, some psychological tests for detecting malingering employ formal scores to measure the patient's claims of having experienced rare or improbable symptoms, such as the Structured Interview of Reported Symptoms.[17] Rare symptoms should be just that – rare. If a patient presents with numerous rare symptoms, the likelihood of malingering goes up substantially.

For use in everyday clinical interviews, Phil Resnick describes a technique he calls the "endorsement of bogus symptoms."[18] With this technique, the interviewer asks the patient if he or she is experiencing a symptom that the clinician knows is highly atypical for the disorder being feigned. If the patient endorses having such a symptom, the likelihood of malingering goes up.

The endorsement of bogus symptoms can be particularly useful when ferreting out psychotic symptoms, for many patients who are feigning psychosis think that almost any "crazy-sounding" process is probably found in disorders like schizophrenia or psychotic manias. As we will see in future chapters, this belief is far from the truth. Psychotic symptoms have distinctive phenomenologies and symptom pictures.

Resnick suggests that questions such as, "When people talk to you, do you sometimes see the words they speak spelled out?" or "Have you ever believed that automobiles were members of organized religion?" may result in positive responses in patients who are malingering, whereas such experiences would be highly unusual in cases of legitimate psychotic process. Resnick emphasizes that such questions must be asked in the context of other questions more typical of psychotic ideation to prevent them from standing out as unrealistic. With malingers who "hear voices," I have found subtle questions such as "Do your voices often slip under the door?" or "Do your voices tend to slam into the back of your head?" to be effective for eliciting malingered responses. Although voices could be experienced in these fashions, it is a rarity.

Here are other examples of the endorsement of bogus symptoms for use in differing disorders:

1. "When you have your flashbacks, do they occur in black and white?" (PTSD: note that patient flashbacks – re-experiences of traumatic incidents – are not typically experienced as black and white images.)
2. "When you have your panic attacks, do they tend to stay with you, hammering at you, for many hours on end?" (Panic attacks are time-limited, seldom lasting in full intensity past an hour or two; they are usually significantly shorter.)
3. "During your most severe periods of depression, do you usually find that you wake up feeling pretty good, but as the day progresses the depression becomes devastating

so that it is frankly hard for you to function, despite your best efforts?" (With major depressions, patients rarely awaken refreshed; indeed they often awaken earlier than they want, barraged by an onslaught of unsettling worries.)

Let us return to Ben, our patient from Video Module 5.1. If you will recall, Ben had presented to our emergency department saying, "I'm really suicidal and crazy." As already noted, at the time of his interview I was suspicious that Ben was malingering, which we now know was later determined to be true subsequent to his admission. In Video Module 5.4, we will see that it was Ben's response to my first use of an endorsement of bogus symptoms that made me strongly suspicious that Ben was indeed malingering.

VIDEO MODULE 5.4

Title: Interviewing Techniques for Uncovering Malingering

Contents: Contains both expanded didactics and an annotated interview excerpt demonstrating the endorsement of bogus symptoms.

Gauging Motivation

Leston Havens developed an interviewing strategy for gauging a patient's motivation to pursue a self-initiated behavior (e.g., pursue a job change) or recommendation from others (e.g., attend alcoholics anonymous). Techniques for improving motivation, as first delineated by Miller and Rolneck,[19] are so important that we devote the whole of Chapter 22 to them. At this point though, Haven's technique – called "soundings" – is an example of an interviewing strategy not designed to increase motivation, but to accurately determine its current level. The following description is adapted directly from Haven's lucid writings.[20]

Curiously, soundings drew its name and its methodology from a most unexpected "clinician," Samuel Clemmons, or Mark Twain as he is more commonly known. Few know that Twain drew his pen name from an everyday process that riverboat captains used to discover the depth of the treacherous Mississippi River.

In unknown waters, a leadsman would throw over a weighted rope until it hit bottom and then call up the depth as indicated by the length of rope, yelling out a phrase such as, "By the mark four!" or "Mark three-and-one-half!" If the depth was found to be 2 fathoms, the boat was in danger of going aground, and the leadsman would urgently call out, "Mark twain!" This measuring process was called "soundings."[21] It was an accurate way of seeing what could not be seen – the bottom of the river. Havens became intrigued by the idea that a similar approach might be of use in helping a clinician to see what could not easily be seen with a patient, the depth of the patient's motivation. With soundings, the interviewer tosses out a series of statements of inquiry, which we first came upon in the Degree of Openness Continuum (DOC; statements of inquiry are statements in which the inflection at the end transforms the statement into something that needs to be addressed by the patient as with, "You found having a child to be more difficult than you had imagined?"). With soundings, this series of statements of inquiry is carefully sequenced in a progressive fashion so as to probe deeper and deeper into the patient's level of motivation. The patient's verbal and nonverbal responses often represent a fairly accurate record of how much the patient agrees or disagrees with the statement proffered by the clinician. With each "sounding," like our riverboat man, the clinician acquires a more accurate feeling for what is hidden.

This strategy is more easily understood by way of an example. Let us take a look a common clinical conundrum – trying to accurately determine a patient's intention to do something that is difficult to do, perhaps leave an abusive marriage. Watch as the clinician in this prototypic conversation below helps both the patient and herself to ferret out the patient's intention. The patient will announce that she intends to leave her husband soon. But what does this really mean? How much intention is behind this statement? The interviewer will toss out a series of soundings, always done with a gentle tone of voice – never in a challenging tone of voice – to see where the depth of the intention actually lies:

> **Pt.:** I really feel that somehow I need to get out of this relationship. I know in my heart, Jim is bad for me. I'll get out soon.
>
> **Clin.:** You dream of this? (a sounding)
>
> **Pt.:** As a matter of fact, I think of it every day. I know that Jim is perhaps my biggest problem.
>
> **Clin.:** You might want to do this then, to leave Jim? (a sounding)
>
> **Pt.:** Yeah, I might need to do it.
>
> **Clin.:** You feel you can do it? (a sounding)
>
> **Pt.:** (patient sighs) Well, I guess so … I think so.
>
> **Clin.:** You feel you will be able to do it within a month or two? (a sounding)
>
> **Pt.:** Well, I doubt that … No I don't think that is in the cards in the near future.

Although often used to determine a patient's motivation to proceed with beneficial activities that may be hard to do, as with following therapeutic recommendations, it can also be utilized to determine activities best not done. For instance, it can be used to determine the depth with which a patient believes in a delusion and may subsequently act upon it.

Let us imagine a patient presenting in an emergency room with a delusion that he is being "constantly watched" by his neighbor who he thinks might be plotting to poison him. The following series of soundings can help the clinician to decide the level of conviction the patient has regarding his delusion, a concept called how much "distance" a patient has from the delusion:

"You may sometimes wonder, can this really be true about your neighbor?"
"You feel that there's too much evidence to doubt it?"
"There doesn't seem any doubt at all in your mind at his point?"

The clinician pauses after each of these soundings to see how the patient responds both verbally and nonverbally.

Later in the interview, when evaluating the level of the patient's intention to act on the delusion (perhaps to violently confront his imagined persecutor), the following soundings might be of use, once again pausing after each one to listen to the patient's response:

"You've thought of doing something about your neighbor?"
"You feel you need to do something about him?"
"You've planned to do something to stop him?"

To such a series of statements of inquiry, the interviewer might discover that a gun has been purchased that the patient plans to bring along, "just in case it's needed," when he confronts his unwary neighbor about his supposed schemes.

Taking a Sexual History

Taking a good sexual history can be uncomfortable for both the beginning clinician and the patient. Some of the techniques described earlier can be of value, but it takes practice with these techniques before one feels progressively at ease. In this regard, the familiarization process can be speeded up by the use of role-playing or practicing the questioning while in front of a mirror. These drills help the clinician to focus on his or her paralanguage and body language, both of which play a pivotal role in helping the patient to relax during the sexual history. The clinician's nonverbal behavior should be identical to his or her nonverbal behavior during the rest of the interview. Sexual questions asked with a calm matter-of-factness are more likely to result in matter-of-fact responses.

Some forms of leading questions can put patients on the spot as well. For instance, the question, "Do you have orgasms about 80% of the time?" may suggest to the patient that a response of less frequency is unusual or abnormal. This unwanted effect can be minimized simply by asking, "How frequently do you reach orgasm during sex, if at all?" But some clinicians feel that this approach, in which no number is proffered by the interviewer, can also generate anxiety, because it leaves the patient alone with his or her projections of what he or she thinks the clinician is expecting. This can be alleviated by asking a question that provides a range without any indication of what is wanted, but communicating, via the range, that any number is fine. By combining this approach with the use of normalization, the question takes on a non-threatening tone as with, "Women vary a great deal on how frequently, if ever, they have an orgasm. What percentage of the time do you think you have an orgasm – 5%, 20%, 80%, or almost never?"

Concerning sexuality, some patients will feel guilt about activities for which there is no reason to feel guilt, caused by cultural stigmatization, such as homosexuality or masturbation. Once again, the clinician attempts to raise the topic in such a way that the patient does not feel awkward. For example, one useful method of approaching possible homosexual orientation is via the developmental history, utilizing normalization, as follows: "As adolescents mature, they frequently experiment with different lifestyles and sexual orientations. When you were an adolescent, did you ever experiment with homosexual contact, perhaps to see what it was like?" One can continue the questioning into adulthood simply by asking, "In the long run, some people discover that the most natural sexual orientation for them is a homosexual or bisexual orientation as opposed to a heterosexual one, or vice versa. At this point in your life, with what orientation have you found yourself to be most comfortable?"

Moving to a different topic, the question of childhood sexual abuse can be difficult to discuss at times. Naturally, the topic will be spontaneously raised by the patient in some instances; however, sometimes there is nothing to suggest its presence. As we saw in our chapter on facilics, and well worth reviewing here, a good way to screen for a history of sexual abuse often presents itself while the clinician is taking the family history for other psychiatric disorders. Suppose it has been uncovered that one of the patient's parents had alcoholism, then the following question, using a natural gate, (with a normalization embedded inside it), can be quite effective, "With your dad's problems with drinking, it is not uncommon for people to tell me that there was also a history of violence in the family or sexual abuse. Was that true in your family?"

Another question for sensitively raising the topic of sexual abuse is, "When you were growing up did anyone in your family, or someone outside of your family, touch you sexually in a way that you felt uncomfortable or wish that they hadn't?" Even a brief pause by the patient may suggest a history of abuse that can be gently uncovered with, "It looks like that question struck a chord with you, what are you remembering?" I sometimes add at this delicate moment, "It can be difficult to talk about such things. Just share what you feel comfortable sharing, it might really help me to help you."

Interview Illustrating the Use of Various Validity Techniques

In this chapter we have explored a large number of validity techniques, from anchor questions to behavioral incidents and shame attenuations. Perhaps, at this point, an interview excerpt can help us to see how an interviewer can intentionally interweave these individual techniques into a graceful tapestry. With patience and skilled timing, the truth of the patient's history will slowly emerge within the fabric of the interview.

In the following dialogue, you can see how the strategic use of validity techniques makes it difficult for the interviewee to distort the truth through processes such as the parsing of words or relying upon an idiosyncratic interpretation of a word such as "hit." Also note the power of the behavioral incident to not only cut away the patient's distortions but also to effectively cut away the interviewer's assumptions and/or projections that can also cast a mist of distortion on the story. We will pick up the conversation well into the body of the interview, at a point when the clinician decided to expand the region of IPV.

> **Pt.:** My wife and I haven't really gotten along well in years (pause). Last weekend we really went at it.
>
> **Clin.:** Tell me what happened. (behavioral incident)
>
> **Pt.:** Well … She just started on me about needing to get a job, that's her big thing now. She wants me to go down to the unemployment office today not tomorrow. Today. So she starts ragging and yelling and I (pause) I just couldn't take it anymore so I lost it on her.
>
> **Clin.:** What do you mean that you lost it on her? (behavioral incident, said gently)

> Pt.: I left. Just took off in a fit of anger. I waited till she went out to the kitchen, and I went out the back door, and I didn't come back for 2 days. I didn't call her. I didn't look for a job. I just bagged it all. Screw her.

I think many clinicians, including myself, would have interpreted the phrase "lost it on her" as probably indicating physical violence. The behavioral incident dismantles this clinician assumption and uncovers a much less disturbing, albeit strikingly passive-aggressive, behavior. Although this assumption would have been in error here, the clinician's intuition of violence will soon prove to be on the mark. The doorway to an exploration of domestic violence is opened through an effectively used "validity triplet":

> Clin.: Sounds like you two really do go at it. At such moments, sometimes people have a hard time controlling their emotions (normalization). With all of the pent-up stress you two have been under (shame attenuation), how many times have you found yourself stressed to the point that you may have lost your temper and perhaps hit her? (gentle assumption)
>
> Pt.: I've not really done that.
>
> Clin.: When you say "not really," what do you mean? (behavioral incident, said in a non-accusatory tone)
>
> Pt.: Oh, I've never actually hit her.
>
> Clin.: Sometimes people mean different things by the same word; to make sure I'm not being confusing here, let me explain what I mean by the word "hit." I'm including anything like using a fist, slapping with an open hand, or pushing her. (clarifying norms)
>
> Pt.: (sighs) Well, (pauses, shrugs shoulders slightly) I guess you could say I slapped her a few times.
>
> Clin.: Did you ever slap her so hard that it caused some bruises? (behavioral incident)
>
> Pt.: Not really (pauses, purses his mouth) Maybe a black-eye once or twice.
>
> Clin.: How many times do you think you have slapped her, 20 times, 30 times, 40 times? (symptom amplification)
>
> Pt.: Not that often. (pauses to reflect) Maybe six, seven times.
>
> Clin.: Has she ever had to get stitches or go to the emergency room? (behavioral incident)
>
> Pt.: Oh no, shit no, never.

At this point, the interviewer is becoming suspicious that the patient may have an antisocial personality disorder and has decided it warrants some further exploration, for the presence of such a personality structure might have important ramifications for designing an appropriate referral for therapy. The problem is that the criteria for an antisocial personality disorder (from childhood problems, such as fire-setting and torturing animals, to adult behaviors, such as problems with the law and chronic lying) can be potentially disengaging to explore in an initial interview. Let's see how this interviewer, with the skilled use of validity techniques, accomplishes this exact task in a surprisingly engaging fashion just as I demonstrated in our video with Ben:

> Clin.: How about outside the house. It sounded to me earlier like you grew up in a really tough neighborhood where you probably had to know how to fight just to survive. (shame attenuation) Is that true?

Pt.:	You better believe it. There were several kids from my high school killed in shootings, probably drug shit, I don't know.
Clin.:	You look like you take pretty good care of yourself. I bet you could hold your own even in a neighborhood like that. (induction to bragging) What types of fights, if any, did you get into back then? (gentle assumption)
Pt.:	Oh, I got into a few fights. Trust me on that one. I didn't pick them, but the guys who did wished they hadn't.
Clin.:	Did you hurt anybody so bad they had to go to the hospital or anything? (behavioral incident)
Pt.:	Nothing like that. But I beat them up pretty good.
Clin.:	Even though someone else started them, (shame attenuation) did you ever end up getting arrested? (behavioral incident)
Pt.:	Nope. Can't say that I have.
Clin.:	Did you ever get into trouble with the law in some way that we haven't talked about? (catch-all question)
Pt.:	Oh yeah, I was picked up for vandalism and that kind of shit, but never arrested. I stopped all that shit as soon as I got out of high school.
Clin.:	I know you got yourself out of that neighborhood as fast as you could, that's for sure, and that was clearly a smart thing to do. How about after you left there, when you moved to Los Angeles, did you have any troubles with the law then? (anchor question, time-focused)
Pt.:	Hmmm. (pauses) Well, I guess you could say so, I got fired once for fighting on the job, and they called the cops then, I wasn't arrested or anything.
Clin.:	Billy, you told me earlier about all the abuse your father did to you, and it sounded like pretty bad abuse to me, do you think it ties in to some of your own angry outbursts, like with your wife or this episode back in LA?
Pt.:	Absolutely. I'm no therapist, but if you get hammered like that in life, you're going to hammer some people back, that wouldn't surprise me. It's just the way it is.
Clin.:	Another thing that some of my patients have told me, who have had very abusive parents like your dad was, is that they had to lie to protect themselves, do you know what I mean by that? (normalization)
Pt.:	Hell yeah. After he'd had a drunk on, you'd tell the old man whatever he wanted to hear. If he asked me if my homework was done and it wasn't, I'd tell him it was all done and then I'd get my ass out of Dodge. If he found out that my homework wasn't done, he'd beat the crap out of me, I mean he'd beat the crap out of me … (pauses) Sometimes I had to lie to protect my mom or my little sister too. Yeah, he was a real bastard.
Clin.:	Some people with similar histories of abuse, especially if they had to keep lying over and over again to protect themselves like you did, tell me that the lying sort of becomes a habit and they find themselves lying even when they are older and sometimes when they don't even realize they are doing it. (normalization) Have you ever found that to be true for you?
Pt.:	(smiles) Well (pauses) … let me put it this way, I've been known to tell a lie or two … if I need to. (smiles again)
Clin.:	Have you become a pretty good liar over the years? (shame attenuation)
Pt.:	(bigger smile) Let me let you in on a secret, Doc. I'm a super good liar. (pauses) And I ain't lying to you. (chuckles)

Clin.: (smiles) Now it also sounds to me like your mother, as well as your father, was abusive to you. She sounds like she was very verbally abusive, did you ever run away from home to get away from it all? (shame attenuation)

Pt.: Yeah.

Clin.: How many times do you think, 10 times, 15 times, 20 times? (symptom amplification)

Pt.: I don't know, maybe around five or six times. But I always came back in a day or two. I don't know why, but I did.

Clin.: To get back at them, (shame attenuation) did you ever do things that you knew would annoy them or frighten them, like set fires?

Pt.: Hell no, he'd have killed me.

Clin.: How about something they couldn't see? Did you ever try to take what you felt was justifiable revenge by hurting something that your parents loved like one of your dad's dogs, you told me he had several dogs? (shame attenuation)

Pt.: You know, I was so afraid of him, I'd have never risked that, but you know, I sort of thought of it, because I did like to tease cats for awhile.

Clin.: What would you do? (behavioral incident)

Pt.: We'd stick a cat in a can and then kick it or sometimes we sprinkled the cat's tail with lighter fluid and then lit it. You should have seen them fly!

Clin.: How do you view those behaviors now when you look back?

Pt.: That was pretty weird. (pauses) I sort of feel bad about it. I don't think I'd do any of that type of stuff now. I've learned that there's no use hurting things in this life, I'm really pretty much of a pacifist. I'm not out to hurt anybody or anything. Just mind my own business.

In this illustration, the clinician is eliciting a powerful history, filled with evidence of antisocial behavior, and yet the patient appears to feel comfortable. Part of this comfort may be related to this patient's innate tendency to not feel guilt, but a considerable part seems to be related to the clinician's skill in exploring sensitive material adeptly. On a disturbing level, some of the uncovered antisocial material hints at true sociopathy (with people and animals being viewed by the patient with a disturbing lack of empathy). Note how the clinician is skillfully able, without any damage to the therapeutic alliance, to raise often highly disengaging topics such as the patient participating in animal torture or fire-setting by tying the topics into the patient's own rationalizations via shame attenuation (e.g., the patient potentially viewing such behaviors as okay to do because of his parent's abuse).

We have concluded our exploration of the four clusters of validity techniques and have covered a lot of ground. It may be useful to summarize what we have learned in each cluster:

Cluster 1: techniques for improving generalized recall (anchor questions, tagging questions, and exaggeration)

Cluster 2: techniques for avoiding miscommunication (defining technical terms, clarifying norms)

Cluster 3: techniques for raising a sensitive or taboo topic (normalization, shame attenuation, induction to bragging)

Cluster 4: techniques for exploring a sensitive topic once raised (behavioral incident, gentle assumption, denial of the specific, catch-all question, and symptom amplification)

We have also examined validity techniques for miscellaneous tasks such as Resnick's endorsement of bogus symptoms for spotting malingering and Haven's soundings for gauging motivation.

Our efforts will not go unrewarded. Through the creative and flexible use of the validity techniques described in this chapter, we will be much better able to help our patients to share sensitive topics about which it is often difficult to talk. We will have gone a great way towards gently cutting through the "mists of words" that Oscar Wilde alluded to in the epigram that opened our chapter. The result will be a clearer picture of the reality of the problems that are facing our patients and the behaviors that may be leading them to cause harm to either themselves or to others, and sometimes both. It is our patients who will be the beneficiaries of our hard work and our studies. The art of interviewing will have taken its much-deserved place as the first step in the art of healing.

REFERENCES

1. Pearson H. *Oscar Wilde, his life and wit.* New York, NY: Harper & Brothers Publishers; 1964. p. 129.
2. Carlat D. *The psychiatric interview.* Philadelphia, PA: Lippincott Williams & Wilkins; 1999. p. 26–7.
3. Sudman S, Budman NM. *Asking questions: a practical guide to questionnaire design.* San Francisco, CA: Jossey-Bass; 1987.
4. Carlat D. 1999. p. 27.
5. Othmer E, Othmer SC. *The clinical interview using DSM-IV,* vol. 1. *Fundamentals.* Washington, DC: American Psychiatric Press; 1994. p. 76.
6. Carlat D. 1999. p. 28.
7. Shea SC. *Psychiatric interviewing: the art of understanding.* 2nd ed. Philadelphia, PA: W.B. Saunders, Inc.; 1998. p. 402–3.
8. Shea SC. 1998. p. 393–5.
9. Othmer E, Othmer SC. 1994. p. 77.
10. Pascal GR. *The practical art of diagnostic interviewing.* Homewood, IL: Dow Jones-Irwin; 1983.
11. Pomeroy WB, Flax CC, Wheeler CC. *Taking a sex history.* New York, NY: The Free Press; 1982.
12. Shea SC. *Psychiatric interviewing: the art of understanding.* 1st ed. Philadelphia, PA: W.B. Saunders, Inc.; 1988. p. 372.
13. Shea SC. My favorite tips from the "clinical interviewing tip of the month." *Psychiatr Clin North Am* 2007;**30**(2):219–25.
14. Davila S. Uncovering unusual methods of suicide. *Interviewing Tip of the Month Archive from the website of the Training Institute for Suicide Assessment and Clinical Interviewing (TISA).* January 2010. <http://www.suicideassessment.com./tips/archives.php?action=prod&id=119> [accessed 23 August 2015].
15. Shea SC. *Psychiatric interviewing: the art of understanding.* 1st ed. Philadelphia, PA: W.B. Saunders, Inc.; 1988. p. 371–2.
16. Shea SC. *Improving medication adherence: how to talk with patients about their medications.* Philadelphia, PA: Lippincott Williams & Wilkins; 2006.
17. Rogers R, Bagby RM, Dickens SE. *Structured Interview of Reported Symptoms (SIRS) and professional manual.* Odessa, FL: Psychological Assessment Resources; 1992.
18. Resnick PJ. My favorite tips for detecting malingering and violence risk. *Psychiatr Clin North Am* 2007;**30**(2):227–32.
19. Rollnick S, Miller WR, Butler CC. *Motivational interviewing in health care: helping patients change behavior.* New York, NY: The Guilford Press; 2007.
20. Havens L. Approaching the mind in clinical interviewing: the techniques of soundings and counterprojection. *Psychiatr Clin North Am* 2007;**30**(2):145–56.
21. Welland D. *The life and times of Mark Twain.* New York, NY: Crescent Books; 1991.

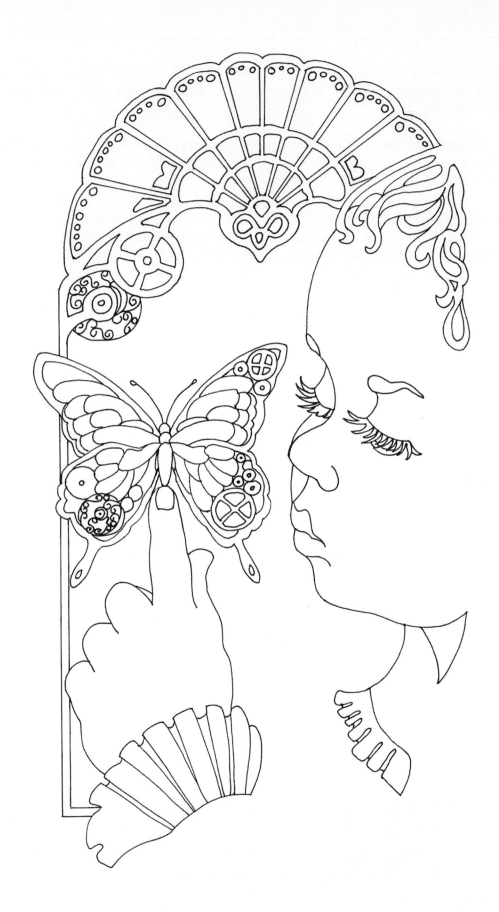

CHAPTER 6

Understanding the Person Beneath the Diagnosis: The Search for Uniqueness, Wellness, and Cultural Context

Every physician must be rich in knowledge, and not only of that which is written in books; his patients should be his book, they will never mislead him ...

Paracelsus, Renaissance alchemist and physician[1]

INTRODUCTORY ILLUSTRATION: THE PERSON BENEATH THE DIAGNOSIS

As the clinician integrates the processes of the first two way-stations on our map of the initial interview – engagement and data gathering – a curious phenomenon emerges. Gradually, the clinician begins to gain an understanding of the world through another person's eyes. This process does not happen suddenly or dramatically. Instead, like the imperceptible clearing of a mist, the clinician's conceptualization of the patient's perspective crystallizes. To return to our analogy of the Victorian room, the nooks and crannies of the environment gradually become more familiar. As interviewers, we are no longer strangers.

Indeed, we have reached the third way-station on our map – a deeper understanding of the person sitting before us. This way-station overlaps with the first two, for an understanding of the patient will not occur unless there is adequate engagement. Moreover, accurate understanding emerges from the facts, feelings, and opinions culled in the process of data gathering. Despite this overlap, from the perspective of person-centered interviewing, the process of understanding warrants a closer examination.

It is our understanding of the unique qualities, circumstances, and cultural determinants of the patient that will lead us not only directly into the fourth way-station on our map – accurate assessment and diagnosis – it will also have a profound impact on the fifth and final way-station on our map – treatment planning. Put succinctly, the success of a treatment plan is ultimately dependent upon the clinician's ability to understand the person beneath the diagnosis. Clinicians arrive at this understanding by uncovering a compassionate, sophisticated understanding of the multiple systems – from biological and psychological to familial, cultural, and spiritual – that continuously coalesce to create the patient, the clinician, and the patient/clinician dyad.

As we shall see in our next chapter, there are a variety of assessment perspectives that serve as nice complements to one another for accomplishing this integrative task, including differential diagnosis using the DSM-5, viewing the patient as a matrix of intersecting and interacting systems (matrix treatment planning), and understanding the patient's core pains. An interviewer can shape a useful formulation of what is right and what is wrong with the patient through a skilled delineation of the information needed to utilize these three assessment frameworks. Indeed, these three frameworks provide the classic foundations for collaboratively developing an initial treatment plan by the end of the interview, and these are good foundations. Consequently, we will examine them in detail in the next chapter.

But if one looks at our interview map (Figure 6.1), one will notice that, in addition to an arrow leading from diagnosis and assessment to treatment planning, there is a second arrow that leads to treatment planning. It is the arrow that originates from the understanding of the patient.

Many a well-intentioned interviewer has been trapped by the inviting misconception that ideal treatment plans can be generated by strict algorithms stemming directly from specific DSM-5 diagnoses. The spirit behind this goal is an admirable one, to improve quality of care by ensuring that the best possible evidence-based therapies are utilized. Unfortunately this concept misses a rather simple, but often-overlooked, reality: an "ideal" treatment plan that doesn't work is not ideal, it is foolish. It is the patient's interest in and agreement with the treatment plan – as well as his or her ability to follow through with the treatment plan – that will determine whether or not the treatment plan will work. One cannot simply look at a DSM-5 diagnosis and conclude that one can

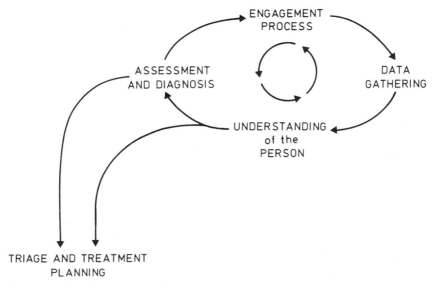

Figure 6.1   Map of the interviewing process.

apply a pre-determined best treatment plan dictated by the diagnosis, for it can't possibly be the best plan for the patient if the patient does not like it and, consequently, will not do it. Treatment plans are created for people, not for diagnoses.

Moreover, effective treatment plans are not really made for people by clinicians, they are co-created by people *with* their clinicians. This fact is true not only in psychiatry, but in all branches of medicine. A clinician cannot help a patient to control diabetes, asthma, or hypertension unless the patient personally chooses, and helps to sculpt, the treatment plan, and is not blocked by external circumstances (lack of money, problematic circumstances, and cultural roadblocks) from following through with the treatment plan that he or she has chosen.

The art of treatment planning achieves its greatest healing power when it is guided by a sophisticated understanding of the person sitting before the clinician. The search for this understanding during the initial encounter will often reveal many factors, including psychodynamic, interpersonal, and cultural factors, that have little to do with the DSM-5 diagnosis *per se*, that can suggest powerful ideas for treatment planning. In addition, it is our understanding of the person beneath the diagnosis that will determine whether or not we can collaboratively create a treatment plan that the patient will embrace during the initial interview and in subsequent therapy. Perhaps an illustration will make this point more clear.

Imagine a clinician at a busy community mental health center who is in the midst of an initial intake. Further imagine that at this particular center the "intake clinician" is supposed to triage the patient to whatever clinical program would best be able to help that individual, ranging from outpatient individual therapy or group therapies to psychiatric care or other specific programs, such as an incest survivor's group, an eating disorders group, or a DBT (dialectical behavioral therapy) group.

Now imagine that the interviewer is quite talented at all of the skills we have been discussing thus far, from engagement techniques to facilic principles for creating flowing conversational interviews. The patient is a young woman of about 18, still living at home, hoping to go to college next year if finances can be worked out, who unfortunately has become fairly seriously depressed; indeed, there is a strong family history of depression. We will call our imagined patient, Jennifer.

As the interview is nearing its closing phase, the clinician has become convinced that Jennifer is suffering from a moderately severe, major depressive disorder from the diagnostic perspective of the DSM-5 system. The clinician is also concerned about the depth of the depression and feels that rapid intervention is indicated, although there is no suicidal ideation. The clinician decides to recommend a combination both of a referral to the psychiatrist for medications and to one of the outpatient psychotherapists. The decision to recommend medications is certainly reasonable considering her diagnosis (which is accurate) and the rapid progression of Jennifer's symptoms and the severity of her pain. Jennifer seems reasonably comfortable with the both recommendations and states she feels she has benefitted from the interview, thanking the clinician in a genuinely warm fashion. There is only one problem: Jennifer never appears for either her meeting with the psychiatrist or her therapist.

Now imagine the exact same scenario with the same patient, but with a different clinician. Once again, this is a talented clinician and empathic interviewer. Indeed, she gathers essentially the same database as our first clinician. She, too, feels the patient meets the criteria for a moderately severe major depressive episode by DSM-5 criteria. She, too, feels that the rapid progression of the depression and the of the depth of Jennifer's pain suggests the wisdom of using an antidepressant.

On the other hand, during the body of the interview, she does one thing differently than our first clinician. It relates to something that she noticed – a piece of jewelry. A cross is hanging from a simple chain around Jennifer's neck. It has some decorative elements that suggest it may be an heirloom; perhaps it's Victorian. Although not expensive, it is clear that the owner of this cross, Jennifer, has taken meticulous care of it:

Clin.: I can't help but notice the cross you are wearing. It's quite pretty, was it a gift?

Pt.: (Jennifer smiles) Oh, oh, thank you. It was a gift. My gran gave it to me on my 16th birthday. It was hers as a child.

Clin.: That's a very wonderful gift.

Pt.: You think so?

Clin.: Sure. You had told me earlier what a kind person your gran was, and to have such a gift from her own childhood I'm sure is special to you.

Pt.: Yeah, I really love her and it's a neat old cross. (Jennifer looks downward and seems to be suddenly a little ill-at-ease)

Clin.: You seem lost in thought. (observed gate) Is there something bothering you?

Pt.: (Jennifer looks up at the interviewer). There's something I probably should have told you, that I really didn't explain very well earlier.

Clin.: What's that? (said gently)

Pt.: Remember when I told you, I was pretty religious?

Clin.: Yes. You told me you had a Christian background. And it seemed to me you had some very reassuring beliefs and had been praying to God for some guidance.

Pt.: Right. And that's all true. But what I didn't tell you is how religious my family is.

Clin.: That's alright. Fill me in.

Pt.: Well, we're all born again. (looks a little sheepish) And here's the part I probably should have told you. My whole family, and I mean my whole family, including Gran, were strongly opposed to me seeing you. I mean strongly opposed.

Clin.: Oh, I bet that was sort of messy. What happened?

Pt.: They spent almost a half-hour trying to convince me not to come. My mom told me that God would heal me, and I needed to just pray harder. I told her I'd been praying for months and God told me that I should seek help.

Clin.: What did she say?

Pt.: She just kinda shook her head. I think she's pretty disgusted with me.

Clin.: I see. Are you still glad you came?

Pt.: Oh yeah (said with genuine enthusiasm). But I tell you, it was tough. Everybody was really angry with me, including my two brothers. Right as I was going out the door, my mom yelled at me, "Mark my words, they're going to tell you to take a medication. That's their answer for everything. It's not God's answer. Whatever you do, don't let them drug you."

When this clinician reached the closing phase of the interview, despite the fact that, on a theoretical level, she felt an antidepressant might help significantly, she said the following, "You know, Jennifer. There's lots of different ways we might be able to help you. But I think a really good way to start is with one of our therapists, you know, a talking therapy. You have been very easy to talk with, and I think you would genuinely enjoy working with one of our therapists. And the two of you could see if talking some stuff out might help with your depression and some of your stresses. How does that sound to you?"

The clinician chose not to mention medications, not because she didn't believe that an antidepressant might help, but because she felt that if she suggested a medication (just as the family had predicted she would), it would never be taken. And, worse than that, it might risk alienating Jennifer, perhaps leading her to not proceed with any recommendations from the interviewer. Instead, she chose a treatment plan that began with psychotherapy, which also has a good track record with the type of moderately severe depression that Jennifer is describing.

In addition, if the psychotherapy did not provide adequate relief in the ensuing weeks, then it would be the psychotherapist who would be suggesting the use of a medication. If Jennifer had bonded well with the therapist, the therapist's recommendation for medication would likely have a more positive reception from Jennifer than the same suggestion made by an initial interviewer. Here is a plan that has a shot at working. It is not an ideal plan from an ivory tower, but a realistic plan from the practical world of the clinical trenches where we all work and in which Jennifer lives. The following week Jennifer appears promptly for her session, a cross reassuringly dangling from her neck and an open mind sitting atop it.

As Paracelsus suggested in our opening epigram, this clinician's treatment plan was implemented by the patient because the clinician used her patient as her book. She read the nonverbal and cultural cues from the pages of this book to collaboratively develop a treatment plan that resonated with the uniqueness of Jennifer's family milieu and her own spiritual story. In this chapter we will focus upon the art of learning to more astutely understand what patients are saying in their book, as well as learning how to read between the lines of what they are saying in that very same book. Our goal is to view not only the patient in isolation but the patient as part of an ever changing set of psychodynamic forces and cultural systems that point to the person beneath the diagnosis. In this way, we adhere to the age-old wisdom to not judge a book by its cover, a misstep that can occur if a clinician relies too heavily on a DSM-5 diagnosis alone.

To effectively undertake this search for a more sophisticated understanding, in this chapter we will look at three topics that help clinicians to understand the patient beneath the diagnosis: (1) phenomena that can hinder this understanding (focusing upon ways to avoid them), (2) phenomena that can further it (focusing upon ways to enhance them), and (3) an introduction to cultural diversity and its role in the initial interview.

PART I: PHENOMENA THAT HINDER THE UNDERSTANDING OF THE PERSON

Parataxic Distortion

It is clear that the initial interview is an interpersonal process. Both the patient and the interviewer develop perceptions about each other that will shape both their trust in each other and their affinity towards each other. One could assume that these interpersonal perceptions are created primarily via conscious and/or preconscious processes in both parties. If only it could be so simple. Unfortunately, the patient's developing image of the clinician and, for that matter, the clinician's developing image of the patient are influenced by unconscious processes as well. Unknown to the clinician, he or she may resemble a family member of the patient or an ex-spouse, or fill a stereotype of a concrete prejudice. As Sullivan put it, "The *real* characteristics of the other fellow at that time may be of negligible importance to the interpersonal situation. This we call parataxic distortion."[2]

This distorting process can affect the patient or the clinician and sometimes both parties. In actuality, parataxic distortion may evolve from the early seeding of both transference and countertransference; as such, its formation and resolution may play a pivotal role in subsequent therapy. But in the initial interview, such undetected early distortions may beleaguer an already fragile alliance. Moreover, parataxic distortion can lead to remarkably difficult roadblocks to understanding the person beneath the diagnosis. Such unconscious distortion by the patient may lead a patient to mistrust the interviewer with a resulting hesitancy to share critical material necessary for a sophisticated understanding of the patient. Parataxic distortion occurring within the clinician can lead to false impressions and inaccurate "gut instincts" about the patient. Either way, an accurate understanding of the patient is made less likely.

Fortunately, intense parataxic distortion is atypical. But when it does occur, it generally displays itself either through unusually poor blending or by atypically high levels of anxiety in the patient, perhaps even frank antagonism. This weakening of the engagement process represents one more area in which monitoring of the blending process can provide important clues to the engagement itself. Once such weak engagement is recognized, the clinician can begin repair work.

The first step in the repair process consists of questioning whether one's own actions are somehow disengaging the patient. At times these interviewer self-defeating behaviors may be related to countertransference issues with the patient (parataxic distortion on the part of the clinician as with a patient who unconsciously reminds the clinician of a patient who was deceitful and antagonistic towards the clinician in the past or reminds the clinician of an abuser from the clinician's own family). In such a situation the clinician may inadvertently "hear" the patient's story differently than it was described, become overtly suspicious of the truth of the patient's story, or be repulsed or judgmental about the views of the patient. These unconscious clinician tendencies can prevent a clear picture of the patient from emerging.

When a clinician finds himself or herself having a strong visceral negative reaction to a patient, two self-directed questions can lead to the uncovering of parataxic distortion at play with the clinician: (1) Does this patient remind me of any previous patients? (2) Does this patient remind me of any of my family members, friends/enemies, employers or public figures? Clinicians must be keenly aware of their own beliefs based upon cultural biases, including racial, religious, and political biases. It is surprising how quickly and powerfully a clinician can develop a dislike for a patient who holds a differing political or religious worldview. I have been disturbed by the intensity of stereotyping I've seen from both ends of the political spectrum with supervisees who are either Progressives or Conservatives when they discover that their patients are of an opposite political persuasion, a problem that has intensified as America has become a more politically divided nation.

If the clinician discovers that he or she is free of such processes, the clinician can then legitimately wonder whether parataxic distortion is at work in the patient's mind. If such distortion is suggested, an open exploration may decrease the growing antagonism. For instance, the clinician can ask, "I'm wondering what you're feeling as we are talking," or "I sense you are feeling a little displeased with the interview so far, and I'm wondering what's going on?"

This type of non-defensive statement may help to defuse the situation, because it brings hostile feelings into the open, where they can at least be approached. Moreover, the clinician should not be afraid to uncover specific feelings of ill will, such as, "I find you very controlling," because these feelings can be tapped for clues of psychodynamic significance, which may be addressed later in the interview with questions such as, "When have you felt similar feelings in the past?" Once again, the emphasis rests upon allowing the patient to openly express his or her view of the world, in this case, of the interview itself. This emphasis upon understanding the patient's view of the world provides the gateway to a better understanding of who the patient really is.

Sullivan, who died in 1949, is viewed as a pivotal innovator in what he called the interpersonal theory of psychiatry.[3] His work pioneered the realization that patients are not social isolates. To understand a person, one must delve into the person's current interactions with family, friends, culture, and even the therapist's unconscious itself. More recently, theorists such as Ogden have expanded the study of the specific interactions occurring unconsciously between the therapist and the patient, a psychoanalytic concept called "intersubjectivity."[4]

Intersubjectivity teases apart the dynamic interplay between the therapist's subjective experience during the interview with the patient's subjective experience, highlighting the fact, as we saw with Sullivan's parataxic distortion, that an interviewer's own unconscious may have the potential to distort both the conscious and unconscious "facts" of the patient's story, thus hiding the real person beneath the diagnosis. Jonathon Dunn, referring to intersubjective theorists, succinctly summarizes as follows:

These theorists see the analyst and the patient together constructing the clinical data from the interaction of both members' particular psychic qualities and subjective realities. The analyst's perceptions of the patient's psychology are always shaped by the analyst's subjectivity.[5]

I love Dunn's use of the words *"constructing* the clinical data," for they serve to remind us that the "facts" garnered in an interview are actually educated guesses of what happened. These guesses are sculpted by the interplay of what really happened with the chisel strokes made by both the patient's and the clinician's unconscious processes. The interviewing instrument in an initial interview – the clinician – is not a thermometer that has been calibrated for accuracy. The interviewer is more of a human eyeglass that may have been fitted by personal history with lenses that are prone to see a world with some distortion. The real patient sitting before the clinician may be a good deal different from the one sitting inside the clinician's head.

Further Problems With Inaccuracy: The Issue of Reliability

In our chapter on validity, we have seen that there are many issues regarding the patient's propensity to relay the truth that can clearly cause problems with developing a realistic understanding of the patient. The problems highlighted by the concept of intersubjectivity actually address a concept similar to validity but distinct from it – reliability. In a statistical sense, reliability can be defined as follows:

> *Reliability is an indication of the extent to which a measure contains variable errors; that is, errors that differed from individual to individual using any one measuring instrument and that varied from time to time for a given individual measured twice by the same instrument. For example, if one measures the length of a given object in two points of time with the same instrument – say, a ruler – and gets slightly different results, the instrument contains variable errors.*[6]

One can translate the above somewhat obtuse concept into practical interviewing terms by remembering that our own interviewing style functions as our measuring instrument. The question then becomes: Does our way of asking questions change from one individual to another and, if so, do we bias patients towards certain answers? Here we see that the unconscious and habitual patterns of the interviewer may not only distort the interpretation of the data, as suggested by intersubjectivity, but may actually change how the measuring instrument is actually used.

This issue of interviewer reliability can be framed within two problem areas, although many other areas also exist: (1) The interviewer changes his or her style of asking a question and is not aware of the impact of this change, and (2) the interviewer has good reliability (asks questions in the same manner from patient to patient) but unfortunately reliably evokes invalid information. We will briefly examine each of these potential pitfalls.

Specific clinical settings predispose to the problem of *unconsciously* changing styles (note that this potentially negative process is distinctly different from the positive attribute of *consciously* and intentionally changing interviewing style to suit the needs of the patient or clinical situation). This problematic unconscious shifting of styles frequently shadows the presence of countertransference or emotional strain in the clinician. For example, if an interviewer feels pushed for time or begins to dislike an interviewee, subtle changes in interviewing style frequently emerge. The interviewer may cut-off the patient's responses or actually cast a disarming scowl. In other cases, in which a clinician might ordinarily have requested a pleasant patient to explain a vague response further, the same clinician might ask for no further clarification from a sarcastic patient, resulting in a shortened interview and a less valid database. In this sense, processes such as parataxic distortion can not only distort patient information but impact directly on how the patient is being asked for information in the first place.

Such changes in style can significantly decrease the reliability of the interviewing instrument, with subsequent deficits in the validity of the data. All clinicians will experience such negative emotions. There is nothing innately wrong with these negative feelings as long as their potential impact is considered and they are not allowed to interfere with the interview process. Indeed, at times an awareness of such emotions may provide us with clues to the inner workings of both the clinician and the patient.

The second area of concern focuses on the knotty issue that I shall loosely label as being "reliably invalid." In brief, it is possible that some interviewers develop habits that consistently increase the risk of obtaining invalid data. Actually, we have already seen an example of this process, because an interviewer who seldom uses behavioral incidents is probably reliably invalid. Furthermore, as normal humans, most of us have developed other rather clever ways of not hearing what we do not want to hear. Such ingenious devices may get us through some touch-and-go dinners with our in-laws, but if unchecked, these habits may cause problems during a clinical interview. In a more precise fashion, I am describing processes such as cajoling desirable answers from patients through choices of words and tone of voice.

Interviewers may not want to hear positive responses to questions concerning sensitive topics such as suicidal ideation, homicidal ideation, child abuse, or even the emergence of certain target symptoms such as depression. The hesitancy to uncover positive replies to such questions probably results from the fact that such responses may demand increased time from the clinician, legal action, or even generate fear or a sense of failure in the clinician. Consequently, as we saw with negative statements of inquiry in Chapter 3, clinicians may unconsciously develop methods of decreasing the risk of a positive reply by including in their closed-ended questions a negative (e.g., "not" or "don't"), as follows:

a. "You don't really feel more depressed, do you?"
b. "You're not feeling any chest pain today, are you?"
c. "You're not having thoughts of hurting yourself, are you?"
d. (Said to your mother or father-in-law) "You're not really thinking of spending the whole week here, are you?"

An "unusually sophisticated" clinician will reinforce the negative bias by adding a subtle shake of the head from side to side. In essence, this negative approach to asking for a "yes" or "no" answer strongly biases the patient to say no. The reason for this negative bias most likely relates to the fact that the patient feels a need to please the clinician with a negative response. This biasing remains one of the most common errors I see during supervision. It represents a particular nemesis when employed around issues of high sensitivity such as sexuality or suicidality, areas in which patients are hesitant to share positive answers to begin with, and answers which clinicians are occasionally afraid to hear.

Another reliably invalid type of questioning consists of habitually asking multiple questions disguised as a single query, the so-called "cannon question." In Chapter 5 we saw how cannon questions can cause problems when trying to finish a list, as when the clinician is using the validity technique of denial of the specific. Cannon questions can also cause problems with simple fact-oriented inquiries as demonstrated below:

> **Pt.:** I just don't feel the same, there's no question about that. Even my weekends seem bland.
>
> **Clin.:** When did you begin to feel depressed, to feel hopeless, to feel like life was not worth living?
>
> **Pt.:** Probably back around May. Everything seemed to be collapsing back then, near our anniversary.

In this excerpt, the clinician has unwittingly set up a confusing situation. He or she does not know if the patient's depression *or* the patient's hopelessness *or* the patient's death wishes began back in May. It is possible, even probable, that the patient's depression began much earlier than the deep sense of hopelessness. Only further questioning could clarify this murky issue that resulted from the use of a cannon question. In addition, cannon questions are frequently employed during a review of physical systems, such as:

> **Clin.:** Are you having any problem with your eyes, ears, heart, or stomach?
>
> **Pt.:** No.
>
> **Clin.:** Have you noticed any coughing, constipation, diarrhea, headache, backache, or change in bowel habits?
>
> **Pt.:** No, I don't think so.

Although time constraints may sometimes lean the interviewer towards cannon questions, it remains important to realize that such questions may be confusing to patients. Only one of the words may stick out in their minds, and such confusion can cause considerable problems with validity.

PART II: PHENOMENA THAT DEEPEN THE UNDERSTANDING OF THE PERSON BENEATH THE DIAGNOSIS

Sullivan's Interpersonal Perspective Revisited

It seems naive to assume a simple causative agent for most examples of human anxiety. For instance, research in neuroscience has unmasked many physiologic as well as psychosocial precipitants to anxiety. In this section we will focus on some of the interpersonal forces at work in the creation of anxiety as it unfolds in an initial interview. Much of the following discussion is borrowed directly from the work of John Whitehorn,[7] as well as further insightful work by Harry Stack Sullivan,[8] both pivotal pioneers of interpersonal psychology.

To begin our discussion, the following question is worth considering as the interview proceeds: "How does this patient feel that he or she is viewed by others?" In many instances, the answers to this question will provide clues to the patient's immediate presence in our office. Guilt, shame, inadequacy, and fear of failure – these concerns are the stuff of neurosis. Many of the paralyzing defenses developed by people are erected to deflect such painful feelings. Whitehorn cogently expressed this idea, "Even in deadly warfare one's greatest apprehension is not of death but of being maimed or of failing in one's duty, and that, in large part, because one dreads the reactions of other persons. This is not to downplay the fear of death but rather to emphasize the fear of life."[9]

In another sense, developmentally speaking, the child appears to incorporate its sense of self-worth through a synthesis of perceived parental and family attitudes towards it. Indeed, persons demonstrating poorly developed personality states, such as the borderline personality and the narcissistic personality, have frequently evolved from chaotic childhoods. These developmental issues highlight the importance of interpersonal issues in the birth and feeding of unpleasant affects such as anxiety and depression. An actress once told me, "I can play any role once I understand what the character feels guilty about."

With regard to the art of understanding the person at a more sophisticated level in the initial interview, these concerns suggest the utility of a sensitive search for answers to the question "How does this patient feel that he or she is viewed by others?" In particular, certain questions concerning the adolescent years may help to open the interpersonal door a bit, such as:

a. "What were some of your teachers like?"
b. "Tell me a little bit about the kids in your neighborhood where you grew up."
c. "What was it like for you to walk home from school or go on the bus?"
d. "Which of your brothers or sisters are you most like?"
e. "Who do you think is the happiest in your family?"
f. "Who do you admire most in your family?"
g. "What do you think are some of your parents' concerns for you?"
h. "What was gym class like for you?"
i. "What was report card day like for you?"
j. "Did you enjoy social networking on the web?"
k. "Did kids say bad things about you or harass you on the web?"
l. "Have you ever been flamed or physically threatened on the web?"

This list could almost be endless, but these questions represent samples of pathways into interpersonal affect related to past and perhaps current symptomatology. Of course, besides these reflections on the past, the interviewer will also pay heed to the patient's immediate concerns about spouse, family members, friends, bosses, and fellow employees, as well as any current harassment problems on the web.

Of even more immediate concern to the interviewer is the generalization of the patient's interpersonal fears to the interview itself. As mentioned earlier, the patient's self-system may be activated by the perceived threat of rejection or disapproval from the interviewer, or problems with parataxic distortion may undermine a newly emerging therapeutic alliance. Whitehorn, once again, crystallizes the idea, "The patient's attitudes are not likely to appear at first, in answer to prepared questions, but later, in reaction to what he feels is the interviewer's response to his statements."[10] In this regard, the clinician may be aptly rewarded by reflecting upon the following two queries: (1) How is this particular patient trying to come across to me? and (2) Why does he or she feel a need to present himself or herself in this fashion?

Some patients may feel that either the clinician or their friends think that they must be weak or "nuts" to be "seeing a shrink." This anxiety can seriously hamper engagement and may be partially alleviated by allowing some ventilation later in the interview with questions such as, "What has it been like for you to come to see a mental health professional?" Such a question may provide reassuring feelings of interpersonal safety for the patient, because he or she realizes that the clinician is aware of the all-too-human anxieties associated with admitting a need for help.

Another possible method of gaining insight into interpersonal issues arises from asking patients to describe their attitudes toward others. As Whitehorn states, "A fruitful field of study lies in a consideration of his sentiments or prejudices, that is, his attitudes toward father, mother, siblings and other significant others, toward church and state, toward his home town and toward secret societies, antisemitism, Socialism, Fascism, and other 'isms'. In the discussion of such matters, the patient reveals more clearly than in response to direct questions the character of his ideals and the way in which he has come to dramatize his role in life."[11]

During an interview with an adolescent boy of about 14 years of age, the wisdom of this approach became apparent to me. The boy was suffering from a severe depression and seemed reluctant to talk about himself, but to my surprise he was not reluctant to talk about others. The request, "Tell me about some of the things you would change at school," led to a long and revealing discussion of complex social issues such as his school's policy towards racial integration and his own contempt for prejudice. Clearly this was not a boy interested only in the next football game or party. His detailed analysis suggested that he was a person preoccupied with powerful moral concerns, which, when on overtime, could transform into harsh superego admonishings. His world was tense and dotted with rights and wrongs, creating an intrapsychic field of land mines.

This boy's interview also raises another pertinent issue, "Can an interviewer probe too much or too quickly?" Generally speaking, when questioning is done sensitively, it infrequently goes too far. But the trick lies in being attuned to the degree of interpersonal guilt generated by the patient's responses. If the questions generate too much guilt, the initial interviewer may find that an impressively thorough database has been gathered but that there is no patient present with whom to discuss this database at the second appointment.

To avoid this problem, the interviewer can watch vigilantly for signs of embarrassment or shame in the patient, perhaps indicated by an averted gaze or a hesitant first step into speech. This awareness is combined with a common sense attitude towards which subject areas typically produce anxiety. When present, these signs may suggest the presence of potentially disengaging guilt, at which point the clinician may opt to reduce the tension by gently asking a question such as, "What has it been like for you to share such complicated material today?"

Asked calmly and sincerely, such questions demonstrate Rogers' unconditional positive regard while allowing patients to ventilate fears of clinician rejection, discovering to their surprise that such rejection is not imminent. The clinician can further decrease tension by positively reinforcing the patient's courage for sharing delicate material with phrases such as, "You've done an excellent job of sharing difficult material. It's really helping me to understand what you've been experiencing."

A combination of these techniques was useful in allaying the intense interpersonal anxieties generated in a man of about 30 years of age who had presented for an initial assessment. Ostensibly requesting self-assertiveness training, he eventually related a striking list of paraphilias, including voyeurism, exhibitionism, and frotteurism (rubbing one's genitals against people in crowded public places). As he spoke, eye contact vanished, while his hands picked at one another. Near the end of the session, the dialogue evolved roughly as follows:

> **Clin.:** John, I've been wondering what it has been like for you to share this material? You look like you're feeling a little upset.
>
> **Pt.:** It's been very unsettling. I have never shared this stuff with anybody, it's so weird, … uh … uh … I, I feel ashamed every time I meet someone new, afraid of … what they might think.
>
> **Clin.:** What have you been afraid I might be thinking?
>
> **Pt.:** Oh, that I'm really sick or disgusting.
>
> **Clin.:** Has there been anything I've done or said that has conveyed that to you?
>
> **Pt.:** (pause) No, no, I can't say there has been.
>
> **Clin.:** Good, because I have a feeling there is only one person in this room who feels you are sick or disgusting, and that person isn't me.
>
> **Pt.:** (patient nods head and smiles gently) That could be. (patient visibly relaxes)
>
> **Clin.:** Why don't we try to find out more about why these unwanted behaviors developed so that we can look at potential ways of changing them. It's important we can talk about them openly and you've done an excellent job so far.
>
> **Pt.:** Oh, that sounds real good to me.
>
> **Clin.:** Tell me what you were feeling the last time you exposed yourself.
>
> **Pt.:** I had had a bad day, I was really angry at a sales clerk …

John went on to be successfully treated using cognitive–behavioral techniques. The above interaction had helped him to dismantle a powerful projection, a projection that threatened to disrupt the therapy before it even began.

As clinicians, we need to consider carefully the impact of our probings, recognizing that certain patients may not be ready to discuss certain issues, whereas others might actually benefit from our exploration. At these moments during the initial assessment, we must rely upon our ever-growing experience to guide us, keeping in mind a most relevant statement made by a wizened monk in the novel *The Name of the Rose* by Umberto Eco: "Because learning does not consist only of knowing what we must or we can do, but also of knowing what we could do and perhaps should not do."[12]

Phenomenological Inquiry

We now have a moment to re-examine the process of engagement and phenomenological interviewing from Chapters 1, 2, and 3. As we have seen, both engagement and its reflection (blending) can be improved by utilizing a style of questioning that can lead directly to a clearer understanding of the patient. This style has its roots in the fields of existentialism and phenomenological psychology, to which the book *Existence*, by Rollo May,[13] remains an excellent introduction. While employing a more phenomenological style, the clinician attempts to see the world as the person experiences it, to literally see the world through the patient's eyes, to understand the phenomenon of being that person.

The emphasis rests upon what Medard Boss called "Daseins-analysis," a German word translatable as "analysis of being-in-the-world."[14] In short, the clinician attempts to know what it *would* be like and what it *is* like to be the person sitting across from himself or herself. To this end, it is often useful to emphasize the world of the senses by asking specifically about what the patient is seeing, hearing, feeling, smelling, or tasting. From this sensate inquiry, doors may open into the patient's feelings, attitudes, and thoughts. To borrow a phrase from Aldous Huxley and William Blake, it is "through the doors of perception" that one may enter a patient's unique way of being, the patient's inner home. Indeed, this home may be turbulent, beautiful, or terrifying, but once experienced, the clinician's understanding cannot help but be clearer.

Moreover, such sensitive questioning can convey to the patient that the clinician is interested in the patient as a person, not merely as a new case or diagnosis. In this regard, in the first interview the clinician may decide to include brief (or sometimes not so brief) forays into the phenomenology of the patient. These dialogues may be similar to the following one involving an overweight woman whose eyes see only deadness:

> **Pt.:** I guess I was just sick of everything … everything … so I wanted to get away, to be by myself away from everybody who can hurt me. So I went into my room and shut off the light. I lit a few candles and I sat there.
>
> **Clin.:** What were you looking at as you sat there?
>
> **Pt.:** Nothing really … occasionally I watched the candlelight flickering, it made the shadows of the vase dance around on the wall.
>
> **Clin.:** Do you remember anything else that caught your eye?
>
> **Pt.:** Uh huh, I remember looking at my high school prom picture.
>
> **Clin.:** And?
>
> **Pt.:** I thought how cruel it was the way relationships have to break up. The person in that picture meant nothing to me now, and I don't think I really meant anything to him ever (patient sighs).
>
> **Clin.:** What else are you feeling in the room?

Pt.: Lonely and empty. I just wanted to crawl up into a tiny ball like a cocoon.

Clin.: What does the world feel like to you in your cocoon?

Pt.: It feels distant, dark, and numb. I feel, feel sort of blank, but I also am angry. I'm angry at my mother for never really caring, for putting me in the cocoon in the first place. I don't ever remember her hugging me (begins crying gently). I remember going away for the summer once to stay with my grandparents. And at the train station I felt very frightened and sad. I kept wondering what my mother would do when she said good-bye – would she hug me or kiss me, and for how long? And you know what she did? She did nothing. She said good-bye.

Clin.: That must have hurt.

Pt.: It really did, it really hurt … (perks up) But that's the way it's always been.

Clin.: Do you expect people to hurt you?

Pt.: … Yes, yes I do, maybe I'm growing accustomed to it, maybe I even like it.

Clin.: Going back to that night in the room with the candle flickering, did you have any thoughts of wanting to kill yourself?

Pt.: Yes, I did. As I sat there it all seemed sort of silly, so I began thinking about taking some pills. I'd stored up some Valium.

Clin.: What thoughts went through your mind?

From this dialogue the clinician can begin to feel the resounding hollowness of this patient's world, the intensity of her pain. One gains a sense of her neediness and her latent expectation of rejection, an expectation that may very well create the very bitterness that seeds actual antagonistic behavior from others put off by the patient's hostility. In any case, the patient seems somehow more "real." Moreover, this phenomenological excursion has provided many hints for the clinician of potentially productive regions of future exploration, another example of intuition guiding further analysis. Indeed, one wonders if this hollow world represents one petal in the abated flower we call a border line personality.

This excerpt began with an active investigation of the room with the patient, moving into associations generated by this phenomenological exploration. When exploring in this way, sometimes the patient will share associations experienced at the time being discussed, while at other times new associations stirred by recounting the experience may surface. In either case, rich material may become accessible to the clinician. Phenomenological inquiries are not necessarily based on questions dealing with the five senses. Frequently the patient's experience of the world is entered by questions exploring attitudes, opinions, recollections, and by an immediate sharing of feelings as they arise within the clinician–patient dyad.

Before leaving this excerpt, a quick perusal reveals an interesting twist. Notice that the clinician switched tenses from past tense to present tense with the phrase, "What else are you feeling in the room?" Such a switch sometimes facilitates a regression in the patient to a point where images become more real and less memory-derived. This type of maneuver can unlock repressed memories and emotions, as witnessed here by the unexpected emergence of anger directed towards a parent figure perceived as cool and distant. If one feels the interviewee cannot tolerate such a regression, as in an unstable patient or a psychotic patient, one would not utilize such a technique. In conclusion, phenomenological inquiry provides one more powerful method by which understanding may be increased.

The Search for Wellness: Patient Strengths, Skills, and Interests

For decades, one of the cornerstone characteristics of client-centered counseling and, more recently, person-centered medicine has been a belief in the importance of uncovering the inherent strengths of the patient, maximizing them, and realizing that the patient brings many healing factors to the table. As noted in Chapter 4 on facilics, in addition to the concept of the "presenting problem," I like to talk about the importance of uncovering the patient's "presenting solutions" as the interview proceeds. This concept recognizes the wellness of the patient as well as his or her illness. Patients have often tried a variety of measures for recovery and problem solving, some of which may have had some degree of success. We want to draw upon these inherent strengths, and capitalize on their utility during our subsequent efforts at collaborative treatment planning during the closing phase of the interview.

Several decades of research on the nature of happiness, spearheaded by researchers such as Seligman, Peterson, and others,[15-19] has evolved into the exciting field of positive psychology. Positive psychology attempts to delineate the characteristics and etiologies of positive states of mind such as happiness, resilience, psychological strength, and social well-being in a somewhat similar fashion that diagnostic systems sculpt out the attributes of psychopathological states. Used together, both approaches form a synthetic balancing of complementary ways for creatively helping patients with difficult times and symptoms.

To me, there are three markers of wellness: strengths, skills, and interests, which we will simply refer to as the "wellness triad." These wellness markers, when skillfully explored by an interviewer, not only help to flesh-out the person beneath the diagnosis, they may immediately provide suggestions for treatment planning based upon the idea of maximizing these wellness attributes to help the patient navigate whatever life circumstances or mental disorders he or she is encountering.

In the following sections I attempt to provide a quick overview of the wellness triad, so that the reader has a familiarization of these areas and the interviewing techniques that can be used to explore them. I refer the interested reader to the many outstanding books on the subject of positive psychology, such as the work of Seligman,[20] and more recently Robert Biswas-Diener,[21,22] as well as my own work on creating resiliency in both ourselves and our patients during difficult times.[23]

Before proceeding, I would like to add a note of reassurance to clinicians early in their careers who, as they have read the chapters in this book thus far, may be struck by the voluminous amount of material that appears to be important to uncover in an initial interview. The amount of material to be covered in an initial interview may seem intimidating at first, and to some degree it is. But it need not be overwhelming. I want to emphasize that I am not suggesting that in an initial interview one can explore all of the areas of the wellness triad, nor ask all of the questions about to be described. It is simply impossible.

In fact, much of the process of uncovering the numerous aspects of the patient's well-ness triad is a part of ongoing therapy. In the real world of a busy clinic, during the initial interview a clinician may only be able to barely touch upon these areas. On the other hand, an awareness of the importance of these wellness markers can help an interviewer to explore them as efficiently as possible, *when possible*, in the initial encounter. Moreover, the questions described in this section can subsequently be utilized in ongoing therapy.

This is also a good time to re-emphasize another reassuring point made earlier. *A clinician could never cover all of the questions or explore fully all of the content regions described in this book during an initial intake and should not try to do so.* By the end of any intake, time limitations will have forced us to leave untapped many questions that we wish we could have covered, from diagnostic questions using the DSM-5, to questions concerning wellness and aspects of social history. It is just a fact of life.

On the other hand, the resulting omissions do not have to be left to the chaotic whims of chance. If left to chance, critical data for helping the patient are often missed, perhaps never to be found, even in subsequent therapy. *Instead, one of the major themes of this book is that a clinician who has become familiar with what topics are most important to explore, and what interviewing techniques are available for sensitively exploring them, can gather a surprisingly sound database in 50 minutes.*

This knowledge of what to ask and how to ask it, coupled with a sophisticated under-standing of the facilics of an interview, can result in conversational interviews that are brimming with the information that is pivotal for successful treatment planning. Clini-cians can, and should, create intentional interviews in which wise decisions are made about what to delete, when to delete it, and how to delete it. With confidence, the inten-tional interviewer can make these decisions while noting what it is they want to further explore in later sessions. Even when time limitations become acute, as in emergency department interviews, the principles of this book allow the clinician to make wise deci-sions as to what to delete, while maximizing both engagement and the information needed for safe triage.

In essence, although we are focusing upon the initial assessment interview in this book, assessment is an ongoing process. A good clinician will continue to perform assess-ment in all succeeding sessions of therapy and/or medication management. Whether we are addressing aspects of the wellness triad or re-thinking our DSM-5 diagnostic formula-tions, the assessment process continues. Even in the last session of psychotherapy, a clini-cian is carefully assessing how the patient is handling termination itself. Indeed, it is only with the soft sound of the door shutting as the patient leaves our office for the very last time that the process of assessment actually ends.

Exploring Component #1 of the Wellness Triad: Patient Strengths

For both interviewer and patient, the concept of strengths can appear to be a nebulous subject, possibly because both parties seldom focus upon the delineation of strengths. In 2004, Peterson and Seligman[24] created an inventory of character strengths called the Values in Action Inventory of Strengths (VIA-IS), which provides a heuristically pleasing and practical listing of 24 potential human strengths, placed in six categories as follows:

Strengths of Knowledge:
1. Creativity
2. Curiosity
3. Love of learning
4. Perspective (wisdom)
5. Open-mindedness

Strengths of Courage:
6. Bravery
7. Persistence
8. Integrity
9. Vitality

Strengths of Humanity:
10. Capacity to love and receive love
11. Kindness
12. Social intelligence

Strengths of Justice:
13. Citizenship
14. Fairness
15. Leadership

Strengths of Temperance:
16. Forgiveness/mercy
17. Modesty/humility
18. Prudence
19. Self-regulation

Strengths of Transcendence:
20. Appreciation of excellence and beauty
21. Gratitude
22. Hope
23. Humor
24. Spirituality

For ongoing work with a patient, a well-validated self-administered assessment survey, which helps patients to spot their own strengths on the VIA-IS using a 240-item questionnaire, is available for free on the web and can be used quite effectively in ongoing counseling (www.authentichappiness.sas.upenn.edu).[25]

For the initial interviewer, the above list serves a slightly different function. I find that the list helps me to recognize patient strengths more readily, for I find it to be surprisingly easy to miss them in an initial interview. Such omissions occur for a natural reason.

Patients present to us not because they intend to discuss their strengths but because they are worried about their weaknesses. As they describe their presenting crises and as we explore the immense database required to provide optimum help during the initial session, it is easy to lose sight of the patient's strengths.

For instance, if I am interviewing a soldier's spouse, the above list can help me "to see" not only the obvious bravery and persistence of the patient's spouse in Iraq, Afghanistan, or wherever the soldier may be deployed, but the less obvious bravery and persistence of the patient in front of me. The patient may be single-handedly maintaining the well-being of the family, while dealing with the intense fear that his or her loved one could be killed at any moment. At times we might also find that we are not the only person in the room who has lost sight of these strengths.

In an initial interview, I find that occasionally I have time to uncover these types of processes through the use of statements that both explore and simultaneously acknowledge the patient's strengths as with the following, "However do you find the toughness to keep everything going at home when your husband is in Iraq and everyday you are dealing with the fear that he might be killed? It's really quite remarkable." Such a sensitive statement can powerfully enhance engagement, while also opening the door to a useful exploration of the patient's strengths and self-image. There is much to be learned if the patient responds, "I don't know. I've never viewed myself as tough."

In a different fashion, a clinician can decide, initially, to mentally file an observed strength, purposefully choosing to relay it later during the closing phase of the interview. Genuine complements provided during the closing phase regarding the strengths one has seen in an interview often pleasantly surprise a patient. They also can be used for treatment planning purposes at that time, as with, "How do you think we could tap your ability to organize material so well, as we develop a plan for helping with your burn-out at work?" Closing on strengths also tends to provide a positive feel to the ending of the initial session, better ensuring that there will be a next session.

In some interviews, one may have the time to ask directly about strengths with open-ended questions such as:

1. "When you look at yourself, what would you view as some of your best strengths?"
2. "What do you think your wife would say are your best strengths?" (insert husband, partner, best-friend, parents, boss or whomever is appropriate)

Some patients may feel a bit awkward about discussing their strengths openly, and some cultures may support such reluctance. Robert Biswas-Dienar has found that the following comment, which acknowledges the cultural taboo of speaking highly of oneself, can create a "local culture" between interviewer and patient in which the patient can feel more free to open up: "I know it may feel strange, like you are bragging, but I assure you I will not take it that way. I am genuinely interested in what you do well."[26]

Exploring Component #2 of the Wellness Triad: Patient Skills

Unlike patient strengths (which represent generalized characterological traits), the concept of patient skills is more specific. A patient skill is an actual ability that can be taught, improved, and consciously used to achieve a specific goal. A thorough listing of potential skills is well beyond the goals of this book and might well fill the remaining pages. On the other hand, it is useful to have a short list that can function as a framework for exploring patient skills both in the initial interview and during subsequent therapy:

Creative Skills:
1. Musical
2. Artistic
3. Mathematical
4. Writing/journaling
5. Reading
6. Web design, app design, or blogging/web journalism
7. Web or console game design

Task Related:
8. Problem-solving skills
9. Organizing skills
10. Marketing skills
11. Selling skills
12. Buying skills
13. Financial planning skills

Interpersonal Skills:
14. Listening to others
15. Providing comfort
16. Nurturing others
17. Teaching and mentoring
18. "Reading" people
19. Interviewing others
20. Being interviewed
21. Public speaking
22. Web-related skills such as social networking

Athletic Skills:
23. Skills in a particular sport
24. Coaching skills
25. Conditioning, nutrition, healthy living, body building, yoga, meditation, martial arts, etc.

Manual Dexterity:
26. Specific craft or discipline such as carpentry, gardening, auto bodyshop work
27. Precision technical expertise such as metal lathe, woodworking, etc.

Specific Career Training:

28. Everything from teaching, to health services, to managing a store, to web marketing

There exist many more categories and each of the above categories could have many other entries. This list gives us a starting point. As was the case with patient strengths, patient skills may indirectly be uncovered when the patient spontaneously raises them or describes situations where they naturally arise. But unlike patient strengths, which might seem a little awkward to directly raise in the initial interview, patient skills are relatively easy to raise in the initial assessment. When exploring the social history, one routinely asks about schooling and job history, thus opening the door to inquiries about specific skills.

Asking about skills is a particularly rich arena for uncovering the person beneath a diagnosis. Not only can it uncover skills that can be directly used as part of collaborative treatment planning, it also provides an open door into the patient's sense of self-esteem, secret ambitions, lost dreams, psychodynamic defenses, and interpersonal pressures from the expectations of others. To enter the region, one can ask directly, as with, "We all vary on what types of skills we have, what would you say are some of your skills?" If a patient seems to be a little hesitant to respond, I might add, "What do you think some of your friends or teachers or family might view as some of your skills if I were to ask them?"

With the right patient (powerfully engaged thus far in the interview, strong ego strengths, and a clear demonstration of humor earlier in the interview), a clinician can sometimes use wit to open the topic of the patient's skills in a rather paradoxical, yet highly effective, fashion. In the following illustration we will see the power of a well-timed use of humor and genuineness, as Egan described the concept in Chapter 2, to swing open the door hiding the patient's skills. What is behind such doors is sometimes unexpected, almost always useful, and, occasionally, of significant psychodynamic interest, as we are about to see.

Let us picture a Black male with smartly styled dreadlocks in his early 20s whom we shall call Jamal. He has presented complaining of depression, which he feels has resulted from his problems finding a job after graduating from college during a deep recession. Jamal wears a matter-of-fact, no-nonsense attitude towards life that protects him from the harshness of reality that he has all too often faced. Tall in stature, he enters the office with a bent posture, as if his depression was pushing downwards on his shoulders.

> **Pt.:** … there is simply nothing I can do right now. There are no jobs. I've been killing myself looking for 7 months now, it's just nuts. My girlfriend Tasha and I are really strapped for money. We're living together and rent is becoming a problem.
>
> **Clin.:** It sounds really tough. You certainly have been tenacious at looking. That is evident from your history. (the interviewer makes explicit an implicit strength from the patient's history in an intentional effort to help the patient see a potentially forgotten positive aspect of himself)
>
> **Pt.:** Yeah, yeah, that's true (pauses and looks towards the interviewer with a somewhat beaten look) – hasn't gotten me much though, but I suppose it's good that I try, not everyone would I suppose.

Clin.:   Absolutely not. I assure you I have many people who sit in that very chair who don't have your strength or persistence (Jamal smiles). You know, one thing you could do that could help me get a better handle on how you might approach the stress of hunting for a job would be if I had a better idea of what you think some of your skills are, you know, what you think you might have to offer on a job market. We all have things we feel skilled at and a few things we feel unskilled at. For fun let's start with the unskilled? What are you terrible at? (said with a straight face followed by a smile)

Pt.:   (patient chuckles) Where do I start? ... You mean it?

Clin.:   Sure, what are you really, remarkably terrible at?

Pt.:   (patient chuckles again) Let me put it to you this way, you don't want to hear me sing.

Clin.:   I guess American Idol is out? (clinician smiles)

Pt.:   (patient laughs out loud) American Idol is definitely out. But, I'm not devoid of any musical ability. I used to be a pretty good drummer.

Clin.:   Oh, what type of drumming?

Pt.:   Different kinds, but my favorite shit is heavy metal.

Clin.:   How good were you?

Pt.:   I was pretty awesome. (catches himself and sheepishly smiles) I wasn't Mike Smith, you might not know him, but he played in a band called Suffocation, now that brother can really play. But I was pretty good. I even won several drumming competitions while I was in high school. (seems lost in thought for a moment) Truth be told, I really wanted to make it as a drummer.

Clin.:   It sounds like you probably could.

Pt.:   Yeah. I probably could have. (shrugs his shoulders) I think I could have made it as a studio drummer. I would have loved that, but I decided to go to college instead.

Clin.:   I'm curious. Did you do that because your parents gave you some pressure to go to college? I ask that because sometimes parents, with all good intentions, try to push their kids away from a career in music, recognizing it's a rough way to make a living.

Pt.:   You know, strangely enough, the answer to that is "no." In fact, my dad thought I was very talented and on several occasions, both before I went off to college and while I was in it, he told me I could take off for a year or two and try to make it as a drummer and he would support that.

Clin.:   I wonder what stopped you?

Pt.:   (more deeply lost in thought for a moment) I don't know. (looks up) I really don't know.

Clin.:   What do you think you might have been afraid of, that made you choose to shy away from your own dream?

Pt.:   I never thought of it that way. But I guess I must have been afraid of something about pursuing the drumming (long pause) ... failure maybe? I don't know, but it's a really good question.

Clin.:   You know Jamal, it doesn't have to be a question about the past. It can be about the future?

Pt.:   I don't follow.

Clin.:   Last time I heard, the world still needs good drummers.

Pt.:	Hmmm (Jamal's eyebrows raise with the look of cognitive surprise). Maybe. At least I'd have plenty of time to practice. (smiles again)
Clin.:	Who knows? You might enjoy drumming again, simply because you seemed to love doing it so much in the past, and your face lit up just now while you were talking about it. It might even help with the depression a bit. I don't know. I'm also wondering if there is anything else you might be able to do with it, even to help with the financial problems you and your girlfriend are having?
Pt.:	You mean, like tutor somebody for money?
Clin.:	I'm not certain, but that's not a bad idea. I really don't know the field, but maybe there's something to be said for checking it out. You seem to really like people, and it's a chance to help some kid who could really use the help. I bet you'd be a good teacher.
Pt.:	Yeah, I sort of like teaching, but never thought of it as something I could do with the drumming. Sort of an interesting idea (pauses) … Tasha and I really, really need the money.

This highly productive exchange is not the norm for an initial interview, but an initial interviewer interested in uncovering patient skills, and trained to do so effectively as this interviewer illustrates, is much more likely to have such encounters. Our clinician has skillfully uncovered a specific patient skill set, clearly enhanced the therapeutic alliance, demonstrated his own competence to the patient, and gently parlayed into an exploration of the psychodynamics of the patient while providing some collaborative ideas on treatment planning. Not bad for 4 minutes of an initial interview, aptly demonstrating that explorations of patient skill can be successfully integrated into the first encounter.

Exploring Component #3 of the Wellness Triad: Patient Interests, Hobbies, and Pastimes

How a human being spends his or her time when not involved in making a living is a direct reflection of not only who may be beneath the diagnosis, but also of how the person beneath that diagnosis may unconsciously wish to be perceived. Beneath hobbies and pastimes, psychodynamic defenses are busily at work.

It is here that the importance of "reading between the lines" of the patient's book often makes itself clear. In the same way that the manner in which a house is decorated reflects the person who is living in the house, hobbies are interpersonal decorations that, in addition to personal interests, often reflect psychodynamic needs such as the need to be loved, to be left alone, or to be special at something. In this regard, the following question sometimes leads to surprising windows into a patient's needs to feel special or appreciated by others, "I'm curious, Anne, what types of photos do you like to post on Facebook (or whatever social media the patient uses)?" Patients reporting an unusually persistent and frequent posting of things they've made, accomplishments in sports, items they've bought, or pictures of their kid's accomplishments are, not infrequently, reflecting their inner needs to be recognized by others.

In this regard, in addition to uncovering what interests the patient pursues, it can be valuable to read between the lines as to what these pursuits may imply about the psychodynamics of the patient. An adolescent or young adult who spends entire weekends engaged in role-playing games at a local comic and manga store may have strong attachments to the group to which such an activity is appealing. The unassuming back-room of that little alley shop may be a place of safety, self-growth, and interpersonal refuge for a student who otherwise would be left alone to deal with the pangs of being an outsider in the hallways of his high school. Hobbies sometimes become identities, whether one is an athlete, biker, or goth. Depending upon the expressed interests of the patient, questions such as the following can lead to revealing dialogues:

1. "Do you view yourself as a 'biker'?"
2. "What do other students think of your goth friends?"
3. "How bad would it be for you, if you couldn't tailgate at the Steeler games?"

Curiously, the same hobby can range from being one that requires highly developed social skills to one that allows a person who is missing such skills to flee social interaction. It is worth finding out how a specific patient approaches a hobby before assuming what it means in a stereotypic fashion about socializing. For instance, one might assume that patients collecting sports cards or vinyl LPs might spend much of their time holed up alone in their homes perusing their treasures or listening to their finds. Yet both of these types of collectors could equally choose to hang out at card shops or attend "record shows" where they eagerly pursue social banter and even enjoy the high-level social exchanges required when wrangling over price, an art that requires not a small touch of ego strength. Web activities also range dramatically in their social interaction. The following type of question can provide some surprising insights in this regard: "When you are playing World of Warcraft online, do you play as a single or do you seek out a party?" If they seek out a party, it can be revealing to find out whether the party consists of friends, family members, strangers, or a combination.

As we saw with both strengths and skills, an exploration of interests can point towards treatment planning ideas based upon already present attributes of the patient that the patient has simply not thought of using to solve current stressors. We saw this earlier with Jamal, who had thought of his drumming neither as a potential antidote to his depression nor as a source of income. As a further example, a person coping with obsessive–compulsive disorder (OCD) who spends much time on Facebook and feels quite comfortable on the web, may not have thought to use these skills to utilize a chat room for people coping with OCD. They might not even know that such chat rooms exist. More and more crisis centers are providing chat and texting arenas, manned by expert crisis providers, for patients who are having suicidal thoughts but may be afraid to talk with someone on the phone.

One can raise the topic of outside interests and hobbies in a variety of straightforward fashions as with, "When you are not working, how do you like to spend your time?", "What types of things do you like to do in your spare time?", "Do you have any hobbies, sports, or things you really like to do a lot, like watch television or go online?", or "Do you like to use Twitter or other social media very much?" In closing, the very act of asking about the patient's interests can enhance engagement. Especially if the patient enjoys a rather unusual hobby or interest, a gentle command such as, "Tell me more about that,

I'm not very familiar with it, it sounds very interesting," when done with a genuine interest, can be surprisingly engaging. Such interludes may even "break the ice" in an interview where engagement has been lukewarm thus far.

PART III: UNDERSTANDING CULTURAL DIVERSITY – ITS VITAL ROLE IN THE INITIAL INTERVIEW

Culture and psyche make each other up.[27]

Richard Shwerder, cultural psychologist

We do not solely interview patients. We interview cultures as well. It is an illusion to believe that a human being exists outside of the culture in which the person developed. Equally, it is an illusion to believe that human cultures would exist without individuals. Thus the pains of our patients are the pains of the cultures in which they were raised and in which they now live. The pains of the culture are the aggregate pains of the people who walk the streets of the culture, abide and break its rules, obey and create its gods.

Kitayama and Cohen elegantly describe this curious paradox of identity in which people and culture exist within one another, a concept technically called "mutual constitution"[28]:

... culture is not a "thing" out there; rather, it is a loosely organized set of interpersonal and institutional processes driven by people who participate in those processes. By the same token the psyche is also not a discrete entity packed in the brain. Rather, it is a structure of psychological processes that are shaped by and thus closely attuned to the culture that surrounds them. Accordingly, culture cannot be understood without a deep understanding of the minds of people who make it up and, likewise, the mind cannot be understood without reference to the sociocultural environment to which it is adapted and attuned.[29]

The answer to the question as to why it is vitally important in person-centered interviewing to understand the role of culture in the initial interview is a simple one: From the perspective of mutual constitution, we cannot fully understand the person beneath the diagnosis unless we understand the culture that shaped, and is still shaping, the mind of the person waiting there. Moreover, to effectively help the patient, the clinician must understand the culture to which the patient is returning, for a treatment plan that does not take into consideration the cultural demands of the person seeking help may very well be doomed to failure by that very same culture. We saw the importance of this principle in the opening vignette of this chapter. The second clinician wisely shaped the initial treatment recommendations for Jennifer to fit the familial and spiritual culture to which Jennifer returned and which gave birth to the simple, yet powerful, cross that dangled from her neck.

To deeply understand, and perhaps equally importantly, to effectively empathize with the concerns of patients, the clinician must understand that the patient's concerns, symptoms, and even their diagnoses will be partially determined by the culture of both the patient and the clinician. At the interface of these two powerful forces – the culture of the patient and the culture of the clinician – the initial interview will unfold. As noted in an earlier chapter, not only the patient will be changed by the initial encounter, so will the clinician. Even more mysteriously, whether aware of it or not, by the end of the hour the patient and the clinician will have subtly changed the culture in which they find themselves, for they are integral elements in its never-ceasing evolution.

This deepening of the clinician's understanding of cultural diversity, a process that will continue throughout the clinician's career, is addressed in a variety of ways through-out the remaining pages of this book. We will later devote an entire chapter (Chapter 20) to the topic of culturally adaptive interviewing, at which point we will look at specific interviewing techniques and strategies for exploring the cultural beliefs of the patient, especially the patient's world view and spiritual frameworks. We will also explore in more detail what we mean by concepts such as "culture" and "cultural competence" as they are applied to interviewing in a practical everyday sense.

In the meantime, throughout the chapters of this book, we will see that processes we have already explored – such as empathy and the therapeutic alliance – are affected by cultural factors. By way of an introduction to this interface, in this chapter we will explore two specific arenas in which the forces of culture clearly impact on the clinician's under-standing of the person beneath the diagnosis: (1) potential misperceptions of each other, by both participants of the interview, created by cultural biases and (2) roadblocks to effective treatment planning, as well as fresh opportunities for effective treatment plan-ning, that are created by cultural factors.

Misperceptions Related to Cultural Biases: Impact on the Initial Therapeutic Alliance

Franz Boas, one of the founders of American cultural anthropology, created a wonderful metaphor – "kulturbrille." Kulturbrille is the set of "cultural glasses" that each of us wears at all times. These cultural glasses, like all lenses, have both the power to clarify the world the patient is describing and the ability to distort the view of that very same world.[30]

Such distortions are far from unilateral in nature. Each participant in the interview dyad peers outwards through his or her own cultural spectacles, potentially unaware of what distortions are being created. In essence, whereas Sullivan's parataxic distortions are caused by the unconscious processes of both parties, "kulturbrille distortions" are caused by the unconsciously created biases of the cultures from which we all grow. If not understood by the interviewer, these bi-directional distortions can damage the inter-viewer's ability to engage the patient, to understand the patient, to collaboratively plan treatment with the patient and, ultimately, to help the patient. It is thus of critical impor-tance for clinicians to understand the impact of both sets of eyeglasses being donned in the initial encounter, even though they may be as invisible as a pair of contacts.

Expectations of "what should happen in therapy" can be discordant, depending upon cultural attitudes. For instance, cultures may vary on how they address the concept of time and timeliness. Compared to a White American's concept of time, a Native American may have a more relaxed attitude towards time (based upon a feeling of how time seems to almost imperceptibly pass during the turnings of a day in Nature as opposed to the tickings of a clock).[31] Consequently, a Native American patient may consistently appear late for appointments. An interviewer not aware that the patient is simply following acceptable cultural norms may misinterpret the patient's behaviors as signs of resistance or irresponsibility. On the flip side, a Native American patient may find a White American therapist's demands for timeliness, as well as their attempts to "pin-down" when subsequent appointments should occur – and for exactly how long (50 minutes) – somewhat puzzling. Both parties may also have different views as to the importance of ending the sessions "right on time." A Native American who perceives a clinician as being overly focused upon such time issues during an initial interview may find himself or herself feeling uncomfortable with the interaction. The patient could even come away with the feeling that this particular clinician is a "pushy" person "who seemed more interested in time than me," a perception that could easily diminish the likelihood of a second appointment. Let us look at a different possible area for a cultural disconnect.

All of the largest racial/ethnic subcultures that might be encountered in the United States (including Asian American, Indian American, White American, African American, Hispanic American and Native American) hold in high regard the quality of trustworthiness. All of these cultures value a person who is honest, a person who stands by his or her word. Thus clinicians – no matter what their culture of origin, from Latino/a to Black to White – also tend to view trustworthiness as an important component for successful therapy.

Of the cultures listed above, all of which value trust, there is a difference in how the cultures approach the seemingly unrelated concept of expressing disagreement, especially when disagreeing with a figure of respect or authority. Yet these two apparently unrelated cultural values can sometimes intertwine to create a curious misperception by an interviewer. Let's see how it might unfold.

We will picture an interviewing dyad composed of an Asian graduate student on a visa sitting with a non-Asian university counselor (the counselor could be Black, White, Latino/a, or Native American, etc.). The patient is suffering from a depressive episode during his first year of graduate school.

This patient's Asian background will provide us with a vivid example of how interviewers naive to cultural norms may inadvertently misattribute negative qualities to a patient. Compared to the cultures of the non-Asian potential counselors mentioned above, many (not all) Asians or Asian Americans may tend to shy away from the direct expression of disagreement and/or confrontation.

Consequently, as the Sommers-Flanagans point out, if an Asian American is hesitant about a specific treatment recommendation, the patient may not directly say so, for it would be viewed, within his or her culture, as a sign of possible disrespect to the therapist with whom they are meeting for the first time.[37] Consequently, the patient may generate the mildest (yet still unwanted) affirmative response available. The mildness of the agreement would be interpreted as a possible or *even a probable "no"* in the patient's culture of origin. But, to the non-Asian therapist, raised in a culture where disagreement is voiced much more readily, it appears quite obvious that the patient has given a "yes" to the treatment recommendation.

When, in the next appointment, it becomes apparent that the patient did not do "what he agreed to do," it is very easy for the non-Asian therapist to view the patient as being, at best, ambivalent in nature and, at worst, unmotivated, irresponsible, or even prone to deceit. Clearly the "cultural glasses" of Franz Boas are at work here. Such kulturbrille distortions can result in a remarkably shaky therapeutic alliance.

For a moment we will stick with this combination of a non-Asian American therapist and an Asian American or recent Asian immigrant or visitor, for it introduces another aspect of culture that can interfere with the accuracy of clinician perception – nonverbal norms. Compared to the other cultures mentioned above, Asians may handle eye contact differently.

The Asian cultures have a rich, and deeply rooted, heritage of respecting elders. Consequently, during the first meeting with an elder, or any respected figure such as a physician or mental health professional, direct eye contact may be relatively minimal. A gently reduced level of eye contact is often the culturally accepted way of expressing deference to a respected person. Direct and persistent eye contact could be viewed as a sign of disrespect.[33] Unaware of this cultural norm, the non-Asian therapist (whether White, Black, Latino/o, etc.) could misperceive the lowered eyes and poor eye contact of the patient as evidence of poor blending, shyness, lack of confidence, or even "attitude" if the patient happened to be an adolescent.

Culture Impacting Directly on Treatment Planning in the Initial Interview

The insights of the anthropologist Ward H. Goodenough shed light on the impact of culture on the process of the initial encounter and the treatment planning created within its confines, for patients come to us as agents of change. As Goodenough highlights, it is culture that may ultimately determine the patients' actual interests in changing and how they approach it:

> *Culture, then, consists of standards for deciding what is, standards for deciding what can be, standards for deciding how one feels about it, standards for deciding what to do about it, and standards for deciding how to go about doing it.*[34]

In our opening vignette with Jennifer, we already witnessed the power of a subculture – a strict fundamentalist perspective by her family – to create concrete roadblocks to treatment planning. As Goodenough suggests, it is not only the treatment options for the patient that may be limited by culture. Such limitations affect all elements of the treatment team, including the clinicians. We all are wearing the kulturbrille spectacles that Franz Boas described earlier. Cultures can limit the ability of the clinician to see viable treatment options that may be appearing in the dialogue of the interview – effective treatment options that would be readily apparent to a clinician familiar with the patient's culture.

As clinicians walk into initial interviews, they enter with distinct biases about treatment planning. Some like to use medications; some don't. Some like psychotherapy; some don't. Those who like psychotherapy may prefer cognitive–behavioral therapies, others may prefer psychodynamic models, and some embrace both. Some routinely involve family members in treatment planning. Others seldom do, except in inpatient settings. Some are open to alternative therapies, others do not believe in them.

Of critical importance to us, as students of the initial interview, is the recognition that these biases (and we are all entitled to our individual beliefs about therapeutic interventions) can sometimes distort what we "hear." At times, clinicians tend to "hear" in the database those bits of data that support their predispositions towards their preferred therapeutic interventions. Such a distorting process is potentially damaging, for it can prevent a clinician from seeing the value of an intervention that is new to the clinician, but perhaps of great importance to the patient's subculture. The success of the therapy, *and even the validity of the database upon which it is based,* may be dependent upon the clinician's ability to spot these kulturbrille distortions.

Cultures and subcultures can provide unique resources for treatment planning purposes, if the clinician is willing to listen to the culture. For example, many clinicians in the United States and Canada find themselves working with the Hmong, who have had a significant immigration to North America. Within this culture, shamans can play a major role in community function and in the approach to healing. Understanding this cultural fact, an interviewer may opt to invite the patient's shaman, if requested by the patient, to consult upon the treatment plan. If one is working within a culture where shamans or medicine men play a major role (such as the Hmong, Native Americans in the United States, and First Nations people in Canada), it can be useful to ask, "Have you talked to a shaman (or medicine man) about your problems?" If the answer is "yes," by then asking "What were his opinions?", unexpected yet useful ideas for treatment intervention may be shared, ideas that the patient is already predisposed to pursue. An open and respectful discussion of the shaman's recommendations by the interviewer can metacommunicate that the clinician is not culturally bigoted or narrow in his or her approach. This metacommunication can be remarkably powerful in securing initial engagement.

After brainstorming on a treatment plan in the closing phases of an intake interview, it can also be wise to ask, "What do you think your shaman might think about our plan?" If there are going to be culturally related roadblocks to treatment planning acceptance, an astute interviewer will want to know about them beforehand, not after the patient returns, having already decided against the treatment plan because of the cultural antagonism with which it was met. Alerted to such a potential impasse, the clinician may be able to prospectively transform it.

As the Sommers-Flanagans point out, some cultures, such as the Asian American culture, tend to downplay the role of individual decision making.[35] Most personal decisions by an individual are viewed as directly reflecting the values, worth, and integrity of the larger family unit. Hence, some Asian American patients may believe that these decisions should be made by the family as opposed to the individual. If this is the patient's belief, it is important to involve family members in treatment planning early on. With almost all young Asian Americans, the following type of question may be both useful and revealing: "What do you think your parents will think of our ideas for using psychotherapy (medications, etc.)?"

Latino/a cultures traditionally place strong emphasis upon the father as the "head of the family."[36] As with the Asian American patient, it may be useful to ask questions such as, "What do you think your father will think of this treatment?" If a father disagrees "back home," the clinician may need to give considerable support to the patient's personal choice for treatment, for such parental opposition can be strikingly intense. The pressures on Latina patients by paternal dictates can be remarkably stressful, literally destroying a treatment plan before it is begun.

Although we have been focusing on situations in which cultural roadblocks to treatment planning may be related to cultural biases, at times clergy and key family members can become strong advocates for beneficial treatment interventions that the patient, and perhaps even the patient's culture, may be wary of utilizing. For instance, a patient lost within the terrors of a psychotic process may be more likely to agree to the use of potentially life-saving antipsychotics, not by the entreaties of a clinician from a different culture, but by the respected words of a trusted figure within the patient's culture.

I would like to end this chapter by sharing one of the clearest examples I have encountered of this exact phenomenon. I believe it nicely illustrates some of the key principles of this chapter. It highlights the importance of trying to understand the patient beneath the diagnosis in the initial assessment, as well as the fact that to do so, one must understand the cultural context of that patient and of the patient's symptoms.

It began when I met Anna for the very first time. Anna had been admitted to an inpatient unit dedicated to helping people with schizophrenia. When I entered the room, I was met by a pair of eyes that had the paradoxical quality of being both piercing and frightened at the same time. Anna was a 24-year-old African American who had been admitted the night before, through the emergency department, suffering from what would prove to be her first break of schizophrenia. She wore a colorful shawl wrapped tightly about her somewhat overweight body, as if she had enveloped herself in a protective suit of magical armor. I would soon learn that she was protecting herself from a hoard of demonic voices and fears of possession.

Anna was strongly opposed to the use of medications. In the initial interview I learned that she belonged to a Pentecostal church in which her own mother was the minister. Her mother was, quite naturally, steeped in the beliefs and rituals of her chosen faith, being quite adept at speaking in tongues and performing exorcisms. I was concerned that her mother's religious beliefs were going to be "problematic" from my viewpoint, in the sense that she might disagree with the diagnosis of schizophrenia and be strongly opposed to the use of an antipsychotic. She would soon prove me to be very wrong indeed.

In a subsequent session alone with Anna's mother, we both shared and listened to each other's beliefs shaped by our respective subcultures about what was wrong with Anna. Her mother had, indeed, been concerned that Anna was possessed and had already performed an exorcism. When I asked about the impact of the exorcism and also the presentation and actions exhibited by Anna since possession, she described her church's efforts in some detail. I asked about other possessions she had seen, other exorcisms that had worked effectively, and what she felt the future would hold for both her daughter and herself. After talking extensively about her previous experiences with exorcism, she paused for moment and then queried, "What do you think is going on?"

I subsequently shared thoughts about the symptoms of schizophrenia, the potential role of the brain and neurotransmitters, and some of the subtle pre-psychotic phenomenology of psychotic process (social withdrawal, problems with sleep, wariness, mild agitation, moments of being lost in thought, all of which often predate for weeks or months the onset of delusions or hallucinations). It was here that Anna's mother seemed particularly interested, nodding on several occasions, the type of nod accompanied by a quiet "hmmm," as if nonverbally acknowledging, "I might have seen that." At one point she gave a little sigh, and asked, "If Anna has this schizophrenia thing, do you think you can help her?" Later she commented, "I'm not so sure she is possessed. It's not like any possession I've ever seen." Apparently, through her careful listening, she had independently arrived at her own personal conclusion that her daughter's behavior seemed to fit the description of schizophrenia better than the possibility of possession.

As she was about to leave my office, she turned and commented, "You know, Dr. Shea, I agree that Anna is probably suffering from what you call schizophrenia, but there is something important for you to know." I asked, "What is that?" She said, "Just keep in mind that Satan causes it. He is always behind our suffering." She smiled, and walked out the door.

Two cultures met, both cultures saved face, and both cultures agreed to join forces. This anecdote serves as poignant reminder that some of the most important culturally powerful interviews are not necessarily the ones with our patients. They are sometimes the ones we have with the people who love our patients.

Anna's mother subsequently convinced Anna to give the antipsychotic a try. The results were exciting, with an excellent remission within 1 month. Interestingly, during this episode of her daughter's illness, Anna's mother was comfortable asking Anna to not attend church services, "until God has healed the chemistry of your brain, for I don't think it's a good idea for you to be around thoughts of possession and exorcism until your brain is working the way God intended it to." Anna agreed.

I am convinced that Anna's suffering would have been remarkably more intense and prolonged (she remained in good remission) had it not been for the interventions of her mother, whose religious beliefs were open enough to a different perspective to decide upon an atypical approach to healing from her culture's perspective. I would like to think that the openness and genuine respect of the interviewer, myself in this instance, of her beliefs and her previous successes at healing, set the tone for her reciprocal openness to my ideas. We will never know for sure.

What I am sure of, however, is that for about 20 minutes, two people – Anna's mother and myself – were able to remove their cultural glasses. The kulturbrille effect was suspended, and each participant saw the other with a more accepting eye. More importantly, it gave us the chance to see that we both shared the same mission – to help Anna with her great pain. And, appropriately enough, it would be Anna who would ultimately gain the most from our clearer vision.

REFERENCES

1. Jacobi J. *Paracelsus: selected writings*. [Guterman N, Trans.] Princeton, NJ: Princeton University Press; 1995.
2. Sullivan HS. *The psychiatric interview*. New York, NY: W.W. Norton; 1970. p. 25.
3. LaFarge L, Zimmer RB. Other early theories. From the chapter: Psychoanalytic theories. In: Tasman A, Kay J, Lieberman JA, editors. *Psychiatry*, vol. 1. Philadelphia, PA: W.B. Saunders; 1997. p. 411–12.
4. Ogden T. The analytic third: working with intersubjective clinical facts. *Int J Psychoanal* 1994;75:3–19.

5. Dunn J. Intersubjectivity. From the chapter: Psychoanalytic theories. In: Tasman A, Kay J, Lieberman JA, editors. *Psychiatry*, vol. 1. Philadelphia, PA: W.B. Saunders; 1997. p. 435–7.

6. Nachmias D, Nachmias C. *Research methods in the social sciences.* New York, NY: St. Martin's Press; 1976.

7. Whitehorn JC. Guide to interviewing and clinical personality study. *Arch Neurol Psychiatry* 1944;**52**:197–216.

8. Sullivan HS. 1970.

9. Whitehorn JC. 1944. p. 197–216.

10. Whitehorn JC. 1944. p. 197–216.

11. Whitehorn JC. 1944. p. 197–216.

12. Eco U. *The name of the rose.* San Diego, CA: Harcourt Brace Jovanovich; 1983.

13. May R, editor. *Existence.* New York, NY: Simon & Schuster; 1958.

14. Hall CS, Lindzey G. *Theories of personality.* 3rd ed. New York, NY: John Wiley; 1978. p. 320.

15. Seligman MEP. *Authentic happiness.* New York, NY: Free Press; 2002.

16. Seligman MEP, Csikszentmihalyi M. Positive psychology: An introduction. *Am Psychol* 2000;**55**:5–14.

17. Peterson C, Seligman MEP. *Character strengths and virtues: a classification and handbook.* New York, NY: Oxford University Press/Washington, DC: American Psychological Association; 2004.

18. Ryan RM, Deci EL. On happiness and human potentials: a review of research on hedonic and eudaimonic well–being. *Annu Rev Psychol* 2001;**52**:141–66.

19. Park N, Peterson C, Seligman MEP. Strengths of character and well-being. *J Soc Clin Psychol* 2004;**23**:603–19.

20. Seligman MEP. 2002.

21. Biswas-Diener R. *Practicing positive psychology coaching: assessment, activities & strategies for success.* New York, NY: Wiley; 2010.

22. Biswas-Diener R. *Positive psychology coaching: putting the science of happiness to work for your patients.* New York, NY: Wiley; 2007.

23. Shea SC. *Happiness is.: unexpected answers to practical questions in curious times.* Deerfield, FL: Health Communications, Inc.; 2004.

24. Peterson C, Seligman MEP. 2004.

25. Seligman MEP. *Authentic happiness* <www.authentichappiness.sas.upenn.edu> [accessed 15 August 2011].

26. Biswas-Diener R. 2007. p. 125.

27. Kitayama S, Cohen D. *Handbook of cultural psychology.* New York, NY: The Guilford Press; 2007. p. xiii.

28. Kitayama S, Cohen D. 2007. p. xiii.

29. Kitayama S, Cohen D. 2007. p. xiii.

30. Monaghan J, Just P. *Social & cultural anthropology.* New York, NY: Sterling Publishing; 2010. p. 52.

31. Sommers-Flanagan R, Sommers-Flanagan J. *Clinical interviewing.* 2nd ed. New York, NY: John Wiley & Sons, Inc.; 1999. p. 379.

32. Sommers-Flanagan R, Sommers-Flanagan J. 1999. p. 383.

33. Sommers-Flanagan R, Sommers-Flanagan J. 1999. p. 383.

34. Monaghan J, Just P. 2010. p. 63.

35. Sommers-Flanagan R, Sommers-Flanagan J. 1999. p. 382–3.

36. Garcia-Preto N. Latino families: an overview. In: McGoldrick M, Giordano J, Pearce JK, editors. *Ethnicity and family therapy.* 2nd ed. New York, NY: Guilford Press; 1996.

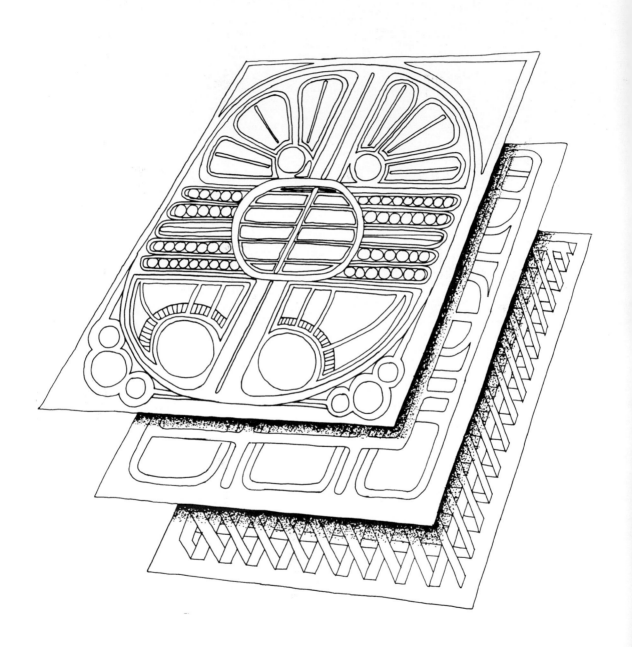

CHAPTER 7

Assessment Perspectives and the Human Matrix: Bridges to Effective Treatment Planning in the Initial Interview

We shall not cease from exploration
And the end of all our exploring
Will be to arrive where we started
And know the place for the first time.

T. S. Eliot
Little Gidding[1]

We have already seen how a deeper understanding of the person beneath the diagnosis can suggest powerful methods for securing a sound initial treatment plan, while simultaneously maximizing engagement and the likelihood of a second meeting. One critical way-station on our map of the initial interview remains untapped – the cognitive art of assessment. By "assessment" we are referring to the fashion in which the clinician "puts all of the puzzle pieces together" from the patient's history. The clinician will arrive at his or her initial formulation of what the problems are, what are the various forces at work contributing to the patient's problems, and what are some of the possibilities for transforming these problems. This fourth way-station in our map is arguably the major gateway to our fifth, and final way-station – collaborative treatment planning (Figure 7.1).

In our first six chapters we have focused upon clinician behaviors as manifested in specific interviewing techniques and strategies. But it is not only the interviewer's behaviors that define an interview; interviewing is also a cognitive art. In this regard, the initial interviewer's mind is alive with assessment possibilities – potential clues to healing.

Much cognitive work is occurring while the interview unfolds, for the interviewer, in addition to gathering the database, must also "listen" to the database as it reveals itself. The ultimate goal of the initial interview – in addition to enhancing the likelihood of a second interview – is to collaboratively develop an initial treatment plan that seeds hope by the end of the interview and, indeed, begins the healing process. It is from the interviewer's and patient's assessment of what is right and what is wrong that treatment options come to mind. It is this cognitive assessment that creates the bridges leading into

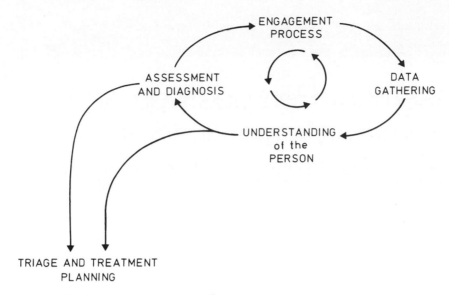

Figure 7.1 Map of the interviewing process.

effective treatment planning. These cognitive skills, utilized throughout the initial encounter, are the focus of this chapter.

I must emphasize that this is not a chapter about how to choose specific therapies and design concrete treatment plans. Such a topic as treatment planning is both complex and vast – well beyond the scope of a book focused on the interviewing process. The interested reader is directed to the many outstanding texts on treatment planning.[2–4] Instead, this is a chapter about the cognitive processes and decisions that a clinician must make *during the interview itself* about what data to gather in the first place and how to use this data to collaboratively develop treatment plan options with the patient. I believe that a fundamental familiarity with the basic principles of treatment planning is an essential part of an interviewing course, for a clinician cannot truly understand how to interview effectively if one does not understand the reason for the interview – what information is needed for a treatment plan and why.

This chapter explores three assessment perspectives by which clinicians can organize, during the interview itself and immediately afterwards, the massive stream of information encountered in an initial interview in such a way that the database provides signposts pointing towards possible treatment options. In essence, a sound assessment perspective can generate a listing, in the interviewer's mind, of possible treatment interventions to collaboratively share with the patient. Such ongoing organization can also significantly enhance the clinician's ability to rapidly create a final assessment document (whether dictated, typed, or written), a skill of marked importance in this age of managed care and tight time constraints, as well as representing the final task of the initial interview.

Frequently I have seen clinicians falter, not because they lack adequate knowledge about the use of specific treatment modalities, but because the use of certain modalities never comes to mind. They become lost in the database, emphasizing certain information while ignoring, or not even obtaining, other pertinent data. We are dealing with an information processing problem, a not unexpected dilemma considering the vastness of the information involved in understanding another person's problems. In this chapter we will study a common-sense approach to creating a realistic list of viable treatment options. No attempt is made to suggest the pros and cons of any specific treatment; rather, the focus is upon bridging from the process of data gathering in the body of the interview to collaboratively creating an initial, albeit tentative, treatment plan in the closing phase of the interview.

This chapter also demonstrates that the treatment opportunities that come to mind for the clinician appear to be directly related to both the data collected and the method of organizing the data. For example, a clinician who does not learn to ask questions concerning the neurovegetative symptoms suggestive of a medication-responsive depression will most likely not think to utilize such a medication. Likewise, a clinician is less likely to think of intervening via social work channels if current stressors are ignored.

To avoid such tunnel vision, clinicians can organize their data into schemata that emphasize conceptualization from multiple viewpoints. In this chapter we will look at three such systems. Through them, the power of a well-organized database to lead to effective treatment planning will become apparent.

We shall look at the following three assessment perspectives: (1) the diagnostic perspective provided by the *Diagnostic and Statistical Manual of Mental Disorders* (DSM-5 version),[5] (2) matrix treatment planning, and (3) the perspective provided by understanding the "core pains" of the patient. Although overlapping at their interfaces, each of these perspectives generates unique clues for treatment planning. Consequently, it is often expedient to create an initial treatment plan utilizing all three perspectives. I have found single-perspective treatment planning to be generally unsatisfactory, akin to beginning a watercolor with only half of the necessary paints. The value of multi-faceted treatment plans, which integrate care longitudinally, has been well described in a variety of areas by authors such as Kim Mueser and Robert Drake concerning dual diagnoses[6] and McKinnis-Dittrich with elders.[7]

Each of the three assessment perspectives provides the following benefits for usefully organizing clinical information:

1. An easy and rapid method of checking, during the interview itself, whether pertinent data regions for treatment planning have been explored, thus decreasing errors of omission
2. A reliable method of reminding the clinician to borrow from different data perspectives when collaboratively formulating a treatment plan with the patient
3. A flexible approach to delineating a list of potential treatment modalities with the patient

In addition, outside of the domain of the initial interview, a clinician who understands how to effectively utilize these three bridges into treatment planning will have learned a set of skills that are invaluable in ongoing treatment planning, especially when there appears to be a roadblock. These treatment-planning perspectives often allow treatment teams to create new and refreshing transformations of stalled moments in ongoing care. We will begin by reviewing a database gleaned from an actual initial interview. Following this presentation, the information from each of the three perspectives mentioned above will be examined, observing the utility in the initial interview provided by each viewpoint.

CLINICAL PRESENTATION: THE INITIAL INTERVIEW

When I first saw Ms. Baker (Debbie) she was sitting in the waiting room. Her eyes were hiding behind a pair of large, pink-framed sunglasses. These frames were bordered by her shortly bobbed brown hair. She had a round face and a rather short frame. She was wearing a neon-pink T-shirt and a pair of freshly washed jeans. Wrapped around her left wrist was a wide leather band with the name Paul tooled into it.

When I asked if she was "Ms. Baker" she pertly looked up, smiled and replied, "Yes, I'm Ms. Baker, but not for long." I asked what she meant, and she replied, "Oh, I'm getting married in a month."

Once in my office, she related a story of a longstanding problem with fluctuating moods. She spoke in a quiet voice, frequently casting her eyes to the floor, as if to avoid seeing the impact of her words upon my face. She displayed no evidence of derailment (loose associations), thought blocking, pressured speech, or illogical thought. She gave no evidence of responding to hallucinations and denied both auditory and visual hallucinations.

With regard to her moodiness, she stated that her moods frequently changed throughout the day. It was not at all unusual for her to feel various moods, including anger and rejection, during the course of a single day. Although she reported intermittent periods of feeling decreased energy, decreased interest in activities, decreased libido, and difficulty falling asleep, she denied any periods of 2 weeks or more in which these symptoms were persistent. She denied manic or hypomanic symptoms past or present.

She lived in a world of imagined fear, persistently worried that she would be abandoned. At night she would become angered if her partner fell asleep first, because she would quickly become engulfed by her fear of being alone. These fears fostered an intense dependency, which she readily admitted was a major handicap. She went out of her way to please her partner, allowing all major decisions to be made by her, including the upcoming wedding plans. This dependency also surfaced with the string of therapists lying in her wake. Her most recent therapist had to have her forcibly removed from his office by the police, an act marking the end of their contact.

As one might have surmised, impulse control was not a strong point. For instance, several years earlier she had managed to toss a picnic table bench through a friend's picture window while enraged. Moreover, she had a history of popping pills in small suicidal gestures about every 2 to 3 months over the past 3 years.

Her relationship with her parents was very strained, and she felt she had always been marked as the black sheep of the family. She had one sister 2 years older than she, who was employed as an accountant and was reported as happily married. One of her earliest memories consisted of standing behind the front door weeping as her father walked away down the stone path. As she cried, her mother shook her violently, pulling her away from the doorway.

To my surprise, the wristband bearing the name Paul had nothing to do with past or present friends or her partner. Instead it referred to herself, for she often fantasized that she was Paul Newman. This vivid fantasy game was indulged by her partner, who would call her Paul when they decided to play this game of pseudo-identity. At no time did Debbie, nor her partner, lose sight that this was merely a fantasy, although she longed to be anyone but herself. When talking of her fantasy identity, she would occasionally cry softly, as if punctuating her story with tears.

THE DIAGNOSTIC PERSPECTIVE OF THE DSM AND ICD SYSTEMS

The Healing Power of Differential Diagnosis

For clinicians, differential diagnosis serves one major purpose – to discover information that may lead to more effective methods of helping the patient. Diagnosis should not be an intellectual game or a pastime used to placate insurance companies. Over the years I have found the DSM systems (*Diagnostic and Statistical Manual of Mental Disorders*), including the DSM-IV and the DSM-5,[8] as well as the International Classification of Diseases (ICD) nomenclatures,[9] to be invaluable in helping me to initiate the healing process, serving as a robust bridge to treatment planning. A formal diagnostic schema provides this bridge to treatment planning in many ways.

Like the common language we have developed for discussing the interviewing process itself, the art of differential diagnosis allows one to conceptualize the complexities of the patient's presentation more clearly, while alerting the clinician to hidden problems. Differential diagnosis can also provide valuable information concerning prognosis, possible treatment modalities, and pitfalls to be avoided in dealing with certain syndromes (i.e., a psychotherapist who has spotted that the patient fits the criteria for a dependent personality disorder in the initial interview will be careful to avoid psychotherapeutic missteps in subsequent sessions that could lead to a pathologic dependence on the therapist).

A particularly important benefit of performing a sound differential diagnosis *with all patients in an initial interview* is the ability of a clinician adept at such skills to uncover a hidden diagnosis that a patient will not share spontaneously because of problems with stigma, embarrassment, or lack of self-awareness that a problem exists. Such a hidden diagnosis, if left hidden, can lead to problems, including severe ramifications such as untreated substance abuse and even suicide, all because the patient was afraid to share the symptoms unless directly asked about them, a surprisingly common phenomenon.

For instance, as we saw in Chapter 2, many patients with obsessive–compulsive disorder (OCD) will develop reactive depressions to the problems caused by having the OCD. Because of fears of appearing crazy or strange, they will present to the therapist complaining only of their depression or marital problems. Likewise, a college student presenting with depressive or anxious symptoms may have severe bulimia or substance abuse underlying it, which is not shared spontaneously secondary to stigma. For these reasons, the art of diagnostic formulation remains a cornerstone of sound assessment during an initial interview.

In my opinion, many treatment failures are the result of such untreated hidden diagnoses. Studies such as the National Comorbidity Survey (NCS) have shown marked comorbidity among commonly presenting mental disorders including depression, panic disorder, OCD, and alcohol dependence.[10] In a community sample, over 56.3% of patients presenting with a major depression had another current psychiatric disorder.[11] The rate of comorbidity is even higher with another commonly presenting disorder – generalized anxiety disorder – where rates of comorbidity have been reported of more than 90% in both a clinical and community sample.[12] By doing a sound differential on all patients, no matter "how obvious" the presenting symptoms may be for a mood or anxiety disorder, one may uncover a disorder that is even more problematic or might even be the root of the patient's problems.

In addition, diagnostic systems such as the DSM-5 and ICD-10 allow both clinicians and researchers the opportunity to share their successful experiences in treating a specific disorder in a common language. When a clinician discovers a treatment plan that is useful in relieving a resistant major depression, these findings may be applicable to a patient being treated by a fellow clinician, who might benefit from the shared knowledge. Formal differential diagnosis is a practical passport to the knowledge housed in journals, books, and the minds of our fellow clinicians.

A clinical vignette will make this abstract discussion more concrete. I was working with a couple whose marriage was riddled with a nasty streak of passive aggression and strained communication. After several sessions, the marital therapy seemed to be bogging down. The husband, a rather narcissistic man, kept insisting that nothing was being done for him. In reviewing my notes, I discovered that the referring clinician had diagnosed the husband as suffering from a dysthymic disorder. I had recently read an article reporting that certain types of dysthymic disorders responded well to antidepressant medication. My patient fit one of these descriptions and consequently was begun on an appropriate antidepressant. He quickly found significant relief.

However, to the chagrin of both the patient and his spouse, their marital friction remained painfully present. Up to this point, he had balked at couples therapy, categorically stating, "My problems are all from my depression. Trust me, there is nothing wrong with my marriage." With marked marital discord remaining despite relief from his depressive symptoms, he no longer had an excuse for avoiding the work of therapy, thanks to the antidepressant suggested by his DSM diagnosis. Suddenly the marital therapy could move ahead more effectively. This vignette illustrates the power of a common diagnostic language to provide a clinician with knowledge discovered by others. Without the diagnosis of dysthymia, and its relation to the article that I had just read, this pivotal treatment intervention would not have been tried.

Let us explore in more detail how diagnoses can be valuable in suggesting possible treatment modalities. For instance, major depressions frequently respond to antidepressants and may also benefit from concurrent psychotherapy or, frequently, from psychotherapy alone. Bipolar disorder (manic phase) is usually approached with lithium, antipsychotic medications, or antiseizure medications such as carbamazepine, lamotrigine, and valproic acid. Phobias are frequently alleviated by using cognitive and behavioral techniques. Mild to moderate forms of major depression can be approached using dynamic and cognitive psychotherapies, behavioral approaches, or numerous counseling techniques. Uncovering the presence of a borderline personality disorder can suggest the use of specific evidence-based interventions such as Marsha Linnehans' dialectical behavioral therapy (DBT)[13] or recent time-limited transference-based therapies.[14] The above list merely represents a terse survey, but it nevertheless highlights the power of a diagnostic system to help in developing a diverse treatment approach.

Finally, diagnosis can play a key role in the healing process from a completely different perspective than the clinician's viewpoint. Correct diagnoses, shared sensitively, can be surprisingly comforting to patients who have had no idea what was plaguing them other than there "must be something really wrong with me" or "I must be a weak person." Underlying biologic disorders such as bipolar disorder or adult attention-deficit disorder not only can destroy effective functioning, they can savage self-esteem and self-image. Such patients often go for years without any knowledge that they have an underlying biologic disruption, which has been the root cause of their ruined marriages, lost jobs, failed grades, and financial collapses. In such cases, patients often view themselves as the sole creators of their distress and failures. These types of self-degrading cognitions can lead to untold suffering and can also provide fertile soil for suicide. Learning that there exists a different explanation for their inability to function – than they had believed – can be powerfully healing, as we saw with the woman who presented with depression but had severe OCD as her primary diagnosis in Chapter 2.

Limitations of Formal Diagnostic Systems Such as the DSM and ICD

Before proceeding, it seems expedient to review some of the important limitations of traditional diagnostic approaches, such as the DSM-5. Only through knowledge of a system's weaknesses can its strengths be utilized safely.

One of the most obvious limitations remains the fact that diagnoses are labels. As labels, they can be abused. One such abuse occurs when clinicians fall into the trap of using diagnoses as stereotypical explanations for human behavior. It should be remembered that a diagnosis provides no particular knowledge about any given patient. It merely suggests possible characteristics that may or may not be generalizable to the patient in question. In addition, as we saw in Chapter 6, it is critical to uncover the person beneath the diagnosis, a point elegantly stated by the gifted physician Sir William Osler, many years ago, when he commented, "It is much more important to know what sort of patient has a disease than to know what sort of disease a patient has."[15]

Moreover, diagnostic formulations are evolving processes and as such should be periodically re-examined. There is a realistic danger that patients can become stuck with inappropriate diagnoses, a problem that can only be avoided through persistent reappraisal. In a similar fashion, the clinician should remain healthily aware of the potential ramifications of certain diagnostic labels with regard to the patient's culture and family. By way of example, the label of schizophrenia can result in the loss of a job or in the development of a scapegoating process within a given family. Considerations of these problematic aspects of diagnosis related to cultural issues should be integral parts of sound clinical care.

In this regard, the kulturbrille effect, introduced in our last chapter, can cause problems such as over-pathologizing, if the interviewer is not aware of cultural norms. For instance, where I trained in medicine at the University of North Carolina in Chapel Hill, it was not uncommon for patients to talk about "root-working," which was a culturally accepted folk belief that some people could perform malicious magic by burying and manipulating certain roots. Obviously, with some people who were suffering with schizophrenia this became part of a delusional belief system. But it was important for clinicians to realize that all patients who discussed root-work were not necessarily psychotic. In some patients it was merely an accepted belief and not evidence of psychopathology. In advanced diagnostic systems such as the DSM nomenclature and ICD, it is stressed that clinicians should be aware of such cultural norms so as to avoid such misattributions.

The issue of the significance of a specific diagnostic label to the patient himself or herself can be of marked importance. For this reason, I frequently ask patients if anyone has given them a diagnosis in the past. If the answer is "yes," one can follow with questions such as, "What is your understanding of the word schizophrenia?" or "Do you think that diagnosis is right?" The answers to these questions can provide valuable insight into the patient's self-image, intellectual level, and previous care.

With these limitations in mind, we can now begin our exploration of the DSM-5 in more detail. In 1980, the DSM-III system introduced many of the innovations, such as multiaxial formulation, that formed the foundation of the contemporary DSM systems. A bridge between the two systems called the DSM-III-R appeared in 1987, and added its own new ideas and refinements. The DSM-IV itself was published in 1994. In 2000, the DSM-IV-TR (Text Revision) was published, which did not change any diagnostic criteria but added much useful information about psychopathology and the subtleties of the diagnostic system to enhance the system as an educational tool, while keeping its material updated to reflect advances in evidence-based research.

It is to the DSM-5 system that we will now turn. We will not attempt to review diagnostic criteria now, because these are discussed in subsequent chapters. Instead we will look at those principles that help to make diagnostic formulation possible in the first 50 minutes. As diagnostic systems evolve they necessarily experiment with various changes, many of which are good, and occasionally, a few are not so good. There are some significant improvements in the DSM-5, but we will begin our study by noting what I, personally, feel is a potential regression in the system. This book focuses on contemporary practice, but I feel that this brief exploration of historical context can help the reader to be a better clinician both now and in the future.

The Loss of Multiaxial Formulation: a Historical Footnote

To me, one of the most compelling aspects of the DSM-III and the DSM-IV-TR was the fact that these systems pushed the interviewer to consider various contextual perspectives while formulating a diagnostic picture. Each perspective was placed upon one of five axes.

On Axis I, clinicians were prompted to delineate the patient's presentation in terms of the classic psychiatric diagnoses such as major depression, bipolar disorder, schizophrenia, anorexia nervosa, OCD, and post-traumatic stress disorder (PTSD). Indeed, all psychiatric disorders – with the exception of personality disorders and intellectual disabilities – were listed on this first axis. It was on Axis II that clinicians were to list personality disorders as well as personality traits, whether the traits were problematic or sometimes beneficial in nature. Medical disorders and other biologic conditions such as pregnancy were placed on the third axis. It was on Axis IV that the clinician could help place the patient into their contextual matrix by addressing processes such as family, friendships, living conditions, financial concerns, and cultural issues. Finally, on the last axis, the interviewer considered in what fashion the above concerns and disorders were impacting on the patient's relatively recent and immediate functioning.

The beauty of the system was the fashion in which it emphasized a holistic approach to conceptualizing the patient's presentation while simultaneously preventing biological reductionism. This multiaxial approach metacommunicated that the field of psychiatry emphasized the importance of a contextual understanding of the patient. Indeed, the multiaxial system demanded that clinicians look at the patient contextually.

The DSM-5 has removed the mutiaxial system and, to my knowledge, is now the only major international diagnostic system that is not multiaxial. I mention it as being odd (a personal opinion) in that it seems to fly in the face of the current emphasis upon person-centered medicine, whether one is dealing with diabetes and cancer or schizophrenia. It should be noted that the final arbiters of the DSM-5 still felt that contextual factors, whether they be cultural, interpersonal, or environmental are important. Indeed, they recommend that such factors be routinely addressed in separate notations with all patients, but this recommendation seems to be undermined by the elimination of specific axes where it was *required* that these factors would be routinely addressed.

I feel that the lack of these axes, especially in our current age of time constraints, may invite a lack of attention to core aspects of care by harried clinicians. For instance, placing personality function and disorders on a separate axis in the DSM-IV-TR reminded clinicians that it is *always* important to understand the personality functioning of the patient and how it might impact on Axis I disorders such as OCD or schizophrenia. It further pushed clinicians to sensitively uncover the unique personality attributes of each patient, for such personality predispositions can be invaluable in understanding how a patient responds to his or her symptoms as well as in collaboratively developing treatment plans that fit the needs of that patient's unique personality traits.

In any case, despite the lack of formal axes in the DSM-5, I myself find it useful when listing the DSM-5 diagnoses to always address the presence or absence of personality disorders and medical disorders separately, to remind myself (and the reader of my clinical assessment) of the importance of such factors. By way of illustration, in the chapters on differential diagnosis in Part II of this book, I will demonstrate how to do so in our clinical vignettes.

Later in this chapter, we will see that factors such as psychological, social, and spiritual aspects are comprehensively addressed in the two other treatment planning frameworks that I suggest routinely employing in addition to the DSM-5: matrix treatment planning and understanding the core pains of the patient.

Major Psychiatric Disorders (Other Than Personality Disorders)

At first glance the DSM-5 may appear confusing because of the large number of diagnostic entities that it contains. But there is little need for concern. The craft in using this system lies in approaching the task by first uncovering the general diagnostic probabilities and then delineating the specific diagnoses (Figure 7.2).

As the initial interviewer listens during the opening phase and the body of the interview, the symptoms of the patient will suggest diagnostic regions worthy of more elaborate expansion. This primary delineation will lead the clinician to one or more of the following easily remembered regions of adult psychopathology:

1. Schizophrenia Spectrum and Other Psychotic Disorders
2. Mood Disorders (including major depressive disorders, bipolar disorders, etc.)
3. Anxiety Disorders
4. Obsessive–Compulsive and Related Disorders
5. Trauma/Stress-Related Disorders (includes acute stress disorder, PTSD, adjustment disorders, etc.)
6. Dissociative Disorders
7. Somatic Symptom and Related Disorders (somatic symptom disorder, illness anxiety disorder, conversion disorder, etc.)
8. Feeding and Eating Disorders
9. Substance-Related and Addictive Disorders
10. Neurocognitive Disorders (delirium, dementia, etc.)
11. Other miscellaneous disorders (gender dysphoria, disruptive and impulse-control disorders, sleep–wake disorders, paraphilic disorders, etc.)
12. Mental disorders due to a general medical condition (e.g., personality change secondary to a frontal lobe tumor, etc.)
13. V-codes and other conditions that may be a focus of clinical attention

Looked at in this simplified fashion, the first step in utilizing the DSM-5 appears considerably more manageable than at first glance. In order to succeed, the clinician must be well grounded in psychopathology, as will be discussed in Part II of this book. This knowledge base will allow the interviewer to quickly determine which of the thirteen areas are most pertinent. As the interview progresses, the clinician can reflect upon whether each of these broad areas has at least been considered, thus avoiding errors of omission.

Once the primary delineation has been made, the interviewer can proceed with the secondary delineation, in which the specific diagnoses subsumed under the broad diagnostic areas are explored and the more exact DSM-5 differential diagnosis is determined. Thus, if the clinician suspects a mood disorder, the clinician will eventually hunt for criteria substantiating specific mood diagnoses such as major depressive disorder, bipolar disorder, dysthymia, cyclothymic disorder, other specified or unspecified depressive

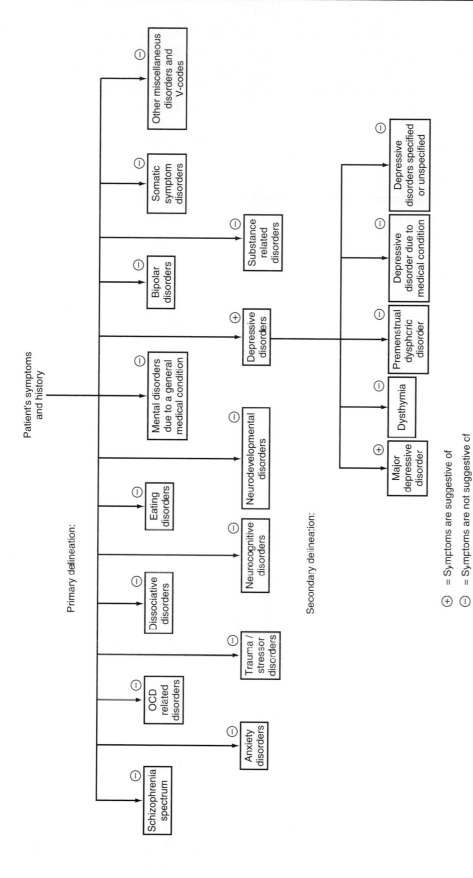

Figure 7.2 Basic approach to diagnostic utilization with adults (patient with a major depressive disorder).

disorders, and other specified or unspecified bipolar disorders. This secondary delineation would be performed in each broad diagnostic area deemed pertinent.

As already described in Chapters 3 and 4, these explorations occur during the main body of the interview. Most importantly, they are done in a highly flexible fashion, always patterning the questioning in the style most compatible with the needs of the patient and the clinical situation. Consequently, the clinician expands these diagnostic regions in a unique fashion with each patient, mixing them with various other content regions and process regions. When done well, the result is an interview that feels unstructured to the patient yet delineates an accurate diagnosis.

V-codes represent conditions not attributable to a mental disorder that might be useful as areas for the focus of therapeutic intervention. Examples include academic problems, occupational problems, uncomplicated bereavement, low interest and follow-through with medications, marital problems, parent–child problems, and others. Sometimes these codes are used because no mental disorder is present, and the patient is coping with one of the stresses just listed. They can also be used if the clinician feels that not enough information is available to rule out a psychiatric syndrome, but, in the meantime, an area for specific intervention is being highlighted. Finally, these V-codes can be used with a patient who carries a specific psychiatric syndrome but for whom that syndrome is not the immediate problem or the focus of intervention. For example, an individual with chronic schizophrenia in remission may present with marital distress.

Personality Disorders

The basic approach to differential diagnosis with personality disorders follows the same two-step delineation that we found to be useful in delineating the non-personality related psychiatric disorders above. In the first delineation, one asks whether the interviewee's story suggests evidence of long-term interpersonal dysfunction that has remained relatively consistent from adolescence onwards. If so, the patient may very well fulfill the criteria for a personality disorder or disorders.

After determining that a personality disorder may very well be present, the clinician proceeds with the secondary delineation in which specific regions of personality diagnoses are expanded. This secondary delineation will result in the generation of a differential from the following list:

1. Paranoid personality disorder
2. Schizoid personality disorder
3. Schizotypal personality disorder
4. Histrionic personality disorder
5. Narcissistic personality disorder
6. Antisocial personality disorder
7. Borderline personality disorder
8. Avoidant personality disorder
9. Dependent personality disorder
10. Obsessive–compulsive personality disorder

11. Other specified personality disorder
12. Unspecified personality disorder

In Chapter 14 we will examine in great detail the many fascinating subtleties involved in exploring personality structure during an initial interview. One area not covered by the DSM-5 but sometimes of great value in understanding personality functioning is the role of defense mechanisms. Defense mechanisms range from those commonly seen in neurotic disorders such as rationalization and intellectualization to those seen in more severe disorders such as denial, projection, and splitting.

Understanding a person's unconscious defense mechanisms (in classic psychoanalytic thought, defense mechanisms are viewed as being generally unconscious) can help the interviewer to uncover a more accurate picture of the person beneath the diagnosis. Defense mechanisms represent unconscious coping skills that protect a person from intense anxiety and/or unconscious ideas, images, or desires that would create intense guilt or shame. A detailed exploration of the various defense mechanisms, as they unfold in ongoing psychotherapy, is beyond the scope of this book, but the interested reader will find an excellent survey of them in the DSM-IV-TR, where a proposed possible axis called "the Defensive Functioning Scale" is outlined.[16]

Non-Psychiatric Medical Conditions

Non-psychiatric medical conditions such as diabetes, hypertension, seizures, etc., were listed on Axis III in the DSM-IV-TR. In the DSM-5, such disorders are now merged into a listing of the psychiatric disorders that are present.

The importance of an awareness of the potential presence of non-psychiatric medical disorders cannot be emphasized too much. In my opinion, all patients who exhibit psychological complaints for an extended time period should be evaluated by a physician, nurse clinician, or physician's assistant to rule out any underlying physiologic condition or causative agent. To not perform this examination is to risk a real disservice to the patient, because entities such as endocrine disorders and malignancies can easily present with psychological symptoms. *The astute clinician will always keep in mind that one can easily misattribute depression or anxiety that is being caused by an undiagnosed medical illness, such as hyperthyroidism, a low-grade encephalitis, or a frontal lobe brain tumor, to a current stressor. Just about anybody who develops a medical illness will have unrelated concurrent stressors in his or her life, for stress is a common aspect of living.*

A person with an undiagnosed, slow-growing brain tumor that is resulting in a moderately severe depression with angry outbursts could be undergoing a severe financial loss with foreclosure that is completely unrelated to the brain tumor. An unwary clinician can quickly ascribe the depression and anger to the foreclosure (because the patient also is ascribing the depression and anger to his finances and loss of his house), thus missing the real cause of the mood disturbance and disruptive behaviors – a potentially fatal brain tumor. Proceeding with psychotherapy, without having uncovered the malignancy via a referral to a medical specialist, will result in precious time lost as the malignancy continues to grow and potentially metastasize. A keen persistence in ruling out the presence of a contributing non-psychiatric medical disorder can help clinicians to avoid such potentially dangerous red herrings.

It should also be remembered that the presence of a serious medical condition such as diabetes or congestive heart failure (even when it is unrelated to any psychiatric symptoms or disorders) represents a major stressor to the patient. Such conditions can significantly impact on the patient's resiliency and ability to cope with his or her psychiatric disorder. Such considerations are of immediate importance in collaborative treatment planning and mobilizing familial/social/medical supports.

In this same light, a medical review of systems and a past medical history should become a standard part of an initial psychiatric assessment. Other physical conditions that are not diseases may also provide important information concerning the holistic state of the interviewee. For instance, it is relevant to know if the interviewee is pregnant or a trained athlete, because these conditions may point towards germane biologic and psychological issues, sometimes indicating potential strengths, such as routine exercise or yoga practice, that can be capitalized upon as parts of the treatment plan.

Psychosocial Context and Stressors

Although there is no specific axis for assessing psychosocial factors in the DSM-5, their importance is emphasized. Indeed, the DSM-5 recommends routinely assessing psychosocial factors and documenting the assessment as a special notation in all diagnostic assessments. Unfortunately, as mentioned earlier, I fear that without the mandate of a specific axis requiring an exploration of these factors, they may frequently be under-explored.

Nevertheless, this exploration, when done well, allows the interviewer to examine the crucial interaction between the patient and the environment in which he or she lives. All too often interviewers can be swept away by the complexities, intrigues, and symptoms of specific psychiatric disorders, failing to uncover the reality-based problems confronting the people coping with these disorders. These reality-based concerns frequently suggest avenues for therapeutic intervention as well as uncovering unexpected support systems.

By way of illustration, an interviewer may discover that secondary to a job layoff, the home of the patient is about to be foreclosed. Such information may suggest the need to help the patient make contact with a specific social agency or may suggest referral to a social worker.

This area of inquiry also remains of paramount importance in the successful use of crisis intervention counseling, time-limited therapies, and solution-focused therapies. Any time a patient presents in crisis, it is generally useful to determine what perceived stressors have brought the patient to the point of seeking professional help. A question such as the following is often useful: "What stresses have you been coping with recently?" or "What was going on for you that made you decide to actually come here tonight as opposed to coming tomorrow or some other time?"

Level of Current Functioning and Impairment

Once again, the DSM-5 has eliminated a designated axis for recording information regarding the patient's level of function (formally Axis V in the DSM-IV-TR). However, the DSM-5 does acknowledge the importance of such explorations. In this regard, the World Health Organization's Disability Assessment Scale (WHODAS) is included in Section III of the DSM-5, but the WHODAS is not easy to use in the tight time constraints of an initial assessment. The absence of a designated axis for requiring a sound assessment of current functioning, to me, invites potentially inferior exploration.

A robust assessment of actual current functioning pushes the clinician to carefully review evidence of immediate coping skills as affected by symptomatology. It is important to utilize behavioral incidents in this exploration, for patients, if merely asked for their opinions, may give misleading answers. By way of example, an acutely psychotic patient who does not want to be admitted to hospital may reply with a simple "not often" when asked, "Are the voices bothering you frequently?" Utilizing validity techniques such as behavioral incidents and symptom amplification as described in Chapter 5, the clinician may find that the dialogue develops more along the following lines:

Clin.: Looking at the last 2 days, how many times have you heard the voices per day, 10 times a day, 30 times a day, 60 times? (symptom amplification)

Pt.: (pausing and glancing away for a moment) Probably, well … maybe a good 30 times a day.

Clin.: What types of things do they say? (behavioral incident)

Pt.: (pause) They tell me I'm ugly. So what else is new.

Clin.: What do you feel when the voices say mean things like that to you? (behavioral incident)

Pt.: It hurts, but I try to push them out of mind.

Clin.: Do they ever tell you to hurt yourself? (behavioral incident)

Pt.: You could say that.

Clin.: What exactly do they tell you? (behavioral incident)

Pt.: They tell me to kill myself because I'm too ugly to live.

By starting with a symptom amplification and then repeatedly using the behavioral incident technique, the clinician has found not only that the voices are bothersome but also that they are frequent and potentially dangerous.

The clinician may find it to be opportune, during the exploration of current functioning, to ask directly about elements of the wellness triad, hunting for strengths, skills, and interests as described in Chapter 6, for all of these attributes may be of value in helping the patient to cope more effectively with their current problems. Also keep in mind with regard to current functioning that sources outside the patient, such as family, friends, roommates, and employers frequently provide more valid information than the patient. Once again, when questioning collaborative sources, behavioral incidents can be used to enhance validity.

Clinical Application of the DSM-5

To begin applying our first assessment perspective, the DSM-5, we must first organize our data. We will then ask ourselves what, if any, treatment modalities are suggested by the diagnoses we have generated. With regard to major psychiatric diagnoses (other than personality disorders), Debbie's presentation suggests several diagnostic entities. The primary delineation suggests that her symptoms are those of some type of mood disorder. Regarding the secondary delineation into the specific mood disorders present, she does not appear to currently fit the criteria for a major depressive disorder, but she may represent a variant of persistent depressive disorder (dysthymia). As mentioned earlier, the presence of this disorder might suggest the short-term use of an antidepressant. Dysthymia can also be approached using a variety of psychotherapeutic modalities, including cognitive–behavioral therapy (CBT) and psychodynamic models.

Her history suggests no strong evidence for entities such as schizophrenia or other psychotic processes, although the clinician may want to explore her vivid fantasy productions in more detail to rule out the possibility of delusional material or dissociative identity disorder. There is no evidence of a neurocognitive disorder such as delirium or dementia. Several areas not well explored are the areas of anxiety disorders, obsessive–compulsive disorders, trauma-related disorders, and dissociative disorders. In a later interview these omissions can be easily addressed.

Here we see how the use of a diagnostic paradigm can help prevent problematic errors of omission. Even the best clinician, and I have encountered this process many times in my own work, will not have time to scan for all potentially pertinent diagnoses because of the tight time constraints under which we all work. Through the use of a diagnostic schema such as the DSM-5, one can quickly, and reliably, spot diagnostic areas that were inadvertently missed, opening up the chance to appropriately explore for potentially hidden diagnoses in the next interview. To miss a diagnosis such as PTSD (possibly related to childhood abuse) in a patient with Debbie's presentation could lead to missed opportunities for treatment intervention, including such opportunities as a survivor's group.

Regarding personality dysfunction, several possibilities are emerging that may provide important clues as to how to proceed. Many of her symptoms, such as her frequent angry outbursts, her numerous overdoses, and her deep fears of abandonment and being alone, suggest the possibility of the diagnosis of a borderline personality and perhaps a dependent personality. Both of these diagnoses serve to warn the clinician that Debbie may be predisposed to becoming overly dependent upon the clinician. Dependency issues may be important areas for focus in the upcoming therapy. Also of importance is the fact that a large body of literature exists concerning the treatment of the borderline personality, literature that can be easily tapped by the clinician. As a triage agent, the diagnostic label of a borderline personality may also suggest the wisdom of not assigning this patient to a newly trained or poorly skilled therapist, because such patients are frequently difficult to manage. Regarding personality dysfunction, one might further explore entities such as a histrionic personality, a schizotypal personality, or an antisocial personality.

As mentioned earlier, all patients should be conceptualized within the context of their personality structures and predispositions, no matter how striking the presenting symptoms of the patient's non-personality related symptoms may be. In this fashion, diagnoses such as borderline personality will not be missed. By not recognizing processes such as the potential for borderline dependency early in therapy, the therapist risks missing the diagnosis until well into therapy, by which time the patient may have already become markedly enmeshed and dependent on the therapist. By this point, much painful acting out may have occurred for the patient, and smooth transitions to other treatment options, such as DBT, will have been made more difficult. All of this pain could be avoided by screening for this diagnosis in the initial interview, as was done with Debbie.

An exploration of possible non-psychiatric medical conditions brings many important points to mind. In the first place, Debbie's depressive symptoms suggest the possibility of a mood disorder due to a general medical condition. She needs a medical examination. If the initial clinician is a psychiatrist, then this clinician has omitted a good medical review of systems. This omission will need to be rectified. Pertinent laboratory work will be ordered, and a physical examination may be indicated.

But the exploration of non-psychiatric medical conditions does not end here. The history of episodic violence may suggest an underlying seizure disorder (caused by head trauma) that may have been routinely missed by previous clinicians. Once again, the interviewer will want to ask questions pertinent to this diagnosis and may consider ordering an electroencephalogram (EEG) or referral to a neurologist. Her worsening of symptoms near her menstrual periods also adds the possibility of a premenstrual dysphoric disorder, which may suggest the use of medications to relieve cramping and an antianxiety agent used for a day or two near her periods to decrease her premenstrual tension or the addition of a low-dose selective serotonin reuptake inhibitor (SSRI) antidepressant.

A final medical consideration concerns Debbie's obesity. One wonders whether there may be an organic etiology for her obesity, such as hypothyroidism or polycystic ovarian disorder. One also wonders as to whether her weight represents a powerful psychological concern, which she was hesitant to discuss because of stigma.

Even though there is no specific axis devoted to assessing psychosocial factors, as mentioned earlier the DSM-5 system suggests that a careful exploration of psychosocial factors should be a part of any evaluation. With regard to Debbie, one questions what the impact of the upcoming wedding will be. Even for the most stable of people, weddings are stressful. Her wedding stresses may be further amplified by cultural bigotries related to same-sex marriage, once again an arena for supportive counseling in future sessions. A review of psychosocial factors also indicates that the interviewer has not explored current stressors very well yet. With regard to triage and the determination of when Debbie should be seen next, it would be useful for the interviewer to have a much clearer picture of the current stressors.

Regarding Debbie's current functioning, the information is sparse here, reflecting a relative weakness in the database thus far collected. Keep in mind that such database weaknesses are common, and inevitable, in initial interviews, for there is not enough time to collect a perfect database. But it is our diagnostic perspective that prompts us to recognize these weak areas, a recognition that will allow us to explore these important topics in future sessions. A more thorough examination of current functioning would be of value in determining disposition. One also wonders what skills Debbie may possess that may be utilized in her treatment. For instance, her possibly overactive fantasy life, if toned down, may represent a fertile imagination, which could be an asset in her development as an individual. Current functioning and the availability of immediate social supports clearly warrant further exploration.

The above discussion illustrates the immense power of diagnostic systems such as the DSM-5 or the ICD-10 as methods of organizing data in a fashion that generates treatment options and also for "pointing out" areas of important clinical information that may have been overlooked. In addition, if utilized as intended, a clinician employing the DSM-5 system should be routinely looking for the person beneath the diagnosis by better understanding the patient's personality functioning, biological health, and the complexities of the patient's psychosocial and environmental stresses.

But these factors may be under-emphasized or overlooked by clinicians because of the absence of specific axes emphasizing their inherent importance in the DSM-5 system. In addition, there are other elements of a holistic assessment (such as spirituality, family dynamics, and cross-cultural nuance) not emphasized by the system. Consequently, even when used as intended, in my opinion, this assessment perspective alone can yield an incomplete picture of the patient. We will now turn to an assessment system that directly focuses upon the areas of relative weakness in the DSM-5, perspectives that may provide us with new insights into Debbie and how to help her.

MATRIX TREATMENT PLANNING

Nothing exists in isolation. Whether a cell or a person, every system is influenced by the configuration of the systems of which each is a part, that is, by its environment.

George L. Engel[17]

Introduction

Matrix treatment planning provides a stimulating and practical method of organizing and utilizing the data gained from the initial interview that complements the DSM-5 or the ICD-10. The term "matrix treatment planning," which I am introducing to the clinical literature in this chapter, is a recent term that I prefer to the more standard and traditionally accepted term "biopsychosocial treatment planning." *They describe the same system.*

Although they describe the same system, as we shall soon see, I believe there are advantages to the newer term and the re-emphasis it places upon the interactional principles behind the biopsychosocial model as it was first delineated.

The goal in this section is to provide the initial interviewer with a reasonable conceptualization of what matrix treatment planning offers, how it is used, and its ramifications concerning what information needs to be gathered in an initial interview (as well as during ongoing psychotherapy). To accomplish this task in the sophisticated fashion that it warrants, we will examine exactly what is meant by matrix treatment planning, including the ideas from which it evolved (the biopsychosocial model) and from which it is still evolving.

As with our exploration of the DSM-5 system, there is no attempt to describe the pros and cons of specific treatment interventions here. Rather, the intention is to describe how to maximize the use of matrix treatment planning during the collaborative planning undertaken with the patient in the closing phase of the interview. Although not the intention of this chapter, I believe the reader will find that these principles will also be of use in long-term treatment planning.

Indeed, initially, our exploration of matrix treatment planning will require a somewhat extended side-trip from our interviewing map. The type of sophisticated understanding that a clinician needs in order to effectively undertake collaborative treatment planning, in the closing phase of the initial interview, will demand a focused attention upon some of the core principles of treatment planning itself.

Before we begin our exploration of the interface between the initial interview and matrix treatment planning, I would like to add a cautionary note to the reader. At times, some of the nuances of matrix treatment planning may appear somewhat complex, perhaps even overwhelming. Truth be told, they are complex. They are also intricate, delicate, and richly practical.

The goal of this chapter is *not* for the beginning student to understand and be able to immediately utilize all of the principles of matrix treatment planning delineated in the following pages. The goal is to leave the reader with a fascination and a genuine appreciation of the power of matrix treatment planning to heal. If successful, the reader will leave the chapter with a lively motivation to learn how to effectively employ the concept of the human matrix.

As you read, you will develop a sophisticated understanding of how matrix treatment planning principles can be elegantly interwoven into the initial intake. I believe it is important, in a beginning course on interviewing, to immediately see how this integration is gracefully achieved by a skilled interviewer, so as to have a model from which to work from the very beginning of your initiation into clinical interviewing.

As you continue into your more advanced years of training, you will participate in a variety of courses, internships, and clinical rotations that will provide you ample opportunities to learn how to implement the principles described in the following pages. Indeed, it is my hope that in the remaining years of your training (and post-training) you will frequently return to this chapter to help you integrate the many new skills you will be encountering.

Thus, sit back and enjoy the ride. The following pages describing the interface between the initial interview and matrix treatment planning are intended to provide an enticing and practical preview of the process. Nothing more. It will hopefully provide, in the years to come, a goal towards which you can work and a model from which you can more easily achieve that goal.

Basic Paradigm and History of the Biopsychosocial Treatment Planning Model

George Engel, an internist in medicine with many interests in psychosomatic medicine, was an elegant proponent of utilizing a biopsychosocial approach to treatment planning.[18] Indeed, he can be viewed as one of the founders of the biopsychosocial model. More recently, many authors, including Glen Gabard and Jacqueline Barkley, have provided cogent reminders of the importance of this approach to treatment planning for clinicians across all mental health disciplines.[19-23] Engel's work was an extension of what can be called systems theory or analysis. The following depiction of matrix treatment planning parallels Engel's work, but applies it directly for use by mental health professionals.

The term "matrix" has several definitions. With regard to treatment planning it refers to the idea that a matrix is the "stuff" from which something, in this case the patient and the clinician, are created. In matrix treatment planning, human beings are seen not so much as static "things" with permanent characteristics but rather as an intertwining series of processes. The patient is viewed as a moment in time, in which various processes intersect and interact to create what we call a human being. In short, the patient and the clinician are both viewed as ever-changing processes, evolving with each passing moment.

Since the various systems of a matrix, by definition, represent fields of interdependent interaction, changes in one system of a matrix almost always create changes in the other systems within the matrix. If a change in one system has a positive effect on another system it is called a healing matrix effect. If a change in one system creates a negative impact on another system it is called a damaging matrix effect. Sometimes a problem in one system of the matrix can cause such marked problems in a different system that it appears to the interviewer that the primary problem resides in this secondary system, when, in reality, this is a misperception – a phenomenon called a red herring effect. Each system of the patient's matrix offers a potential wedge for therapeutic intervention.

Guided by such a theoretical understanding, an initial interviewer understands at once the importance of gathering information from all the systems impacting upon the patient. To not do so, the interviewer risks making misjudgments as to what is right or wrong with the patient during their initial encounter. Moreover, the patient may feel as if he or she is being viewed as an object or mere diagnosis taken out of context, a feeling that can result in significant disengagement.

In addition, the matrix perspective – because it emphasizes that changes in one wing may cause unexpected changes in other wings – alerts the clinician that beneficial matrix effects from unexpected fields of the patient's matrix may be waiting to be tapped. In addition, it simultaneously cautions the initial interviewer to carefully weigh finalizing recommendations until the ramifications of such interventions on more distant fields of the patient's matrix can be more accurately assessed.

In matrix treatment planning, each person is viewed as representing the conjunction of the following six progressively larger systems: (1) the biologic system, (2) the psychological system, (3) the dyadic system (including intimate relationships), (4) the family system, (5) the cultural, societal, and environmental system, and (6) the patient's worldview or framework for meaning. Each smaller system is subsumed by the system above it. In matrix treatment planning, each of these systems is known simply as a "wing" of the matrix. Each of these wings can be used as a level in which to organize data and subsequently develop a list of potential treatment modalities. The six wings of the human matrix are illustrated in Figure 7.3.

The original biopsychosocial model, as envisioned by innovators such as Engel and as implemented extensively by pioneers in the fields of social work, clinical psychology, and nursing, emphasized that changes made in one system often created changes in the other wings, whether intended or not. In fact, Engel's original delineation focused heavily

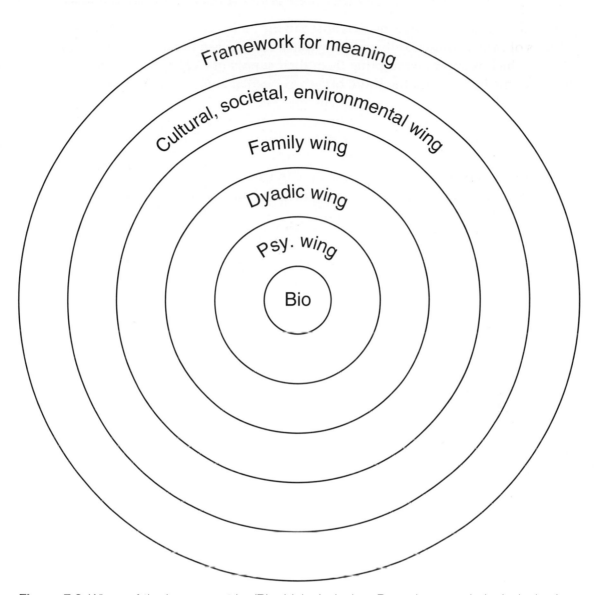

Figure 7.3 Wings of the human matrix. (Bio, biological wing; Psy. wing, psychological wing.)

upon the idea that treatment planning, at a sophisticated level, often found ways of transforming a problem in one wing of the matrix by making changes in another wing of the matrix.

A clinical example from Engel's world of internal medicine brings this interactional quality to life. Picture a man in his mid-50s and his wife presenting to an emergency room at 2:00 A.M. on a drizzly Saturday, the man having been awakened by a crushing sensation in his chest. We shall call our hypothetical patient Mr. Franklin. On this particular night, Mr. Franklin, whose belt cannot quite adequately contain his belly, is wiping away the profuse sweat pouring from his forehead, a rather odd phenomenon for such a cool October night.

As the triage nurse rapidly assesses the situation, she accurately recognizes that Mr. Franklin is suffering from an acute heart attack and must be triaged rapidly to advanced care. A life-threatening emergency has arisen in the biological wing of Mr. Franklin, where millions of cardiac muscle cells are being starved for oxygen because one of his coronary arteries, which is supposed to bring them their supply of oxygen, has abruptly clogged. The faster his heart beats, the more oxygen is needed and the more cells will abruptly die from lack of oxygen. If enough cells die, Mr. Franklin dies. Here we clearly see a problem that is solely related to the biological wing of Mr. Franklin's matrix. Or is it?

The phenomenon that innovators of the biopsychosocial model, whether internists, nurses, or social workers, found to be fascinating had to do with what happened next. A palpable anxiety and urgency engulfed the triage room. It could be seen in the eyes of the triage nurse, the sudden rapid movements of the emergency room staff, and the increasingly frightened questions of both Mr. Franklin and his wife, "What is happening? What's going on?" Terse answers were provided by rushing staff, for all staff recognized the need for rapid intervention. Both Mr. Franklin and his wife became progressively more agitated and frightened as the environmental wing of their matrix – the emergency room triage area – erupted into an anxiety-provoking blur of intervention. As Mr. Franklin was wheeled away, he called out, "I want my wife with me, I need my wife with me." His entreaties, however, rapidly vanished behind the fluttering curtains of the emergency room as he was whisked off to receive what would prove to be excellent biologically oriented emergency room care.

But therein lies the problem. Non-biological processes were now negatively interacting with the biological wing of Mr. Franklin. Curiously, these damaging matrix factors were inadvertently triggered by the actions of the treatment team. The ramifications of these factors could prove to be deadly. Complicating the situation was the fact that these non-biological factors were completely hidden from the treatment team. Let us examine the situation in more detail.

The fear, on the psychological wing of Mr. Franklin's matrix, generated by the medical staff's rushed behaviors, on the environmental wing of Mr. Franklin, had created a change on the biological wing of Mr. Franklin. His heart was beating wildly, triggered by his ever-growing fear and anxiety. More and more oxygen would be needed to keep his heart cells alive because of their sharp increase in activity, yet no increase in oxygen could pass through the blocked artery. Consequently, the area of the heart attack was growing larger. Thousands of Mr. Franklin's heart cells were now unnecessarily dying, and Mr. Franklin was more than a few steps closer to death.

The last thing that any emergency room team would want for a man suffering from a heart attack would be a rapid increase in his heart rate. Yet it was the unintended actions of the team that were creating this exact result in Mr. Franklin. A more compelling example of a damaging matrix effect may be hard to come by – a problem on the environmental wing (the urgent behaviors of the staff) was creating a damaging matrix effect on the psychological wing of Mr. Franklin (fear), and this fear (on his psychological wing) was now creating a second damaging matrix effect on his biological wing (a dangerous increase in his heart rate). The emergency room staff were creating, inadvertently, the exact opposite change in Mr. Franklin's heart to what they intended.

From the perspective of matrix treatment planning, some creative proactive measures could be taken that might prevent this damaging matrix effect from unfolding. What if emergency rooms had volunteer staff available, trained to rapidly and effectively impact on the environmental wing of the matrix, exactly in such life-threatening situations. Such trained volunteers could quickly intervene, providing, in a calming voice, immediate information to both Mr. Franklin and his wife. They might be making comments such as, "I'm going to be here for you Mrs. Franklin, throughout the night, to let you know how things are going and to be a support for you," and, addressed to Mr. Franklin, "Don't worry Mr. Franklin, I'll take good care of your wife. And the team of doctors and nurses you are about to meet will take good care of you. I know them personally and they are really great." With such interventions, there is a reasonable chance that the heart of Mr. Franklin, and the hearts of thousands of other Mr. Franklins around the world in similar emergency rooms, would be beating a good deal more slowly. The chance for Mr. Franklin to see the light of a new October morning just became a good deal more likely.

Here a change made on the environmental wing of Mr. Franklin produced healing matrix effects on the interpersonal wing of the worried couple, as well as on the psychological wings of both Mr. Franklin and his wife. More remarkably, these psychological changes created a healing matrix effect on the biological wing of Mr. Franklin. Quite literally, a change on the environmental wing caused a profoundly important change on the biological wing of a precariously poised heart. By adding the calming influence of a well-trained volunteer, the heart of Mr. Franklin was beating a good deal more slowly, a potentially life-saving consequence. From the biopsychosocial perspective, even in the sterile confines of an emergency room, we do not treat hearts, we do not even treat people, we treat systems. *Everything interconnects in matrix theory.*

Note that in the original biopsychosocial model, clinicians look for two types of clinical interventions: (1) *intra*-wing interventions (interventions occurring within the same wing as the identified problem) and (2) *inter*-wing interventions (healing interventions implemented on an entirely different wing than the identified problem). In the first category, *intra*-wing interventions, the clinician surveys each wing of the patient's matrix, and if a problem is found, then an intervention is considered that occurs directly in that wing. Thus, if one finds there is a problem with hypertension on the biological wing, then one uses a biological intervention (a medication).

In the second category, *inter*-wing interventions, the clinician surveys each wing of the patient's matrix, and if a problem is found, then an intervention is used from a different wing of the matrix that indirectly changes the wing where the problem is occurring. Thus, if one finds there is a problem with hypertension on the biological wing, then one uses a technique from a different wing of the matrix such as meditation or stress reduction (psychological wing) to impact on the biological problem. In the original biopsychosocial model, as aptly demonstrated in our above illustration from an emergency department, there was a heavy focus upon *inter*-wing interventions as a means of jump-starting stalled treatment plans and maximizing as many useful interventions as might help the patient.

It has been my observation that over the decades this original emphasis upon interaction between wings has sometimes deteriorated among treatment teams. Instead, the emphasis is often upon *intra*-wing matrix interventions. Is there something wrong on the biological wing and, if so, is there a medication we can use? Is there something wrong on the psychological wing and, if so, should we use individual psychotherapy? Is there something wrong on the dyadic wing and, if so, should we use couple's therapy? Is there something wrong spiritually and, if so, should we refer the patient for spiritual counseling or to a clergy? This *intra*-wing initial treatment planning is excellent in its own right for it ensures a holistic approach, but it is only a part of the biopsychosocial model as originally designed, for it has left out the second step involving interventions done between different wings (*inter*-wing interventions) that was the hallmark of the original model.

By staying true to the original model's emphasis upon interventions implemented between differing wings, an entire array of new interventions may come to mind to the treatment team, as well as the patient. Such "out of the box" solutions arise if the following types of questions are routinely asked: If there is a problem on the biological wing, is there something we could do on the psychological wing that might change the biochemistry of the brain (such as CBT changing the pathophysiology of the brain in OCD)? If there is a problem with a couple's marriage, is there something we might do on the biological wing to one member of the couple that could help to save the marriage (as with a medication alleviating a severe depression in one-half of a couple, thus helping to heal the relationship)? Such creative thinking is at the very heart of the original biopsychosocial model.

With true matrix treatment planning, where there is an emphasis on tapping *inter*-wing healing matrix effects as well as intra-wing interventions, an almost innumerable number of fresh treatment ideas can be developed. With its renewed emphasis upon inter-wing interventions, *the matrix treatment model* is filled with hope and possibilities. It helps patients, initial interviewers, and the treatment teams they are a part of, to view each potential roadblock to healing as a new beginning for brainstorming. I am reminded of the wise words of the Zen master, Shunryu Suzuki:

In the beginner's mind there are many possibilities, but in the expert there are few.[24]

Matrix treatment planning allows us, even as experts, to once again become "beginners" who see many possibilities. To a clinician trained to be a matrix treatment planner, for every roadblock encountered on one wing of the patient's matrix, there is the potential that a solution may be found on a different wing of the patient's matrix. In this sense each problem is usefully viewed as a new beginning, for it opens the door to searches for solutions on new wings. It also allows us to share the optimism of this beginner's mind with our patients as we collaboratively treatment plan.

Over the decades, there has been another change in the biopsychosocial model – this time a positive one. There has been a greater recognition of the importance of both cultural and spiritual aspects in the formation and functioning of an individual, as was emphasized in the last chapter. A variety of authors have delineated the importance of this framework for meaning, or as Alan Josephson coined the term, "worldview." Indeed, it is now common to refer to "biopsychosocialspiritual treatment planning." Josephson and Peteet elegantly emphasize this point, as well as provide a cogent example of an *inter*-wing intervention, in an article of direct relevance to the initial interview, "Talking with Patients about Spirituality and Worldview: Practical Interviewing Techniques and Strategies" (complete article available in Appendix IV):

Simply put, inquiry in this area [spirituality and worldview] has the potential to enhance how we can help people and improve our treatment planning. The term "biopsychosocial-spiritual" reflects the fact that spirituality may, along with biologic, psychological, and social factors, impact a variety of issues related to clinical care including contributing to the risk of developing clinical disorders and serving as protective factors ... For example, could an intervention consistent with the patient's spirituality (e.g., meditation or listening to Gregorian chant) have a positive impact on the patient's biology, perhaps accentuating or replacing the use of an antianxiety agent?[25]

An innovative matrix-based model of treatment planning has been developed by Danilo E. Ponce that highlights the importance of cultural/societal and worldview factors in treatment planning. Ponce describes how to adapt the matrix model of treatment planning to the unique needs of a specific culture – Filipino – in his insightful book *Caring, Healing, and Teaching.*[26]

One of the advances made by Ponce is his concept that when addressing each wing of the patient's matrix, clinicians and case managers can conceptualize their interventions as embracing three clinical functions: (1) caring, (2) healing, and (3) teaching. In his model, the interviewer looks at each wing of the patient's matrix as suggesting possibilities for intervention from these three standpoints: First, from the caring perspective (safety and security) the clinician looks at each wing of the matrix as to how it can be utilized to provide basic needs (food, clothing, shelter) and a basic sense of human safety and security (some degree of certainty, continuity, and predictability in the patient's everyday experience) held together by a basic sense that this clinician/team "cares about me." Second, from the healing perspective (wellness) the clinician looks at each wing of the matrix through the lens of providing physical, psychological, social, and spiritual alleviation of disease, distress, disability, dysfunction and disorder. Finally, from his third perspective – teaching – Ponce urges clinicians to look at each wing of the matrix as a potential avenue for enhancing the patient's sense of self-respect and competence by teaching specific skills, attitudes, and knowledge bases that provide an ever-improving sense of mastery and trust that one can function reasonably well in the world.

A Revitalizing Change in Language

Language counts. Words shape how clinicians view and interpret the clinical world and what they attempt to uncover during the initial interview itself. Terms such as biopsychosocial can become "tired" in usage. Once this occurs, clinicians can become less enthused about a system, no matter how useful the principles of the system may be, for the system appears to be "same-old, same-old." Each generation benefits from a language that resonates with the gestalt of that generation.

This need for an ongoing renewal in language is why I prefer the term "matrix treatment planning" to "biopsychosocialspiritual treatment planning," for I believe the latter term has become a tired one. First, if we are honest with ourselves, the term "biopsychosocialspiritual treatment planning" doesn't exactly roll off the tongue. Moreover, it is often a relatively awkward terminology to use with patients, potentially sounding abstract and cold. Second, the term does not emphasize the original spirit of the model, which is creating interaction between the wings. Indeed the term tends to highlight each wing as if it were a separate silo from the other wings. In sharp contrast, the term "matrix," by its very definition, indicates a set of interlacing systems. It reminds all clinicians of the importance of seeking out creative *interactional* opportunities while both interviewing and collaboratively treatment planning.

Moreover, I have found the term "matrix" to be immediately recognized and understood by millennial, and even younger, clinicians. Indeed, to anyone under the age of 35, the term "matrix" immediately triggers images of a guy bedecked in a black trench coat and shades bending backwards like a Gumby on acid, his body deftly avoiding a hail of hissing bullets. Nevertheless, these very same millennial clinicians know exactly what a matrix is from their understanding of the exploits of Neo in the Hollywood blockbuster *The Matrix*. They immediately view the concept of a matrix as a cogent reminder that the world is a not exactly what it seems to be – a world of separate objects and individuals. Instead they are reminded that the world is perhaps better conceived as a unified and interlaced set of interactional fields where a change on one wing of the matrix invariably causes changes in the other wings. They recognize that healing in the biochemistry of the brain may not always mean the use of medications (CBT causing beneficial changes in the cytoarchitecture of the basal ganglia in OCD), and that, in some instances (the psychotic hyper-religiosity in schizophrenia), damage in the spiritual wing may be repaired through the use of medications.

We can turn to the wisdom of C. Robert Cloninger, who applies the importance of such a worldview to psychology:

> *The science of well-being is founded on the understanding that there is an indissoluble unity to all that is or can be. The universal unity of being is recognized widely as an empirical fact, as well as an essential organizing principle for adequate science. The universal unity of being is not an arbitrary philosophical assumption, and it is not an optimistic assumption. Rather the universal unity of being is the only viewpoint consistent with any coherent and testable science ... Psychology, like particle physics, must postulate a universal field in which all aspects of each person are bound together at the same nodal point in space and time.*[27]

As we shall soon see, the matrix model of treatment planning shows interviewers and clinicians exactly how to navigate the exciting possibilities envisioned by Cloninger's world of therapeutic interaction. Indeed, matrix treatment planning (both its name and its methods) dovetails nicely with contemporary perspectives on the reality of the universe, such as quantum mechanics and the particle physics mentioned by Cloninger. Such contemporary schools of science view the world as unified interlacing fields of potential interaction in which each field interacts with all other fields. In addition, the advent of the web, social media, and wireless interconnectivity allows changes on one wing of the human matrix to impact on other wings in a remarkably fast fashion.

It is always nice when a term, such as the term "matrix" fits with the gestalt of a culture. In addition, I have found that patients find the concept of collaboratively "changing their matrix" to be understandable, exciting, and self-empowering. Moreover, when clinicians utilize the concepts of matrix treatment planning, the possibilities generated can subsequently be translated into actual applications for teams of clinicians and multidisciplinary teams. This process is in line with the concept of "integrative care," where the practical implementation of matrix interventions must be communicated and coordinated effectively over time between all persons/organizations involved in addressing the patient's problems. Thus matrix treatment planning is a valuable first step in the creation of truly integrated care that underlies all person-centered health care. In any case, we will use the term "matrix treatment planning" throughout this book to refer to this re-vitalized concept of the biopsychosocialspiritual model.

We have now completed our historical, theoretical, and contextual side-trip regarding matrix treatment planning. We possess the information needed to see how we can effectively apply this material to the clinical interview. Indeed, it is time to see how it was applied to Debbie herself in the real world of a busy outpatient clinic.

Matrix Treatment Planning: General Clinical Principles and Specific Applications to Debbie in the Initial Interview

As the interview proceeds, the clinician asks himself or herself whether enough information, if any, has been gathered in each of the six wings of the human matrix. Such self-reflection minimizes errors of omission while maximizing the usefulness of the database as a treatment-planning platform. Even as the information from a given wing is revealed, treatment options – both intra-wing and inter-wing – may "pop into the mind" of the interviewer. Just as was the case with the diagnostic assessment perspective of the DSM-5, if the clinician carefully listens to the patient's problems, the problems begin to suggest their own solutions. It is the organization of the data that provides this momentum. Let us examine each wing in order.

First Wing of the Matrix: Biologic

On the first wing of the matrix, the interviewer focuses on the biological makeup of the patient. This wing overlaps with the DSM-5 system. In it the clinician hunts for evidence of biologic wellness and illness, as well as the presence of symptoms suggesting that somatic treatments may be of value.

Biological Intra-Wing Interventions

From the perspective of intra-wing interventions, possible biological interventions include antidepressants, antipsychotics, other medications including herbal approaches such as St. John's wort in the case of mild to moderate depressions, antianxiety agents and mood stabilizers, hormonal replacements in the case of diseases such as hypothyroidism, addressing nutrition and healthy diet, or electroconvulsive therapy (ECT). Note that all of these interventions are biological interventions being utilized when one suspects biological disruption. The matrix model offers little difference from the DSM-5 assessment approach from this *intra*-wing matrix perspective, both assessment systems providing valuable frameworks suggestive of treatment interventions.

Biological Inter-Wing Interventions

However, on the *inter*-wing perspective – interactions between wings – matrix treatment planning opens a door into a room filled with new potential treatment interventions for the interviewer and interviewee to collaboratively explore. To open these doors, interviewers can ask themselves two questions during the interview itself, after the interview, and in subsequent treatment planning sessions: (1) Could there be interventions on the biological wing that may have healing matrix effects on other wings? and (2) Could there be interventions on a non-biological wing that could heal the pathophysiology of the brain itself?

Question #1: Healing Matrix Effects Arising From the Biologic Wing

Over the years, I have consistently noticed how patients who do not seem to be benefiting from psychotherapies on the psychological wing (individual therapy), dyadic wing (couples therapy), or group/societal wing (group therapy) are actually often floundering because of biological depressions. Once an antidepressant or biologically active herbal remedy is utilized, the patient's ability to effectively benefit from these therapies sometimes strikingly improves – a nice example of a biological intervention having a healing matrix effect on a non-biologic wing, in this instance enhancing non-biologic interventions themselves. In fact, to expect a patient with a severe biologic depression, beleaguered by an intense loss of energy, drive, and motivation, to be able to effectively utilize family therapy, is often unrealistic, in my opinion. Many a marriage or employment situation has been saved by the judicious use of medications and other biological interventions, which have helped not only the underlying biologic dysfunction, but have also "jump-started" a stalled psychotherapy on the psychological wing of the patient.

With regard to Debbie, perhaps the use of a mood stabilizing medication, such as Depakote, might decrease her tendency for affective lability, a potentially key trigger to her angry exchanges on the interpersonal wing of the matrix – an example of a biological intervention producing a healing matrix effect on the interpersonal and family wings of Debbie's matrix. Such mood lability and anger (she had to be forcibly removed by police from a previous therapist) could naturally disrupt her ability to benefit from psychotherapy. Hence, the mood stabilizer might help her to optimize her individual psychotherapy.

Question #2: Healing Matrix Effects to the Biologic Wing From Other Wings

We can now turn our attention to our second inter-wing question: Could there be interventions on a non-biological wing that could change the pathophysiology of the brain? In some instances, wellness interventions on the psychological or worldview wings of the matrix may actually change brain physiology.[28] Examples could include the healing matrix effects of interventions such as meditation,[29] relaxation techniques and biofeedback,[30] and disciplines from the spiritual wing of the matrix, such as prayer[31]; it has been documented that these psychological and spiritual techniques can have significant changes on brain function.

To give just one example of the multitude of interventions that inter-wing matrix treatment planning could bring to the table with regard to changing pathophysiology, let us return to Debbie's problems with rage. On a speculative and theoretical level, the more often her neuronal circuits fire with regard to anger and rage, it is possible that synaptic plasticity and pruning may be resulting in the emergence of increased synaptic production in these circuits, resulting in an increased propensity for the firing of these very same maladaptive circuits, a potentially maladaptive positive feedback loop. In this instance, some of the psychological techniques inherent in therapies such as CBT, DBT, and mindfulness-based therapies, by decreasing the firing of these circuits, may actually result in decreased synaptic production in these circuits changing the neurocircuitry itself – in short, a healing matrix effect (psychological intervention changing the biologic wing of the matrix).

Second Wing of the Matrix: Psychological

In the second wing, the psychological system, one enters an area that only partially over-laps the DSM-5 in relation to considerations of personality development. Consequently, it suggests many interventions not as readily suggested by the DSM perspective.

Psychological Intra-Wing Interventions

At this level the clinician attempts to understand the patient both in a phenomenological sense as a unique human and in a psychodynamic sense as a product of past develop-ment. Each interviewer will have preferences for which psychological theories seem rel-evant, whether they be Freudian, Jungian, Rogerian, behaviorist, interpersonal, or some combination of the numerous viewpoints available. But the important point remains that the clinician attempts, once again, to understand the person beneath the diagnosis. In this wing of the matrix, interviewers expand their lists of treatment options by con-sidering the use of individual psychotherapies or counseling techniques.

As the psychological wing of Debbie's matrix is explored, including her psychological symptoms, a more personalized view of Debbie emerges as she becomes at once more complicated and more human. Several conflictual issues are readily apparent, including: (1) fears of abandonment, (2) problems with anger and impulse control, (3) ongoing problems with low self-esteem, (4) non-lethal self-harming behaviors, and (5) problems with identity and sense of self. By beginning to delineate these areas during the first interview, the clinician can begin to generate options for treatment on the intra-wing of her psychological matrix – psychological interventions for psychological problems.

For example, in addition to the CBT and DBT interventions already mentioned, from an analytic viewpoint, one could look at disturbances in her sense of self as indicating the potential usefulness of specific psychotherapeutic approaches developed by clinicians such as Kohut, Kernberg, or Masterson. In a similar vein, Debbie's low self-esteem and difficulties in accepting herself may bring to mind the usefulness of psychotherapies such as Acceptance and Commitment Therapy (ACT).

Furthermore, a survey of the information garnered in her psychological matrix reveals that not much psychogenetic data has been garnered yet, a deficit that can be addressed in future sessions. Here we see the application of a matrix perspective *during an initial interview* functioning as a method to help the interviewer spot, and perhaps alleviate, potential omissions of useful data for treatment planning. The important point remains that by conceptualizing in the psychological wing, interviewers prompt themselves to consider areas of intervention utilizing individual psychotherapy, as well as checking to see if this region of highly pertinent information has been adequately tapped.

Psychological Inter-Wing Interventions

Once again, the *inter*-wing perspective of matrix treatment planning is ripe with potential interventions. In each wing of the matrix, the same two questions can be asked by the interviewer of himself or herself. With regard to Debbie's psychological wing: (1) Could there be interventions on the psychological wing that may have healing matrix effects on other wings or therapeutic modalities being used on other wings? (2) Could there be interventions on a non-psychological wing that could change Debbie's psychological matrix?

Question #1: Healing Matrix Effects on Other Wings Arising From the Psychological Wing

In a generic sense, recent research has shown progressively more robust evidence that classic forms of psychotherapy may impact on brain pathophysiology. One of the most striking examples being the power of CBT to impact on the biological dysfunctions related to OCD. Research has shown the power of CBT to change pathophysiology, with resulting symptom improvement in obsessions and compulsions in OCD, as illustrated in the patient self-help book *Brain Lock* by Schwartz,[32] which I highly recommend. There is growing hope that some forms of CBT may decrease the frequency of auditory hallucinations in diseases such as schizophrenia, or dampen the intensity of the patient's response to hallucinatory phenomena, once again perhaps related to changes in neuronal circuitry prompted by a decreased firing of circuits related to CBT response-prevention techniques.

With regard to Debbie, one could look at the potentially precarious nature of the strength of her dyadic wing of her matrix, involving tremendous strains on the relationship with her partner. Naturally, one can address these intimacy strains directly on the dyadic wing with couple's therapy. In addition, from a matrix perspective, one could focus upon psychological techniques for shoring up Debbie's fragile sense of self-esteem, for these psychological problems may be fostering the extreme dependency needs that threaten the very heart of her relationship with her partner, a classic example of a damaging matrix effect. It is her lack of self-esteem and sense of a core self that may be at the center of her oddly angry responses to her partner's going to sleep first. Changes on the psychological wing – the enhancement of her self-esteem – could have major healing matrix effects on the intimate wing of Debbie's matrix.

Question #2: Healing Matrix Effects to the Psychological Wing From Other Wings

Could there be interventions on a non-psychological wing that could change Debbie's psychological matrix? As already mentioned, the use of medications can often have marked healing matrix effects on psychological functioning. Other wings can also be creatively tapped. For example, with Debbie, on her spiritual wing she was re-kindling her interest in her Christian beliefs and she was also being influenced by Eastern thought.

Knowledge of her evolving worldview could lead a clinician to see if participation in a more structured spiritual outreach might kindle an understanding of compassion and its role not only in accepting others but in accepting herself (a healing matrix effect on her psychological wing). This might also cause better acceptance of the needs of her partner (resulting in a healing matrix effect on the dyadic wing of her matrix as well). Cloninger provides insight into the pivotal role that such self-acceptance often plays in the initial stage of healing, describing such self-acceptance as, "It is being willing to see what we are in reality without wanting to become something else."[33]

Third Wing of the Matrix: Dyadic

When we move to the third level, the dyadic wing, the patient is viewed as one component of the numerous two-person interactions that fill the patient's day-to-day communications, including highly supportive and intimate relationships as with a spouse, partner, or parent. The patient's interpersonal skills are assessed.

Dyadic Intra-Wing Interventions

Does the patient have adequate verbal skills and social skills? Some patients suffering from schizophrenia or schizoaffective disorder may act oddly or may share their delusions with others without realizing the disengaging impact of these activities. Such patients may benefit from social skills training. In a similar vein, people with problems along the autistic continuum or with permanent deficits in intellectual functioning represent another category of patients with whom social skills training may yield gratifying results.

The interviewer should also bear in mind that the patient's interaction with the interviewer provides direct and immediate information concerning the strengths and weaknesses of the patient in this wing of the matrix. Unfortunately, this immediately available direct evaluation of the patient's interpersonal skills is frequently overlooked by clinicians. Reminding oneself to examine each wing of the patient's matrix helps to prevent such important omissions.

In the case of Debbie, the dyadic system focuses attention on her style of relating to other individuals. One wonders if her angry outbursts may be reactions to a chronic style of passively deferring to the needs of others. Such a situation may suggest the utility of self-assertiveness training.

This wing refocuses attention on the impact of the patient's physical appearance and behavior. Debbie's loud sunglasses and T-shirt may indeed strike an unappreciative chord in some people upon first contact. Debbie may be unaware of the ramifications of her behavior, and social skills training may be useful at some point.

In the end, all of these interpersonal issues are of relevance to her relationship with her partner. Upon my first contact with Ms. Baker in the waiting room, the importance of her relationship with her partner immediately emerged, as she quickly announced her upcoming wedding and change of her name. It was as if she could hardly wait to shed her identity, washing her hands of her own name with a brisk shrug as she first met me. On a positive note of wellness, her relationship with her partner had endured for several years and may represent a potentially powerful resource in therapy. To increase light on their relationship, the clinician might consider the use of a joint assessment session with the couple and perhaps the ultimate use of couple's therapy.

Dyadic Inter-Wing Matrix Effects

Once again, inter-wing matrix effects may prove to be invaluable, both healing matrix effects to other wings arising from interventions on her dyadic wing, to healing matrix effects on her dyadic dysfunction coming from interventions on other wings of her matrix. A change in a possibly pathologic interdependency, on her dyadic wing, between the two partners might lead to healing matrix effects on other wings such as a new willingness by Debbie to spend time on community activities or new relationships with friends, family members, church members, or participation in an outpatient support group or day hospital. At the time of the initial interview, she was shying away from such interactions because she wanted to spend all of her time with her partner. Moreover, matrix treatment planning reminds the interviewer of the importance of uncovering hallmarks of wellness (the strengths, skills, and interests of the "wellness triad" from the last chapter), as well as the possible psychopathology of her partner, who might herself be suffering from a biologic depression or psychological trauma, which if addressed could have major healing effects not only for the partner but for Debbie as well.

Fourth Wing of the Matrix: Family

As we look at the fourth wing of the human matrix, the family, we come upon one of the most powerful systems affecting all humans. To conceptualize patients during an initial interview without considering the dynamics of their family is to see half a picture at best. To plan treatment without considering the needs and opinions of the patient's family invites treatment failure.

Moreover, whether interviewers like to admit it or not, the patient's family is psychologically present in any interview, representing a powerful determining force on the patient's behavior. The interviewer should always consider the utility of a family assessment or eventual employment of family therapy.

Familial Intra-Wing Interventions

Ideally, a clinician may actually be presented with an opportunity to interact with the family as a unit in a joint interview. For example, in an emergency room situation, the patient is frequently accompanied by family members. On these occasions the clinician can directly observe the process of family interaction.

But even within the confines of an individual assessment, an enormous amount of information can be gained concerning family dynamics by gently probing. Pertinent data will emerge simply by learning some of the background facts and pieces of demographic information. The clinician can begin a familiarization with the family matrix by inquiring into where various family members have chosen to live. It is probably not merely chance that leads to a situation in which all the children have moved thousands of miles away from Mom and Dad. Nor should one ignore the implications of a family in which most members have chosen to live on the same block.

I remember a young woman seeking help for severe marital discord, who complained that she could not get her mother "to mind her own business." Later in the interview I was surprised to find that the patient had recently moved back into the same apartment complex where her parents lived, ostensibly for convenience. The issue of inappropriate attachment to her parents appeared as a psychodynamic theme throughout the remaining therapy.

Another important area reveals itself when one inquires about which people are living under the same roof with the patient. Such questioning may uncover unexpected findings, such as a domineering grandparent whose ideas of discipline clash with the concepts of the parents.

On a more specific level, further questioning may directly begin to unravel the complexities of the family, such as:

a. "What were holidays like at your house?"
b. "What kinds of things did your brothers or sisters like to do?" (often yields clues to sibling rivalry)
c. "Describe the physical appearance of your brother." (another nice gate through which to explore sibling rivalry)
d. "Whom do you share secrets with in your family?"
e. "Who makes the decisions in your family?"
f. "Who do you think you are most like in your family?"
g. "Tell me a little about what kinds of things your parents used to argue about."
h. "Did you go to the same schools as your brother? (and if so, "what was that like?")
i. "Did you share a room with any siblings?" (and if so, "what was that like?")

With questions such as the above, the initial interviewer can begin to determine whether a family assessment may be indicated.

An analysis of the family system is not emphasized in the DSM-5, once again highlighting the utility of applying several assessment grids when planning treatment. Further discussion of this critical area of assessment would take us away from the topic of this book, but the interested reader may find the writings of Stephen Fleck useful in building a foundation for a more specific approach to family assessment.[34,35]

In addition to learning more about the patient contextually as shaped by family processes, matrix treatment planning also reminds us of the added mission of helping to relieve the pain of family members and other loved ones who have family members suffering from severe mental disorders, from schizophrenia to PTSD, OCD, and bipolar disorder. Indeed, there is an entirely different "initial interview" that we all undertake – our first meeting with family members. An enormous amount of good can be done in these sessions, which benefits not only the patient but also the patient's family. Murray-Swank and colleagues have written an elegantly practical article of direct significance to the initial interview, "Practical Interview Strategies for Building an Alliance with the Families of Patients who have Severe Mental Illness" (complete article available in Appendix IV).[36]

Turning towards the impact of her nuclear family, Debbie's poignant early memory of being tugged away from the door as her father vanishes conveys the sense of a deeply troubled childhood. Clearly, more information in this region will be enlightening, and the clinician is reminded, once again, of the potential utility of family assessment or therapy.

Cultural issues can play major roles in understanding the family matrix in an initial interview. For example, powerful control is often exerted by men over Latina women, both with spouses and with daughters. While being careful not to stereotype, it is important that, as treatment possibilities are touched upon in the closing phase with a Latina patient, questions such as "What do you think your father (or boyfriend) might think about this idea?" are considered by the interviewer. In such instances, even a nonverbal such as the hint of a patient rolling her eyes may speak immeasurably of the powers at work in her family matrix.

Another important cultural issue may be at work in some immigrant families when considering the family matrix: In many cultures, the parental generation commands respect and has implicit power assigned to it, simply because the parents have more experience and familiarity with day-to-day life, culture, and stresses. However, in families in which the parental generation does not feel comfortable integrating into the new culture and society, it is the children who may know more about the family's new environment. These children will have gained much insight from listening to popular music, utilizing street language, actively engaging friends and strangers on social media, and interacting with peers regarding moral, sexual, and ethical expectations. Suddenly, a 15-year-old may actually be a better authority on the surrounding culture than the father, mother, or grandparents living in the same house. Such a reversal of informal power can lead to a profound disruption in the family matrix.

Familial Inter-Wing Matrix Interventions

As with previous wings of the matrix, interviewers should keep an open mind to various healing and damaging inter-wing matrix effects. When reviewing this chapter with a noted innovator in the care of patients with autism and related disorders, Larry Welkowitz,[37] he offered the following example of such a healing matrix effect, related to an understanding of both familial and cultural diversity issues:

One of his patients of a Hispanic background, who was coping with Tourette's syndrome, would often find a marked increase in Tourette's symptomatology when his family visited from Columbia. Upon questioning, it was discovered that his parents and siblings expressed a culturally normal exuberance and affective intensity common to Latin cultures, with much hugging, joking, dancing, and close interpersonal spacing. Apparently, this cultural and familial exuberance seemed to trigger the patient's Tourette's symptoms. A careful and gentle explanation of the possible link communicated by the therapist to the patient's family members resulted in a subtly, but noticeably, quieter interpersonal milieu upon visits. The result was a striking decrease in the patient's Tourette's symptomatology, a result greatly appreciated by both the patient and his family. Here we see an intervention, by a savvy clinician, on the family wing of the matrix that impacted directly on the biological and psychological wings of the patient, resulting in a decrease in disruptive behaviors.

Fifth Wing of the Matrix: Cultural, Societal, and Environmental

In the fifth wing, the cultural, societal, and environmental wing of the matrix, the interviewer investigates the patient's ability to function within groups outside of the family. In particular, one looks at the patient's relationships at work, school, and with networks of friends, including the society at large and the patient's everyday living and online environment.

Cultural, Societal, and Environmental Intra-Wing Interventions

A pivotal issue concerns the patient's abilities to handle authority figures such as employers. The clinician keeps an eye open for evidence that the patient is generalizing feelings from family members onto other relationships, such as sibling rivalry reappearing as intense competitiveness at the workplace.

It is also valuable to search for subcultures to which the patient may look for values and support. Such cultures could include the drug culture, the club culture, the jock culture, or problematic ideologic entities such as the Ku Klux Klan. An ignorance of a patient's cultural subgroup can lead to major errors in treatment planning. Substance abuse treatment will probably serve little purpose if the patient immediately returns to the club scene for a rendezvous with designer-drug buddies. While contemplating this wing of the matrix, the interviewer should consider whether group therapy might be of value. Moreover, it is important to remember that one can utilize subcultures for therapeutic effect, such as recommending Alcoholics Anonymous or tapping veteran peer-to-peer programs. While reviewing the information gathered at this level concerning Debbie, the clinician is reminded of the possible advantages of group therapy or perhaps a day hospital or drop-in center. On a behavioral level, as therapy progresses, it may be beneficial to steer her towards rewarding group activities such as volunteer work.

Another critical subculture, as discussed in our last chapter, is the web and social media. In this chapter, I want to emphasize the amount of interpersonal abuse that is now occurring on the web and via smart phones. Despite the numerous gifts electronic media have provided, one serious problem has been the use of smart phones (via texting) and the web (through social media such as Twitter and Facebook) to provide abusers with an almost constant access to their victims. This type of ongoing wireless harassment is frequently focused on various personal aspects of victims, such as sexual orientation, looks, social status, intelligence, social awkwardness, and their cliques. As initial interviewers, especially with adolescents and young adults, this damaging aspect of social media, including harassment by posting damaging YouTube material, including sexual photos or videos of the target of the harassment or flaming, is critical to a sound assessment of the cultural, societal, and environmental wing of the matrix.

Patients, especially adolescents, may be hesitant to share such harassment because of shame unless directly asked with questions such as:

1. "Do you like using social media?"
2. "Does anybody post mean or degrading comments about you on Facebook or Twitter?"

3. "Has anybody ever made fun of you or posted a demeaning video of you on YouTube?"
4. "Does anyone send you vicious or disturbing texts?"

At the end of the initial interview, little was known about the functioning of Debbie at a group level. Indeed, the absence of her mentioning friends piques our interest, perhaps suggesting problematic relationships or none at all. There also seems to be a conspicuous absence of support groups or outside activities.

As introduced in our last chapter, the power of culture and social forces is immense in understanding the person beneath the diagnosis. Matrix treatment planning pushes the interviewer to always look for the various social forces shaping the patient's functioning within the community. These forces include economic, political, institutional, and social class factors.

As Engel's quotation at the beginning of this section suggests, the patient's environment should always be considered. For some patients this will include issues relating to immediate environment and safety (akin to Abraham Maslow's first level of needs) such as availability of adequate food, shelter, and personal safety (as compromised by a dangerous neighborhood, a war zone, or a region of genocide). All of these conditions are intimately related to the political climate of the patient's county, federal, and state governments.

It is also possible that a patient's society is problematic, disabling the patient through prejudice or violence related to race, religion, sex, and/or sexual orientation. By way of example, I find it of use to ask any patient of an Islamic background if they, or their loved ones, have experienced any problems with harassment since 9/11 and the rise of ISIS. Similarly, it is of value to ask Jewish patients if they have or are currently encountering prejudicial treatment. Depending upon geographic location in the world, anti-Semitism remains very active. Even in the United States, according to the Hate Crime Statistics compiled by the FBI, the highest rate of hate crimes against religious members in the United States are perpetrated against people of the Jewish religion (such crimes being committed at five times the rate towards Jews than any other religious group).[38]

Once again, the interviewer must remember not to focus solely on individual dynamics, because the patient is part of many different systems, any one of which may be malfunctioning. It remains a basic tenet of assessment interviewing that one must understand the patient's culture in order to understand the patient's behavior.

In this light, the issue of Debbie's sexual orientation warrants an understanding of her culture. Interviewing in both the initial and subsequent meetings (*re-emphasizing that matrix assessment is impossible to complete in one session and represents an ongoing process that is simply begun within the opening meeting*) revealed that a possibly powerful support system had not been well tapped by either Debbie or her partner. They were not well integrated into the local resources of the LGBT (lesbian, gay, bisexual, and transgender) community. From an intra-wing perspective, helping both parties to explore the possibilities of support in their local LGBT community could be well worth considering.

Within the societal and environmental wing, one other crucial system is worth noting when planning treatment, namely, the mental health system itself. The clinician needs to be aware of the actual resources available for follow-up. It is useless to recommend behavioral therapy to a patient if there is no behavioral therapist available to the patient. Indeed, such "pie in the sky" thinking can frustrate patients, hanging false hopes before their eyes. Similarly, a common error at academic centers is the tendency to generate complex treatment plans for patients referred from community centers that these centers cannot implement when the patient returns to them. Such state-of-the-art treatment planning is, in reality, an example of poor assessment formulation, because its impracticality breeds frustration in the patient and anger in the treating clinicians.

To finish our discussion of the societal system, an important mental health resource for Debbie was uncovered by further interviewing. An excellent day hospital had been providing intermittent support for Debbie over the past year or so. As we will soon see, this community system suggested a future area for more intensive support.

Cultural, Societal, and Environmental Inter-Wing Matrix Interventions

We will use this arena to look at a specific matrix effect that we hinted at earlier, but have not yet had a chance to examine in detail. A healing matrix effect on one wing of the matrix may have unexpected consequences on other wings, often good, but occasionally bad – a damaging matrix effect. This fact highlights a key aspect of matrix interviewing in the initial interview: caution is required when first designing treatment interventions until one has explored what the impacts on other wings might be.

Further interviewing revealed that Debbie and her significant other had been forced to deal with considerable ostracism within their apartment building and neighborhood related to their sexual orientation. At first glance, this ostracism seems totally at odds with Debbie's further development, but there is a curious paradox here. In essence, this easily identified enemy had served as a common threat around which Debbie and her significant other had mobilized, thus stabilizing their relationship.

A clinician might prematurely suggest that immediately moving to another neighborhood could be beneficial, but such a suggestion could be a serious miscalculation. One of the most powerful glues for this relationship could be their unified need to protect each other from this community's psychological attacks. If placed in a new and more benign community prematurely, the relationship could begin to collapse, fulfilling Debbie's great fear of abandonment. In this example, it might be better to get the relationship on more solid ground before suggesting such a move.

A real-world example of such an unexpected damaging matrix effect can help to illuminate the effect more clearly. At the end of a recent presentation on matrix treatment planning, a workshop participant related the following. She was a clinician in an innovative Veteran's Affairs (VA) system. They had developed an outstanding program addressing the growing problem of homelessness in veterans returning from Iraq and Afghanistan and it was helping many veterans. She commented, "I wanted to share an unexpected impact on one of our vets that demonstrates the importance of 'being on the lookout' for unexpected damaging matrix effects that you were just talking about." (As an aside, I cannot emphasize enough how impressed I am with these programs. The following example is provided merely to illustrate an example of where matrix awareness during the initial interview can help any team to generate person-centered solutions.)

In this example, the program had unexpectedly backfired with a specific vet, whom we shall call Ted. Shortly after finding Ted an apartment, his condition deteriorated. He became seriously depressed, essentially apartment-bound, and developed suicidal thoughts. When homeless, Ted had been living with a group of vets who had pitched makeshift tents near a bridge. Ted later reported that the tent city had reminded him, in a strangely reassuring fashion, of how he had been living in Afghanistan (providing a sense of community on the patient's societal and environmental wing of his matrix). It also offered a sense of familiarity and hence safety, as Ponce talks about in his "caring" aspect of matrix treatment planning. There were several vets less fortunate than himself that he enjoyed helping on a daily basis (providing a sense of mission on the wing devoted to his worldview and framework for meaning). He had also developed some very good friends (the most powerful driver of his dyadic wing), as well as a sense of group camaraderie (the glue for the cultural, societal, and environmental wing of his matrix).

His nice apartment, a real find during the difficult financial problems of the times, was unfortunately many miles away from the "bridge community." In addition, for whatever reason, Ted intensely disliked public transportation such as the bus system and the subway (perhaps related to some PTSD phenomenon), so he was unwilling to travel to a local center that had been set up as a day center for returning vets. The result: with one single "positive" move (finding a home for a homeless man), severe damage occurred on almost all other wings of his matrix, resulting in the collapse of the "moment in time" we call Ted. He was now sitting "at home" in a dimly lit room, television flicker flashing across the lenses of his glasses hour after hour, reflecting the harsh reality that with the procurement of improved housing, Ted's real home had been lost.

One of the advantages of matrix treatment planning is that it gives new meaning to the concept of understanding the person beneath the diagnosis. Diagnoses (or labels) are not limited to systems such as the DSM or ICD. Words such as "homeless," "lonely," and "survivor" are all "diagnostic labels" of a sort. But, of course, all homeless people are not identical, and the solution to homelessness in each case may not be as simple as "this patient will benefit from our homeless program." Once again, it becomes important to uncover the person beneath the diagnosis of "homeless" – to understand the invariably interdependent impacts of the patient's uniquely intersecting matrices. Oftentimes this can enable us to sculpt programs collaboratively with the patient, beginning in the initial interview itself.

A useful question for interviewers to ask themselves when collaboratively treatment planning during the closing phase of an initial interview is, "What are some of the potential impacts on other wings of this person's matrix if we do this intervention?" This internal question transforms into a useful external question for patients, which I like to call the "matrix question." The matrix question can have many variants, but in all its variations it does not slant the patient towards consideration of healing or damaging matrix effects, it merely finds out what the patient imagines may result from a proposed intervention. In the resulting discussion, a patient's hopes and concerns about the proposed intervention frequently emerge in a naturalistic fashion. One of my favorite variations of the matrix question is perhaps the simplest: "How do you think your life might change if we find you an apartment (add an antidepressant, invite your husband to join us next session, get you into our eating disorders group, get you food stamps – whatever the proposed intervention might be)?"

For a moment let us imagine a clinician using the matrix question during the closing of his initial mental health intake with Ted at the VA. We will enter the interview a few minutes after the clinician had first mentioned the program, an idea that initially seemed very appealing to Ted:

> **Pt.:** You know this program could really help me out. It's gonna get cold, real cold, real fast, soon enough.
>
> **Clin.:** Oh yeah, we have helped a lot of vets with this program. How do you think things will change for you if we get you a place to live? (matrix question)
>
> **Pt.:** For the better, that's for sure. I'm not looking forward to winter and it would be amazing to have a shower. (pauses) …You know, will this apartment be near the bridge?
>
> **Clin.:** What bridge do you mean?
>
> **Pt.:** You know, the one where we've pitched our tents?
>
> **Clin.:** Oh … (pauses) … it could be, but probably not. I can't tell you for sure where the apartment will be, they're sort of all over the city, but it will be nice. It will have a shower, trust me (smiles).
>
> **Pt.:** Good. (looks a bit introspective) Will I be moving with a group of the vets, you know, sort of together.
>
> **Clin.:** We often try to do that. It's not always possible. Are you worried that you might not be seeing some of your buddies?
>
> **Pt.:** (Ted looks up immediately) … Yeah, that's sort of something that might bother me a little.
>
> **Clin.:** You don't have to worry about that, we have several centers set up around the city that are right on the bus line, where vets can hang out during the day. They are very popular.
>
> **Pt.:** Hmmm (pauses) … I guess it's better than living under a bridge, that's for sure.
>
> **Clin.:** You have really developed some great friendships under that bridge haven't you?
>
> **Pt.:** Oh yeah, these are my guys. They're my family.
>
> **Clin.:** Ted, could I make a suggestion.
>
> **Pt.:** Sure.
>
> **Clin.:** Well, I think we should try to get you on our waiting list for our housing program. But you know what, I think we should note that you really want to wait and move only with a group of vets into a shared apartment or shared apartment building. Now I got to tell you, that could drop you on this list for quite a while. If I'm honest with you, it could take us well into the winter months. But, I don't know. I sense this is pretty important to you, to be near your friends, I mean.
>
> **Pt.:** (looks a lot brighter) Oh yeah, I would really prefer that plan. I don't really like buses too much either, so I'm willing to wait, if that's okay with you.
>
> **Clin.:** Sounds good to me (smiles). We better look into getting you a parka, if you know what I mean.
>
> **Pt.:** (chuckles) Don't worry, it got plenty cold at night in the desert.

From this exchange one can see the value of using the matrix perspective as an organizing lens, even in the first interview. Hopefully it cogently demonstrates why an understanding of treatment planning is so important in a book on initial interviewing, for the two processes are entwined. Here, a well-timed use of the matrix question in an initial intake might have resulted in a profoundly different outcome for Ted.

Sixth Wing of the Matrix: Worldview (Framework for Meaning)

On the sixth level, the interviewer examines the patient's framework for meaning or what Josephson and Peteet call the patient's "worldview." Although in actuality this wing of the matrix could be conceived of as part of the psychological wing already discussed, it is so important that it is best viewed separately. To understand the patient more fully, it becomes necessary to understand his or her religious beliefs, philosophical beliefs, and ethical standards as part of the patient's cultural milieu, once again emphasizing the importance of culture and diversity in understanding the patient. At times the patient's symptoms may be directly related to unrest within the patient's worldview.

Worldview Intra-Wing Interventions

Josephson and Peteet emphasize that the concept of worldview is multi-tiered. It can include concrete philosophical belief systems such as religious affiliation, agnosticism, or atheism. But in a broader sense it includes what can be called spirituality, which may have no affiliation with a specific religious system. In an even broader sense they emphasize that it can include any belief systems that provides a framework for understanding the world and/or a personal sense of mission. In this light, the patient's worldview can include patriotism, his or her family, an organization such as Alcoholics Anonymous, or an identification with a street gang or a sports team.

Josephson and Peteet suggest a variety of nuanced and specific interview questions and strategies for exploring worldview in their article, mentioned earlier, "Talking with Patients about Spirituality and Worldview: Practical Interviewing Techniques and Strat- egies"[39] (complete article available in Appendix IV). We will also address the realm of spirituality in great detail in Chapter 20: Culturally Adaptive Interviewing: The Challenging Art of Exploring Culture, Worldview, and Spirituality.

One way of conceptualizing the patient's worldview is to ask yourself "what are the beliefs that make this patient tick?" I have found this exact concept, when phrased as the following question, to be an excellent doorway into this wing of the matrix: "What is it that make you tick?" The open-ended quality to this question allows it to touch upon all tiers of Josephson's concept of worldview, with answers ranging from family and/or country to specific religious beliefs and "my relationship with God?"

Information uncovered when exploring this wing of the patient's matrix may suggest the utility of individual psychotherapy slanted towards ethical or spiritual issues. It may also serve to remind the clinician of the availability of clergy and pastoral counselors in the treatment of the patient. Sometimes one of the most powerful interventions available to clinicians is the ability to help patients re-unite with a religious or spiritual discipline that has become dormant over the years or to separate from one that has proven to be a problematic match for the patient.

Worldview Inter-Wing Matrix Interventions

With regard to inter-wing matrix effects, I have seen changes in the spiritual wing of the patient's matrix lead to profound healing matrix effects, at times on numerous wings of the matrix from biological to family.

In the initial interview, this region was left relatively poorly explored in the case of Debbie. Later interviews revealed a paucity of religious and philosophical supports at this level, although her interest in her Christian upbringing and Eastern thought was emerging as an important avenue for change, as mentioned earlier.

Conclusion: Matrix Treatment Planning Redux

But every man is more than just himself; he also represents the unique, the very special and always significant and remarkable point at which the world's phenomena intersect, only once in this way and never again. That is why every man's story is important, eternal, and sacred ...

Herman Hesse
from the preface of *Demian*[40]

We have now concluded a brief survey of the six levels used in matrix treatment planning. Although there exists some obvious overlap with the DSM-5, a matrix analysis provides many new areas in which to deepen an understanding of the person beneath the diagnosis from the perspective of person-centered interviewing, as well as suggesting new areas of intervention. The concept of the human matrix also provides a more realistic picture of the patient as one process inextricably woven among the other systems of the world at large.

Two books for advanced reading on the concepts of the human matrix (one for clinicians and one for patients) may be of interest to the reader. For a compelling clinical exploration of the science and ramifications of different systems on the development of human behavior (essentially a book about the human matrix), I find *Feeling Good: The Science of Well-Being* by C. Robert Cloninger to be a remarkable synthesis of current scientific, clinical, and philosophic knowledge on how we are created by the interactions of the processes around us. As a bonus, it is also a remarkably compelling read.[41] For patients, *Happiness Is: Unexpected Answers to Practical Questions in Curious Times* was written by myself to provide insights on how people (both the general public and people currently in therapy) can use the knowledge of healing matrix effects, damaging matrix effects, the red-herring principle, and other nuances of the human matrix model to solve everyday problems, stresses, and crises.[42]

Before we move to an exploration of our third assessment perspective – the patient's core pains – I would like to revisit a working premise of this chapter. Throughout this chapter I have tried to illustrate the importance of addressing the *basic* principles of treatment planning when teaching interviewing itself. Hopefully I have effectively shown the three benefits of this understanding for the early trainee, as outlined at the beginning of this chapter. Our assessment approaches provide the following three bridges into treatment planning for the initial interviewer:

1. An easy and rapid method of checking, during the interview itself, whether pertinent data regions necessary for effective treatment planning have been explored, thus decreasing errors of omission
2. A reliable method of reminding the clinician to borrow from different data perspectives when collaboratively formulating a treatment plan with the patient
3. A flexible approach to actually delineating a list of potential treatment modalities with the patient

Yet there is one more utility to introducing *basic* treatment planning principles (as we have done in this chapter) simultaneously with clinical interviewing itself (keeping in mind that the actual specifics of treatment modalities and the advanced principles for treatment planning are to be addressed by their own courses later in training). As trainees learn the basics of creating an effective initial interview, they do not want to learn bad habits, only to have to "break" them later in their graduate training or in subsequent clinical practice.

Thus, learning the art of how to think about treatment planning *while one is concurrently moving through the various stages of the initial intake*, in my opinion, should be an integral part of the clinician's way of functioning. It should be introduced in the very first course on clinical interviewing and refined with each successive course in graduate training. To view treatment planning as an "afterthought" that occurs once the interview is done, or only during treatment planning sessions, is unrealistic, for the database collected and the structure of the interview itself are dependent upon how the interviewer intends to treatment plan. To view the interview and treatment planning in such an artificial fashion, as if they were separate silos, is, in my opinion, a potentially bad habit.

Moreover, especially when using matrix treatment planning (which requires a good deal of analytic thought and mental discipline), the clinician is able to see the patient in a critically holistic and contextual fashion. The real person beneath the diagnosis emerges. Sometimes this process of seeing the person beneath the diagnosis is viewed as being solely the result of the interviewer's innate empathy and intuition. It is not. Naturally there exist clinicians gifted with intuition, but even such clinicians are not bound by the limits of their "gifts." Their innate skills can be enhanced.

I am often asked, "Can intuition be taught?" My answer is a simple, "No." Nevertheless, I am convinced that it can be nurtured. James Carse, when describing the poetical power of Robert Frost, makes a point of significance to us as clinicians:

Frost was a master builder of word walls. He had learned the assorted techniques of putting words together in a way that made them poetry. But learning the techniques of poetry does not by itself make great poetry any more than building a well guarantees the vitality of a spring. Just as the poet has to let the ego step aside, technique too must be abandoned at just the right moment, allowing the poetic to enter on its own terms.[43]

Part of the art of interviewing is the clinician's ability to "let go" of techniques at just the right moment and to allow oneself to move purely with intuition. To be able to do so effectively, like Frost, one first spends enormous energy on learning techniques. Whether one is a poet, a martial artist, or a clinician, it is the disciplined practice of techniques and their analytic application, over and over again, that allows the techniques to become part of oneself. Paradoxically, it is at that moment that the poet, martial artist, or clinician will be able to "let go" of these very same techniques.

Here we come to a clinical paradox of sorts. I believe that by *consciously* applying the matrix perspective over and over again, from the first patient to the last, the process of thinking about the matrix becomes ingrained into the clinician. It becomes absorbed into the very essence of the clinician. It is taught as part of the beginner's mind so that it eventually becomes a part of the expert's soul. This is why basic treatment planning from a matrix perspective, in my opinion, is best begun as part of early training. It is why it appears in the first section of our book on core principles, not in our last section on advanced principles.

If done in such a disciplined fashion, I assure you that your rewards will be great. From years of the disciplined analysis of seeing people through the lens of the human matrix, one's intuition will be sharpened until one creates interviews like Frost wrote poetry. As with Frost, such a clinician will have moments in the initial interview when his or her technique, related to matrix treatment planning, will drop away. At those moments, they will feel or see something that other clinicians may not have felt or seen. The clinician, because of years of disciplined matrix thinking will "get it" – perhaps recognizing a matrix effect that others would have missed. It may be a matrix effect that is about to trigger an imminent suicide attempt or create the dangerous undertow of an emerging psychosis, or it may be the intuitive hint of a patient scarred by childhood abuse.

At such moments a curious reciprocity occurs between clinician and patient. Not only will the clinician "get it," but the patient will know that the clinician "gets it" – that this particular clinician sees what others have missed, that this clinician "sees the real me" that others glanced past, that this clinician sees my life as a complex interplay of processes that others may have felt to be unimportant. At such moments, the alliance will be made vibrant. Healing will begin. A second meeting will be secured. It is the type of moment in clinical interviewing that somehow goes beyond words. I don't want to sound too magical, but truth be told, there is something magical about such moments.

ASSESSMENT OF CORE PAINS

I can see behind everyone's masks. Peacefully smiling faces, pale corpses who endlessly wend their tortuous way down the road that leads to the grave.[44]

Edvard Munch, 19th century expressionist painter

Although Munch depicts a somewhat grim picture of human existence, he was a man keenly aware of the pains that all of us endure by our very nature of being human. His ability to intuitively sense underlying pain represents a gift that all clinicians hope to possess. Indeed, this ability to understand pain provides a major gateway through which therapeutic trust is born.

Throughout this book, an emphasis is placed on combining intuition and analysis, and the relationship between the two as just described. Many times the clinician will be able to intuitively sense the pains of the interviewee, but this intuition is enhanced when guided by an increased awareness of underlying themes. One of the more fascinating themes is the co-existence of the complexity of human nature with the simplicity of that same nature. Nowhere is this curious paradox more conspicuous than with the issue of psychological pain. Patients frequently present with complicated histories and concerns, sometimes even involving bizarre delusions and idiosyncratic perceptions. But the underlying pains from which these patients are fleeing are few in number.

Skilled clinicians possess the knack of cutting through the complexities until the bare wounds, the core pains, are understood. An understanding of these core pains is a powerful clinical tool. This empathic understanding can suggest avenues for treatment planning. Even more important, it can also guide the interviewer towards methods of navigating the patient's hesitancies that can develop during the interview itself, because the seeds of such hesitancies are often attempts to avoid these core pains by the patient. We have already had a glimpse of this process when we discussed methods of transforming communication breakdowns and patient fears in the opening phase of the interview in Chapter 3.

In any case, an understanding of core pains, and the increased sensitivity such an understanding can bring, provides an assessment perspective that complements both the DSM-5 and matrix treatment planning. It is based on the principle that clinicians should intermittently ask themselves, "What are the core pains that are hurting this patient at this time?" Or as Edvard Munch would have it, what is behind the mask?

The relevance of the concept of core pains was made plain to me by a psychotic patient when I was least expecting it. The patient was a young woman in her mid-20s who presented violently and was riddled with terrifying delusions. During the initial interview she described her sincere belief that aliens were speaking directly into her mind, taunting her sanity. Her world was convulsed with a pricking sensation of paranoia. She had become convinced that the aliens were about to kidnap her to a distant world. Her affect was intense, and she spoke in a disorganized fashion with a loosening of associations.

At this point, I asked her why she felt the aliens were coming for her. To my surprise she looked at me as if I had not been listening. Her affect calmed, her speech became coherent, and she said, "Don't you understand? I am alone here. No one cares for me. I have no family, no friends. And I have no reason to be here. Wouldn't you want to leave this horrid place if you were me?" At which point she promptly popped back into her psychotic language and refuge.

In a sense she was right concerning my inadequate listening, because I had become overly involved in diagnosis and systems analysis. A balancing perspective was needed – a sense of her pathos on a human level. She provided me with a lesson that led me to think more carefully about the presence of core pains and methods of conceptualizing them more clearly even as the interview itself proceeds.

Towards this goal, one can generate a list of core pains that singly, or in combination, appear to be driving any given individual. Each clinician may have a unique list. The following serve only as a platform for discussion. To me the core pains are as follows:

1. Intense loneliness
2. Feeling worthless or bad

3. Feeling rejected or wronged
4. A sense of failure
5. Loss of external control
6. Loss of internal control
7. Fear of the unknown
8. Loss of meaning

With Debbie in mind, one can survey these pains, examining their usefulness in both treatment planning and in understanding the dynamics of the interview itself.

The fear of being ultimately alone remains one of the most powerful and common pains. In the case of Debbie, it appears to be surfacing in one of its frequent guises, intense dependency. As such, it serves to remind the interviewer that some patients may seek an unhealthy dependency on the clinician even during the initial interview. Debbie would be one such person in whom this process could occur, as reflected by her intense feelings of abandonment when her significant other goes to sleep.

Her dependency needs may be intimately related to the second core pain, a sense of worthlessness or of being a bad person. Debbie was convinced of her ultimate inability to cope with life. In this sense, she probably avoids situations in which she could modestly succeed, thus depriving herself of the positive reinforcement needed to gain a sense of mastery. With these factors in mind, the clinician might consider assigning Debbie small, easily accomplished homework tasks, resulting in a gradually increasing sense of worth. In addition, the clinician might employ problem-solving skills therapy. Such therapy may not only improve her ability to navigate life's difficulties, it might have a marked impact on her self-esteem as she moves from a sense of inadequacy to, "You know, I've really learned something about how to cope with life and problem solve." In addition, a cognitive therapy approach might reveal that Debbie has a distorted self-image (perceiving herself as a bad or defective person, not uncommon in people coping with borderline process) maintained by tendencies for negative thinking and inappropriate self-blame. In this light, techniques such as cognitive restructuring might be of use.

Like its predecessor, this core pain appears to lead naturally into a discussion of the next core pain, a sense of rejection or being wronged. This fear reared its head throughout the interviewing process. Debbie demonstrated poor eye contact and frequently commented, "That's a stupid thing for me to say." Such anxieties can hamper the progress of the initial interview as the patient expends inordinate amounts of attention attempting to please the interviewer. Alert to this situation, the interviewer may purposely reassure the patient. For instance, the clinician might choose to say, "You are doing a very good job of discussing difficult material. It's really helping me to get a clearer picture of what has been going on." Even such a simple statement can make a patient such as Debbie feel considerably more comfortable, decreasing her fear of imminent rejection.

The fourth core pain, a feeling of failure, overlaps with a sense of worthlessness, but has an intensity all its own. The initial interviewer needs to attend to this particular pain, because the patient may bring it into the initial interview. Specifically, the patient may predict an impending failure in therapy and consequently decide not to appear for follow-up. If left as a hidden issue, the risk of losing the patient is real. In the closing phase of the interview, the clinician may opt to bring this fear to the surface with questions such as, "Now that we have talked about possible therapies, I'm wondering what you think about their usefulness for you?" or "If you tried outpatient therapy, how do you think it would go?" The interviewer may be able to cite the patient's success in handling the initial interview as evidence that the patient has the necessary abilities to succeed in therapy.

The fear of losing external control, the fifth core pain, can be extremely frightening to patients, because suddenly it seems as if nothing they can do will alter their situation. This combination of fear and anger can present a fertile field for suicidal ideation. A feeling of "being trapped" is viewed as one of the significant warning signs for suicide in recent work by Van Orden and company.[45] If one listens to the steelworker laid off indefinitely or the Detroit factory worker who watches the closing of an automobile plant, the roar of this pain can certainly be heard. While interviewing elderly patients or patients coping with chronic illnesses, one should bear in mind that they may be dealing with a sense of the ultimate loss of external control, death itself. When this core pain appears particularly prominent, the initial interviewer can make an effort to consciously increase the patient's sense of control within the interview itself by using statements such as, "At this point what do you think would be the most important area we should focus our discussion on?" Such modest, yet timely, intervention can significantly return some feeling of control to the patient.

The sixth core pain, the fear of loss of internal control, surfaces in patients who are becoming increasingly frightened of their own impulses, such as drives towards suicide or violence. I doubt that this pain could be more vividly portrayed than in patients who are moving into progressively more psychotic or manic behavior. In Debbie's case, her history of episodic violence, as evidenced by her throwing a picnic table bench through a picture window, suggests that this core pain may be a frequent motivator of her behaviors. Fortunately, in her initial interview she appeared to be in good control.

In other situations, the interviewer may find a patient who reports feeling imminently unstable. In such cases, it is generally, if not always, sound to attend to these fears on the spot. If the interviewer chooses to ignore these feelings, he or she risks driving the patient to an act of violence. Ironically, the patient's own increasing fears of losing control may act to spur further anxiety, perhaps pushing the patient even closer to a loss of control. The clinician can gently probe to see what the patient is afraid may happen and ask the patient if, indeed, he or she feels in control. The appearance of this core pain may suggest the usefulness of an antipsychotic medication.

We now come to the seventh element in the assessment of core pains, the fear of the unknown. As described in Chapter 3, most patients are probably experiencing this pain during the interview itself, because they are frightened of what the results of the interview will be. As mentioned earlier, a few minutes spent performing a sound introduction can greatly relieve the patient's unnecessary fears. In Debbie's case, her fear of the unknown may add to her dependent patterns, making her reluctant to try things on her own. With regard to treatment planning, one sometimes finds that patients such as Debbie do not have the communication skills or the assertiveness to find out what the future may hold, thus locking them into the paralysis of the moment. Their lack of assertiveness may prevent them from asking appropriate questions, even of the interviewer. The presence of this core pain should alert the clinician to the potential use of assertiveness training and social skills work, as well as to the need to address unasked questions.

The eighth and final core pain, loss of meaning, addresses the type of material addressed in the worldview wing of matrix treatment planning. The loss of a framework for meaning is a common precipitant of anxiety and depression, or it may appear in response to an ongoing psychiatric disorder such as schizophrenia or bipolar disorder. Patients may have a variety of differing ways of searching for meaning. With Debbie, we had already discussed some of her burgeoning interests in her religious roots as well as Eastern thought. But there was another endeavor that would prove to be powerfully important in her search for meaning – her interests in creating poetry and artwork.

We have now reviewed our third assessment schema. I have not explored the use of this system in detail; we will do this in upcoming chapters. Instead I have tried to survey this assessment system, which provides yet another set of pathways toward treatment planning. *This particular schema provides more on-the-spot information pertinent to altering the course of the interview itself than either the DSM-5 or the human matrix model, for it suggests various engagement strategies that can transform patient hesitancy or fear before it consolidates.* Together, these three assessment perspectives complement each other, helping the interviewer change a potentially impotent mass of data into a crisp and practical formulation, bridging directly into the treatment planning process.

As the clinician becomes familiar with using these three systems, one of their most appealing aspects surfaces – their speed. Once familiar with their use, after the interview the clinician can assess the known database while generating a powerful list of treatment options in about 5 to 10 minutes. This rapid integration of a large database can be a godsend in a busy clinic or private practice. Furthermore, the clinician can review the ongoing treatment plan quickly and with a fresh perspective as time passes.

Before wrapping up this chapter, it may be gratifying to review the course and ultimate outcome of Debbie in therapy, while also looking at the actual selections that were made from the lists of potential treatments generated by the above perspectives.

REVIEW OF THE CLINICAL COURSE OF MS. BAKER

In the first place, despite her chaotic history, Debbie brought to therapy a variety of healthy coping skills. She displayed motivation, intelligence, and a keen capacity for self-reflection. She also possessed the often-too-rare quality of compassion. Indeed, it was her apparent inability to recognize and accept her strengths that stood as one of the major obstacles to her development. In a large measure, therapy consisted of an attempt to help Debbie develop the attributes hinted at during her moments of high functioning.

The rest of her eventual treatment plan evolved directly from the data gathered in the initial interview. Regarding psychiatric disorders, she did not fulfill the criteria for a major depressive disorder. She did appear to meet the criteria for dysthymia, which, as mentioned earlier, may respond to antidepressant medication. In her case, I opted to forgo an antidepressant at first, hoping that psychotherapeutic measures would be more effective. In particular, because of her long-established pattern of self-debasement and a sense of worthlessness, I was concerned that she would immediately deny any credit for improvement if an antidepressant could be pointed to as the curative agent. If she had developed a major depressive episode or if the chosen treatment track had failed, I would most likely have promptly added an antidepressant. In the long run, the goal was to enable her to gain an increasing sense of self-worth and mastery over her environment.

Her problems with the development of a stable self were reflected by her primary diagnosis of a borderline personality disorder. She also met the criteria for a dependent personality. In any case, these diagnoses suggested the need to attend to her dependency issues quickly, a generalization extrapolated from the diagnosis and borne out by her long history of dependent relations (police being called to remove her from her last therapist's office). Consequently, in the closing phase of the initial interview, the issues of possible dependency upon me were discussed openly and mutually decided upon as a major concern to be avoided.

To sidestep a maladaptive dependency upon myself, she was seen only on a weekly basis. Moreover, we agreed to adopt a long-term treatment plan built around the concept of meeting for 3-month periods in which we focused on a specific problem list generated by her. At the end of each 3-month period, we would break from therapy for progressively longer periods of time as she began functioning more and more independently. These successful breaks from therapy allowed her to discover for herself, by practicing her new-found skills, that she was indeed improving and gaining a gently evolving sense of self-mastery.

This treatment approach characterized by intermittent stretches of therapist-free time was only possible because of considerations made with regard to the cultural/societal/environmental wing of her matrix. Specifically, it was discovered that a day hospital was available that could offer appropriate support when needed, as she underwent the pangs of separating from me. Thus she received enough support to gain the additional sense of independence offered by successfully navigating her loss of me. Only through the cooperation received from this agency of the mental health system could the treatment plan be made operational, a nice example of the power of integrated care, as emphasized in person-centered health care.

During her 3-month period of active therapy, specific tasks were assigned as homework, which she mastered easily, increasing her sense of worth. She also became adept at utilizing cognitive restructuring, which helped her to decrease her tendency for overgeneralization, splitting, and inappropriate self-blame. These cognitive techniques were implemented while simultaneously considering the psychodynamic issues of the development of her core sense of self. These cognitive and psychodynamic techniques all represent *intra*-wing treatment approaches in which psychological problems (low self-worth/weak self-identity) were addressed with psychological interventions (psychodynamic and cognitive–behavioral therapies).

It was here that an interesting *inter*-wing intervention would prove to have a major healing matrix effect on Ms. Baker's sense of self-identity. As I mentioned earlier, one of her main pathways for finding spiritual stability was her ongoing creation of poetry and artwork. I decided to place some increased emphasis on this well-established strength with the hope that further successes in this arena might provide her with a stronger sense of accomplishment and self-respect using the spiritual wing (artwork) to make a healing matrix effect on her psychological wing (self-identity).

When first entering this part of the therapeutic process, Debbie would timidly show me some of her artwork. One could see her fears of rejection, reflected by her almost sheepish looks for approval and the hesitant handing over of her artwork to a perceived "master judge." Even more striking was the signature on the painting, "Paul." If you recall, she liked to fantasize that she was Paul Newman. She always used her fantasy identity when signing her artwork or poetry. As therapy continued, much positive feedback was provided by both myself and the staff at the day clinic on her artistic progress. Indeed, her skills improved at a brisk pace.

One day, several years into the therapy, Debbie handed me a piece of her artwork. She presented it with a quick and confident gesture, commenting, "I like this one a lot, Dr. Shea." She passed it to me looking me directly in the eye. I looked down, impressed by its quality. I then looked down more intently. When I looked up, she was smiling broadly, "Yeah, it was done by me." She had signed it "Debbie." It's the type of moment in therapy that one does not easily forget.

Furthermore, as therapy proceeded she stopped wearing her wristband with the false identity, a behavioral change paralleled by a significant decrease in her fantasy activity. Several years after her therapy was completed, I saw one of her poems in the local paper. Her real name sat quietly at the bottom.

Another *inter*-wing matrix effect was used by utilizing a biologic intervention (medication) to impact on her anxiety and poor impulse control during her premenstrual unrest (psychological wing). Specifically, small doses of the antianxiety agent Xanax (alprazolam) were used as deemed necessary by Debbie, and carefully monitored by me, during her premenstrual phase. The medication proved efficacious. Moreover, she was pleased by her ability to wisely use the medication in a limited fashion and felt good about herself that she was maturely controlling a behavioral problem that had previously been highly problematic. In addition, a behavioral system (an intra-wing intervention), in which she played a major role in developing, was employed to help her to prevent suicidal and violent activity. The emphasis remained on her to help herself, using her decreased need for my "parenting," as reinforcing evidence of her ability to manage independently.

A further area for intervention appeared in the family assessment. To this end, a session was arranged for Debbie and her partner (dyadic wing of her matrix). By explaining to her partner certain aspects of the overall plan for increasing Debbie's independence, her partner was better able to support progress. It was also discovered that her partner appeared to be a loving and dependable support system. This session also served to decrease her partner's anxieties concerning the therapy itself, thus decreasing the risk of resistance generated by her partner. During the course of therapy, several joint sessions with her partner proved to be valuable. These interventions all demonstrate *intra*-wing interventions.

With regard to her relationship with her partner, greatly strained by Debbie's demands on her partner's time, a decision was made to partially heal the relationship by using an *inter*-wing intervention. Specifically, an attempt was made to relieve Debbie's dependencies on her partner by nurturing group relationships at the community day hospital. Group therapy was utilized successfully in this regard. Her relationship with her partner strengthened considerably as she spent more time with others, while developing more mature social skills. These interventions on the "group wing" of her matrix had healing matrix effects both on the dyadic wing with her partner but also on her psychological wing where she began to view herself as a more worthwhile and capable person.

By 2½ years into the therapy, Debbie had been involved in three 3-month therapy courses separated by increasingly large interludes. Her mood shifts had stabilized markedly, as had her relationship with her partner. She had only two minor suicidal gestures in this time period. In the subsequent year and a half, the length between courses of therapy increased with an eventually uneventful termination of therapy. Needless to say, police intervention was not required.

CONCLUSION

In this chapter we have looked at the process of effectively organizing the information gained from an initial interview. It has become apparent that the methods chosen for conceptualizing data can greatly affect the ultimate usefulness of the data. The three organizational methods discussed here – the diagnostic perspective of the DSM-5, matrix treatment planning, and an understanding of the patient's core pains – when deftly combined can provide a practical and flexible method for generating a list of viable treatment options during the interview itself. These three assessment systems also establish a reliable method of noting pertinent gaps in the database.

In the long run, the major reason for performing an assessment interview remains the generation of a sound treatment plan. Unlike T. S. Eliot in our opening epigram, we are not undertaking an exploration to know a place, we are undertaking an exploration to try to know a person. But like T. S. Eliot, "we come to know the place for the first time" by arriving where we started, the words of the patient during the interview itself. The treatment plan arises from our attempt to understand the patient and the ever-changing matrix from which the patient evolves. Ultimately, this understanding must come from our ability to sensibly organize what the patient is trying to communicate through his or her words. Once we have gained this ability to quickly organize the seemingly chaotic information coming our way, treatment plans naturalistically come to mind; it almost seems as if the database speaks for itself. Our task becomes one of learning to listen, for the patient's past history points towards the patient's future healing.

REFERENCES

1. Eliot TS. Little Gidding. In: *Collected poems of T. S. Eliot*. Pennsylvania, PA: Franklin Center, The Franklin Library; 1976. p. 201.

2. Seligman L, Reichenberg LW. *Selecting effective treatments: a guide to treating mental disorders.* 4th ed. Hoboken, NJ: Guilford Press; 2011.
3. Anthony MM, Barlow DH. *Handbook of assessment and treatment planning for psychological disorders.* 2nd ed. Hoboken, NJ: Guilford Press; 2011.
4. Adams N, Grieder DM. *Treatment planning for person-centered care: the road to mental health and addiction recovery.* Waltham, MA: Academic Press; 2004.
5. American Psychiatric Association. *Diagnostic and statistical manual of mental disorders.* 5th ed (DSM-5). Washington, DC: American Psychiatric Publishing; 2013.
6. Mueser KT, Noordsy DL, Drake RE, Fox L. *Integrated treatment for dual disorders: a guide to effective practice.* New York, NY: Guilford Press; 2003.
7. McInnis-Dittrich K. *Social work with elders: a biopsychosocial approach to assessment and intervention.* Boston, MA: Allyn and Bacon; 2005.
8. American Psychiatric Association. 2013.
9. World Health Organization. *The ICD-10 classification of mental and behavioural disorders: clinical descriptions and diagnostic guidelines.* Geneva: World Health Organization; 1992 <http://apps.who.int/classifications/icd10/browse/2015/en>; [accessed 9 June 2015].
10. Kessler RC, Berglund P, Demler O, et al. Lifetime prevalence and age-of-onset distributions of DSM-IV disorders in the national comorbidity survey replication. *Arch Gen Psychiatry* 2005;**62**(6):593–602.
11. Blazer DG, Kessler RC, McGonagle KA, Swartz MS. The prevalence and distribution of major depression in a national community sample: The national comorbidity survey. *Am J Psychiatry* 1994;**151**:979–86.
12. Turk CL, Mennin DS. Phenomenology of generalized anxiety disorder. *Psychiatr Ann* 2011;**41**(2):72–8.
13. Koerner K, Linnehan M. *Doing dialectical behavioral therapy: practical guide (Guides to individualized evidence-based treatment).* New York, NY: Guilford Press; 2011.
14. Yeomans FE, Clarkin JF, Kernberg OF. *A primer of transference focused psychotherapy for the borderline patient.* New York, NY: Jason Aronson; 2002.
15. Cushing H. *Life of Sir William Osler.* Oxford: Clarendon Press; 1925.
16. American Psychiatric Association. *Diagnostic and statistical manual of mental disorders.* 4th ed – Text Revision (DSM-IV-TR). Washington, DC: American Psychiatric Publishing; 2000. p. 807–13.
17. Engel GL. The clinical application of biopsychosocial model. *Am J Psychiatry* 1980;**137**(5):535–44.
18. Engel GL. The need for a new medical model: A challenge for biomedicine. *Science* 1977;**196**:129–36.
19. Gabbard GO, Kay J. The fate of integrated treatment: whatever happened to the biopsychosocial psychiatrist? *Am J Psychiatry* 2001;**158**:1956–63.
20. McClain T, O'Sullivan PS, Clardy JA. Biopsychosocial formulation: recognizing educational shortcomings. *Acad Psychiatry* 2004;**28**(2):88–94.
21. Kay J. Integrated treatment: an overview. In: Kay J, editor. *Integrated treatment for psychiatric disorders: review of psychiatry,* vol. 20. Washington, DC: American Psychiatric Press; 2001. p. 1–29.
22. Barkley J. Biopsychosocial assessment: why the biopsycho and rarely the social? *J Can Acad Child Adolesc Psychiatry* 2009;**18**(4):344–7.
23. Christ G, Diwan S. *Section 2: the role of social work in managing chronic illness care.* From the Geriatric Social Work Initiative created by the Council on Social Work Education. Release date 09.11.09. <www.cswe.org/File.aspx?id=25465>; [accessed 9 June 2015].
24. Suzuki S. *Zen mind, beginner's mind.* Boston, MA: Shambhala; 2006. p. 1.
25. Josephson AM, Peteet JR. Talking with patients about spirituality and worldview: practical interviewing techniques and strategies. *Psychiatr Clin North Am* 2007;**30**(2):181–97.
26. Ponce DE. *Caring, healing & teaching: fundamentals of a ministry for human services.* 2nd ed. Makati City, Philippines: Society of Filipino Family Therapists; 2011.
27. Cloninger CR. *Feeling good: the science of well-being.* Oxford: Oxford University Press; 2004. p. 317.
28. Newberg A, Waldman MW. *Born to believe: God, science, and the origin of ordinary and extraordinary beliefs.* New York, NY: Free Press; 2007.
29. Davidson RJ, Kabat-Zinn J, Schumacher J, et al. Alterations in brain and immune function by mindfulness meditation. *Psychosom Med* 2003;**65**(4):564–70.
30. Cade CM, Coxhead N. *The awakened mind: biofeedback and the development of higher states of awareness.* Shaftesbury, UK: Element Books; 1989.
31. Newberg A, Pourdehnad M, Alavi A, d'Aquili EG. Cerebral blood flow during meditative prayer: Preliminary findings and methodological issues. *Percept Mot Skills* 2003;**97**(2):625–30.
32. Schwartz JM, Beyette B. *Brain lock: free yourself form obsessive–compulsive behavior.* New York, NY: Regan Books; 1996.
33. Cloninger CR. 2004. p. 87.
34. Fleck S. Family functioning and family pathology. *Psychiatr Ann* 1980;**10**:17–35.
35. Fleck S. A holistic approach to family typology and the axes of DSM-III. *Arch Gen Psychiatry* 1983;**40**:901–6.
36. Murray-Swank A, Dixon LB, Stewart B. Practical interview strategies for building an alliance with the families of patients who have severe mental illness. *Psychiatr Clin North Am* 2007;**30**(2):167–80.

37. Welkowitz L. *Personal communication*. 2011.
38. FBI Hate Crimes Registry. <https://www.fbi.gov/about-us/cjis/ucr/hate-crime/2014/topic-pages/victims_final.pdf>; 2014 [accessed 15 April 2016].
39. Josephson AM, Peteet JR. 2007. p. 181–97.
40. Hesse H. *Demian*. New York, NY: Bantam Books; 1974.
41. Cloninger CR. 2004.
42. Shea SC. *Happiness is: unexpected answers to practical questions in curious times*. Deerfield Beach, FL: Health Communications, Inc.; 2004.
43. Carse JP. *Breakfast at the Victory: the mysticism of ordinary experience*. San Francisco, CA: HarperSanFrancisco; 1994. p. 152.
44. Stang R. *Edvard Munch: the man and his art*. New York, NY: Abbeville Press Inc.; 1977. p. 107.
45. Van Orden KA, Joiner TE, Hollar D, et al. A test of a list of suicide warning signs for the public. *Suicide Life Threat Behav* 2006;36(3):272–87.

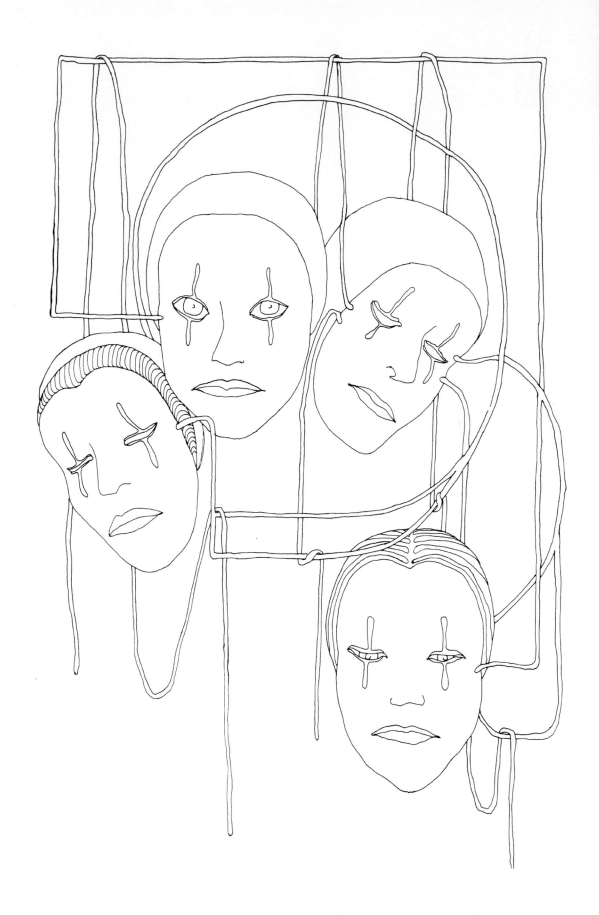

CHAPTER 8

Nonverbal Behavior: The Interview as Mime

And now a dark cloud of seriousness spread over her face. It was indeed like a magic mirror to me. Of a sudden her face bespoke seriousness and tragedy and it looked as fathomless as the hollow eyes of a mask.

Herman Hesse
Steppenwolf[1]

INTRODUCTION

In this chapter we will explore the intricate processes known as nonverbal behavior. Few studies are more intriguing or more pertinent for the clinician. It is only fitting that as we wrap up our review of the fundamental principles of clinical interviewing in Part I, we should address nonverbal behavior, for nonverbal processes have an impact on all of the way-stations delineated on our map of the clinical interview. Nonverbal cues play an obvious and critical role at way-stations such as engagement, data gathering, and in understanding the person. They even indirectly impact assessment processes, such as diagnosis, as well as enhance our ability to communicate as we collaboratively treatment plan in the closing phase of the interview. We will also see that nonverbal behaviors play a vital role in deciphering and effectively utilizing cross-cultural cues during the initial interview.

Our study will include not only body movements but also those elements of verbal communication that are concerned with *how* the words are spoken. In the early 1980s, one of the pioneers in the study of nonverbal behavior, Edward T. Hall, speculated that communication is roughly 10% words and 90% "hidden cultural grammar." He states, "In that 90% is an amalgam of feelings, feedback, local wisdom, cultural rhythms, ways to avoid confrontation, and unconscious views of how the world works. When we try to communicate only in words, the results range from the humorous to the destructive."[2] A decade later, a review of the more recent research on nonverbal behaviors by Burgoon showed that Hall's speculations foreshadowed what would eventually be validated by a more empirical evidence base, which has suggested that 60–65% of social meaning is derived from nonverbal behaviors.[3]

The practical relevance of Hall's words can be readily seen in the following clinical vignette. During an afternoon of supervision, I had the opportunity to watch two interviewers interact with the same patient in back-to-back interviews. The patient, a male in his early 20s, sat with a slumped posture, his head seemingly pulled to his chest by an invisible chain. His legs were open, and his hands lay resting quietly on his lap.

The first interviewer was a young woman, who spoke in a quiet but persistent voice. The blending between the two was weak at best, provoking an occasional upward nod from the patient, rewarding the starved interviewer with a momentary scrap of interest.

When the second interviewer entered the room, an intriguing process unfolded. Within 5 minutes, the patient sat more alertly in his chair. Eye contact improved significantly and was accompanied by some actual animation in his voice, albeit mild. By the end of the interview, the conversation was proceeding naturally, and a reasonably good therapeutic alliance had been formed. Both interviewers were relatively young women, both of whom conveyed a caring attitude. One wonders what factors resulted in the clearly more powerful blending of the second interview.

Some of the answers may lie in the communication channels each of these interviewers used in an effort to engage the patient. The first interviewer spoke in a quiet tone of voice intermixed with numerous nods of her head. Such head nodding frequently appears to facilitate interaction. Unfortunately, visual cues lose their impact if the patient refuses to look at the clinician. In short, her facilitating efforts were on the wrong sensory channel. In contrast, the second interviewer spoke in a more lively tone of voice, which appeared to grab the patient's attention. More important, her words were frequently punctuated with auditory facilitators such as "uh huh" and "go on." The first interviewer verbalized few such auditory facilitators. The patient had been stranded in the room, responding with detachment to the clinician's monotone voice. Like the first clinician, the second interviewer also utilized head nodding, but her nods became progressively more effective as the patient met her eyes more frequently.

This example demonstrates the usefulness of flexibly employing different communication channels depending on the receptiveness of the patient. If the patient's head is down, one can increase the number of facilitatory vocalizations. With a deaf patient, one can increase head nodding. Perhaps more important, this example emphasizes the overall influence of the interviewer's nonverbal communication on the patient. It suggests that we may be able to consciously alter our nonverbal style in an effort to create a specific impact on the patient – yet another example of intentional interviewing.

This possibility brings us to one of the most important challenges of this chapter. In order for interviewers to flexibly alter their styles, they must become familiar with the baseline characteristics defining their own styles. From such a position of self-understanding, flexibility emerges.

Thus, study of nonverbal behavior provides two distinct avenues of exploration. First, as the opening quotation from *Steppenwolf* suggests, one can learn an immense amount about the patient by studying their nonverbal cues. This aspect of nonverbal behavior is the most commonly acknowledged. Hesse's protagonist quickly perceives his companion's change of affect as "a dark cloud of seriousness spread over her face." Second, as our clinical vignette illustrates, one can discover the impact of one's own nonverbal behavior on the patient and subsequently alter it as appropriate.

The goal of this chapter is to provide concrete examples of how to use a knowledge of nonverbal behavior to effectively navigate the above two avenues in a busy clinical setting. In addition, my hope is to provide an appropriately sophisticated understanding of the theory and language used to describe nonverbal behaviors by experts in the field. Such a knowledge will enable the reader to rapidly and effectively explore the fascinating literature on nonverbal behaviors outside the pages of this book – a literature rich with clinical implications.

Basic Terminology of Nonverbal Behavior

Before proceeding, it may be expedient to examine the definition of nonverbal behavior, for this term can have different meanings. In their excellent book, *Nonverbal Communications: Science and Applications*, Matsumoto, Frank, and Hwang provide a lively, descriptive definition:

> *Nonverbal behaviors intrigue us. We see the way a person looks, the way he or she moves, and how he or she sounds. Nonverbal messages are transmitted through multiple nonverbal channels, which include facial expressions, vocal cues, gestures, body postures, interpersonal distance, touching and gaze. We call these channels because, like channels on a television, they are each capable of sending their own distinct message."*[4]

Operationally, in our book we will view nonverbal behavior as the general category of all behaviors displayed by an individual other than the actual content of his or her speech. Note that, as Matsumato and colleagues state, various factors can impact upon nonverbal behaviors, including such elements as the speed and intensity of a person's movements, interpersonal distance, and the pacing, loudness, and tone of voice used when speaking. To effectively address these elements from a clinical perspective, I have found it useful to split the broad category of nonverbal behavior into two general subcategories: (1) nonverbal communications and (2) nonverbal activities.

Nonverbal Communications (Emblems)

In the first category, nonverbal communications, the patient is using a commonly accepted symbol associated with a specific meaning. You will sometimes see the word "emblem," as coined by Ekman and Friesen,[5] used as a synonym for nonverbal communications.

An irate American football fan "throwing the finger" to the quarterback of the visiting team is displaying a piece of rather vivid nonverbal communication. Entire subcultures or organizations may develop a set of emblems for internal use. To once again use American football as a reference, the referees use a complex set of emblems to communicate the various penalties that have been committed by the players. Emblems may also be used in situations where speech is not possible (skin diving) or where it might not be practical (raising a hand for a question in a classroom).

Generally speaking, nonverbal communications (emblems) are relatively easy to interpret, for they evolved to communicate specific messages, but a word of caution is in order, which is of immediate importance to initial interviewers: Different cultures may attach significantly different meanings to the same nonverbal communication.[6]

The American "okay sign," which indicates that one approves of the current suggestion or situation, is viewed as somewhat vulgar in Brazil, and in France simply means "zero." On the other hand, in Arab countries the exact same "okay sign" is viewed as a rude sexual gesture. An initial interviewer using an okay sign to indicate to a patient in the closing phase of the interview that the patient has nicely understood a complex recommendation could result in a puzzling or discordant communication if it is to an Arab patient who is naive to the use of this emblem in American culture.

The Arab culture also provides a bridge into our second word of caution, which relates to the ease with which nonverbal activities can be misinterpreted as being forms of nonverbal communication. For example, a non-specific nonverbal *activity* from the clinician's culture may be seen as a quite specific nonverbal *communication* in the patient's culture or vice versa. For instance, Americans cross their legs frequently in everyday conversation, a nonverbal activity that often results in their companions seeing the bottom of their foot. Indeed, if a clinician crosses his or her legs with one ankle on the opposite leg's knee, the bottom of the clinician's foot may be facing the patient at times. Unfortunately, in the Arab culture, showing the bottom of one's foot is viewed as an extreme insult, representing a quite specific emblem. Even when interviewing an Arab patient familiar and comfortable with the Western interpretation of such a posture, a wise clinician may choose to avoid it – for why risk a possibly deep-seated unconscious negative response in the patient?

A basic principle for clinicians evolves from these caveats on nonverbal communications. If a clinician has moved to a different culture or has begun to practice in a part of the country in which a large immigrant population is being served, it is advisable for him or her to ask experienced clinicians in that setting to describe the relevant cross-cultural emblems as soon as possible. Some early, and unnecessary, missteps in engagement may be averted from such a simple survey.

Nonverbal Activities

In the second, vastly larger category – nonverbal activities – the overt behavior does not have a single commonly agreed upon meaning, and the sender may not be consciously trying to convey a message. Hand gesturing, facial expressions, and even more directive acts such as chain-smoking cigarettes all represent nonverbal activities. A nonverbal activity, such as fidgeting with a pen, may indeed be usefully interpreted by the observer as having a meaning, perhaps indicating anxiety; however, this interpretation is inferred and may be wrong. In short, nonverbal activities may have numerous meanings.

Ekman and Friesen categorized *nonverbal activities* into four classes: illustrators and regulators (which, respectively, play a direct role in either descriptive gesturing or the regulation and flow of speech) and adaptors and affective displays (both of which may convey secrets to underlying emotions, feelings, and attitudes).[7]

Illustrators are hand gestures used to complement, expand, and clarify spoken language. Deictic illustrators are used to point at an object while speaking about it. A different style of illustrator (iconic) involves using the hands to outline or suggest an object that is being described. With the use of iconic illustrators, a person can suggest characteristics such as size and shape. Gifted public speakers are masters of iconic illustration. Sign language, as used with the hearing impaired, partially evolved from iconic illustration and, in my opinion, often achieves a gracefulness deserving of the term "art."

Regulators consist of facial movements, hand gestures, and body movements that serve to control, adjust, and sustain the flow of a conversation. Bente and colleagues have referred to these behaviors collectively as "dialog functions."[8] They describe specific uses of regulators such as turn-taking signals (eye contact) and managers of communication flow (such as head nods, suggesting the speaker should go on and that they are being understood).

Adaptors are behaviors that are performed, for the most part without conscious intention, to allow oneself to feel more comfortable. They can include various hand behaviors such as stroking the face, picking at ones nails, or rolling a pen, as well as more generalized body movements such as changing posture, stance, or position in a chair. As with all nonverbal activities, adaptors may mean many things. On a mundane level, they may simply indicate that the person needed to change position for the person's body was simply growing tired or strained in a particular position. On a more psychodynamic level, they may indicate various underlying feelings or attitudes, from anxiety to a feeling of being socially uncomfortable, perhaps a tell-tale sign of patient deceit, as we shall see later.

Affective displays are generally facial movements (furrowing the brow, tensing the jaw, intense staring) that tend to spontaneously occur when a human is feeling a particular emotion. Learning to read affective displays is a critical skill for any interviewer. Prominent affective displays are usually fairly easy to read, for they often have an almost universal meaning that can generally be inferred regarding emotions such as anger, disgust, fear, happiness, sadness and surprise (Ekman's original list of core emotions),[9] as well as more subtle emotional states including amusement, contempt, contentment, embarrassment, excitement, guilt, pride in achievement, relief, satisfaction, sensory pleasure and shame (Ekman's expanded list of core emotions). Some highly skilled clinicians are naturally adept at "picking up" on subtle affective displays, a skill that is often viewed as intuition. On the other hand, interviewers can learn methods for more rapidly and accurately spotting affective displays, a highly useful skill for any clinician. For the interested reader, such behaviors are nicely described and illustrated by photographs in Paul Ekman's book, *Emotions Revealed.*[10]

A Cautionary Note on Interpreting Nonverbal Behaviors and Nonverbal Research

As clinicians we are interested in understanding the significance of both nonverbal communications (emblems) and nonverbal activities (illustrators, regulators, adaptors, and affective displays). *It is important to keep in mind that nonverbal activities are generally multiply determined.* It seems unwise to begin assuming that one "knows" exactly what any given nonverbal activity means. Even nonverbal activities generally viewed as obviously representing a specific mood state, such as laughter, can be misinterpreted, depending upon the interpersonal and cultural context of the laughter. The kulturbrille effect can be quite striking here.

For instance, in the Japanese culture laughter generally means what it does in Western culture – the patient is finding something to be humorous. But this common affective display has several uncommon uses, from a Western interviewer's perspective, in the Japanese culture. It can be utilized as a way of covering up or controlling displeasure, as well as concealing embarrassment, confusion, and shock.[11] An interviewer unaware of these uses of laughter could view a Japanese patient who is laughing intermittently in an initial session to be demonstrating a powerful degree of blending, when, in reality, the patient is feeling highly uncomfortable and will not be making a second appearance with this particular clinician.

In this regard, Wiener and associates criticized some psychoanalytically oriented researchers as immediately positing unwarranted unconscious meanings to nonverbal activities.[12] Considering this context one is reminded of the old psychoanalytic saw in which the astute clinician detects that the patient is experiencing severe marital discord because she is playing with her wedding band. Such interpretations of nonverbal activities are invaluable if kept in perspective. However, the clinician needs to think about other possible causes of the stated activity. For instance, this patient may be playing with her wedding band because she feels intimidated by the interviewer. She releases her anxiety by playing with objects in her hands. Normally she rolls a pencil back and forth, but because no pencil is available, she twists her ring. Other interpretations may be equally correct. To ignore these other possibilities while assuming the marriage is troubled is to ignore sound clinical judgment. On the other hand, having considered the various possibilities, the experienced clinician may gently probe to sort out which is correct and may indeed uncover marital discord.

From this discussion, it is reasonable to make the following generalization: Nonverbal communications are relatively easily deciphered (but even here there are caveats), whereas nonverbal activities should be cautiously interpreted, because more than one process may be responsible for the behavior. This point deserves emphasis because both in clinical and popular literature, the idea that exact meanings of nonverbal activities can be directly read is put forward by some authors. They imply that one can read a person like a book. In a similar vein, the concept of "body language" suggests that nonverbal activities are more codified than they actually are.

A similar degree of caution is required as one surveys the research concerning nonverbal behavior. The body of research appears both vast and promising, but there exist many limitations. Nonverbal interactions are so complex that it remains difficult to successfully isolate variables to study. For instance, suppose a piece of research was designed to prove that it was the paralanguage (how the words were said) of the second interviewer in our opening clinical vignette that directly increased blending. An attempt to isolate this single variable would prove difficult, for a variety of other variables could have had an impact, such as the interviewer's physical attractiveness, the distance between seats, and even the fact that there were two interviews.

Even when one successfully isolates the relevant variables, the very act of isolation poses serious problems. Nonverbal elements seldom function as isolated units.[13] Instead, the various nonverbal elements exert their influences jointly, making the findings of research based on single channels such as paralanguage or eye gaze somewhat artificial. A different approach, the functional approach, attempts to study the various nonverbal elements as they function in unison.

Finally, two cultural elements of academia impact on the quality of nonverbal research. First, the most common sampling methods used in many studies tend to focus upon Western cultures, and even within that sample it is common practice to recruit subjects from undergraduate students – hardly a group that is representative of the general population.[14] Second, like many other research arenas, research in nonverbal behavior has a paucity of replication studies, i.e., where published research is repeated to ensure that the results are valid. In fact, much of the research has not been duplicated for a variety of reasons including: funding agencies are sometimes unwilling to support replication studies; researchers often do not want to replicate the work of others, but would rather "do their own research"; and academic institutions tend to value and reward "original research" more highly. Thus, in both the academic and popular literature, findings about nonverbal communication are sometimes cited as being "evidence based," when the research may have been of poor quality and/or may never have been replicated.

These research issues are worth mentioning because it is important for the clinician to realize that relatively limited knowledge exists on nonverbal behaviors that can be called "factual." It is safe to say that this body of exciting research is still in its adolescence. In this regard, the material of this chapter is best viewed as opinion concerning an evolving craft or art. The material itself is culled from a variety of sources, including clinical work, supervision, research literature, personal communications, and even popular literature[15,16] if it seems to shed light on clinical issues. But despite the lack of an extensively validated evidence base, I want to reassure the reader that my trainees and I have found the following material on nonverbal behavior to be invaluable, both in interviewing and in ongoing psychotherapy.

Organization of the Chapter

The chapter is divided into three sections. In Part 1, the classic fields of study in nonverbal behavior will be briefly surveyed, emphasizing those theoretical foundations that are immediately clinically relevant. As with previous chapters, we shall develop a concrete language through which to study the phenomena in question. The following three areas will be addressed: (1) proxemics (the study of the use of space), (2) kinesics (the study of body movement), and (3) paralanguage (the study of how things are said).

Using our understanding of these three cornerstones of nonverbal study, in Part 2 we shall adopt a functional perspective, carefully investigating the interplay of these areas as directly applied to clinical practice. The broad clinical tasks studied include assessing the nonverbal behaviors of patients, actively engaging patients, and calming potentially violent patients.

In Part 3, we will wrap up the chapter by exploring a remarkably exciting new arena for clinical interviewing, the web and its associated world of wireless connectivity, from texting to chatting. We will find that, within this world, many of the possibilities and limitations are directly related to nonverbal issues.

PART 1: CORE FIELDS OF STUDY IN NONVERBAL BEHAVIOR

Proxemics

Edward T. Hall was quoted at the beginning of the chapter. Few people would be more suitable for introducing the topic of nonverbal behavior, because Hall coined the word "proxemics," a term that defines one of the major topics of interest in the field of non-verbal communication. It was in his book *The Hidden Dimension* that he defined proxemics as "the inter-related observations and theories of man's use of space as a specialized elaboration of culture."[17]

Proxemics deals with the manner in which people are affected by the distances set between themselves and objects in the environment, including other people. As Hall notes, humans, like other animals, tend to protect their interpersonal territories. As humans move progressively closer to one another, new feelings are generated and new behaviors are anticipated. Hall postulates that people learn specific "situational person-alities" that interact with the core traits of the individual, depending on the proximity of other individuals. This set of expected behaviors and feelings can be used by the clini-cian to improve blending. By observing the patient's use of space, the clinician may even uncover certain diagnostic clues.

Hall delineated four interpersonal distances: (1) intimate distance, (2) personal dis-tance, (3) social distance, and (4) public distance. With each of these distances, different sensory channels assume various levels of importance.

At the intimate distance (0 to 18 inches), the primary sensory channels tend to be tactile and olfactory. People feel at home with the specific scents they associate with lovers and children. At these close distances, thermal sensations also play a role, especially when making love or cuddling. Visual cues are of diminished importance. In fact, at the inti-mate distance, most objects become blurred unless specific small areas are focused upon. Voice is used sparingly. Even whispered words can sometimes create the sensation of more distance.

As one moves to the personal distance ($1\frac{1}{2}$ to 4 feet), kinesthetic cues continue to be used and olfactory and thermal sensations diminish in importance. With their decline, the sense of sight begins to assume more importance, especially at the further ranges of this interpersonal space.

Upon arriving at the social distance (4 to 12 feet), we have reached the region where most face-to-face social interchange occurs. Touch is less important, and olfactory sensa-tions are markedly less common. This region is the play-land of the voice and the eyes. Most conversations and interviews unfold within the range of 4 to 7 feet.

At the public distance (12 feet or more), vision and audition remain the main channels of communication. Most important, as people move further and further away, they tend to lose their individuality and are perceived more as part of their surroundings.

A respect for these spaces is of immediate value to the initial interviewer. In general, people seem to feel awkward or resentful when strangers, such as initial interviewers, encroach upon their intimate or personal space. With this idea in mind, it is probably generally best to begin interviews roughly 4 to 6 feet away from the patient. If an interviewer is by nature extroverted, by habit the interviewer may sit inappropriately close to the patient, intruding upon the patient's personal space. Obviously, such a practice can interfere with blending and should be monitored.

It should be kept in mind that patients do not determine a sense of interpersonal space by slapping yardsticks down between themselves and clinicians. As observed by Hall, it is the intensity of input from various sensory channels that creates the sensation of distance. An interviewer with a loud speaking voice may be invading a patient's personal space even when seated at 6 feet. Once again, clinicians must examine their own tendencies in order to determine how they come across to patients.

To emphasize the point that it is sensory input, not geographic distance, that determines interpersonal space, one need only consider the impact of a patient who seldom bathes upon friends, family, and strangers (even clinicians). Such patients frequently create a sense of resentment, because, in essence, olfactory sensations are supposed to occur only at intimate and personal distances. These patients invade the intimate space of those around them even when seated at a distance. The same principle can explain why even pleasant odors such as perfume can also be resented if they are too strong.

If a clinician intrudes into a patient's personal space, the clinician can set into motion the same awkward feelings and defenses commonly encountered in elevators. The artificial intimacy created by invading the patient's space results in a shutdown of interactive channels, so as not to further the intimate contact. Like a person in an elevator, the patient will avoid eye contact and move as little as possible. The patient's uneasiness may even predispose the patient to decreased conversation. In effect, the clinician might just as well be conducting the interview in an elevator, hardly the image of an ideal office. This "elevator effect" can also occur if the clinician ignores cultural differences.

Hall's distances were determined primarily for White Americans. These distances may vary from culture to culture. One piece of research found that Arab students spoke louder, stood closer, touched more frequently, and met the eyes of fellow conversants more frequently.[18] Sue and Sue relate that Latinos, Africans, and Indonesians like to converse at closer distances than do most Anglos.[19] They go on to describe that when interviewing a Latino, a White American interviewer may feel a need to back up, because the interpersonal space feels crowded. Unfortunately, this need for distance by the clinician could be perceived as an element of coolness or indifference by the patient (a kulturbrille effect). In a similar light, the clinician may make the mistake of immediately feeling that the patient is being socially invasive, when in reality the patient is merely interacting at the appropriate distance for a Latino/a culture.

Race may also play a role during the interview. Research suggests that Black Americans may prefer greater distances than White Americans.[20] Moreover, Wiens discusses the finding that the sexes of the participants can affect the preference for interpersonal distance.[21] One study demonstrated that male–female pairs sat the closest, followed by female–female pairs. Male–male pairs sat the furthest apart. More recent work has suggested that psychological gender is a better indicator of the patient's feeling of comfortable seating distance. People with a feminine orientation tended to interact at closer interpersonal spaces no matter what their biologic sex.[22]

Kinesics

Kinesics is the study of the body in movement. It includes "gestures, movements of the body, limbs, hands, head, feet, and legs, facial expressions (smiling, frowning, furrowing the brow, etc.), eye behavior (blinking, direction and length of gaze, and pupil dilation), and posture."[23] In short, kinesics is the study of how people move their body parts through space with an added attempt to understand why such movements are made. Both nonverbal communications and nonverbal activities are broadly subsumed under the term kinesics. As a field, it is a natural companion to proxemics. Like proxemics, it had its own avatar, Ray T. Birdwhistell, who first elaborated his work in 1952 with the book *Introduction to Kinesics: An Annotation System for Analysis of Body Motion and Gesture*.[24]

Birdwhistell was an anthropologist and emphasized understanding body movements in the context of their occurrence. He also pioneered the study of videotapes in an effort to decipher the subtle nuances of movement. Through his microanalysis he attempted to define the basic identifiable units of movement. For instance, he coined the term "kine" to represent the basic kinesic unit with a discernible meaning.[25]

Albert Scheflen, a student of Birdwhistell's, expanded these notions to the study of broad patterns of kinesic exchange between people. In this context, Scheflen postulated that kinesic behavior frequently functions as a method of controlling the actions of others.[26] By way of example, hand gestures and eye contact may be used to determine who should be speaking at any given moment in a conversation ("regulators" as defined by Ekman and Friesen).

Kinesics plays a role in all interviews. Specific activities may shut down or facilitate the verbal output of any given patient. Early kinesic studies emphasized the accurate description, delineation, and definition of facial/body movements and gestures (the explicit aspects of kinesics). More recently, researchers and clinicians have come to realize that "how" movements are done may be as important as "what" movements are done. This newer aspect of kinesic study has been called the "implicit behavioral qualities" of movement.[27] Some studies suggest specifically that dynamic qualities such as speed, acceleration, complexity, and symmetry of body and facial expressions may have a great impact on how nonverbal behaviors are interpreted (both how we interpret our patients and how they interpret us).[28] A smile done with abruptness by a harried clinician when first meeting a patient in the waiting room may be far more disengaging than engaging.

Both explicit and implicit kinesic factors can greatly change the meaning of the words spoken by either the patient or the clinician. Once again cross-cultural factors may lead to significant misunderstandings if the kinesic norms of a culture are not understood. A poignant example of this kinesic kulturbrille effect is described by Elizabeth Kuhnke:

Maria was working in Japan with a Japanese colleague, preparing a patient presentation. She asked him if he was pleased with the work they had done together. He told her that, yes, he was. A couple of days later Maria heard through the grapevine that her colleague wasn't happy with the result and wanted to rework the presentation. When she asked him why he'd told her that it was all right when it wasn't, he replied: "But I told you with sad eyes, Maria."[29]

Besides yielding information that may help the clinician to foster engagement, the study of kinesics can provide valuable insights into the feelings and thoughts of patients. Freud phrased it nicely when he stated, "He that has eyes to see and ears to hear may convince himself that no mortal can keep a secret. If his lips are silent, he chatters with his finger-tips; betrayal oozes out of him at every pore."[30]

Paralanguage

The study of paralanguage focuses on how words are delivered. It may include elements such as tone of voice, loudness of voice, pitch of voice, rhythm and fluency of speech.[31] You will sometimes see paralanguage called vocalics or paralinguistics in the literature.[32] The power of paralanguage is immense and popularly acknowledged. Phrases such as, "It's not what you said, but the way you said it, that I don't like," are considered legitimate complaints in our society. Moreover, actors and comedians are well aware of the power of timing and tone of voice as it impacts upon the meaning of a statement. The comedian Jon Stewart is phenomenally adept at changing meaning through the use of paralanguage, transforming a statement that sounds complementary, at first glance, into a wickedly funny sarcastic slight, with a delightful twist in his tone of voice.

By way of illustration, the phrase "that was a real nice job in there" appears complimentary at first glance. But one cannot determine its meaning unless one hears the tone of voice used in its conveyance. It could be far from pleasant if it was said with a sarcastic sneer by a displeased supervisor following an interview observed via a one-way mirror.

Besides the tone of the voice, speech is characterized by a number of other vocalizations. Although not words *per se*, vocalizations can play an important role in communication. One set of vocalizations consists of "speech disturbances."[33] Under the heading of flustered or confused speech, these disturbances include entities such as stutters, slips of the tongue, repetitions, word omissions, and sentence incompletions, as well as familiar vocalizations such as "ah" or "uhm." Such disturbances occur roughly once for every 16 spoken words. As would be expected, under stressful conditions these disturbances increase significantly. Thus they can serve to warn the clinician of patient anxiety as the interview proceeds.

There is more to vocalizations than just their appearance or lack of it. Some vocalizations serve to enhance blending, as seen with the frequently used facilitatory statements "uh huh" and "go on." But, once again, the way in which these vocalizations are used can significantly alter their effectiveness, as shown in the following vignette.

The interviewer in question possessed a pleasant and upbeat personality. He was a caring clinician, but he found patients shutting down at times during his interviews.

Videotape analysis revealed an interesting phenomenon. As he listened to patients, he frequently interspersed his silences with the vocalization "uh huh." His "uh huhs" were said quickly with a mild sharpness to his voice. He also used vocalizations such as "yep" and "yeah," also stated with a curt tone of voice.

The net result was the creation of the feeling that he was in a hurry, wanting just the facts. And that is exactly what his patients gave him. This habit, combined with a tendency to over-utilize note taking, fostered a business-like persona, despite his natural warmth in daily conversation. It was a habit well worth breaking and once again highlights the power of paralanguage.

Cross-cultural differences also affect paralanguage. Sue and Sue describe the variations in paralanguage that can interfere with the blending or assessment process when working with people outside the clinician's culture. For instance, silences are frequently interpreted as moments when the patient, for conscious or unconscious reasons, is holding back. Silence may also signal that the patient is ready for a new question. At other moments, silence can create a feeling of uneasiness in both interviewer and interviewee. But, as Sue and Sue clearly state, the obvious may be too obvious, once again demonstrating the potentially disruptive power of the kulturbrille effect.

> *Although silence may be viewed negatively by Americans, other cultures interpret and use silence much differently. The English and Arabs use silence for privacy, whereas the Russians, French, and Spanish read it as agreement among parties. In Asian culture silence is traditionally a sign of respect for elders. Furthermore, silence by many Chinese and Japanese is not a floor-yielding signal inviting others to pick up the conversation. Rather, it may indicate a desire to continue speaking after making a particular point. Oftentimes, silence is a sign of politeness and respect rather than lack of desire to continue speaking. A counselor uncomfortable with silence may fill in and prevent the patient from elaborating further. An even greater danger is to impute false motives to the patient's apparent reticence.*[34]

Immediacy and Context: the Delicate Interface of Proxemics, Kinesics, and Paralanguage

Immediacy

Immediacy is a term describing the sensation that one is in the immediate presence of another person and the positive or negative feelings of warmth, closeness, involvement, and acceptance experienced in that presence, as created and/or reflected by their nonverbal behaviors. It is a major component (in addition to the actual words being exchanged) of what we have been calling blending. As such, the ability to interpret and use the nonverbal cues of immediacy is one of the keys to identifying the underlying *real* engagement of our patients.

One can argue, and indeed, Peter Andersen, the author of one of the core textbooks on nonverbal communications, has done so, that the most central function of nonverbal behavior is the exchange of immediacy.[35] Immediacy results from the interface of factors from all three of our core elements of nonverbal behavior (proxemics, kinesics, and paralanguage). Immediacy can be communicated by how close we sit or how far forward we decide to lean (proxemics). Our emblems, illustrators, regulators, adaptors, and affective displays all play a marked role in the conveyance of immediacy (kinesics). Tone of voice, loudness, and pacing of speech further sculpt the sensation of immediacy (paralanguage).

A variety of nonverbal behaviors impact on immediacy.[36] Eye contact, and even pupil dilation, contribute to it. In a classic study, Hess and Goodwin[37] showed subjects pictures of mothers holding their infants. The pictures were identical except for one small detail – in some photographs the mother's pupils had been retouched to appear larger. The response by the subjects was remarkable, with an overwhelming number perceiving that the mothers with enlarged pupils loved their babies more. This phenomenon has not gone unnoticed by marketers, who frequently increase the size of the pupils of individuals in their advertisements using Photoshop, in an effort to entice the consumer into a "closer relationship" with the model or celebrity who is plugging their product.

Other immediacy behaviors include smiles, head nodding, hand gestures, synchronicity of nonverbal behaviors between conversants, and paralanguage. Touch remains one of the most powerful indicators of immediacy and, consequently, should be used very cautiously by clinicians, a topic we shall address later in this chapter.

As we saw with empathic statements, one can ascribe a *valence* to immediacy behaviors ranging from low valence (the behaviors are not particularly powerful at communicating immediacy) to high valence (the behaviors strongly communicate immediacy). As with empathic statements, there is a time and place for both low- and high-valenced immediacy behaviors, a critical principle for understanding how to effectively engage patients battling with paranoid process or on the brink of violence, another topic we shall soon examine in detail in Part 2 of this chapter.

Nonverbal Context

Immediacy provides a natural bridge into the role of context in nonverbal behaviors. We can see from our discussion that immediacy generally is the result of the constellation of many nonverbal factors, simultaneously interpreted by the patient. Even a culturally accepted emblem may be received quite differently, depending upon the context in which it occurs. A close friend of many years might "throw the finger" in a joking fashion at a friend, following a playful criticism. A variety of other nonverbal activities (such as smiling, a twinkle in the eye, and a joking tone of voice) indicate that this emblem should not be interpreted in its normally aggressive fashion, because it was delivered in a humorous context.

Many experts feel that context is one of the most important concepts for understanding and effectively using nonverbal communication. Ekman includes the following elements as crucial to understanding context: the nature of the conversation, the history of the relationship, whether the nonverbal behavior is occurring while speaking versus listening, and how well the identified behavior is congruent with other simultaneous nonverbal activities such as facial expressions and tone of voice.[38]

Arguably, this last factor – the congruence among all simultaneous nonverbal activities – has been viewed as one of the most significant determinants of meaning in actual practice.[39] Take for example a smile by a patient. A genuinely warm smile is not limited to facial movement near the mouth. A genuine smile often has significant muscular movement around the eyes, with the appearance of smile lines beneath and at the corner of the eyes, and a narrowing of the lids. Sometimes a genuine smile is also accompanied by a gentle nodding of the head up and down. But there are many other types of smiles including the smiles of anxiety or of discomfort with a topic, as well as more hostile smiles, as seen with repressed irritation, anger, or contempt. During deceit, if the deceiver feels that a smile is indicated, a weak version of a smile may be consciously attempted. In contrast to a genuinely warm smile, all of the latter may have minimal contextual movements of the muscles around the eyes or head, allowing a clinician to more adeptly recognize that all is not as it seems.

As clinicians, another major factor regarding context is the impact of psychopathology. A well-intentioned, genuine smile from a clinician can be interpreted as hostile (by a person coping with paranoid psychotic process) or as flirtatious (by a person with an underlying histrionic personality structure).

PART 2: CLINICAL APPLICATION OF NONVERBAL BEHAVIOR

Section A: Assessment of the Patient

Nonverbal Hints of Hidden Psychopathology

Sir Denis Hill made the following observations during the 47th Maudsley Lecture in 1972:

> *Many experienced psychiatrists of an earlier generation believed that they could predict the likely mental state of the majority of the patients they met by observations within the first few minutes of contact before verbal interchange had begun. They did this from observation of nonverbal behavior—the appearance, bodily posture, facial expression, spontaneous movements and the initial bodily responses to forthcoming verbal interaction.*[40]

Sir Denis Hill was concerned that the ability to observe nonverbal behavior astutely represented a skill that had fallen by the wayside. Let us hope this demise is not the case, because experienced clinicians today as much as yesterday need to utilize nonverbal clues throughout their clinical work. The knowledge available today concerning nonverbal behaviors is significantly more advanced than 40 or 50 years ago. It is to this knowledge that we now turn our attention.

Uncovering Hidden Psychotic Process

To begin our discussion, we will look at another statement by Sir Denis Hill: "An important difference between the disturbed mental states which we term 'neurotic' and those we term 'psychotic' is that in the latter, but not in the former, those aspects of nonverbal behavior which maintain social interactional processes tend to be lost."[41] An awareness of these potential deficits in the psychotic patient can alert the clinician to carefully probe for more explicit psychotic material in a patient whose psychotic process is subtle.

Perhaps an example will be useful at this time. I was observing an initial assessment between a talented trainee and a woman in her mid-20s. The patient had been urged to the assessment by her sister and a close friend. Apparently the patient's mother was currently hospitalized with major depression.

By the end of the 50-minute intake, the clinician seemed aware that the patient was probably also suffering from major depression or some form of a mood disorder. But the severity of the patient's condition did not seem to have registered and the clinician was about to recommend outpatient follow-up. However, the patient's nonverbal behavior was telling the clinician to take another look.

In the immediately subsequent second interview, which I performed, the patient disclosed a recent weekend brimming with psychotic terror. She had felt that her long-dead father had returned to the house to murder her. She was so convinced of this delusion that she had shared her secret with several young siblings, not a good idea if one is trying to get baby brother and sister to sleep. Eventually she ran from her house to escape her father's wrath. Even in the interview she could not clearly state that her father's return was an impossibility, although she hesitatingly said she thought it was.

Let us return to the interview in order to uncover the nonverbal cues that suggested the possibility of an underlying psychotic process. The patient, whom we shall call Mary, answered honestly and appeared cooperative. She displayed no loosening of associations or other overt evidence of thought process disorganization, but she demonstrated some oddities in her communicational style. With regard to paralanguage, she demonstrated long pauses (about 4 to 8 seconds) before beginning many of her responses. This gave her a somewhat distracted appearance as if muddled by her thinking. This effect was heightened by a mild slowing of her speech as well as a flattening of the tone of her voice.

As we have seen, silences, especially of this length, are generally avoided in daily conversation. Everyday social protocol would ordinarily pressure Mary to answer more quickly. This breakdown in normal communicational interaction was one suggestion that all was not well and represents a disruption of the empathy cycle. Her body also spoke to her internal turmoil.

Although for the most part she had reasonably good eye contact, there existed protracted periods of time when she looked slightly away from the interviewer in a distracted fashion, whether she was talking or listening. This lack of "visual touching" during conversation is unusual.[42,43] In fact, if one had a sound understanding of nonverbal communications, it would have been apparent that Mary was displaying difficulties in her dialogue function, as displayed by an odd use of the nonverbal activities Ekman called regulators. As stated earlier, these regulators provide the cues for the timing of everyday back-and-forth conversation.

Frequently, before beginning to speak, the intended speaker glances away briefly. As he or she looks back, speech will begin. While talking, the speaker will frequently look away. But as the end of the speaker's statement is reached, the speaker will look towards the listener. This glance signals to the listener that the speaker's message is over. The speaker and the listener glance at each other's eye regions for varying lengths of time, usually between 1 and 2 seconds, the listener giving longer contact. This complex eye duet was frequently missing with Mary. In depression, the eyes are frequently cast downward, but it was the peculiar manner in which Mary tended to stare past the clinician that hinted at the possible presence of psychotic process. As Sir Denis Hill had suggested, Mary had lost some of the nonverbal cues that maintain social interaction.

Mary was also showing disruption of other aspects in her dialogue function. In this case, the problem with "marking her speech"[44] was related to her dysfunctional use of her hand gestures as conversational regulators. For instance, hand gestures are generally made as one initiates words or phrases. As the speaker finishes commenting, the hands tend to assume a position of rest. To keep one's hands upwards, in front of oneself, can indicate that one is not done speaking or will soon interrupt.

In Mary, these hand regulators were generally diminished. She sat stiffly with her feet flat on the floor. Her head seemed to weigh her body down as she sat slightly hunched over with her fingers interlocked. She displayed little hand gesturing, leaving the interviewer with the odd sensation that it was not clear when Mary was going to start or stop speaking. Most likely, Mary's lack of movement was an associated aspect of her major depression, but it may also have been a ramification of her psychotic process.

A more striking nonverbal clue to the degree of Mary's psychopathology lay in her method of dealing with unwanted environmental input, in this instance the questions of the interviewer. Apparently Mary had been concerned for some time that she might be "just like her mother," who was currently in the hospital. In addition, her sister had experienced a psychotic depression approximately 6 months earlier. Mary had been attempting to hide from herself the evidence of her own psychotic process, while the fear of an impending breakdown nagged at her daily. During the interview, as questions directed her back into her paranoid fears, she began to realize the extent of her problems. At this moment she did something out of the ordinary.

Mary leaned forward slowly, her elbows perched upon the tops of her knees, with her head cupped between her hands. In this position her hands literally covered her ears, as if keeping out unwanted questions or thoughts. All eye contact was disrupted. Mary remained in this position for a good 5 minutes, answering questions slowly but cooperatively. She appeared detached from the world around her. This type of nonverbal adaptor has been studied under the rubric of "cut-offs."[45] Cut-offs represent nonverbal adaptors made to dampen out environmental stress. When exaggerated to the degree of appearing socially inappropriate, as was the case with Mary, they may be indicators of psychotic process. Indeed, catatonic withdrawal represents a prolonged and drastic cut-off.

One must also attempt to compare nonverbal activities to the patient's baseline behavior. Mary was normally a high-functioning secretary and most likely possessed better than average social skills. In this light, her preoccupied conversational attitude, and in particular her prolonged cut-off, represents very deviant behavior for her. A subsequent interview with Mary's friend revealed that Mary had been observed at work sitting and staring at the phone for long periods.

For a moment I would like to take a brief sidetrack on the issue of cut-offs. We have been discussing dramatic forms of cut-off behavior, which may indicate underlying psychotic activity; however, mild forms of cut-off behavior occur routinely in our work with nonpsychotic individuals and frequently do not hint at psychopathology *per se*. These more subtle forms of cut-off are not without meaning and warrant some discussion. Morris[46] described four such visual cut-offs, to which he attaches some descriptively poetic names.

With the "Evasive Eye," the patient shuns eye contact by looking distractedly towards the ground, as if studying some invisible object. It can create the feeling that the patient is purposely not attending to the conversation and may frequently accompany the speech of disinterested adolescents. In the so-called "Shifty Eye," the patient repeatedly glances away and back again. With the "Stuttering Eye," the patient now faces the interviewer directly, but the eyelids rapidly waver up and down as if swatting away the clinician's glance. Finally, in the "Stammering Eye," the patient once again faces the clinician but shuts the eyes with an exaggerated blink, sometimes lasting as long as several seconds.

These four eye maneuvers represent nonverbal activities whose meaning may be multiple. They may indicate that the patient at some level no longer wants to communicate. Perhaps a specific topic has been raised that is disturbing to the patient, resulting in a nonverbal resistance. At such moments, a simple question such as, "I am wondering what is passing through your mind right now," may uncover pertinent material. Such cut-offs may also represent objective signs of decreased blending and movement into a shut-down interview. Exaggerated examples of these cut-offs can also be part of a histrionic presentation and in this sense could also be seen in both wandering and rehearsed interviews.

Nonverbal Hints of Classic Psychiatric Diagnoses

Returning directly to the topic of nonverbal hints of psychopathology, investigators have also looked at the promising possibility that nonverbal activities could provide even more specific diagnostic clues, but at this point the research results remain tentative.[47,48] Moreover, the results appear to be in accordance with what common clinical sense would predict.

Concerning the classic psychiatric diagnoses, schizophrenia appears to be accompanied by some distinctive nonverbal behaviors. Studies show that schizophrenic presentations are marked by a tendency for gaze aversion. A flattening of affect with decreased movement of the eyebrows is noted (which can alternatively be secondary to antipsychotic medication). Patients' postures are slumped, and they have a tendency to lean away from the interviewer. Naturally, the type of schizophrenia and the stage of the process can significantly affect the type of nonverbal behavior present, emphasizing a cautionary note to these generalizations.

Depressive disorder has also been investigated. Researchers have noted that nonverbal behaviors vary depending on whether one is observing an agitated depression or a withdrawn depression. In subgroup 1 (agitated depression), patients demonstrated "a puzzled expression, grimacing and frowning, gaze aversion, agitated movements, a crouched posture, and body leaning towards the interviewer. Subgroup 2 (withdrawn depressions) showed some increase in gaze, slowed movements, self-touching, an emotionally blank expression, and a backward lean away from the interviewer."[49] In many respects, these findings have limited usefulness, because they simply seem to confirm the obvious.

But at a different level, especially with depressive patients, these findings emphasize the importance of nonverbal behaviors as clinical indicators of improvement.[50] The return of routine hand gesturing may herald an oncoming remission even before the patient admits to much subjective improvement. As the clinician becomes more aware of such behaviors as spontaneity of facial expression, smiling behavior, and eye contact, the informal monitoring of such cues to improvement can become a routine element of clinical follow-up.

Nonverbal Hints of Specific Personality Diagnoses

With regard to personality disorders, less research is available. Consequently, we will emphasize principles derived from clinical observations. Observations made during the 7 or so minutes of the scouting phase may provide important diagnostic clues. In this sense, these cues can help determine which diagnostic regions to emphasize in the body of the interview, for, in the limited time available, it is generally not feasible to explore all areas of personality dysfunction. The following three clinical vignettes illustrate the usefulness of nonverbal activities in suggesting the presence of possible character pathology.

In the first example, I was observing an interview performed by a psychiatric resident during morning rounds on an inpatient unit. The patient was an adolescent girl with a head of curly light-reddish hair. The interviewer was sitting on a couch in a group activity room. The patient pertly entered the room and promptly plunked down beside the clinician. At first she leaned towards him with her right arm straddling the back of the couch behind his shoulder, but she quickly withdrew the arm. Her final perch was with her right knee up on the couch resting a few inches from the clinician's body.

In a proxemic sense, she had positioned herself well within the personal distance zone and actually very close to being within the clinician's intimate zone. Her speech was bright and snappy, percolating from a face rich with expressions and playful eyes. All this activity occurred in a matter of a few seconds. The clinician immediately responded by leaning away from the patient and crossing his legs by placing his left ankle over his right knee. This brief territorial excursion by this patient is not a typical initial interaction, even with adolescents, who frequently feel more comfortable with "chummier" interpersonal distances. Instead, this type of interpersonal game is sometimes seen in people with underlying histrionic personality traits or borderline personality traits. This observation in no way indicates that this patient had these traits. It merely suggests that it might be worthwhile to do more specific diagnostic interviewing within these specific diagnoses.

In the second example, the patient was a woman in late middle age, with graying hair pulled back in a bun. Before the interview she had had to wait longer than usual before entering the room. Initially, the clinician gently apologized for the inconvenience with a warm smile on his face. She made cool eye contact. Her lips did not so much as consider returning his smile. She fluctuated between a baseline of mildly cooperative answers, with a reasonably lengthy duration of utterance (DOU), to brusque shut-down remarks.

A peculiar piece of body movement gradually evolved as she continued with her acerbic tone of voice. She tended to lean back in her chair and gradually proceeded to stretch her legs out in front of her towards the interviewer. The movement was ingeniously slow but as steady as a barge pulling into a dock. As usually happens, the dock was gently bumped – by her feet bumping against the interviewers – at which point she did not pull away. Instead, the "dock" recoiled – with the interviewer quickly tucking his feet beneath his chair.

Her nonverbal activities may be multiply determined, but one possibility well worth exploring would be underlying passive-aggressive traits. Later historical information from the interview tended to further substantiate this diagnostic hunch.

The third and final example is a patient who carefully orchestrated a relatively unappealing opening gambit. She was a tall woman in her mid-20s with long black hair hanging limply about her body. She was dressed in jeans and a black pullover sweater. Her first noticeably unusual action consisted of reaching over to pull up a second chair, which she promptly used as a footstool. She stretched her body out, making herself conspicuously at home. This settling in did not signify the beginning of an easy engagement, because she proceeded to visually cut the female interviewer off throughout most of the interview. She would look down at her hands, frequently using the Evasive Eye movement described earlier.

All of this display was topped with a convincingly dour facial expression. Concerning paralanguage, she managed to push through her disinterested facial mask an equally disinterested and mumbling voice. Her attitude visibly disturbed the interviewer. She also demonstrated one other nonverbal communication with a set meaning. Specifically, she held her coat on her lap throughout the interview, perhaps communicating an eagerness to leave.

Her collection of behaviors, all present during the first few minutes of the interview, suggested a variety of personality traits worth exploring later. Her lack of concern for making the interviewer feel more at ease could suggest a possible hint of antisocial leanings. Along similar lines, her obvious attempt to display disinterest could be part of the manipulative trappings of a borderline personality or perhaps of a narcissistic personality. And, as we saw with our previous example, some passive-aggressive tendencies may be present. Her behaviors in no way prove that she has any of these disorders, but they do provide suggestions as to which disorders warrant additional consideration, further highlighting the importance of noting nonverbal behavior. *It is also critical to remind ourselves that we must be exquisitely careful not to interpret cross-cultural differences in nonverbal behavior as hints of psychopathology.*

Nonverbal Indicators of Anxiety

One of the most well-known indicators of increased anxiety remains the activation of the sympathetic nervous system, the system geared to prepare the organism for fight or flight. During the activation of this system, a variety of physiologic adaptations occur that can serve as hallmarks of anxiety. The heart will beat faster and blood will be shunted away from the skin and gut to be preferentially directed towards the muscle tissue that is being prepared for action. This shunting accounts for the paleness so frequently seen in acutely anxious people, who look like they have seen a ghost. Saliva production decreases, and the bowels and bladder are slower to eliminate. Breathing rate increases, as does the production of sweat.

This last sign, increased sweating, reminds me of one of the more striking and humorous examples of autonomic discharge I have encountered. A medical student was doing one of his first physical examinations on a real patient, which can truly be an upsetting experience, as the student frequently feels painfully inept. In this case, the patient was a child about 9 years old, who could be generally classified under the label "brat." As the exam labored onward, with the worried mother looking increasingly fretful, the student began to sweat profusely. As the student leaned over to listen to the child's heart, a bead of sweat fell from his forehead directly onto the child's chest. Being a subtle kid, he immediately looked the student in the eye and in a loud voice said, "What's a matter with you, you're sweatin' all over me!"

As if the poor student was not already stressed enough, that little proclamation did it. He sheepishly turned to the increasingly upset mother and produced a quick-witted white lie, "Don't worry, I've got a thyroid condition." I know this story all too well because I was the poor panic-stricken medical student. It clearly shows the truth that the autonomic system does not lie. With our patients, subtle signs of anxiety such as sweating, damp palms, and increased breathing rate can help us detect anxiety. If the anxiety represents evidence of poor blending, we may be able to purposely attend to the patient's fears. If it represents the presence of unsettling thoughts, we may be inclined to probe deeper.

If the sympathetic system is not presented with a chance to actually get the organism into action soon enough, the parasympathetic system may try to counterbalance with a discharge of its own. In these cases, one may find a sudden urge to urinate or defecate, as people frequently feel before public performances or job interviews. If a patient begins a session by immediately requesting the need for a restroom, this may represent a clue to a higher anxiety level than the patient may verbally admit.

Desmond Morris believes that one type of nonverbal adaptor, which he refers to as "displacement activities," can be a good indicator of anxiety.[51] These displacement activities are those body movements that release underlying tension. I recently watched a businessman waiting for a meeting. As he sat in the lobby, he nervously tugged at his tie and picked at his clothes. He then hoisted his briefcase onto his lap and meticulously unloaded it piece by piece, after which he gingerly repacked the case, carefully feeling each object as he delicately reassembled his "peripheral brain."

These behaviors were accomplishing very little in the way of needed physical functions, but they offered a calming effect of some sort for the businessman. Other typical displacement activities include smoking, twirling one's hair, picking at one's fingers, nail-biting, playing with rings, twitching one's feet, tugging at the ear lobe, self-grooming activities, tearing at paper cups, and twirling and biting pens. The list could certainly be extended. For instance, Morris points out that serving drinks and holding them in one's hands at cocktail parties probably serve to decrease people's anxiety, as they "have something to do."[52]

Clinically speaking, displacement activities are worth noting during both the initial interview and subsequent psychotherapy. Each patient seems to display a unique set of displacement activities. Once decoded by the clinician, these activities can be fairly reliable indicators of patient anxiety. When suddenly increased, they may represent a more reliable indicator than the patient's facial expression or verbal response that an interpretation was on the mark or that the patient is feeling ill-at-ease with the interviewer or the topic.

Morris also views another sub-category of nonverbal adaptors as being suggestive of possible underlying anxiety or fear, which he calls auto-contact behaviors. Auto-contact behavior consists of movements involving self-touching.[53] Such behaviors may consist of grooming behaviors, defensive-covering behaviors, and self-intimacies.

Self-intimacies are defined as, "movements that provide comfort because they are unconsciously mimed acts of being touched by someone else."[54] These self-intimacies appear frequently during interviews. Patients may hold their own hands or sit with their knees pulled up to their faces, arms literally hugging their own legs. In regressed patients, one can see even more extreme forms of self-hugging as patients lay in tightly curled fetal positions.

According to Morris, with regard to frequency, the most common self-intimacies in order of most to least frequent are as follows: (1) the jaw support, (2) the chin support, (3) the hair clasp, (4) the cheek support, (5) the mouth touch, and (6) the temple support. With hair touching, there is a 3:1 bias in favor of women. Temple touching demonstrates the opposite bias with a preference towards men of 2:1. Sometimes these kinesthetic comforters can be tied into other sensory modalities as well. I remember one patient who would pull her hair across her cheek. She would simultaneously gently sniff at her hair, which she related as being very comforting. Such activity was a sure sign of her underlying anxiety, much like a displacement activity.

In this manner, nonverbal activities such as adaptors (including displacement activities and auto-contact behaviors) may serve to alert the interviewer that the patient is feeling pained or anxious. It can cue the interviewer that the patient may need some verbal comforting, perhaps prompting an empathic statement. *It can also alert the clinician that powerful affective material is being approached, possibly suggesting the need for further exploration.*

It is also of interest that anxiety will sometimes display itself not through the appearance of adaptors but through their conspicuous absence. When engaged in an active conversation, most people will display a normal amount of periodic displacement activity and auto-contact. If these suddenly stop or are not present from the beginning, then the person may be experiencing anxiety. In a sense, the person may be trying to avoid mistakes by doing nothing.

This "still-life response" frequently appears when people are filmed or interviewed in public. It seems to afflict interviewers even more than patients. Supervisors need to be aware that this response may be more of an artifact than a stylistic marker of their supervisees.

Another area of interest revolves around facial clues that the patient is visibly shaken or on the verge of tears. I am sure the reader is well aware of the faint quiverings of the chin and glazed quality of the eyes that frequently indicate that a patient is close to tears. But a fact not as well publicized is the tendency for people to demonstrate extremely fine muscle twitches across their faces when stressed. These frequently occur beside the nostrils and on the cheek. In people who demonstrate this tendency, these fine twitches can be extremely accurate indicators of tension.

By way of example, I was working with a young businesswoman during an initial interview. She had been referred to me for psychotherapy. She was attractively dressed with a bright disposition and her speech was accompanied by a collection of animated gestures. When asked to talk about her history, she launched into a detailed review of her life since age 16. Of note was her striking avoidance of any events prior to age 16.

When I brought to her attention that she had avoided this earlier timeframe, she responded that she did not know why and had not noticed it. I asked her if any aspects of her life seemed different before the age of 16. She commented, "Not really, although I spent more time with my father back then." At that point a few muscle twitches appeared by her left nostril. I commented that I had a feeling she was feeling upset, and she burst into tears. Subsequent therapy revealed a complex and ambivalent relationship with her father and other male figures. Throughout therapy, these faint twitches were a sure sign of tension.

Nonverbal Hints of Deception

The issue of tension and tension release leads directly to another important aspect of nonverbal behavior, the detection of deception. Indeed, the nonverbal clues that often seem to accompany deceit might be less specific to deception than they are generalized indicators that the deceiver is feeling anxious, worried, embarrassed, or frightened while lying.

In one of the early pieces of research into the nonverbal indicators of deceit, led by one of the true pioneers in this arena, Paul Ekman, to whose work we have already referred, a group of nursing students were asked to participate in a study in which they would be asked to deceive a person.[55] They were told that gentle deceptions were sometimes needed in clinical work, as when comforting frightened patients. Thus the nurses felt a need to perform well in the testing situation.

In the experiment the nurses were exposed to two different types of films. Some films were pleasant in nature, such as an ocean scene, and other films depicted unpleasant scenes such as a burn victim and a limb amputation. After seeing the pleasant film segments, the nurses were asked to describe their feelings to the listener. This task was obviously not problematic. But after viewing the unsettling film, in one experimental design the nurses had to convince the listener that the gory film was pleasant and enjoyable to watch. This task was not so easy. Indeed, it so reproduced the sensation of lying that some nurses dropped out of the study.

All of these interactions were videotaped. Segments of these videotapes were then shown to subjects who were asked to determine from the visual images which of the nurses were lying. It was an ingenious experiment and represents the foundation work upon which further research on deception proceeded.

Ekman and his colleague Friesen predicted that subjects would state that while lying they would focus on making their faces "look natural." This prediction proved to be true. The deceivers did attend to their faces more, which suggested that nonverbal activities from the neck down may provide a better lead concerning deception. Interestingly, trained observers could pick up clues of deception from videotaped facial expressions. These micro-expressions may represent accurate clues but are often too difficult to pick up routinely.

In recent years, Ekman has become increasingly fascinated by the presence and importance of micro-expressions.[56] He feels that many emotions, when being hidden by a patient, are "given away" by the presence of minute movements of facial muscles frequently lasting 1/15 to 1/25 of a second, which may be reflections of the person's underlying concealed emotion, be that anger, sadness, or disgust. He believes that observers can be trained to notice these micro-expressions, resulting in an enhanced ability to spot both deceit and the presence of subtle emotions.

Ekman emphasizes that in these situations patients may be consciously withholding information or that unconscious defense mechanisms – such as repression – may be at work. Such moments of withholding may prove to be of critical importance when uncovering suicidal intent or moments where episodes of incest or intimate partner violence are being hidden. In this regard, the ability to spot micro-expressions allows a clinician to recognize that the patient may be withholding material, but it does not necessarily indicate why. The clinician will need to further explore to determine whether the concealment is conscious deceit or the product of unconscious processes.

At such moments, two questions suggested by Ekman may be of value: "Is there anything more you want to say about how you are feeling?" and/or "I had the impression you were just feeling something more than what you said?"[57] Ekman's questions are obviously also of possible value anytime the nonverbal behaviors of the patient suggest that the patient is having a hard time sharing an emotion. For the reader interested in learning how to spot micro-expressions, Ekman has developed an innovative training package, the micro-expression training tool (METT), that is available online (www.ekmaninternational.com).[58]

As mentioned above, the body of the deceiver often has a tendency to betray its own head, so to speak, and further research has substantiated many of the initial findings as described in Ekman's fascinating book, *Telling Lies*.[59] Apparently, changes in below-the-neck movements may be of the most practical significance for accurately detecting deception, unless one has been trained to spot and interpret micro-expressions.

Nonverbal communications (emblems) can sometimes be useful indicators of deceit. You will recall that emblems represent nonverbal behaviors that carry a distinct meaning within a culture, from specific messages such as "throwing the finger" to nodding a yes or no with the head. Just as slips of the tongue may betray hidden feelings, slips of the body via the unconscious use of emblems can occur. With the nursing students in the above study, many felt a helpless sensation that they were not hiding their feelings well.

This feeling was sometimes inadvertently conveyed by a shrugging movement, a subtle yet common emblem of helplessness as in "I don't know what to think or say or do."

When representing indicators of nonverbal leakage, emblems usually appear in parts. Thus only one shoulder may partially rise or one palm may turn up during a shrug. Another good indicator that an emblem represents a deceitful mannerism is the display of the emblem in an unusual placement. An angry fist will not be raised towards an antagonist but will quietly appear by the side of the patient.

Hand gestures, such as illustrators (used to point out or outline an object) or even regulators (used for communicating conversational dialogue) may tend to decrease when deceit is under way. This decrease is particularly true if the patient has not had time to rehearse the lie and must carefully attend to what is being said. The clinician can monitor behaviors such as those described above while exploring regions in which resistance and deceit may be high. For example, when eliciting a drug and alcohol history from a typically active interviewee, a sudden decrease in associated hand movements may suggest that deception is occurring.

On the other hand, nonverbal adaptors, such as displacement activities and auto-contact seem to be one of the most powerful correlates of deception.[60] Although not all studies have confirmed this finding, a variety of comprehensive statistical summaries on deception research, as well as some more recent studies, support the idea that such adaptors, including fidgeting, are correlated with deception.[61-64] Several other studies have also found supportive evidence for the idea that below-the-neck clues are best for detecting deceit on a practical level.[65,66]

Popular literature on nonverbal behaviors has suggested that two of the most prominent adaptors that signal *possible* deception are: (1) touching or partially covering the mouth and (2) touching the nose.[67] Touching the nose while lying has been coined the "Pinocchio Response." It is believed that the release of catecholamines, triggered by the stress of lying, results in the swelling of nasal tissues followed by relief of this itch by a quick scratch. I have not been able to find this material documented in the research literature. On the other hand, it is interesting to note that during his Grand Jury testimony regarding the Monica Lewinsky sex scandal, President Clinton touched his nose 26 times when answering questions on particularly sensitive material. During questions of a more mundane nature, the hand and nose did not meet.

Besides kinesic indicators of deception, the clinician can look for paralanguage clues that deceit is occurring.[68] For instance, a higher pitch to the voice has been associated with deception as well as emotions such as fear. Correspondingly, lower pitches have been associated with the observation that a subject is more relaxed and sociable. Another possible clue to deception involves the response time latency (RTL). Deceptive subjects were found to demonstrate a longer RTL and to give longer answers when in the act of deceiving.

It should be kept in mind that most, if not all, of the kinesic and paralanguage clues to deception mentioned so far represent nonverbal activities, rather than nonverbal communications. Thus, it is important to remember that these behaviors are usually multiply determined and do not in any way guarantee that the patient is being deceitful. In many cases, they may simply indicate that the patient is feeling more anxious. Each activity must be interpreted in the interpersonal matrix in which it was produced. The nonverbal concept of context is critically important when interpreting nonverbal clues to deceit.

By way of example, one researcher found that an increased latency of response could be interpreted in different fashions. If it was followed by a self-promoting comment, then it was often interpreted as being an indication of deception. On the other hand, if the pause was followed by a self-deprecating comment, it was often registered in the opposite direction as evidence of a truthful remark.[69]

If one notices a variety of potential nonverbal indicators of deception, the following strategy may be of value. Once the area in which deception is suspected is passed, carefully note the patient's subsequent nonverbal behaviors, including adaptors and paralanguage clues. Then sensitively return the conversation to the area in which deceit is suspected and look for a return of the nonverbal indicators of deceit. If done multiple times during the interview, and the deceptive patterns continue to disappear (during benign discussion) and re-appear (during areas in which deceit is suspected), this pattern should certainly raise the suspicion of patient concealment.

It is probably best to conclude the discussion of cues of deception at this point. Clearly the research is somewhat tentative, but it suggests that some changes in the baseline behavior of the patient may provide useful hints that deception may be at hand. Caution is certainly indicated. Peter Andersen encapsulates the state of the art well as follows:

1) no foolproof means of detecting deception through nonverbal behavior exists now or is likely to exist in the future; 2) nonetheless, some commonalities in deceptive behavior can aid in its detection; and 3) a complex mixture of unconscious and strategic processes produce subtle changes in behavior during deceptive communication.[70]

Two practical points warrant mentioning. First, as the interview proceeds it is generally a good idea to ascertain the baseline body movements that are typical of the patient. Second, during sensitive inquiries, such as the elicitation of suicidal ideation and intent (an area in which the ability to detect concealment may literally be life saving), it is best to avoid any note taking (whether on paper or by keyboard). Note taking can markedly diminish the ability of the interviewer to observe the subtle nonverbal clues that may be the only warnings of deception. It also markedly limits the ability of the interviewer to deepen engagement through the use of his or her own eye contact and other nonverbals.

In the same sense that nonverbal activities may indicate that the patient may be deceiving the clinician, a variety of important mixed nonverbal messages may be sent to an interviewer. These mixed messages are not necessarily deceptions. Instead, they may represent hallmarks of patient ambivalence and confusion.

Nonverbal Correlates of Patient Ambivalence and Discordance

In order to explore this fascinating area, the work of Grinder and Bandler[71] offers a wellspring of practical and sound clinical observation. Although controversy has arisen over their later work, their first two books provide some pioneering insights into engagement techniques.

Their work follows naturally from the principles we have been discussing thus far. Put simply, they state that as a person communicates a message, the message is transferred through a variety of communication channels simultaneously. The patient's message may be conveyed through the content of the spoken words, the tone of voice, the rate of speech, the amount and type of hand gesturing, the posture, and the facial expression. These messages are termed paramessages. When all paramessages have the same meaning, the paramessages are said to be congruent. But if some of the channels convey discordant information, then the paramessages are said to be incongruent.

The underlying theory is simple; perhaps that is why it proves to be so powerful therapeutically. People who consistently communicate with an incongruent style can frequently create a confusing impression. Their incongruence may make the people around them feel ill-at-ease and uncomfortable. If the clinician can detect this self-defeating interpersonal style, he or she may be able to help the patient modify it. In a more immediate sense, incongruent paramessages may indicate underlying mixed feelings of which the patient is unaware. Once again, the interviewer may be able to cue off this incongruence, leading the patient into an exploration of the uncovered mixed feelings.

More germane to the topic of the initial interview, episodes of incongruent communication may alert the clinician to areas worthy of more immediate investigation or perhaps regions pertinent to explore in later sessions.

I am reminded of a woman in her early 30s whom I was evaluating for possible psychotherapy and/or medication use. Ms. Davis, as we shall call her, was coping with a variety of stresses, not the least of which was the loss of her mother several months earlier. For years she had been her mother's caretaker and verbal whipping post. Ms. Davis was mildly overweight with stocky legs, offset by a face embraced by a full head of black hair. As she spoke, her conversation turned to her bitter relationship with her boyfriend, who apparently enjoyed her sexually but found marital ceremonies not to his liking. She commented, "I hate him, I'll never go back to him. He's not worth it."

Harsh words, but one should be wary of taking them too seriously, for Ms. Davis's body spoke differently. The words were spoken with a tone of pained resignation, not biting anger. They had the quality of the child-like pout, "Daddy's not bringing home a present from his vacation." Not only did her voice lack indignation, but her hands intimated a martyr's role. Rather than the more typical pointing and jerking movements of an angry accusation, they were held low towards her lap with the palms upwards. This type of hand positioning is frequently associated with an attitude of supplication and need.

Put more precisely, Ms. Davis was communicating with an incongruent set of paramessages. As Grinder and Bandler point out, all of these messages may have elements of truth to them. In Ms. Davis's case, she certainly did have angry feelings towards her boyfriend, as suggested by the content of her words. But she also had extremely powerful needs to be accepted by him; indeed, these needs bordered on a masochistic willingness to be verbally beaten by him. Her tone of voice and hand gestures suggested her strong need for acceptance. Her breathing rate did not increase or become more spurt-like, as is frequently seen when someone becomes increasingly angered. This set of incongruent messages was one of the first clues to her deeply rooted problems concerning hostile dependence, which became central working issues in the remaining therapy. Indeed, in this regard, her relationship with her boyfriend was no different from her relationship with her mother.

In any given initial interview, periods of incongruent communication may occur. If noted, they can serve as road signs that effectively guide the interviewer towards a deeper understanding of the patient.

Nonverbal Signals During Collaborative Treatment Planning

As we have discussed in earlier chapters, during the closing phase of the initial interview, the patient and clinician will collaboratively develop an initial treatment plan. Such treatment planning will usually continue during the next several sessions and, indeed, will remain an intermittent aspect of ongoing treatment, whether the treatment involves psychotherapy, medications, or other matrix related interventions.

Positive nonverbal signs of patient interest and agreement, such as natural eye contact, an excitement to the tone of voice, a forward lean, and positive head nodding, make it easy to intuit when a patient is comfortable with a proposed treatment plan. The problem arises when the patient gives a verbal positive to a treatment plan, yet does not really want to proceed with it or has significant unstated misgivings about it. Such a situation is easily understandable, for patients are dealing with intense pain, have not had any time to reflect alone on what has passed during the interview, and may have appropriate difficulties with processing information caused by the amount of information coming their way and the newness of the therapeutic environment.

In this regard, in addition to asking the patient for his or her suggestions while collaboratively treatment planning, clinicians can routinely ask patients questions such as, "How do you feel about these ideas?" The use of such questions is an excellent technique for collaboratively treatment planning. But sometimes these questions are surprisingly ineffective. Why? Because a patient feeling hesitant about the proposed plan of action may feel unintended social pressure to respond positively so as to appear respectful and cooperative, *especially if they have liked the interviewer.* Sometimes a clinician will pick up on this ambivalence and follow up with, "Are you sure this is okay?" Curiously, even this more direct question may not result in an honest answer. In fact, I have frequently seen ambivalent patients respond even more positively at such moments, with statements such as, "Oh yeah, this sounds like a good plan." What gives?

I believe that patients respond in this paradoxical fashion because the clinician's question ("Are you sure this is okay?") prompted further concern by the patient that they were being perceived as being difficult or "resistant." The overly affirmative response was parlayed to please the clinician, a person whom the patient both likes and perceives as a sorely needed source of help.

It is in such situations that our ability to spot discordant nonverbals may help us to better identify patients who have concerns about the treatment plan. Put proactively, when collaboratively treatment planning, it pays off to be on the look out for the discordant paramessages of Grinder and Bandler.

Kuhnke describes a series of discordant paramessages that may help us to recognize hesitancy in a patient, in some instances even hostility.[72] When people are feeling relaxed and "on board" with the conversation, they often gesture fairly frequently and their gestures frequently have open palms. As one inquires about interest in various treatment plan options, hesitant patients may have their fingers closed over their palms, no matter where they have placed their hands (on their lap, by the side of their legs, etc.). Some patients will fold their hands together, in effect holding in their own tension or anxiety. Even when listening intently, a patient who, at heart, does not like what he or she is hearing may fold their arms or cross their ankles. There may be a subtle, or not so subtle, leaning back in the chair. All of these movements, occurring while a patient is verbally agreeing with a treatment plan (an example of discordant paramessages), may suggest the patient has real doubts about the plan. It is important to uncover these doubts for two reasons: (1) the patient might have very good reasons, being missed by the clinician, as to why this is not a good treatment plan and (2) even if it is theoretically a good treatment plan, as we emphasized in earlier chapters, if the patient doesn't like it, it is not going to work.

According to Kuhnke, three other adaptors are worth noting: (1) patients placing their hands to their cheeks; (2) patients resting their chins on their hands; and (3) patients placing a thumb under the chin while pointing the index finger up the side of the face.[73] These three adaptors may indicate that the patient is actively contemplating what is being said. At such moments the patient may be aware of his or her own hesitancies. Indeed, the patient is often actively weighing the pros and cons at the time of such gestures. I have found it to be an opportune time to ask directly about the patient's weighing of the options with questions such as, "What are your thoughts on the pros and cons of using cognitive–behavioral therapy?" or "What are your thoughts on the pros and cons of trying an antidepressant?" It can be surprising how well the strategic use of such questions, based upon an astute observation of these three nonverbal clues, can open up communications, greatly increasing the likelihood that a truly collaborative treatment plan is unfolding.

Nonverbal Behaviors Functioning as Social Scripts

In a similar fashion, the work of Scheflen, whom I mentioned earlier, deserves more detailed examination, because it too focuses on the nonverbal interactions that serve as communication scripts for people.[74] Scheflen discusses the idea that humans, like other animals, engage in certain shared behaviors that tend to escalate into specific actions. Such actions include fighting behavior, mating behavior, and parenting behavior. Frequently, certain mutually recognized behaviors serve to eliminate the need to engage in the final actions. In this way, animals will frequently avoid actual combat by undergoing a territorial display of sorts. Scheflen calls such escalating patterns of behavior "kinesic reciprocals."

Kinesic reciprocals can frequently be seen in clinical interactions. If the patient begins the reciprocal, the clinician may inadvertently continue the process. I have certainly seen this process occur within the realm of the "courting or mating reciprocal," as Scheflen refers to flirtation. Although Scheflen's term sounds a bit dated, there is no doubt that there is a bit of kinesic dance that occurs when two people are looking for a sustained partner or even merely a "hook-up" in our contemporary culture.

Early in my career, I remember watching a videotape of a session of psychotherapy. The patient was a young woman interacting with her therapist, who was a relatively young man with about 7 years of clinical experience. The patient sat pertly forward, cigarette hanging aesthetically from her fingers. The therapist, who was dressed casually in a sport shirt, sat rakishly back, also with a cigarette in hand. Their voices possessed a spritely coyness. It was unclear whether I was watching the beginning moments of a therapy session or the opening sequences of a romantic comedy.

In any case, the therapist and his patient were engaging in the courting reciprocal. Inadvertent participation in such reciprocals can create a variety of problems. Obviously it can stimulate an erotic transference. Moreover, if initiated unconsciously by the therapist and then reciprocated by the patient, it can lead the therapist towards the inappropriate perception that the patient is histrionic.

I am reminded of a talented trainee whom co-workers felt tended to be pleasantly flirtatious and buoyant with staff. She was surprised, yet concerned, when, after several of her initial evaluations, a male patient asked her out. On videotape the answer was obvious. She noted, with some surprise, that she was displaying some mildly flirtatious qualities during her clinical interviews, which she was able to quickly eliminate.

Scheflen describes the types of kinesic behaviors utilized by both sexes in the courting reciprocal. According to Scheflen, males have a variety of kinesic actions that they take to enhance sexual attractiveness. The male attempting to draw attention sexually will move from any type of slumped position into a stance emphasizing his height and musculature. Indeed, the male may unconsciously employ many of the same kinesic clues as are used to display dominance, such as jutting the jaw slightly, sucking the belly in, raising the shoulders, and perhaps standing more closely than normal social protocol would suggest.

The reciprocal behaviors by women are equally well known, as characterized in popular culture as reflected in advertisements, films, and graphic novels. According to Scheflen, a woman who is interested in attracting sexual attention may hold her head high and at a slight angle, perhaps viewing the potential partner from the corner of her eye with an inviting glance. The upper body will be lifted to emphasize breasts. Legs may be crossed "around each other" so as to emphasize the calf musculature and extension of the foot. In addition, she may intermittently present her hands with her palms up, a highly affiliative act, in a variety of ways as when pushing back her hair, when smoking, or when she covers her mouth while coughing.[75]

During flirtation, another common kinesic reciprocal commonly occurs – tentative incursions into the intimate proxemic space of the intended partner. At one level this simply may occur by sitting closer or occasionally leaning forward to whisper into the ear of the other over the din of the bar. At a different level, one participant may gently touch the other on the hand, arm, shoulder, or back. If viewed with favor, a reciprocal touch may be shown, and the dance begins.

Other reciprocal behaviors besides the courting reciprocal can occur in an initial interview. A striking example was provided by a video made of an initial interview for use in supervision.

The interviewer was a young woman. Across from her, the patient, a woman just turning 20, sat with eyes occasionally cast downwards. As the interview unfolded, the patient produced a folded piece of paper, and she asked the clinician to read the paper before proceeding. Her voice seemed to step meekly away from her lips. In the meantime, the patient began fumbling with the microphone. She had correctly wrapped it around her neck but had problems attaching it to her blouse. Noticing her problems the clinician looked over and asked if she needed help. The patient did not look up for a moment as she continued to fumble. Then with her head cocked downwards, she innocently glanced upwards nodding her head "yes." She gazed with the helpless eyes of a little girl and said not a word. The clinician promptly leaned over and fixed the microphone.

The parenting reciprocal had emerged as naturally as if enacted between a true mother and her child. In this brief vignette, the power of the first few minutes of the scouting period to provide clues for further diagnostic probing is once again amply demonstrated. This patient's helpless style and dependent behavior suggested the possibility of some form of character pathology. Indeed, further interviewing revealed a mixed personality disorder with histrionic, passive-aggressive, and dependent characteristics. Apparently this patient had perfected the art of eliciting parental responses as a method of garnering attention.

In Section A, our focus has been on the power of the patient's body to convey information to the perceptive clinician. In Section B we will now explore the reverse situation, those moments when the clinician uses his or her nonverbal knowledge and behaviors to engage the patient.

Section B: Utilization of Nonverbal Behaviors to Engage Patients

Seating Arrangement and Proxemics

One of the exercises undertaken in our interviewing class concerns the use of seating arrangement. Two of the trainees sit in the middle of the room on easily rolled chairs. They are given a simple task, to situate themselves so that they feel the most comfortable with regard to conversing with one another. In about 90% of the cases, the participants choose a similar position. They sit roughly 4 to 5 feet apart. They are turned towards each other but do not quite directly face one another. Instead, they are turned about a 5- to 10-degree angle off the line directly between them, both in the same direction, as shown in Figure 8.1A. Only about 10% choose to face each other directly.

If the participants are asked to turn directly towards each other, they complain of feeling significantly less comfortable. Some will even push their chairs back a bit. The discomfort is related as feeling "too close," the sensation of nonverbal immediacy is too intense. Many of the trainees complain that the head-on position forces eye contact, making it difficult to break eye contact without undertaking a significant head movement. This head-on position fosters a sensation of confrontation.

On the other hand, the preferred position readily allows for good eye contact but also makes it easy to break contact without awkwardness. In my own practice, I have certainly found this position to be the most comfortable and the most flexible interviewing position for me. The last part of this statement is important, because it emphasizes that the most comfortable position may be different for each interviewer and indeed for each interviewing dyad. Each clinician needs to discover a comfortable position, keeping in mind that the clinician must also be willing to alter this position depending on the needs of the patient.

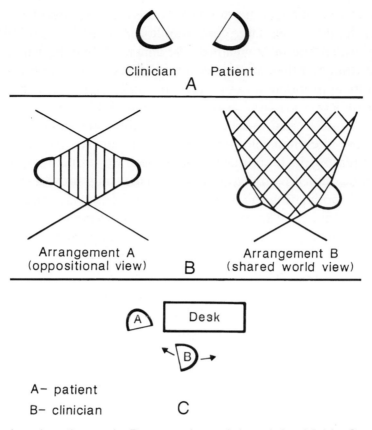

Clinician   Patient

A

Arrangement A
(oppositional view)

B

Arrangement B
(shared world view)

A- patient
B- clinician

C

Figure 8.1 A, Preferred seating angle; B, comparison of shared visual fields; C, utilization of desk.

In addition to the non-confrontational feeling provided by the position described above, another phenomenon may be enhancing its comfortableness. From the perspective of person-centered interviewing, one of the key processes that enhances blending is the ability of the clinician to convey a sense of seeing the world through a shared perspective.

If one looks at the actual fields of vision available to each participant in the interview, an important relationship readily becomes apparent. When two people are directly facing each other, the fields of vision overlap very little. What overlap does exist lies directly between the two participants. This situation tends to foster the sensation that "You are over there, and I am here." It seems to work against the sensation of "We are here together." On the other hand, when the two participants are turned slightly away from each other, so that they are subtly facing the same direction, then the feeling that "We are here, and the rest of the world is out there" naturally emerges.

Thus, in a phenomenological sense, the feeling of confrontation is decreased, while the sense of blending is given a gentle boost, as illustrated in Figure 8.1B. It should be noted that the directly oppositional arrangement may be preferred by some people. Indeed, some interviewing experts recommend it,[76] but I myself do not, for the reasons provided above.

The concept of seating raises the more general issue of furniture arrangement. Some clinicians prefer the use of two large comfortable chairs, away from their desk. Another alternative is to utilize the desk creatively. In general, I believe a desk should not sit between the clinician and the patient, because this places the clinician in an authoritarian position, more appropriate for chief executive officers, not therapists.

However, the desk can be placed as shown in Figure 8.1C, with only a corner protruding between the clinician and the patient. If the clinician's chair rides on wheels, the clinician can move the chair, altering the resultant interpersonal distance either by increasing or decreasing the amount of desk between the participants. I find that such a desk arrangement, coupled with the use of a wheeled chair, provides me with a remarkably quick way of modulating the immediacy of the dyad, an ability that can pay big benefits depending upon the immediacy needs of the patient, needs that might even fluctuate over the course of an interview. A paranoid patient may require more distance from the clinician, which can easily be accomplished by moving only a short way, because the desk quickly provides a protective barrier. With a well-engaged patient, the clinician can easily move to a point where essentially no desk intervenes. Another advantage of this seating arrangement is the fact that, whether one is taking rough notes with a clipboard or a laptop, the note-taking medium can be moved back and forth from lap to desk unobtrusively.

The overall concept of the clinical setting warrants attention. When designing a private office, an effort should be made to provide a comfortable and professional atmosphere. The office represents an extension of the clinician's persona, and the patient's first impression in the scouting period may be significantly affected by the decor of the clinician's waiting area or office. Calming prints or photographs, accompanied by several diplomas and shelves of books, provide a reassuring and pleasant environment.

Trainees are faced with limited financial resources. But three or four unframed art posters and a few plants can be bought very reasonably, producing a sometimes-startling change in the atmosphere of the room. There is no need for a trainee's room to look like a prison cell. On the contrary, part of the training experience is learning to consider the principles behind creating an appropriate private office.

Outside the office, situations can be a bit more difficult, because the clinician faces crowded hospital rooms and disorganized emergency rooms. It remains important in these situations to consider the comfort of both the patient and the clinician. While performing a consultation in a crowded hospital room, there is nothing wrong with saying, "Before we start, would you mind if I slide your bed over, so both of us can have more room to talk."

This discussion of seating arrangements leads to the issue of determining an optimum distance between the clinician and the patient, which will vary for each interviewing dyad. There does seem to exist a small region in which the clinician's presence respects the patient's sense of personal space while still allowing the movements of the clinician to have an immediate impact on the patient. This zone of effective interpersonal space in which the patient feels comfortable with the immediacy sensations of the interaction may be referred to as the "responsive zone" (RZ).

If the clinician moves out of the RZ towards the patient, then the interviewer risks frightening the patient or creating a sense of discomfort. On the other hand, if the interviewer leaves the RZ by moving too far away from the patient, then the movements of the clinician may have little impact on the patient. For instance, the act of gently leaning forward towards a patient, which can enhance communication during particularly sensitive moments of an interview, may have no effect if done outside the RZ.

Two examples may help clarify the importance of establishing an RZ that seems most comfortable for each patient. First, if one intuits that a patient may be feeling paranoid, it is useful to remember that such patients may require a larger space around them in order to feel more comfortable. In these cases, the RZ is larger and it may be wise to begin such interviews sitting further from the patient than one normally would sit. Another option is to position oneself with the corner of a desk or table between yourself and the patient, for the paranoid patient may feel safer with such a small, yet noticeable, "protective barrier." As the interchange proceeds the clinician may find that the distance can be gradually decreased; hence the RZ frequently may change as the blending waxes or wanes.

Second, one looks at the problem of accurately eliciting a formal cognitive examination in elderly patients who are seriously depressed and withdrawn. To attract and maintain their attention, the interviewer might need to sit considerably closer than normal. This more intimate RZ may help decrease the likelihood of obtaining poor cognitive results secondary to the patient's lack of attention or interest. If a patient is not interested in answering, then the risk of getting artificially low scores becomes very real indeed. In such cases, the tendency to suspect a real dementia when only a pseudodementia is present can become a true dilemma.

Another way of obtaining the withdrawn patient's attention during the cognitive examination is to speak more loudly, effectively moving closer without moving one's chair. At times it is also important to ensure attention by literally asking the patient to look at the clinician as the questions are asked. For instance, the interviewer can gently but firmly make statements such as, "It may help you to do well on these questions if you watch me as I actually say the digits to you." In the last analysis, if a withdrawn patient is looking down at the floor as the clinician performs the cognitive mental status, the validity of the results are certainly questionable.

The concept of increasing the validity of the cognitive examination also raises the issue of touching patients. Touch remains one of the, if not *the* most, powerful of immediacy behaviors, for it instantly places one inside the patient's intimate zone as described by Hall. As we saw earlier, touch is also part of the courting reciprocal. Consequently, it can both be misinterpreted by patients easily and be harshly disengaging with paranoid or angry patients. It must be used with caution and, in my opinion, only if necessary to achieve a certain effect on engagement.

If you are going to touch a patient, you should get in the habit of asking yourself two questions before proceeding: (1) What do I want to accomplish by touching this patient? (Is it being done from the perspective of intentional interviewing or is it being done merely by habit or from interviewer needs?) (2) Does the act of touching fit with the patient's needs for immediacy and the nonverbal context of this specific moment in the interview?

On the other hand, some clinicians seem to have a block against the idea of ever touching a patient. Although it is not frequent for me to touch a patient during an initial interview (except for handshakes), I sometimes find touching useful and poignant. With regard to the cognitive examination, some depressed and withdrawn patients may ignore the clinician's attempts to make eye contact and attend to the task at hand. In such instances, one can touch the arm of the patient, offering comments such as, "I know it is difficult for you to concentrate right now, but it really is important." At such times, the patient may glance up at the interviewer and more effective contact will have begun.

Of course, touching, a method of entering the patient's intimate space, may also be used at points at which the patient may benefit from some simple comforting, in which case the clinician's decision to touch the patient fits with the both the patient's sense of immediacy and the context of the interview. I am reminded of a sad, middle-aged man whom I interviewed as he was entering the hospital. For all of his life he had been a kind and hard-working mill worker. Unbeknown to himself he was being exposed to an extremely toxic industrial poison. Over the years he experienced gradual changes in his behavior, including irritability and occasional violent outbursts, which frightened him and produced extreme guilt. Simultaneously, he underwent marked changes in his intellectual functioning, to the point that he had problems dealing with everyday activities. Only recently had he learned that his problems were secondary to brain damage.

As we neared the end of the interview, he told me that he was afraid of the hospital-ization because "people say mean things to me, they think I'm stupid. Please let me come in, I promise I won't hurt anybody, I promise, and I'm not that stupid." At which point he began to weep. It seemed only natural to reach over and grasp his arm while reassuring him that I believed what he said and that we would help him make the transition to the hospital.

Outside of the types of situations described above, touching patients is not common during initial interviews. As mentioned earlier, touch is a powerful communication that may carry numerous connotations, not all of which are appropriate. Patients may mis-interpret touch as an erotic gesture or, at a minimum, as a sign of implied intimacy. Although the clinician may intend the gesture as a sign of caring, a psychotic patient or a patient with a histrionic personality may receive a considerably distorted message.

Indeed, if a clinician finds a routine need to touch patients during initial interviews, it would be wise for the clinician to determine why such a need is arising. Usually it is not from clinical considerations. Such clinicians frequently have a desire to be perceived as "comforting angels." Ironically, this drive to be perceived as "comforting" may get in the way of effective care giving. Such self-exploration may also reveal flirtatious traits or histrionic qualities in the clinician. Unchecked, these types of clinician traits can open the door to sexual misconduct.

At this point we can turn our attention to another aspect of nonverbal behavior, which frequently emerges if the clinician has effectively determined the appropriate RZ for the patient. At such times, the appearance of certain nonverbal behaviors can suggest that the blending process is proceeding well. As mentioned in Chapter 1, several verbal signs, including an increased DOU, may indicate the presence of improved engagement. In a similar fashion, nonverbal activities may also be used routinely to monitor the blending process, for the spontaneous appearance of immediacy behaviors in the patient indicate that the patient is feeling more and more comfortable, safe, and accepted by the interviewer.

For instance, as blending increases, the patient may begin to make progressively better eye contact, while spontaneous arm gestures and "talking with one's hands" may increase. Along similar lines, if a patient in a shut-down interview begins to talk more with his or her hands, this may be a hint to pursue the present topic more fully in order to further strengthen the engagement process. The clinician can also frequently see the patient turn more towards him or her as blending increases. Relaxation is also shown by an asymmetry in posture, while tense posture is frequently seen with a person who feels threatened.[77]

We have been discussing the nonverbal activities that may suggest powerful levels of blending. It is important to return to a topic approached earlier, namely, the differences seen cross-culturally regarding eye contact, for, in a proxemic sense, eye contact can change how close the patient feels in space from the interviewer. With regard to the African American culture, eye contact is not considered as important in conveying attention to a listener as in some other cultures.[78] Just being in the room or close to the speaker may be considered enough to convey that attention is being given.

Direct eye contact may be considered disrespectful in certain cultures, such as with Mexican Americans and with the Japanese. In this context, a clinician could be making a serious error in judgment by interpreting poor eye contact with members of these ethnic groups as an indication of rudeness, boredom, lack of assertiveness, or poor blending.

Another process that may emerge more frequently when one has successfully found the RZ is the surprising phenomenon of postural echoing.[79] In postural echoing one finds that two people who are communicating effectively tend to adopt similar postures and hand gestures. At a café, two lovers may sit across from each other, both heads perched in their hands, as they animatedly stare into each other's eyes.

A frequent phenomenon seen in interviewing occurs when one member of the dyad suddenly shifts position and relaxes. Simultaneously, the other person will also shift and relax. Moreover, microanalysis of videotapes has suggested that as blending increases, the minute movements of the interviewer and the interviewee tend to parallel each other as if a miniature minuet were being performed. During moments of discordant interchange, this reciprocity decreased.

At one level, these findings suggest that the appearance of postural echoing may serve as a clue to the clinician that the blending process is on the right track. In a slightly different vein, the clinician can subtly match some of the patient's postures in an effort to actively increase blending. For example, if a male clinician is interviewing a steel worker who is crossing his legs with his ankle over one knee, the therapist may cross his leg in the same manner, as opposed to crossing his leg at the knees (the latter could be misconstrued by the interviewee as "feminine"). By adopting a style similar to that of the patient's mini-culture, the metacommunication conveyed is that "we do certain things similarly and we may not be as different as one might first suppose." This discussion of the use of postural echoing in an effort to actively engage the patient leads to a consideration of other methods of nonverbally increasing the blending process.

Intentional Use of Head Nodding and Other Facilitative Techniques

As a clinician, it is worthwhile becoming consciously aware of one's use of immediacy behaviors, which you will recall are those nonverbal behaviors that convey warmth, involvement, and engagement. We all enter our residencies and graduate training programs with our own habits regarding immediacy behaviors, which have generally served us well in our everyday encounters. But in clinical work, depending upon the unique needs of a specific patient, as well as the unique interpersonal context inherent to a clinical interview, interviewers may find it useful to intentionally utilize or alter their immediacy behaviors. It has been shown that counselors who demonstrate good eye contact, smiling, and frequent gesticulation, are viewed as significantly more persuasive than counselors who do not.[80] Another commonly encountered immediacy behavior consists of a body lean of about 20 degrees towards the patient.[81]

One of the most well-recognized immediacy behaviors is the simple head nod. Morris[82] makes the interesting observation that the vertical head nod indicates a "yes" or "positive" response in all cultures and groups in which it has been observed, including Caucasians, African Americans, Balinese, Japanese, and Inuit. It has been observed in deaf and blind individuals as well as in microcephalic people incapable of speech. He relates that the head nod may convey different types of "yes" messages, such as the following:

The Acknowledgment Nod: "Yes, I am still listening."
The Encouraging Nod: "Yes, how fascinating."
The Understanding Nod: "Yes, I see what you mean."
The Agreement Nod: "Yes, I will."
The Factual Nod: "Yes, that is correct."

Interviewers should make an attempt to learn the frequency with which they typically head nod. This frequency can vary significantly among interviews. From my own observations, it appears that interviewers who are particularly adept at engaging patients tend to head nod numerous times during any several minutes of an interview. As obvious as the utility of the head nod may appear, I have found that approximately 20% of professionals I supervise tend to underuse it. A few barely head nod at all.

The power of the head nod became apparent to me in an unexpected fashion during a session of psychotherapy. I had been working with a middle-aged male patient for several months. I decided to try a brief exercise in which I would purposely stop my typical head nodding for several minutes, in order to see what this practice would feel like to me. To my surprise I found it difficult to do, because it had become habitual. But more to my surprise, the patient broke off his spontaneous conversation after about 2 minutes and asked, "What's wrong? Somehow I feel that you don't like what I'm saying." This vignette emphasizes the power of nonverbal cues during clinical interaction.

Nonverbal Techniques for Engaging Guarded or Paranoid Patients

If ever there was an art to interviewing, there is an art to engaging actively paranoid patients. In Chapter 1, when we were discussing the use of empathic statements, we discovered that with guarded or paranoid patients, certain changes in approach could enhance engagement. Other changes could result in a sharp decrease in engagement known as the paranoid spiral. In particular, certain verbal approaches that were particularly effective with trusting patients could be potentially disengaging with guarded patients. For instance, paranoid patients frequently respond better to empathic statements with a low valence of intuition rather than empathic statements with a high valence of intuition, for such statements might suggest to the paranoid patient that this clinician is "inside my head." Some paranoid patients respond best to no empathic statements.

Understanding these nuances in *verbal* interaction is important for effectively working with paranoid patients. But over the years, I have come to realize that the use of nonverbal behaviors probably plays an even larger role in effectively engaging patients with guarded and paranoid process. The secret to the art seems to lie in a sound understanding of the nonverbal concept of immediacy. In short, paranoid patients don't want it.

As with the verbal use of empathic statements, the nonverbal use of immediacy behaviors can be "too much" for the typical person wrestling with paranoid process. We noted earlier in the chapter that, much like empathic statements, immediacy behaviors can have a valence, as manifested by their power to communicate warmth and intimacy to the patient. Paranoid patients generally don't want warmth and intimacy upon first meeting a stranger. *Thus, the golden principle for engaging paranoid patients is, at least in theory, a simple one: tone down immediacy behaviors.* In practice this principle can be significantly more complex, for it often requires us to intentionally change our habitual immediacy behaviors to a striking extent; when first being learned, this may feel quite odd to the clinician. During my residency, it took me quite a while to get the hang of it. Let's look at the principle put into practice.

As mentioned earlier, from the perspective of proxemics, patients coping with paranoia often prefer much more interpersonal distance in order to feel safe. Chairs are consequently best set up with more distance between them. If one senses that a new patient is displaying paranoid process, it is a cue to gently wheel ones chair back so as to place more of the corner of the desk between oneself and the patient, thus decreasing the patient's feeling of immediacy and increasing the patient's sense of safety and space.

Specific immediacy behaviors, when done too frequently, may prove disruptive to the paranoid patient. I have heard paranoid patients comment that they have disliked frequent eye contact, for what is meant to convey the attentive gaze of a "good listener" becomes twisted into being perceived as the stark gaze of a potential persecutor. In this context, I have found it useful to purposely break eye contact more frequently with paranoid patients, providing them with more visual space. You may find it useful to increase the turn of your chairs so that now the angle is about 10 to 45% off the line directly between the patient and yourself, further decreasing oppositional gaze. It is part of the lore of interviewing that the great interviewing innovator, Harry Stack Sullivan, who was viewed as remarkably adept at engaging paranoid patients, would sometimes turn his chair so that he and the patient were sitting with their chairs facing the same direction.

Even head nodding and arm gestures, both of which tend to increase a sense of immediacy, which trusting patients like, can be unsettling when done too frequently with guarded or paranoid patients. I vividly remember one patient whom I interviewed in an emergency room. He was an intoxicated male, about 30 years old, who wore a perpetual sneer. He challenged me frequently with not-so-subtle sniping remarks, such as, "I bet you think you're a good listener Doc." And at one point he suddenly began mocking my head nodding by aping it, with his jaw jutting outwards while repeatedly grunting out loud "Uh huhs." This was not one of my more rewarding interviews. While waiting for his disposition, he later spontaneously attacked one of our safety guards.

This patient also illustrates the point that if the clinician finds a patient giving negative responses to typically engaging nonverbal behaviors, then he or she should consider the idea that the patient may be guarded, hostile, or potentially violent.

Immediacy paralanguage must also be toned down in valence with paranoid patients. I tend to speak fairly quickly and slightly louder than the norm in everyday life. I have learned that it is important that I intentionally speak more softly and slowly with paranoid patients. Thus, to make the necessary adjustments to their immediacy behaviors, clinicians are required to become more aware of their own nonverbal behaviors, the topic of our next section.

Clinician's Self-Awareness of Paralanguage

Each clinician has a unique personality, much of which shows itself by how we speak. Clinicians will vary on parameters such as tone of voice, rate of speech, and loudness of voice. It is important for clinicians to discover their own typical way of coming across. This knowledge is of value, because certain patients, as we just saw with paranoid process, may respond better to different approaches. An understanding of one's own natural style offers the clinician the chance to modify it, if necessary, to enhance the blending process.

With this idea in mind, it is useful for clinicians to practice exercises such as speaking more gently and slowing down their rate of speech. If an interviewer tends to speak loudly and quickly, a toning down of these parameters may prove more effective with a frightened or guarded patient as already noted, but it may also be important in a more general sense.

By way of example, as mentioned earlier, my own personality is somewhat upbeat, with a mild pressure to my speech and a slightly louder voice than many people. When beginning interviews, I purposely adjust to a calmer middle ground until I understand the specific needs of the patient. Adjustments can then be made as deemed necessary in either direction. In instances when I have not made this adjustment, I have certainly come on too strongly for certain patients. In a similar light, if we are experiencing a hectic day, it can be surprising how speeded up our speech (as well as gestures) have become as we rush to meet the next patient in the waiting room. Armed with a self-awareness of our paralanguage, we can catch this process and slow it down before walking into that waiting room.

There exists another area in which tone of voice can frequently disengage a patient. Specifically, when talking with elderly patients, clinicians often unconsciously adopt a rather distinctive tone of voice. They talk as if they were speaking to a helpless child. This tone of voice, which is often mildly slowed, can easily be perceived as condescending. It is an extremely frequent phenomenon, and clinicians must guard against it carefully. It is sometimes even done with psychotic patients and adolescents. In all these cases, the clinician is flirting with trouble.

The Impact of Clinician Gestures and Facial Expressions on the Patient

We are generally well trained to observe the behavior of others, but the value of observing our own gestures and facial expressions is frequently underplayed in supervision. As we have seen, the interview represents a dyadic process in which an understanding of one component depends on an understanding of the impact of the other component. The clinician's nonverbal activity always has the potential to significantly alter the behavior of the patient, as we have seen in our discussion of reciprocal behaviors.

With regard to gestures and other kinesic activities, as with paralanguage, clinicians need to develop a sound sense of their natural nonverbal style. One exercise that helps clinicians in developing self-awareness consists of repeatedly picturing a mirror descending during the interview itself. This imagined mirror is to drop into place between the clinician and the patient. Such a visualization exercise rather rudely awakens clinicians to the fact that their every move is potentially an object of scrutiny to an inquisitive patient. As a complement to this visualization exercise, video recording provides invaluable objective self-observation.

The clinician should foster an awareness of those nonverbal activities that may inadvertently decrease blending. I am reminded of an interview that I supervised of an adolescent boy. The patient sat in a pool of brooding preoccupation. He wore a worried expression more suited to a 60-year-old man coping with an agitated depression than to a boy beginning adolescence. Curiously, he had referred himself to the evaluation center and did not want his mother to be contacted.

During the interview he moved about anxiously in his chair and had considerable difficulty looking at the interviewer. He had a rounded face framed by a bowl of sandy hair, which was neatly clipped around his ears. It was about one of these ears that the discussion soon focused. Apparently he had the misfortune of watching a television documentary on cancer several days earlier. Since then he had become fixated on a small bump on his right ear, to which he gingerly pointed. He was convinced that he had developed a malignant tumor. This gnawing obsession, which may very well have reached delusional proportions, was nestled amidst a variety of depressive symptoms and difficult life circumstances.

As the interview proceeded, the boy became progressively more ill-at-ease. At several points he stopped talking, asking the interviewer, "You don't understand, do you?" To this, the interviewer responded in a reassuring fashion that he was trying to understand and wanted to hear more. This type of response generally might have decreased the tension, but in this case it seemed of no avail.

What the interviewer did not realize was the message conveyed by his own face. Each time the boy discussed his "tumor" the clinician furrowed his brow in a not-so-subtle fashion, forming two small vertical lines between his eyebrows. Apparently the patient interpreted this facial gesture as a look of disbelief or condemnation. The clinician had no conscious awareness of this particular expression, which frequently cropped up as a habit during his interviews. It is just this type of habit that can lead to recurrent problems with poor blending.

These habits are difficult to recognize unless the clinician is directly supervised or video recorded. They are also sometimes hard to accept. The clinician above seemed unimpressed with my explanation for the poor engagement until several weeks later. He approached me sheepishly and said, "You'll never believe what a patient just did. In the middle of the interview he cut me off and asked me why I was frowning. My God, I must actually do it!"

One of my own habits illustrates another category of clinician movement that can become problematic. As I become anxious, I begin to twist my hair behind my ears. This nonverbal activity represents what we have discussed earlier as a displacement activity. These displacement activities can be used to monitor patient anxiety, but on the flip side, they can be a useful self-monitor, indicating anxiety in the clinician.

During an interview, clinicians may not even be aware of the presence of their own stress nor recognize that the intensity of their stress may be distracting them from attending effectively to the patient. But the appearance of numerous displacement activities can alert them that such is the case.

At these points of self-awareness in the interview, it can be useful for the clinician to explore the origins of the tension. Sometimes the interviewer may discover that they are fretting about personal matters not related to the interview, such as problems at home or at work. At other times, the clinician may be experiencing countertransference tensions, intuitively registering patient hostility or even sensing well-hidden psychotic process. In any case, the recognition of clinician displacement activities can provide yet another avenue for understanding one's internal frame of mind.

Another good reason for studying displacement activities concerns the eradication of potentially disengaging gestures. For the most part, displacement activities are natural and help to create a feeling of spontaneous communication. As such, there is no need to eliminate them; indeed, they may actually foster good blending. But there exist certain displacement gestures that are probably best eliminated. We can return to my own habit of twisting my hair. This displacement activity has the potential to be disengaging. To some patients it may appear effeminate, because, as mentioned earlier, women touch their hair three times more frequently than do men. To others, it may simply be distracting. In either case, it serves no purpose and is probably best discarded.

Similarly, certain categories of patients may not respond well to demonstrations of increased anxiety in the clinician. The immediate category that comes to mind includes patients escalating towards violence. These patients are frequently frightened that they are about to lose control. If they see the clinician becoming progressively more tense as well, they may become even more agitated. The same holds true for paranoid patients, who may appear almost ludicrously hyperattentive to their environments. I remember an older man with marked paranoid process who once asked me why I had just scratched my head. When I said I had an itch, he did not seem particularly reassured.

Two other clinician displacement activities warrant discussion. The first activity is smoking. Although forbidden in clinics and hospitals, some clinicians choose to smoke in a private practice setting. I personally do not believe that clinicians should smoke cigarettes or even the proverbial "Freudian pipe" while interviewing patients. My bias evolves from the feeling that smoking, at the very least, represents a possible distraction to the patient. More likely, it may actually function as an irritant. Even if one asks permission from the patient, many patients who do not like smoking may find it difficult to convey such concerns. Pipe smoking is so stereotypic of "a shrink" that it may bias transference or simply turn some patients off.

The second displacement activity is much more of a mixed blessing, because it clearly serves some useful purposes. I had never even viewed it as a displacement activity until I had asked one trainee what his most common displacement activities were, and he replied, "That's easy, I'm constantly scribbling notes."

A Few Notes on Note Taking

There exist many good reasons for taking detailed notes, such as making process notes to be shared with a psychotherapy supervisor. On the other hand, I have become more and more convinced that much of note taking in initial interviews represents a displacement activity that frequently distracts both the clinician and the patient. No matter how one views it, a clinician looking down at his or her keypad or clipboard while recording information cannot possibly be attending to the fine nuances of a patient's nonverbal behavior as described in this chapter. Thus, there is a price to be paid for note taking. Let us look at this price in more detail.

First, we should make a clear distinction between taking "rough notes" as opposed to creating the finalized electronic health record (EHR), also sometimes called the electronic medical record or electronic clinical record. By taking rough notes, I am describing typing or jotting down bits of information, mostly *not* in complete sentences, for the primary purpose of reminding the clinician of important information that might have been forgotten by the time the clinician is creating the finalized note for the EHR, which is typed, written, or dictated *after* the patient leaves.

This finalized note (the EHR) is our main way of accurately communicating both benign and critical information to future clinicians, some of which, as we shall see in our chapter on suicide assessment, might actually save a patient's life. In my opinion, we owe it to our patients to produce an accurate and comprehensive permanent record. It should also be noted that this final note will be meticulously read by opposing lawyers in any malpractice suit. In short, the creation of the finalized electronic record requires close to 100% attention. From both the standpoint of good care, and from the standpoint of sound forensic documentation, I do not see how one can create such a document during the interview itself.

In addition, and in my opinion even more importantly, I do not believe one can effectively attend to the critically important verbal, nonverbal, and cognitive processes necessary to effectively engage the patient, sensitively uncover a valid database, attend to nonverbal issues, be aware of one's own internal feelings and psychodynamics, generate a diagnostic formulation, problem solve, and create a treatment plan while simultaneously typing or writing complete, polished sentences and paragraphs. Sound clinical interviewing requires sound listening. It too requires close to 100% attention.

Also, for every second of time and attention focused upon typing the patient's EHR during the interview itself, that time is lost from the patient's hour. As we have seen, the information that can be used to rapidly and most effectively help our patients in the initial interview is massive. In my opinion, there is no time to waste pretending that we are well-trained transcriptionists.

Doing a sensitive interview is a human event. Creating a finalized document from the information garnered in that interview is a mechanical one. Both processes are important. Both processes require our best attention. Both processes require their own timeframes. Let me summarize, I do *not* believe, whether typing or writing, that the finalized note (e.g., the permanent medical/health/clinical record) should be created *during* the interview itself. In my opinion, the *only* notes that should be taken during the interview itself are rough notes, whether typed or handwritten.

With regard to rough notes, once again I am sharing a bias that some clinicians might disagree with, I feel that rough note taking should be fairly minimized in the initial interview as well. Whether you prefer to take your rough notes on a laptop or handwrite them, they should be utilized to jot down hard-to-remember details such as dates, medication dosages, previous treatment histories, and family trees. By minimizing the amount of rough note taking, a clinician can maximize his or her attention to the needs of the patient and the complexities of the unfolding dyadic relationship – and its clinical complexities – as they unfold in real time.

In particular, during the scouting phase, I believe it is much better to do little, if any, note taking unless you are taking some demographic background. At this early stage, the emphasis should be on actively engaging the patient. To this end, I find that patients are more responsive to clinicians who seem more interested in them than in a keyboard or a clipboard.

In addition, I strongly advise against any note taking (even the taking of rough notes) when raising or exploring highly sensitive material such as suicide, incest, or domestic violence, where it is critical to attend to any nonverbal indications that a patient may be withholding information. During such delicate explorations, I find it expedient to place down upon a nearby table or on the floor my means of rough note taking, whether it be a clipboard or a laptop.

I frequently do not even begin taking rough notes until well into the interview. When I do begin, as a sign of respect, I often say to the patient, "I'm going to take a few notes to make sure I'm remembering everything correctly. Is that all right with you?" Patients seem to respond very nicely to this simple sign of courtesy. This statement of purpose also tends to decrease the paranoia that patients sometimes project onto note taking, as they wonder if the clinician is madly analyzing their every thought and action. Along these lines, I advise against *any* note taking when interviewing actively paranoid patients.

How many rough notes should you take? The answer is simple – as many as you need to accurately type up the EHR after the patient has left. This amount may vary among clinicians. I supervised a trainee, with a "photographic memory," who created beautiful finalized notes but took almost no rough notes during the interview itself. The amount of rough notes taken may even vary with a single clinician, depending upon how hectic the clinician's schedule. If the clinician is able to type up the finalized EHR immediately after the interview is completed (an ideal situation), the clinician may need few rough notes. If the day is hectic, requiring the clinician to wait till later in the day to type up several initial intakes, then the clinician will probably need to take more rough notes than usual.

If you choose to use your laptop to make your rough notes, remember that the fields of your EHR should *never* dictate the sequencing of your questions or topics. As we saw in Chapters 3 and 4, the goal is to flexibly structure the various regions and questions of our interviews to meet the unique needs, concerns, and defenses of our patients. Only then can we optimize engagement and the subsequent validity of the information garnered in the interview.

One of the most effective methods of taking rough notes on a laptop – if you so choose to do so – I was taught by a resident. She would sit with both feet on the ground with her laptop open on her lap. She only typed rough notes, for purposes of recall, as we have described. *Consequently, she was actually typing only about 10–15% of the time during the interview itself.* Most strikingly, and cleverly, any time she stopped typing for a significant period, she gently, yet obviously partially closed her laptop to the point where it was clear to the patient that the clinician could not possibly see the keyboard. In addition, she would gently lean slightly forward, over the semi-closed laptop lid. The meta-communication to the patient was immediate and powerful: "I'm not interested in taking these notes, I'm interested in listening to you." Furthermore, if she was not going to be taking notes for an extended period of time, she would set the laptop on the ground or on a desk or table to her side.

I have found that a significant number of contemporary clinicians, especially if they are fast typists, prefer to write their rough notes on a clipboard. It gives them more flexibility with how they can sit and lean during the interview and subsequently provides a quick set of reminders with which they can rapidly type and move through the fields of the EHR itself after the patient has left. I, myself, have found this to be preferable. But you will need to discover for yourself which method of taking rough notes (laptop versus clipboard) works best for you. As demonstrated above, both can be used quite effectively in my opinion.

Nonverbal Aspects of Calming Potentially Violent Patients

Recognizing Contextual Clues of Impending Violence

Interacting with a patient who is escalating towards violence presents the clinician with one of the most difficult of clinical situations. Although it would be nice to think that violent interactions are rare, the facts speak otherwise. Tardiff reports that approximately 17% of psychiatric patients reporting to an emergency room are potentially violent. He further states that roughly 40% of psychiatrists have reported being assaulted at least once in their careers.[83]

Obviously, it is to the clinician's benefit to review the various approaches that may de-escalate an angry patient. In particular, the nonverbal characteristics of potentially violent dyads are of considerable importance, because issues concerning proxemics, kinesics, and paralanguage can all be of value in handling these situations. The interaction with the potentially violent patient provides an excellent topic with which to close

Part 2 of this chapter, for the craft of utilizing nonverbal behavior is seldom put to a more critical test.

I would also like to emphasize that violence is frequently a dyadic process. The clinician and the patient represent a two-person system, and it is this system that becomes violent. Clinicians may inadvertently, with their nonverbal behavior, further escalate an already agitated patient. Fortunately, this cycle, representing a "violence reciprocal" as per Scheflen, can frequently be broken.

To begin with, I am reminded of a curious story related by an anthropology professor during my undergraduate education. He described an interspecies encounter in which violence was averted by the quick thinking of a field anthropologist. This anthropologist had been extensively studying the behaviors of a baboon troop. One day he accidentally startled a mother baboon and her baby. Within seconds the squawkings of the alarmed mother attracted a swarming bevy of guard males. One can assume their intent was not of a social variety. Indeed, baboons are both intelligent and ferocious when provoked. The appearance of an ugly white ape with a mustache and safari hat was more than ample stimulus to prompt a display of their virility. Indeed, the baboons could have quickly disposed of the anthropologist.

Having observed baboons demonstrating submissive behavior within the troop, he purposely replicated their submissive gestures, which apparently involved lowering oneself and making certain jaw movements. To his relief, the baboons grunted and snarled but waved off their attack.

Besides being a delightful tale with which a college professor can regale wide-eyed undergraduates, the above story has a valuable message: A group of animals were about to interact violently. The violence was prevented by the use of specific nonverbal behaviors that functioned as true nonverbal communications (emblems). Like these baboons, the human animal possesses a repertoire of nonverbal communications and nonverbal activities that signal the intent to attack and the intent to submit.

The signals of impending attack, when recognized in a patient, can quickly alert the clinician that something needs to be altered in the interpersonal dyad before a violence reciprocal ensues. Through a knowledge of the signals of submission, the clinician may alter behavior in a fashion that appears less threatening to the paranoid or intoxicated patient. In many instances, these alterations can break the dyadic cycle of violence as effectively as the anthropologist placating the baboon warriors. It should be kept in mind that in rare instances, no matter what preventive actions are undertaken, violence will erupt. The goal is not to eliminate violence but to decrease its likelihood.

Towards this endeavor, the clinician should assess whether the clinical situation indicates that violence is a possibility. In the first place, diagnosis can alert the clinician to an increased likelihood of aggression. Most psychotic patients are not violent, but psychotic process as manifested in schizophrenia, bipolar disorder, paranoid disorder, and other atypical psychoses may predispose the patient towards aggression. This is especially true when paranoid delusions are simmering beneath the patient's social facade. If frightened, these paranoid patients may go to great extremes to protect themselves, as we would if we shared their vision of the world. It is always important to remember that such patients may believe that they are literally fighting for their lives.

Other types of psychosis or poor impulse control may present problems. For instance, patients suffering from organic brain disease, as seen in frontal lobe syndromes, deliria, and various dementias, may be predisposed towards aggression. The possibility of violence should arise in the clinician's mind when interacting with people under the influence of various drugs, including speed, bath salts, hallucinogens, and phencyclidine (PCP). Alcohol intoxication remains a major factor in the instigation of violence, especially in settings such as emergency departments. Because we frequently deal with alcohol intoxication in social settings in our culture, it is easy to be lulled into underestimating the potential for violence when dealing with an intoxicated patient. Such patients can quickly move from jovial jesting into a fit of rage.

Diagnoses do not tell the clinician that any specific patient is about to be violent. Most people suffering from schizophrenia are not violent, but the diagnosis does alert the clinician to the possibility of aggression. This consideration may represent the first step in preventing violence. In addition, the clinician may note that a patient has a history of assaultive behavior. In such instances, the clinician is well advised to take appropriate precautions, such as having safety officers unobtrusively nearby and aware of the situation.

Besides diagnostic and historical factors, the clinician may be part of a situation in which violence is more likely. If the clinician has been asked to participate in the evaluation of a patient who is being committed involuntarily, then caution is always advised. There are probably few life situations more frightening than to have one's freedom taken away. In this situation, patients should always be considered as potentially violent.

I remember one instance in an emergency department late at night. The patient, an agitated woman of about 30 years of age, was being committed. Safety officers had been called down and were appropriately nearby. The patient appeared to have calmed and was quietly sitting with family members by her side. Everything seemed in control. The clinician began to move away from the patient and turned her back as she headed for the staff room. In a matter of seconds the patient was ferociously choking the clinician, for no apparent reason. I mention this vignette because it highlights the need to think cautiously while evaluating committed patients. It also reminds one of the old adage that when working in an emergency department one should never turn one's back on a patient, an adage as true today as when it was first coined.

One other clinical situation to keep in mind arises when patients are agitated and accompanied by family members. In such situations, the clinician should attempt to determine quickly whether the family member is calming or upsetting the patient. In emergency rooms, a common mistake is to not separate feuding family members until it is too late. It is often best to separate the antagonistic family members quickly, and have different staff members attempt to calm and understand the perspectives of both parties.

I have strayed from the topic of nonverbal behavior. However, in a practical sense, the first step in utilizing nonverbal behavior with violent patients consists of recognizing the violent situation in its infancy, not its adolescence. If the clinician is aware of the potential for violence, then the following nonverbal techniques can be brought into play.

We will first look at various nonverbal activities that can alert the clinician that violence may be incubating. Subsequently, we will look at ways to change our own behaviors in an effort to avoid confrontation.

Nonverbal Clues of Impending Violence

The nonverbal signs of impending aggression can be loosely grouped into two categories – early warning signs and late warning signs. Although it is extremely difficult to predict whether a patient will engage in violence in the future, it is not particularly difficult to tell when a patient may be headed towards immediate violence.

The early warning signs consist of behaviors that suggest emerging agitation. In the simplest examples, one may notice the patient beginning to speak more quickly with a subtly angry tone of voice. These paralanguage clues may be augmented by a display of sarcastic statements or challenges, such as, "You think you're a big shot, don't you!"

These types of early warning signs may appear obvious, but this is exactly the reason they warrant mentioning. As clinicians, we may inadvertently ignore these signs – in the process unintentionally escalating the patient. This seems to occur during periods of intense time pressure or when the clinical situation has become increasingly hectic, as in a busy emergency department or inpatient unit. Such obstinacy can unfortunately return as an unwanted gremlin. When these early warning signs are present, it is very important to crystallize in one's mind what the patient's needs may be. If the clinician can move with the patient's needs, hostility will frequently decrease.

Kinesic early warning signs consist of actual evidence of agitation, such as pacing and refusing to sit down. If patients refuse to sit, it is frequently useful to gently request them to return to their seat. One can use phrases such as, "It might help you to relax some if you sit over here," or "Let's sit down and see if we can sort some things out." If the patient fails to sit in response to these comments, one can quietly, yet firmly state, "I'd like you to sit over here so we can talk." Some clinicians might quietly add, "It's difficult to have to keep staring up. I think we'll both be more comfortable if we sit." If these maneuvers fail, then it is probably best to let the patient walk around freely, while recognizing that this patient may be seriously impaired with regard to impulse control. In short, the patient may be on the way towards violence, and appropriate steps should be taken.

If no one is aware that the clinician is alone with such a patient, it is generally best to let someone know what is going on. It is relatively easy for a clinician to make an excuse for leaving the room at such points. It may not be so easy 10 minutes later. Along these lines, if the clinician is at all suspicious of possible violence, the clinician should carry a "safety button" or know where the safety button is located in the interview room, so that other staff can be alerted if problems arise.

Other kinesic early warning clues include rapid and jerky gesturing. Of particular note is the action of vigorously pointing one's finger at the clinician to "make a point." Such a gesture may be a harbinger of impending hostility. Increased and intense staring may also suggest anger. Finally, the appearance of suspiciousness or other increases in psychotic process, such as an increasing disorganization of thoughts and/or behaviors, should alert the clinician to the possibility of violence.

As a person comes closer to overt violence, specific behaviors may serve as reliable indicators that aggression is imminent. Just like the charging guard baboons with their bared teeth, humans have evolved symbolic signs of threat.

Morris has described behaviors known as intention movements.[84] These intention movements consist of those small gestures that suggest impending actions. For instance, when people intend to rise from a chair, they frequently lean forward grasping the arms of the chair. This is a clear signal that they want to rise, signaling that the conversation is about to end. The intention movements suggesting possible violence include activities such as clenching of the fists, whitening of the knuckles while tightly grasping an inanimate object, and even a snarling as the lips are pulled back from the teeth. People may not be as different from baboons as we would like to think.

Perhaps the most common intention movement of attack is the raising of a closed fist over the head. Overhand blows delivered from this position are the most frequent blows seen in street brawls and riots, despite the unlikelihood of hurting one's opponent in this manner. This behavior may be instinctive in nature, because it is frequently seen in children who are fighting.

Morris also describes vacuum gestures. These are gestures that represent complete violent actions, but they are not actually carried out on the enemy. Frequent vacuum gestures include shaking the fist, assuming a boxing stance, gesturing as if strangling the opponent, and the pounding of the fist into the opposite palm. Both intention movements and vacuum gestures serve as late warning signals that violence is near at hand.

It should also be noted that verbal threats or statements that one is about to strike out often accompany the nonverbal behaviors described above. When the above late warning signs are present, violence is a distinct possibility. At this point, an application of nonverbal skills may help to prevent aggression.

Nonverbal Techniques for Calming a Potentially Violent Patient

Scheflen describes dominance and submission reciprocals.[85] In our story of the baboons, the anthropologist refused to participate in the dominance reciprocal. If he had, he might very well have been killed. Instead he chose to begin the submission reciprocal, which his would-be attackers fortunately agreed to follow. In a similar fashion, humans can engage in either of these reciprocals.

When faced with a hostile patient, the trick is to avoid engaging in the dominance reciprocal while utilizing some submissive behavior. One avoids the dominance reciprocal by not demonstrating any of the early or late warning signs of aggression. Although this appears to make an obvious point, it is striking to watch the maladapative behavior of clinicians when faced with an agitated patient. The fear generated by the patient's hostility frequently results in unconscious behaviors that may threaten the patient. The clinician's voice may be raised. At times, the actual movements of the clinician speed up as the waiting area is hurriedly cleared of furniture and other patients. Even frankly antagonistic remarks may emerge. In this respect, it is not an exaggeration to say that sometimes clinicians actually precipitate violence.

There exist no absolute rules for interacting with a patient on the verge of violence, but there are some principles that can help guide the clinician. In the first place, the clinician should appear calm. The speaking voice should appear normal and unharried. It is particularly important to avoid speaking loudly or in an authoritarian manner. With regard to kinesics, the clinician wants to avoid an excessive display of displacement activities, which may be misinterpreted as aggressive displays. Moreover, exaggerated displacement activities may create an increasing atmosphere of fear, stoking the patient's own fears of an impending loss of control.

Eye contact should probably be decreased, and the hands should not be raised in any gesture that may signify an intent to attack or defend oneself. To the contrary, it can be useful to keep the hands low, by the side, and with palms upwards when gesturing. Upwardly open palms are a submissive signal to many primates including humans. Unfortunately, probably related to nervousness and fear, some clinicians will place their hands behind their backs (a soothing auto-contact behavior), a gesture that may raise fears in the patient that a weapon is being hidden. With regard to posture, one can purposely stoop one's shoulders slightly in an effort to appear smaller, because humans, when about to attack, frequently raise their shoulders and chests in a slightly gorilla-like display. In this regard, I have found it to be very valuable to bend my knees slightly, so as to decrease my height, when near a potentially violent patient. Similarly, it is probably also wise to remain in front of the patient, because an approach from behind or from the side may startle an agitated patient.

One of the most important principles concerns an issue mentioned earlier when discussing proxemics. At least one study has suggested that potentially violent patients may have significantly altered buffer zones.[86] Specifically, they will feel that their intimate body space is being invaded at distances that are much greater than for most people. These patients may feel that the interviewer is "in my face" while standing a full 6 feet away. In general, the agitated patient needs more room and interpersonal space. This can be a tough principle to remember, because some good-hearted clinicians feel a desire to calm the angry patient by touching them. This desire usually goes away after a few unfortunate encounters with feet or fists.

If these principles are followed, accompanied by an intelligent use of safety officers and medication as needed, many violent encounters can be avoided in emergency rooms, on inpatient units, and in other settings. With regard to avoiding dangerous situations, another point warrants mentioning. When sitting in an emergency department examination room with a patient whom one does not know, it is probably wise to arrange the chairs so that the clinician is closer to the doorway, while not obstructing the patient's pathway to the doorway. With this arrangement one can always get away if the patient becomes threatening or produces a weapon. It is naive to think that these situations do not arise, especially in emergency departments. To pretend that they do not probably represents a defensive denial that prevents the clinician from fully thinking about these situations in a manner that could help prevent them in the first place.

In conclusion, nonverbal processes are core elements of human communication during violent interactions. A sound knowledge of these processes can help the clinician to calm an angry or frightened patient. Helping patients to regain a sense of internal control remains one of the fine points of the art of interviewing. It also increases the chances that the clinician will be around to practice his or her art.

PART 3: BOLD NEW FRONTIERS – THE NONVERBAL IMPACT OF TECHNOLOGY, THE WEB, AND MOBILE CONNECTEDNESS ON INTERVIEWING

It is both remarkable and exciting to be addressing a topic that did not even exist as a topic when I wrote the last edition of this book. As the new century was approaching, the web was powerfully establishing itself, but it essentially had no connection to clinical interviewing. How times have changed.

The web is bringing many new opportunities and channels for communicating clinically, some of which will hopefully allow us to both transform and save lives. In my role as a member of the Standards and Training Committee for Lifeline (the national organization in charge of certifying and training crisis line staff), it has been my privilege to see some of these dynamic developments. These developments are occurring because the web offers certain characteristics that traditional face-to-face (and even traditional telephone crisis) intervention does not offer.

For instance, one of the great attractions of the web is anonymity.[87] There is no way of recognizing the voice, let alone the face, of a person with whom we are chatting online; neither is it possible to be "tracked down" by such a person in the real world. For some patients who are contemplating suicide, this anonymity is appealing. For them, it is easier and more comfortable to contact a nonprofessional support system, or even a crisis line professional, by using the web. This anonymity creates a sensation of safety. This sense of safety may foster an enhanced sharing of sensitive, intimate, or dangerous material. It may have also been the deciding factor that led an ambivalent patient to make contact in the first place. In addition, the geographic anonymity that prevents the police from easily being contacted by a crisis clinician to do an active intervention on an imminently dangerous caller is actually appealing to some callers in whom a fear of such an intervention is intense.

In addition, chatting, texting, and instant messaging are second nature to the generation that grew up using the web, many of whom are the readers of this book. Consequently, both with veterans and with college students, suicide crisis centers have been developed that are completely web-based. Whether it is the result of anonymity, second nature, or both, it is hoped that potentially suicidal patients who might never have gone to an emergency room, nor called a telephone crisis line, will make contact via these new web-based centers. *It is then hoped that a skilled web-based clinician can subsequently convince the more potentially suicidal patients to seek out a face-to-face interview (college counseling center, emergency department after hours, etc.), where a more effective risk assessment can be accomplished.* I think that many lives may be saved as a result.

All of these crisis contacts are initial interviews of a sort, yet they have a common factor not seen in the interviewing situations described thus far in this book – a scarcity of nonverbal interaction. One wonders what impact this might have and how our understanding of these nonverbal deficits might help us perform these "interviews" more effectively. Indeed, most readers of this book will be involved in clinical interviews in which there is minimal nonverbal communication, including handling our own patients' crisis calls, covering by phone the crises of the patients of our colleagues who are on vacation or ill, and performing tele-video interviews, psychotherapy sessions, and medication checks on patients living in isolated rural areas in whatever country we might live.

In order to most effectively use the advantages of any new technology, we must be familiar and open to the idea that there may be disadvantages and limitations to that very same technology. This is a chapter that explores some of these limitations, in the hope that we will better be able to tap the many promising advantages of online and mobile connectedness, as well as other communication advances such as improved teleconferencing.

Interactive Audio-Visual Technology (IATV) and the "Phantom Presence Effect"

The ability to communicate with people remotely, in real time, both visually and aurally, is a reality made possible only by recent technological advances. It was the stuff of *Star Trek* only 40 years ago. At first, such communications were created via traditional video-conferencing. Today, it is being revolutionized by the web, through Skype and similar platforms. With the advent of apps that can create IATV for smart phones and other devices, it will undoubtedly become commonplace in the very near future.

IATV offers us the chance to provide sound clinical assessments for patients who might not otherwise be able to reach help. With the use of IATV, we have entered the world of telepsychiatry and telecounseling as performed via computer link-up. Ofer Zur summarizes some of these circumstances nicely:

> *IATV offers tremendous advantages for working with those who are in remote areas with limited access to in-person services; those who are home-bound (e.g., those with agoraphobia or a physical disability); those in the LGBT community, who are reluctant to discuss their concerns with local psychotherapists or counselors; those in jails and prisons, where mobility of prisoners and access to care are surmountable problems; and those who need professional services outside usual business hours. Indeed, for some individuals in-person treatment may not be a possibility due to personal, physical, psychological, financial, or cultural issues, and IATV may be a viable treatment option for them … Then there are people who simply prefer the distance and control of the setting that is provided by video technologies in comparison to in-person meetings.*[88]

In order to more effectively utilize IATV, it is important to realize that although it allows for more nonverbal communication than telephone work or purely verbal electronic communication (as with e-mail, texting, and chat rooms), it is still limited in scope, as anyone can attest who "attends" an all-day lecture series by videoconferencing. Such educational formats often seem dull and very long, even when watching a talented speaker. Although such dullness provides a wonderful opportunity for texting friends, playing web games, checking e-mail, sending an Instagram or two, or catching up on the writing of progress notes, one is stuck with the question of "Why this dullness"? Why is watching a talented speaker much less enjoyable when participating by videoconferencing as opposed to attending the training?

I believe that by revisiting the concept of immediacy we will find our answer. Although the positive feelings of immediacy are partially communicated by factors easily seen by the use of videoconferencing (facial expressions, head nodding, and gestures), much of immediacy appears to be related to something else. Part of the "something else" is the role of proxemics, and for proxemic factors to be felt, there must be a palpable presence of "the other" in the same room. There is no such presence in videoconferencing or other forms of IATV, such as skyping. Let us examine this phenomenon in more detail.

With IATV, many of the nonverbal indicators of immediacy, such as facial expressions and gesturing, are clearly visually present. Consequently, it is surprisingly easy for us, as clinicians, to be lulled into the perception that we are a real presence to the patient in the room. But we are not. Our "presence" is merely an image, not a concrete reality. Patients do not *feel* our presence in the room as they would in a face-to-face interview. We are a mere image – a talking head of sorts. To the patient, we are a phantom presence and vice versa.

Our lack of real presence has many powerful nonverbal implications that can limit the quality of the assessment process. This lack of the sensation of the presence of another person in the room, and its resulting problems with creating immediacy, is a phenomenon I like to call the "phantom presence effect." Because of this phantom presence effect, the ramifications on our ability to create an engaging sense of immediacy will impact not only our proxemic interactions with the patient but key kinesic interactions as well.

We have seen earlier in this chapter that people adjust interpersonal distance while communicating. People (and cultures) can be keenly aware of changes in interpersonal distance. When doing interviews using IATV, clinicians must be aware of two facts: (1) The interviewer will not have any of the nonverbal proxemic clues to blending that are normally provided by the patient's spontaneous use of space as engagement either improves (patient tends to move closer or leans forward) or deteriorates (patient is experiencing disagreement, anger, guardedness, or paranoia, resulting in moving away or "keeping at a distance" from the interviewer). (2) Similarly, the interviewer will not have the ability to impact on the patient by his or her use of interpersonal distance (moving closer to a patient during a particularly sensitive or painful moment or "yielding" to an angry patient by moving away).

Another powerful variable in immediacy that is hampered significantly by the phantom presence effect is the ability to make eye contact effectively. Once again, we lose clues to blending and engagement because of this decrement. As with proxemics, we also lose the ability to have an impact on the patient through our own intentional use of eye contact.

Even at surprising distances, eye contact and interaction are important creators of the feeling of immediacy and listener interest. When providing training events, whether nationally or internationally, I have learned that making eye contact with the members of my audience can significantly impact on their engagement. I can read both their interest level and their "buy-in" to what I am saying (some participants return good eye contact and supplement it with head nodding and even a smile, others look blandly on or stare). In addition, these immediacy behaviors also show that the audience member is keenly aware of my presence and of the possibility that I will personally interact with them by engaging them with eye contact. Such an expectation of contact on the audience member is literally "felt," as evidenced by the fact that some participants will quickly look away and not return my eye contact. When I pick up on the uncomfortableness of such an audience member, communicated by his or her nonverbal cues, I know to avoid such eye contact for the rest of the talk with that particular participant, thus shaping the use of my eye contact to the unique needs of the audience member.

I mention this non-clinical setting to highlight the importance of eye contact in engagement and the ability to perceive whether or not someone agrees with you. If I can have an impact on an audience member at a distance of 50 feet, imagine the power of eye contact when interviewing at a distance of 5 feet or when trying to recognize the degree of wariness in an actively paranoid patient. Much, although not all, of this is lost in IATV interviewing. It also suggests that during the collaborative treatment planning undertaken in the closing phase, an IATV clinician may be missing some of the important nonverbal indicators of the patient's agreement or disagreement.

Considering the great limitations to the effectiveness of eye contact when using platforms such as Skype to undertake interviews, one will want to maximize whatever remains of the impact on the patient via eye contact. Elisa Rambo offers a useful insight in this regard. She points out that we tend to naturally look patients in the eye intermittently throughout an interview, "but if you peer straight at your patient's eyes on the computer screen, from her perspective you then appear to gaze downwards. Looking upward, into the camera, seems more like eye contact from her end."[89] Rambo further suggests reminding oneself to look straight at the computer's camera at least every 10 seconds or so.

Our discussion of the nuances of a decrease in eye contact suggest that something even more intriguing may be at work in the generation of the phantom presence effect itself. This generating factor is a matrix phenomenon, impacting both participants in the interview. The phantom presence effect may be caused not only by changes in both parties' abilities to read and impact on each other, but by fundamental changes in how intensely each individual is attending and preparing to respond to the environment – the activation level of each person. The degree to which a person is spontaneously interested in an environment probably impacts on how easily engaged the person may be with parts of the environment, such as a clinician. Let us look at this idea in more detail.

As we have already discovered, to effectively gain a feeling of immediacy, there is a pre-requisite: a person must be aware that another human being is in the room. Once this awareness occurs, it is my belief that biological and psychological processes that help an organism to "be alert" and to "remain alert" are probably triggered. They are triggered to monitor the safeness of the environment and to allow the organism to take appropriate action if threatened by the other presence.

Thus a major psychological component and pre-requisite of powerful immediacy is the unconscious and conscious awareness that the other person may "try to interact with me at any moment." Likewise, the person may become aware that the other individual in their environment may force them to interact by speaking to them, moving closer, or touching. All of these factors unite to create a more alert organism, whether it be the presence of a sales assistant in a shop or a patient sitting in our office. This *perceived potential* for face-to-face speakers to cause interaction (making eye contact with an audience member or spontaneously asking a question to a specific audience member) may help to explain why live talks are often more interesting than videoconferences – immediacy (hence alertness) is activated by the very potential for uninvited interaction by the speaker.

As clinicians, we must remember that this powerful precursor of immediacy – the activation of an alerted state caused by the recognition by the patient of the actual presence of another person in the room – is not available when communicating via IATV. This activated alertness, and resulting readiness to interact, can be an important part of the engagement process. With some patients, its absence may negatively impact the engagement process, placing an increased emphasis upon the content of what we are saying (such as an increased need for empathic statements) to generate the same level of engagement we would have achieved in a face-to-face interview.

Curiously, yet logically, if one thinks about it, we may discover that IATV is preferred by some patients (perhaps those patients with intense social anxiety or with paranoid process), for the exact same reason that makes engagement more challenging – the lessening of immediacy – because they don't like the sensation of immediacy. To their great relief, the feeling of immediacy will be significantly decreased by IATV. There is no way that a clinician many miles away can "touch me or do bad things to me."

Another important possible limitation with IATV interviewing is the question of intuition. We do not know exactly what allows us to be intuitive, a skill of particular importance in many aspects of clinical interviewing, from recognizing when to use an empathic statement to recognizing acute suicidal intent. Most likely many factors contribute in an interactive fashion, some of which we have already alluded to earlier in the book. I personally feel that our own sense of immediacy, while interviewing, plays a significant role. Consequently, when undertaking an interview via IATV, it is important for the clinician to recognize that his or her intuitive abilities may be compromised, a realization that can have important ramifications when assessing for suicide or trying to spot patient deceit.

Closing on a minor, yet still significant, point, it is important to recognize the effects of the decreased size of the patient's image in most IATV interviews. The limited size of IATV images (sometimes as small as the screen of a smart phone) can significantly hamper our ability to see or recognize the visually available nonverbal behaviors of our patient, such as the patient's facial expressions, head nods, and gestures (many of which may be off-screen).

Interviewing on the Telephone

We will now visit a more traditional technology. Telephone work has some advantages. Once again, the relative anonymity (more than IATV but less than text-based web communication) and the geographic distance from the clinician (with a resulting decrease in immediacy) are appealing to some patients. In certain instances these factors probably foster an increased sharing, the so-called "bartender effect" in which people tend to open up to total strangers. But overall, telephone work is difficult.

In contrast to IATV, telephones more radically diminish nonverbal behaviors. Indeed, all nonverbal behaviors are absent except for paralanguage cues. The ramifications are significant and well acknowledged by anyone performing telephone intakes or handling crisis calls. In this brief section we will examine two difficulties in this type of work.

Problems Assessing Patients on the Phone

Off the bat, all of the problems in assessment described for IATV interviews are equally present in telephone interventions. Indeed, problems with understanding the patient's sense of engagement and immediacy are further heightened, for nonverbal clues to immediacy (such as facial expression, eye contact, head nodding, body lean, and gesturing) have vanished. In the absence of these nonverbal clues, clinicians need to recognize that their clinical intuitions on highly sensitive assessments such as determining suicidal intent, dangerousness to others, presence of deceit, and genuine interest in follow-up may be impaired. This impairment does not mean we should avoid tapping our intuitions on these topics; it simply means we should trust them less, once tapped.

Confronted with such difficult clinical challenges, when we are on the phone, we must make our clinical formulations of suicide risk with an increased reliance on analytically processing the information we have garnered. If something does not add up, it is important to continue the call and try to uncover any missing information that might help, as opposed to intuitively thinking, "Well, I think he sounds okay." If one is bothered by the situation, one needs to find out why. This is true in all suicide assessments, including face-to-face ones, but one could argue it is even more true in telephone work, where the lack of nonverbals may hinder our intuition.

Paralanguage becomes critically important in telephone work. You will recall that it includes elements such as tone of voice, loudness of voice, pitch of voice, rhythm and fluency of speech. One of the most important skills, especially if taking a call from a patient in crisis, is learning to *purposely* get a feel for the caller's paralanguage traits early in the interview, especially when they seem to be talking openly and freely. This familiarity with the caller's typical speech characteristics is important, for they may change when the caller is hiding material that is sensitive, such as incest, domestic violence, drinking and drugging behaviors, and suicidal thoughts, behaviors, and intent.

It has also been suggested that problems with speech and language, such as more errors in speech, repeating words and phrases, and taking longer to respond (increased RTL) appear to be indicators of both anxiety and deceit.[90] Good telephone clinicians learn to listen carefully for such changes in the patient's speech.

In addition, hesitancies and silences are almost always useful to note, keeping in mind that they are nonverbal activities that may be multiply determined. A silence before answering a question could be caused by something benign (as with a patient carefully thinking through an answer or perhaps being caught off-guard by a question) to something more troublesome (as when the silence indicates disengagement, hesitancy to share sensitive material, or deceit). At such moments one can gently ask, if the alliance seems reasonable, "You seemed to hesitate a bit before answering that question, what was going through your mind?" When timed well, the answers can be quite revealing.

A brief note on training is in order. To acquire a good handle on assessing the paralanguage clues of patients, I believe it is useful to do role-playing exercises that are done back-to-back. Such back-to-back role-playing better simulates the real world of clinical practice when interacting with the patient over the phone.

Problems Engaging Patients on the Phone

The loss of all nonverbals except paralanguage poses some unique challenges when we are performing phone assessments. The first thing to remember is that the patient is also limited in his or her ability to read our nonverbals. Thus, the patient may place a remarkably high importance to our paralanguage, such as our tone of voice and speed of speech.

Clinicians must become aware of these parameters in their normal interviewing style through supervision, input from fellow trainees, and observation. I think it is very useful to not only be video recorded but to also be audiotaped (or to turn away from a video while listening only to ones voice). If a clinician discovers that his or her tone of voice or speech rate occasionally communicates haste, terseness, disinterest, or a judgmental attitude (when heard in isolation from kinesic and proxemic cues) it is well worth noting.

In everyday face-to-face practice, a clinician's potentially disengaging paralanguage traits may be nicely counterbalanced contextually by other immediacy behaviors, such as smiling warmly, head nodding, and naturalistic gesturing. But when this same clinician interviews over the phone, all of these counterbalances will be missing. Only his or her paralanguage characteristics will remain. *The patient's nonverbal impressions of the interviewer will be made solely on how the interviewer sounds.* If you have a terse voice, then you will probably be viewed as a terse person over a phone. If you speak quickly, you may be viewed as busy or pushy; and so it is for the other paralanguage traits. Naturally, when on the phone one wants to learn to speak in a naturalistic, engaging fashion, attempting to convey a quiet warmth and a genuine concern.

I have come across some clinicians who were very talented at engaging patients in face-to-face interviews, being greatly surprised that they were not perceived as warm on the phone. These trainees possessed great visual immediacy behaviors that powerfully facilitated engagement in a face-to-face context. But their paralanguage traits were merely run-of-the-mill with regard to communicating warmth and empathy. Once spotted in supervision, I have seen such trainees make significant improvements in their paralanguage skills.

In addition, it is important to realize that when we are on the phone, our verbal communicators of empathy can be put to good use. Empathic statements, as well as "empathic grunting" and facilitative phrases (such as "Go on" and "Uh-huh") can, and should, be intentionally increased.

In closing on this topic, there is one caveat to be aware of: humor is great on the phone, but use it carefully. There are many visual nonverbal behaviors that cue people that a statement is to be taken humorously. These visual cues are totally absent over the phone. I do not recommend the use of humor by phone with angry, disengaged, or paranoid patients. In addition, with many people, sarcasm and "kidding comments" may be misinterpreted over the phone, for we communicate that they were meant in jest primarily by visual cues made immediately after such comments. A patient previously unknown to the interviewer may not find such a comment to be funny. Even a more familiar patient can misinterpret such comments when stripped of their visual envelopes.

The Ultimate Nonverbal Challenge: Interviews Done by Chatting, Instant Messaging, and Texting

As stated earlier, it is hoped that programs such as internet-based crisis chat rooms may save many lives by offering people who might not otherwise seek help the opportunity to reach out, because they feel more familiar and/or more comfortable with the anonymity of online communication. Initial responses to such programs with college students and vets appear to be promising in this regard.

While developing such programs, it is important to keep in mind that we are entering uncharted territory that will undoubtedly hold surprises, many of which are related to nonverbal behaviors, or the lack thereof. With chat, instant messaging, texting, and e-mailing, the last vestiges of nonverbal interaction fall by the wayside. Even paralanguage cues are absent. All natural nonverbal clues that are used to determine the patient's engagement, emotions, level of anxiety and agitation, and clinical state are suddenly gone. In the non-clinical world of everyday web communication, an attempt to compensate for the loss of nonverbal interaction has given rise to emoticons and contextual acronyms (e.g., LOL), but they prove to be painfully inadequate in this arena.

There is no doubt in my mind that an interviewer's abilities to rapidly understand and read patients is hampered by this great loss in nonverbal behavior. In addition, even more dramatically than we saw with IATV and telephone interviewing, the interviewer must cautiously assess the accuracy of his or her intuition.

In addition, there is no ability for clinicians to use their own nonverbal behaviors to impact their patients. Kinesic immediacy behaviors, such as head nodding, eye contact, and gesturing are unavailable for use in engaging the patient and building a sense of safety. Powerful proxemic behaviors, such as leaning forward and moving closer, are now empty shells. The clinician's ability to modulate tone of voice and pace of speech are also of no utility.

Keeping in mind that research has shown that roughly 60 to 65% of social meaning is communicated by nonverbals, a lack of nonverbal interaction between patient and clinician can leave interviewers feeling distinctly ill-at-ease. This unpleasant disquietude, created when a clinician is stripped of the use of nonverbal interaction, I like to call the "naked communication effect." Normally, we clothe all of our everyday words with nonverbal communications and activities. Their sudden absence can be surprisingly unsettling. As one might logically suspect, when the interviewer is performing complex assessments that carry critical ramifications (such as suicide assessments), the naked communication effect can be truly unnerving to some clinicians.

Moreover, novel stresses that one might not as easily have anticipated can be experienced by clinicians who are performing such delicate tasks via chat programs. For instance, useful hesitancies in vocal speech and silence, often indicators of patient affect, anxiety, and even deceit are absent, which further amplifies the naked communication effect. But curiously, a new form of "silence" is causing problems.

When chatting online or instant messaging, people don't always answer questions immediately. They can wait minutes, hours, or simply not answer the clinician's question at all by signing off. One can imagine the potential stress of such delays on a clinician. Picture a patient who has communicated to an interviewer that he has pills in his hand. Imagine the psychological strain on the interviewer if the patient did not respond for an hour in response to the following question, "Are you thinking of overdosing right now, are you okay?"

The tendency of some patients to not answer immediately when chatting or texting is creating another unexpected clinical challenge, never before encountered. In traditional telephone crisis work, clinicians stick with the caller until the call is completed and then handle the next crisis call. In chat room crisis work, because some patients may demonstrate many delays before answering, many interviewers must learn to handle multiple assessments simultaneously. If one or more of the "calls" is particularly "dicey" with regard to risk, this need for the interviewer to multiprocess can be quite stressful. It is not everybody's cup of tea.

It should also be kept in mind that the patient's slowness in responding may indicate that the patient is also multitasking. The patient may even be chatting or texting with someone else while being assessed for suicide by the clinician. They can even be asking a friend or friends what they think of the interviewer's responses and suggestions (e.g., "This guy thinks I should go to the emergency room for assessment, what do you think?"). It is truly a new world of interviewing.

One benefit for web interviewers, and it may prove to be a very significant one, is the ability to engage in ongoing contact, via phone or web, with a supervisor during a difficult call. This supervision can even be enhanced by the fact that complex exchanges, or ambiguous statements, occurring earlier in the intervention can be referenced immediately with total accuracy, for they can be pulled up on screen or downloaded.

I believe that research in this arena, which is desperately needed, will skyrocket in the years to come. Some excellent research has already begun to shed some useful light. With regard to instant messaging, Zhou has shown that liars tend to pause more briefly than truth tellers. In addition, they tend to spontaneously correct their text less frequently.[91] Andersen suggests that these results may not merely reflect unconscious processes. They might be the result of conscious manipulation by the sender. The deceitful sender might assume that long pauses or numerous corrections could be perceived as evidence of lying. Consequently the sender intentionally decreases both.[92]

In the final analysis, it is hoped that for those patients presenting with difficult suicide assessments, the web-based interviewer will be able to persuade the patient to meet with a clinician face-to-face. In the presence of a caring and skilled interviewer, an even more effective assessment can then be undertaken, enhanced by the richness of communications provided by the nonverbal behaviors of both participants.

As we wrap up this section, the interested reader can find some excellent resources regarding the use of the web as an interviewing medium. A variety of articles are insightful,[93-99] and the chapter by John and Rita Sommers-Flanagan is a rich resource for further practical tips.[100]

CONCLUSION

In this chapter we have reviewed the basic principles of proxemics, kinesics, and paralanguage. It can readily be seen that these processes are at the very root of effective communication. As such integral parts of human interaction, they remain pivotal in the creation of a successful interview. I can think of no better way to close our chapter than with a statement by Richard Frankel, the noted researcher on the patient–physician relationship. It captures the essence of our chapter admirably: "Most physicians in training spend at least the early part of their careers interacting with their books. The book doesn't care what facial expression you have when you are reading it, but patients care a lot."[101]

In Part I of this book we have reviewed many of the basic principles of both verbal and nonverbal behaviors as they apply to the initial interview. We are now ready, in Part II, to explore the various mental disorders and symptoms that cause the intense suffering of the patients seeking our help. We will learn how to better understand these symptoms and what they mean to both our patients and those who love them. From the painful world of depression and bipolar disorders to the puzzling and frightening world of psychosis, we will hunt for better ways to interview our patients so that they can share their pain and their symptoms more easily. Such an exploration will quickly move us into some of the most complex and fascinating aspects of clinical interviewing.

REFERENCES

1. Hesse H. *Steppenwolf*. Norwalk, CT: The Easton Press; 2005. p. 87.
2. Hall ET. Excerpts from an interview conducted by Carol Travis. *GEO* 1983;**25**(3):12.
3. Burgoon JK. Nonverbal Signals. In: Knapp ML, Miller GR, editors. *Handbook of interpersonal communication*. Beverly Hills, CA: Sage; 1994. p. 229–85.
4. Matsumoto D, Frank M, Hwang H. *Nonverbal communication: science and applications*. 1st ed. Washington, DC: SAGE Publications Inc.; 2012.
5. Ekman P, Friesen WV. Detecting deception from the body or face. *J Pers Soc Psychol* 1974;**29**(3):288–98.
6. Kuhnke E. *Body language for dummies*. Chichester, England: John Wiley & Sons, Inc.; 2007.
7. Ekman P, Friesen WV. 1974. p. 288–98.
8. Bente G, Kramer NC, Eschenburg F. Is there anybody out there? Analyzing the effects of embodiment and nonverbal behavior in avatar-mediated communication. In: Konijn EA, Utz S, Tanis M, Barnes SB, editors. *Mediated interpersonal communication*. New York, NY: Routledge; 2008. p. 131–57.
9. Ekman P, Friesen WV. The repertoire of nonverbal behavior: categories, origins, usage, and coding. *Semiotica* 1969;**1**:49–98.

10. Ekman P. *Emotions revealed: recognizing faces and feelings to improve communication and emotional life.* Revised ed. New York, NY: St Martin's Griffin; 2007.
11. Kuhnke E. 2007. p. 254.
12. Wiener M, Devoe S, Rubinow S, Geller J. 1972. p. 185–214.
13. Edinger JA, Patterson ML. Nonverbal involvement and social control. *Psychol Bull* 1983;**93**(1):30–56.
14. Heine SJ. *Cultural psychology.* New York, NY: W.W. Norton; 2008. p. 35.
15. Morris D. *Manwatching: a field guide to human behavior.* New York, NY: Harry N. Abrams; 1977.
16. Kuhnke E. 2007.
17. Hall ET. *The hidden dimension.* New York, NY: Doubleday; 1966.
18. Watson OM, Graves TD. Quantitative research in proxemic behavior. *Am Anthropol* 1966;**68**:971–85.
19. Sue DW, Sue D. Barrier to effective cross-cultural counseling. *J Couns Psychol* 1977;**24**(5):420–9.
20. Baxter JC. Interpersonal spacing in natural settings. *Sociometry* 1970;**33**:444–56.
21. Wiens AN. The assessment interview. In: Weiner I, editor. *Clinical methods in psychology.* New York, NY: John Wiley; 1976.
22. Uzell D, Horne N. The influence of biological sex, sexuality, and gender role in interpersonal distance. *Brit J Soc Psychol* 2006;**45**:579–97.
23. Knapp ML. *Nonverbal communication in human interaction.* New York, NY: Holt, Rinehart, and Winston; 1972.
24. Birdwhistell ML. *Introduction to kinesis: an annotation system for analysis of body motion and gesture.* Louisville, KY: University of Louisville Press; 1952.
25. Harper RG, Wiens AN, Matarazzo JD. *Nonverbal communication: the state of the art.* New York, NY: John Wiley & Sons Inc.; 1978. p. 123.
26. Scheflen AE. *Body language and social order.* Englewood Cliffs, NJ: Prentice Hall; 1972.
27. Bente G, Kramer NC, Eschenburg F. 2008. p. 136.
28. Grammer K, Honda M, Juette A, Schmitt A. Fuzziness of nonverbal courtship communication unblurred by motion energy detection. *J Pers Soc Psychol* 1999;**77**(3):487–508.
29. Kuhnke E. 2007. p. 254.
30. Freud S. Fragment of an analysis of a case of hysteria. In: Freud S, editor. *Collected papers,* vol. 3. New York, NY: Barri Books; 1959 [originally published in 1925].
31. Arnold E, Boggs K. *Interpersonal relationships: professional communication skills for nurses.* Philadelphia, PA: Elsevier Health Sciences; 2015.
32. Andersen PA. *Nonverbal communications: forms and functions.* 2nd ed. Long Grove, IL: Waveland Press Inc.; 2008. p. 56.
33. Wiens AN. 1976, p. 27.
34. Sue DW, Sue D. 1977. p. 427.
35. Andersen PA. 2008. p. 191–3.
36. Andersen PA. 2008. p. 193–206.
37. Hess EH, Goodwin E. The present state of pupilometrics. In: Janisse MP, editor. *Pupillary dynamics and behavior.* New York, NY: Plenum; 1974. p. 209–46.
38. Ekman P. 2007. p. 215–16.
39. Bente G, Kramer NC, Burg F. 2008. p. 136.
40. Hill D. Non-verbal behavior in mental illness. *Brit J Psychiatry* 1974;**124**(0):221–30.
41. Hill D. 1974. p. 227.
42. Wiens AN. 1976. p. 33.
43. Morris D. 1977. p. 75.
44. Scheflen AE. 1972. p. 46.
45. Morris D. 1977. p. 164.
46. Morris D. 1977. p. 165.
47. Pansa-Henderson M, De L'Horne DJ, Jones IH. Nonverbal behavior as a supplement to psychiatric diagnosis in schizophrenia, depression, and anxiety neurosis. *J Psychiatr Treat Ev* 1982;**43**:489–96.
48. Jones IH, Pansa M. Some nonverbal aspects of depression and schizophrenia during the interview. *J Nerv Ment Dis* 1979;**167**(7):402–9.
49. Pansa-Henderson M, De L'Horne DJ, Jones IH. 1982. p. 495.
50. Jones IH, Pansa M. 1979. p. 402–9.
51. Morris D. 1977. p. 181.
52. Morris D. 1977. p. 109.
53. Morris D. 1977. p. 102.
54. Morris D. 1977. p. 102.
55. Ekman P, Friesen WV. Detecting deception from the body or face. *J Pers Soc Psychol* 1974;**29**(3):288–98.
56. Ekman P. 2007. p. 214–40.
57. Ekman P. 2007. p. 230.
58. Paul Ekman homepage. <http://www.ekmaninternational.com/> [accessed September 2015].

59. Ekman P. *Telling lies: clues to deceit in the marketplace, politics, and marriage.* 3rd ed. New York, NY: W.W. Norton; 2009.
60. Andersen PA. 2008. p. 56.
61. Caso L, Maricchiolo F, Bonaiuto M, et al. The impact of deception and suspicion on different hand movements. *J Nonverbal Behav* 2006;**30**:1–19.
62. Caso L, Vrij A, Mann S, De Leo G. Deceptive responses: the impact of verbal and nonverbal countermeasures. *Legal Criminol Psych* 2006;**11**:99–111.
63. DePaulo BM, Lindsay JL, Malone BE, et al. Cues to deception. *Psychol Bull* 2003;**129**:74–118.
64. DePaulo BM, Stone JI, Lassiter GD. Deceiving and detecting deceit. In: Schlenker B, editor. *The self and social life.* New York, NY: McGraw-Hill; 1985. p. 323–70.
65. Littlepage GE, Pineault MA. Detection of deceptive factual statements from the body and face. *Pers Soc Psychol Bull* 1979;**53**(5):325–8.
66. McClintock CC, Hung RG. Nonverbal indicators of affect and deception in an interview setting. *J Appl Soc Psychol* 1975;**5**:54–67.
67. Kuhnke E. 2007. p. 268.
68. Edinger JA, Patterson ML. 1983. p. 42–3.
69. Kraut RE. Verbal and nonverbal cues in the perception of lying. *J Pers Soc Psychol* 1978;**36**:380–91.
70. Andersen PA. 2008. p. 286.
71. Grinder J, Bandler R. *The structure of magic II.* Palo Alto, CA: Science and Behavior Books; 1976.
72. Kuhnke E. 2007. p. 147, 174–175, 118.
73. Kuhnke E. 2007. p. 163.
74. Scheflen AE. 1972.
75. Scheflen AE. 1972. p. 16.
76. Egan G. *The skilled helper: a problem-management and opportunity-development approach to helping.* 10th ed. Belmont, CA: Brooks/Cole Publishing Company; 2013.
77. Wiens AN. 1976. p. 35.
78. Sue DW, Sue D. 1977. p. 420–9.
79. Morris D. 1977. p. 83.
80. La Crosse MB. Nonverbal behavior and perceived counselor attractiveness and persuasiveness. *J Couns Psychol* 1972;**19**:417–24.
81. Hasse RF, Tepper D. Nonverbal component of empathetic communication. *J Couns Psychol* 1972;**19**:417–24.
82. Morris D. 1977. p. 68.
83. Tardiff K. The violent patient. In: Guggenheim F, Weiner M, editors. *Manual of psychiatric consultation and emergency care.* New York, NY: Jason Aronson; 1984.
84. Morris D. 1977. p. 173.
85. Scheflen AE. 1972 p. 173.
86. Wiens AN. 1976. p. 28.
87. Chayko M. *Portable communities: the social dynamics of online and mobile communication.* Albany, NY: State University of New York Press; 2008.
88. Zur O. *Utilizing interactive tele-video technologies (IATV) to provide telementalhealth, e-counseling, or e-therapy.* Zur Institute, online publication, <www.zurinstitute.com/telehealth_IATV.html> [accessed January 2012].
89. Rambo E. Ethical considerations in the practice of telepsychiatry. *The Carlat Report* 2014;**3**(6):5–8.
90. Andersen PA. 2008. p. 294.
91. Zhou L. An empirical investigation of deception behavior in instant messaging. *IEEE Trans Prof Commun* 2005;**48**:147–59.
92. Andersen PA. 2008. p. 294.
93. Mallen MJ, Vogel DL, Rochlen AB, Day SX. Online counseling: reviewing the literature from a counseling psychology framework. *Couns Psychol* 2005;**33**(6):819–71.
94. Lampe LA. Internet-based therapy: too good to be true? *Aust NZ J Psychiatry* 2011;**45**(4):342–3.
95. Graff CA, Hecker LL. E-therapy: developing an ethical online practice. In: Hecker L, editor. *Ethics and professional issues in couple and family therapy.* New York, NY: Routledge/Taylor & Francis; 2010. p. 243–55.
96. Hanley T. The working alliance in online therapy with young people: preliminary findings. *Brit J Guid Couns* 2009;**37**(3):257–69.
97. Bernard M, Janson F, Flora PK, et al. Videoconference-based physiotherapy and tele-assessment for homebound older adults: a pilot study. *Act Adaptat Aging* 2009;**33**(1):39–48.
98. Yoshino A, Shigemura J, Kobayashi Y, et al. Telepsychiatry: assessment of televideo psychiatric interview reliability with present and next-generation internet infrastructures. *Acta Psychiatr Scand* 2001;**104**(3):223–6.
99. Yuen EK, Goetter EM, Herbert JD, Forman EM. Challenges and opportunities in internet-mediated telemental health. *Prof Psychol Res Pr* 2012;**43**(1):1–8.
100. Sommers-Flanagan J, Sommers-Flanagan R. *Clinical interviewing.* 5th ed. Hoboken, NJ: John Wiley & Sons Inc.; 2014. p. 505–26.
101. Frankel R. <http://thinkexist.com/quotation/most-physicians-in-training-spend-at-least-the/1429925.html> [accessed September 2015].

Part II

The Interview and Psychopathology: From Differential Diagnosis to Understanding

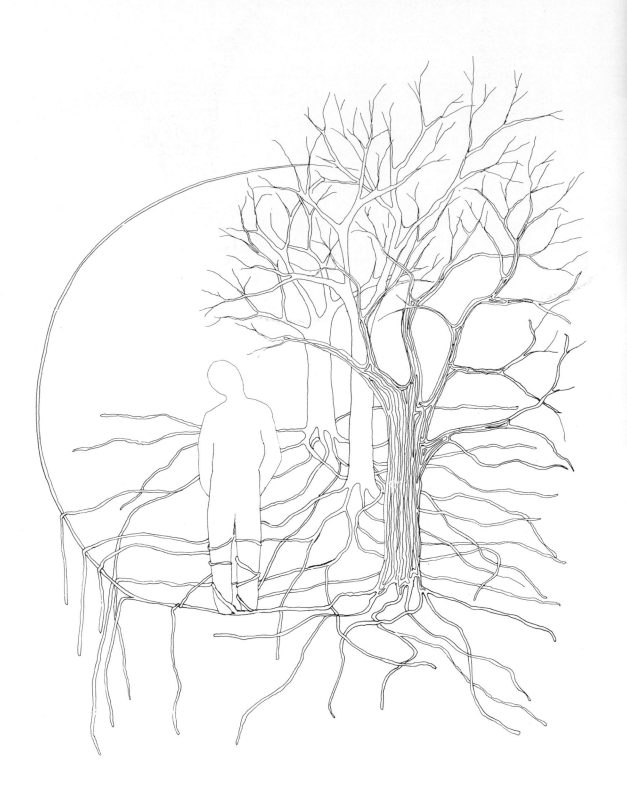

CHAPTER 9

Mood Disorders: How to Sensitively Arrive at a Differential Diagnosis

I wander thro' each charter'd street,
Near where the charter'd Thames does flow
And mark in every face I meet
Marks of weakness, marks of woe.

William Blake
London[1]

INTRODUCTION

In the early 1800s as Blake wandered the drab lanes of London, his eyes met the face of depression at every corner. Depression stalked among merchants, seamen, and prostitutes alike, because depression impolitely ignored the proper boundaries of social class. Today, whether on Fifth Avenue in New York or at a community mental health center in rural Nebraska, mental health professionals encounter faces strongly reminiscent of those that William Blake described centuries ago. As in Blake's time, depression masquerades in many costumes and clinical presentations.

As an illustration of this diversity, I remember working with a woman of about 40, who had been a successful interior designer. In the midst of a severe economic downturn, she found herself jobless. Her confidence and self-esteem were affronted with each passing day. Her belief in herself insidiously weakened as if she were an invalid who decided that there was no hope. Anxiety attacks punctuated her daily routine. Despite her pain she continued her frantic job search, terrified by each job interview. Her days became compacted cells of anxiety neatly delineated by bars of self-doubt.

How different this woman's presentation appears when contrasted with a strikingly white-haired woman I met in North Carolina. Although only 50 years old, this woman's face was branded by thick wrinkles. She had been extremely dependent on her father, a caricature of "Daddy's little girl." Following his death 4 months earlier, she had felt as if her skin had emptied. She was no longer whole. The sight of his face could not comfort her. His touch could not reassure her. She was brought into the hospital on an involuntary commitment. According to the police she had been found wandering a local cemetery with a butcher knife in hand. She related that her father's voice was pleading with her to join him.

These people were obviously experiencing life very differently, yet both were suffering from depressive symptoms. I highlight this diversity of presentation to emphasize that depression, as well as bipolar disorder and other disturbances in mood, are not "things." They are constantly evolving processes. Being processes, mood disorders become a way of living. They are unique for each individual and create damaging effects throughout the wings of each individual's matrix.

Nevertheless, there are many similarities in the presentations of mood disorders that enable the clinician to recognize them despite atypical patterns. This dual capacity of mood disorders to appear both foreign and familiar provides the interviewer with the first inkling that sensitively uncovering mood disorders requires many levels of understanding.

As we have already noted, gifted intentional interviewers integrate the process of differential diagnosis with the continuous art of understanding, incessantly searching for the person beneath the diagnosis. Only when a patient feels the intensity of his or her clinician's drive for such an understanding is it likely that the clinician's help will be accepted, whether it exists in the form of psychotherapy, medication, or other interventions within the patient's matrix.

To this end, in this chapter we will explore interviewing tips and strategies that will allow us to more deftly and sensitively perform a differential diagnosis regarding mood disorders. At the same time it will provide a sound introduction to the psychopathology and symptoms of these disorders.

In addition, by learning how to sensitively explore depressive and manic symptoms, you will be learning interviewing principles and diagnostic strategies that you can generalize to the differential diagnosis of other major psychiatric disorders (such as anxiety disorders, substance abuse disorders, eating disorders, and trauma disorders, which are not included in this book due to size limitations). Indeed, in the video modules at the end of this chapter, you will have an opportunity, if you so choose, to not only watch me utilize the interviewing techniques described in this chapter for exploring a major depressive disorder, but to also watch me utilize the same interviewing techniques to explore other disorders not addressed in this text (such as panic disorder and adult attention-deficit disorder).

This chapter on differential diagnosis will also provide us with yet another bonus of sorts, for as we explore the nuances of the psychopathology and the differential diagnosis of mood disorders, our explorations will bring us face-to-face with several complex everyday interviewing tasks (such as delineating an accurate history of the presenting disorder, taking a past psychiatric history, and uncovering a family history) that are of practical use in all initial assessments. We will also get a chance to address important cross-cultural issues inherent in the understanding of the differential diagnosis of mood disorders.

But before we can begin our exploration of differential diagnosis in this chapter, it is important that we first examine a topic that will be critical for our understanding of all of the diagnostic entities discussed, not only in this chapter but in the rest of Part II of this book. Specifically, we need to briefly address the principles of how diagnostic systems are designed, for how they are designed can create limitations in how effectively you and I can use them.

To understand these practical and clinical limitations – and the design elements that created them – we must focus our attention on some of the principles and terminologies that describe diagnostic design itself. I must admit that when I first encountered these concepts and terms (such as face validity, inter-rater reliability, categorical versus dimensional design) I found them to be somewhat abstract and off-putting. My goal in the following few pages is to create a quite different initial experience for you. I want to provide you with a simple, brief, easily understood, and enjoyable introduction to these pivotal concepts – an introduction that was not available to me. At the same time, I hope to do so with the appropriate level of sophistication that befits a well-trained mental health professional.

In the last analysis, our ability to do differential diagnosis sensitively and effectively will be directly related to the sophistication that we possess regarding the limitations of whatever diagnostic system we have chosen to utilize. A diagnostic system employed without a knowledge of its limitations is a diagnostic system that has the potential to do harm. By the end of the next few pages, I believe we will have the sophisticated knowledge that we need to avoid this trap. We will then be able to effectively use differential diagnosis to help kick-start the healing process.

DIAGNOSTIC SYSTEMS: THERE HAS NEVER BEEN A PERFECT ONE AND THERE NEVER WILL BE

> *The human brain craves understanding. It cannot understand without simplifying, that is, without reducing things to a common element. However, all simplifications are arbitrary and lead us to drift insensibly away from reality.*
>
> Lecomte du Nouy
> Biologist, and author of *Human Destiny*

The Nature of the Dilemma for Front-Line Clinicians

Validity Versus Reliability

At its simplest, the "validity" of a diagnostic system is its ability to describe accurately the person or phenomenon it is delineating. Designers of diagnostic systems feel that highly valid systems are often the most useful in helping patients, for such diagnostic systems accurately capture the symptoms and problems that a patient is experiencing. Such an understanding can provide a sound framework for collaborative treatment planning and intervention.

At first glance, one would think that it would be best to always design a diagnostic system that is maximally valid. But there is a catch. Diagnostic systems that are extremely valid are not necessarily easy to use or even capable of being effectively employed in the real world of clinical practice, because they may require too much time to perform or be so complex as to hinder their acceptance by clinicians.

From this practical perspective, it is essential that a diagnostic system be constructed in such a fashion that different interviewers who interview the same patient will arrive at the same diagnosis, and in a timely fashion, a characteristic called inter-rater "reliability." Without reliability, a diagnostic system is essentially useless in a clinical setting. Without reliability, a single patient could be given radically different diagnoses by different clinicians, either because the clinicians were confused by the too-numerous criteria or were not able to explore the criteria within the tight time constraints of everyday practice. Furthermore, with such difficulties in terms of definitions and diagnoses, clinicians could not effectively communicate with one another and research would also grind to a halt.

An ideal diagnostic system would exhibit extremely high validity and extremely high reliability, while simultaneously being easily completed in an initial interview and easy to learn. The problem lies in the fact that the requirements for validity and reliability are often conflicting and require different approaches. Specifically, they often demand an intentional change in interviewing technique.

Consequently, all diagnostic systems experience a tension between these two desirable traits. The more reliable a system, often the harder it is for it to be valid, and vice versa. An old metaphor may be helpful here: You don't want to miss the forest for the trees. To use this analogy, the tension in designing diagnostic systems is often between gaining accuracy on all the trees (validity) versus simply and quickly identifying the overall nature of the forest (reliability). Truth be told, both are very important, yet neither can be completely maximized in any given diagnostic system.

Thus, whether one is using the DSM-5 (or a future variant) or the ICD-10 (or upcoming ICD-11), one is never using a perfect tool. But the designers of both of these systems have done their best to arrive at a compromise that can help guide collaborative treatment planning with the goal of relieving the greatest amount of pain in our patients in the fastest way possible.

Construct Validity, Face Validity, and Descriptive Essence

Validity, itself, is comprised of subtypes. For instance "construct validity" defines whether a diagnostic system appears to be *constructed* upon previously delineated clinical/design principles that are viewed as being useful by experts and clinicians and logically follow one from the other. A system with high construct validity should adhere to the best evidence base available at the time of development.

"Face validity" describes the degree to which a diagnostic system, or a specific diagnosis within a system, appears "on the face of it" to make sense. Do the diagnostic categories and their criteria fit with how patients with these disorders actually present in the real world of clinical experience?

It is to a special aspect of face validity that I want to now draw our attention, for it has direct ramifications as to whether a diagnostic system will be of immediate use to us during the interview itself. This aspect is a concept I call "descriptive essence." A diagnosis will have high descriptive essence if:

1. As a clinician reviews the diagnostic criteria, the key characteristics of the diagnosis that delineate it from other diagnoses are immediately apparent. (In less technical terms: Do the real-life hallmarks of this disorder jump out at the reader as the diagnostic criteria are scanned?)
2. When an interviewer reads or hears the name of the disorder, the diagnostic label clearly suggests the essence of the disorder. (In less technical terms: Does this diagnostic tag seem to resonate with the symptoms of a typical patient presenting with this disorder?)

From a practical standpoint – and so from the viewpoint of an everyday clinician – descriptive essence is of immense importance. There are a great number of diagnoses and diagnostic criteria in both the DSM-5 and the ICD-10. It is critical that they are as easy to remember as possible. If the criteria seem to fit the fashion in which a clinician pictures people presenting with the diagnosis in question (the diagnosis possesses high descriptive essence), then it is much easier for the interviewer to remember what questions to ask.

Categorical Diagnostic Systems Versus Dimensional Diagnostic Systems

Categorical Diagnostic Systems

In a categorical diagnostic system, the items, phenomena, or behaviors to be classified are placed into discrete categories as one might expect from the name. Thus, the resulting disorders are *qualitatively* different from one another. In the DSM-5, for example, a patient's behaviors and experiences are ultimately classified into discrete diagnostic categories (such as Schizophrenia Spectrum and Other Psychotic Disorders, Bipolar and Related Disorders, Depressive Disorders, Anxiety Disorders, and Personality Disorders).

Each diagnosis within a categorical system contains a set of criteria or an overall cluster of attributes that must be present for the diagnosis to be made. For instance, in the DSM-5 there are nine criteria for satisfying the diagnosis of a major depressive disorder (such as depressed mood, loss of interest or pleasure, and insomnia) of which five or more of the symptoms must be present for the diagnosis to be made.

Generally speaking, with a categorical system, if it is well designed the criteria have excellent descriptive essence, making them relatively easy to remember. Because the criteria are specific and easily recalled, the diagnoses can frequently be made relatively quickly. In addition, the more specific the criteria, the easier it is for different clinicians to arrive at the same diagnosis when interviewing the same patient. Thus, categorical diagnostic systems tend to have relatively high reliability, ease of use, and practicality in everyday clinical situations. If designed well, they will also show good validity. On the down side, it can be hard to design them well, and it is the validity that suffers.

Dimensional Diagnostic Systems

In contrast, dimensional diagnostic systems view phenomena, symptoms, and experiences as not being easily placed into discrete, unrelated categories. Dimensional systems take into account the difficulty of fitting shifting processes such as symptoms and behaviors – that do not have discrete borders – into tightly delineated diagnostic labels (as might occur in a categorical diagnostic system) and that doing so is inherently artificial in nature.

From this perspective, the complexity of a human behavior, personality, and psychopathology cannot be accurately portrayed by fitting it into a box of characteristics *that are present or not present.* Instead, it is more accurate (increased validity) to look at all of the individual behaviors, symptoms, and traits of a person, ascertain which characteristics are present, and subsequently determine how intense and frequent the characteristics may be. Dimensional systems even speculate that characteristics may vary over time and situation.

In a purely dimensional system, it is not so much that a person *has* (meets the criteria for having) such and such a symptom, experience, or trait, it is more that people vary on how much they display symptoms, experiences, and traits *that are shared by most, if not all, people but not to the same degree.* Thus, from the perspective of a classic dimensional system, all people can show anger, but this can range from appropriate anger to inappropriate rage and aggression as seen in an episode of dysphoric mania.

Dimensional systems often require an interviewer to survey a large number of experiences, behaviors, symptoms, and traits in great detail. Often these characteristics are ranked by number (or a severity level) as to how problematic they might be. Generally speaking, the more experiences, behaviors, symptoms, and traits a dimensional system delineates, the more accurate the resulting picture of the person will be (increased validity).

In my opinion, there is no doubt that a well-designed dimensional diagnostic system can result in a highly accurate portrait of a patient, more accurate than a comparable categorical diagnostic system can produce. There is also no doubt that, depending upon the number of characteristics a clinician is expected to explore and the extent to which the interviewer is expected to explore them, a dimensional system can be unwieldy and impractical.

A Pivotal Step Forward in the DSM-5

The DSM-5 remains a diagnostic system that is primarily categorical in nature for ease of use, but it is a system that has added important dimensional qualities. The addition of these dimensional qualities, in my opinion, is one of the most significant advances of the DSM-5 from its predecessor, the DSM-IV-TR. In essence, the DSM-5 has maintained the ease of use of a categorical system and yet has increased validity through the use of judicious dimensional criteria. The DSM-5 even offers an alternative, hybrid categorical/dimensional system (which emphasizes dimensionality) for delineating personality disorders that can be officially used in everyday practice if the clinician prefers a more dimensional approach to personality differential diagnosis.

Dimensional diagnostic characteristics allow one to paint a more individualized picture of a given patient's experiences that better captures both the pain of the patient and the immediate impact of the symptoms on the patient and his or her functioning.

The DSM-5 has accomplished this advance by expanding the "specifiers" that one can add to any specific diagnosis.

For instance, experienced clinicians know all too well that some people afflicted with obsessive–compulsive disorder (OCD) can develop obsessions that truly reach psychotic proportions (i.e., the patient is absolutely convinced that they have dangerous germs all over his or her hands and will die if hand washing is not done). This is, indeed, a very different individual to a patient with OCD who feels his or her fear of germs is not normal and wishes that he or she could stop the incessant hand washing for it is not necessary. In the DSM-IV-TR there was no way to paint this description accurately; in the DSM-5 the clinician can note whether the patient has one of three levels of insight: (1) good or fair, (2) poor, or (3) absent or delusional in nature. Naturally, the presence or absence of insight may have significant implications for both treatment and, equally important, methods for securing the patient's interest in that treatment.

With regard to mood disorders, many specifiers can be utilized. It is beyond the scope of this book to review these in detail, but I urge the reader to become familiar with them, for they can help one to more accurately uncover the phenomena being experienced by the patient and communicate that distress more accurately to fellow clinicians.

By way of example, in the DSM-5, Depressive Disorders have the following specifiers: (1) with anxious distress (including a severity dimension from mild to severe), (2) with mixed features (allows one to include manic symptoms being concurrently experienced by the patient), (3) melancholic features, (4) atypical features, (5) psychotic features, (6) the presence of catatonia, (7) with peripartum onset (if the symptoms emerge during pregnancy or 4 weeks postpartum), (8) seasonal patterns, (9) the presence of remissions, and (10) severity (from mild to severe). In my opinion, the added dimensionality of the DSM-5 has given it an even higher "descriptive essence" than previous DSM systems.

Throughout the chapters on differential diagnosis in Part II of this book, the role of dimensionality will be addressed in those aspects where it can help us to provide better care through better diagnostic acumen. We will soon see that it can play a critical role in achieving a better understanding, recognition, and treatment of bipolar disorder in particular for, I assure you, not all people who have manic episodes experience them in the same fashion.

FIRST STEPS IN THE DIFFERENTIAL DIAGNOSIS OF MOOD DISORDERS

For the sake of discussion, let us assume that the material described in the following clinical presentations has been elicited after roughly the first 40 minutes of an initial interview. As the reader reviews this material, two points will become obvious: (1) all of these people are in significant psychological pain, and (2) all of them appear depressed. The next question facing the clinician is whether all of these people should be diagnosed as having a true major depressive disorder or some other mood disorder such as bipolar disorder or persistent depressive disorder (dysthymia). The following clinical illustrations will focus on the various lines of questioning that an interviewer might use to sort out this sometimes-difficult differential diagnosis.

In the first place, in order to diagnose accurately the clinician needs to be thoroughly familiar with the basic criteria of DSM-5. This familiarization does not mean that the clinician should obsessively memorize hundreds of criteria. On the contrary, this suggests a working knowledge of what material is necessary to clarify the major diagnoses. This diagnostic familiarization allows the clinician to focus on the art of eliciting the necessary material while successfully engaging the interviewee. The establishment of a sound therapeutic alliance, as usual, remains of paramount importance.

The diagnostic criteria for two of the most common depressive mood disorders in the DSM-5 are reviewed below.[2,3] Later in the chapter we will be addressing DSM-5 criteria for other common mood disorders, such as bipolar I disorder, bipolar II disorder, and cyclothymic disorder. The DSM-5 defines major depressive disorder and persistent depressive disorder as shown below.

DSM-5 DIAGNOSTIC CRITERIA FOR MAJOR DEPRESSIVE DISORDER

A. Five (or more) of the following symptoms have been present during the same 2-week period and represent a change from previous functioning; at least one of the symptoms is either (1) depressed mood or (2) loss of interest or pleasure.

Note: Do not include symptoms that are clearly attributable to another medical condition.

1. Depressed mood most of the day, nearly every day, as indicated by either subjective report (e.g., feels sad, empty, hopeless) or observation made by others (e.g., appears tearful). (**Note:** In children and adolescents, can be irritable mood.)
2. Markedly diminished interest or pleasure in all, or almost all, activities most of the day, nearly every day (as indicated by either subjective account or observation).
3. Significant weight loss when not dieting or weight gain (e.g., a change of more than 5% of body weight in a month), or decrease or increase in appetite nearly every day. (**Note:** In children consider failure to make expected weight gain.)
4. Insomnia or hypersomnia nearly every day.
5. Psychomotor agitation or retardation nearly every day (observable by others, not merely subjective feelings of restlessness or being slowed down).
6. Fatigue or loss of energy nearly every day.
7. Feelings of worthlessness or excessive or inappropriate guilt (which may be delusional) nearly every day (either by subjective account or as observed by others).
8. Diminished ability to think or concentrate, or indecisiveness, nearly every day (either by subjective account or as observed by others).
9. Recurrent thoughts of death (not just fear of dying), recurrent suicidal ideation without a specific plan, or a suicide attempt or a specific plan for committing suicide.

B. The symptoms cause clinically significant distress or impairment in social, occupational, or other important areas of functioning.
C. The episode is not attributable to the physiological effects of a substance or to another medical condition.

Note: Criteria A–C represent a major depressive episode.
Note: Responses to a significant loss (e.g., bereavement, financial ruin, losses from a natural disaster, a serious medical illness or disability) may include the feelings of intense sadness, rumination about the loss, insomnia, poor appetite, and weight loss noted in Criterion A, which may resemble a depressive

episode. Although such symptoms may be understandable or considered appropriate to the loss, the presence of a major depressive episode in addition to the normal response to a significant loss should also be carefully considered. This decision inevitably requires the exercise of clinical judgment based on the individual's history and the cultural norms for the expression of distress in the context of loss.

D. The occurrence of the major depressive episode is not better explained by schizoaffective disorder, schizophrenia, schizophreniform disorder, delusional disorder, or other specified and unspecified schizophrenia spectrum and other psychotic disorders.

E. There has never been a manic episode or a hypomanic episode.

Note: This exclusion does not apply if all of the manic-like or hypomanic-like episodes are substance-induced or are attributable to the physiological effects of another medical condition.

DSM-5 DIAGNOSTIC CRITERIA FOR PERSISTENT DEPRESSIVE DISORDER (DYSTHYMIA)

This disorder represents a consolidation of DSM-IV-defined chronic major depressive disorder and dysthymic disorder.

A. Depressed mood for most of the day, for more days than not, as indicated by either subjective account or observation by others, for at least 2 years.

Note: In children and adolescents, mood can be irritable and duration must be at least 1 year.

B. Presence, while depressed, of two (or more) of the following:

1. Poor appetite or overeating.
2. Insomnia or hypersomnia.
3. Low energy or fatigue.
4. Low self-esteem.
5. Poor concentration or difficulty making decisions.
6. Feelings of hopelessness.

C. During the 2-year period (1 year for children or adolescents) of the disturbance, the individual has never been without the symptoms in Criteria A and B for more than 2 months at a time.

D. Criteria for a major depressive disorder may be continuously present for 2 years.

E. There has never been a manic episode or a hypomanic episode, and criteria have never been met for cyclothymic disorder.

F. The disturbance is not better explained by a persistent schizoaffective disorder, schizophrenia, delusional disorder, or other specified or unspecified schizophrenia spectrum and other psychotic disorder.

G. The symptoms are not attributable to the physiological effects of a substance (e.g., a drug of abuse, a medication) or another medical condition (e.g., hypothyroidism).

H. The symptoms cause clinically significant distress or impairment in social, occupational, or other important areas of functioning.

Note: Because the criteria for a major depressive episode include four symptoms that are absent from the symptom list for persistent depressive disorder (dysthymia), a very limited number of individuals will have depressive symptoms that have persisted longer than 2 years but will not meet criteria for persistent depressive disorder. If full criteria for a major depressive episode have been met at some point during the current episode of illness, they should be given a diagnosis of major depressive disorder. Otherwise, a diagnosis of other specified depressive disorder or unspecified depressive disorder is warranted.

For the novice clinician, after reviewing the above criteria, the first step is to ensure that one can readily recall them during the interview itself, a task that can appear a bit daunting at first glance. Cary Gross at Massachusetts General Hospital coined a mnemonic for easily remembering the symptoms of depression, which was popularized by Danny Carlat in his outstanding primer on clinical interviewing.[4] The mnemonic is based upon a well-known Latin abbreviation ("SIG") found on all prescription pads for medication (prescribers write how the medication is to be taken, as with once a day or twice a day directly after the Latin word "SIG"). The idea is that the mnemonic represents a "prescription" for recalling the symptoms of depression. The mnemonic is as follows – **SIG**: Energy **CAPS**ules. I find that for many prescribing clinicians, the acronym is easy to remember because of their familiarity with this abbreviation. Interestingly, for many non-prescribing clinicians it is equally easy to remember for the exact opposite reason, its oddness. See what you think. Each letter represents one of the classic symptoms of a major depression as follows:

Sleep disorder (either increased or decreased)

Interest deficit (anhedonia)

Guilt (worthlessness, hopelessness, regret)

Energy deficit

Concentration deficit

Appetite disorder (either decreased or increased)

Psychomotor retardation or agitation

Suicidality

Let us now proceed to our clinical presentations, for no one can better teach the nuances of depression and bipolar disorder than the people experiencing their destructive power. *Note that, as in the rest of this book, all patient names are fictitious.*

Clinical Presentations and Discussions

Clinical Presentation #1: Mr. Evans

Mr. Evans is a 61-year-old White single man who retired from a prestigious administrative job at the police department 1 year ago. He is accompanied by his fiancée. With her help he hopes to open a bar in the next 6 months if they can get a liquor license. Mr. Evans is well groomed and dressed in a simple flannel work shirt and corduroy trousers. He appears very sad and relates, "It seems strange, but I can't really cry." He speaks softly and slowly, taking a while before answering questions as if the act of thought required immense effort. On occasion, he tries to manage a smile. His eyes study the floor, seldom meeting the eyes of the interviewer. His fiancée chimes in, "Nothing cheers him up. Lord knows, I try. But nothing." Mr. Evans complains of severe depression, of not being able to enjoy anything, sleep disturbance, loss of appetite and libido, and severe loss of energy. In the past 3 weeks he had held a loaded revolver to his head on several occasions. He spontaneously reports seeing no future. Before she left the room, his fiancée, although obviously concerned, appeared to be somewhat irritated and commented to the interviewer. "He just won't help himself no matter how much I try to help him. Now I've got to meet with the Liquor Control Board agent alone next week."

Discussion of Mr. Evans

The Painful World of Anhedonia: Its Role in Diagnosis

Major depressive disorders are common. In any given year in the United States about 7% of the population will meet the criteria for a major depressive disorder. Generally speaking, beginning in adolescence, females experience a 1.5- to 3-fold higher rate of depression. Interestingly, there is also a marked increase in prevalence in adolescence and young adulthood, with 18–29 year olds having a threefold higher rate of major depressive disorder compared to individuals 60 years and older.[5] It is a disorder not to be taken lightly, for up to 15% of patients with this disorder die by suicide.[6]

Mr. Evans demonstrates many of the classic symptoms of a major depression. In the first place, Mr. Evans states clearly that he has a persistently depressed mood, thus fulfilling one of the first two symptoms of criterion A needed for a diagnosis of major depression in the DSM-5. *It is important to note that one does not need to feel "depressed" to fulfill criterion A, because one needs the presence of either Symptom A-1 or Symptom A-2 for making a diagnosis of a major depressive disorder.*

You will recall that Symptom A-2 reads "Markedly diminished interest or pleasure in all, or almost all, activities most of the day, nearly every day." Symptom A-2 is essentially an undeclared definition of anhedonia. The word "anhedonia" is a derivative of the Greek word "hēdonē," referring to pleasure, as also seen in the English word "hedonism." In anhedonia, one demonstrates a decreased ability to experience or to anticipate pleasure or to develop interest. This alteration in the experience of pleasure is a common symptom of depression warranting a careful search in the initial interview.

One of the ways in which to sensitively explore anhedonia is to discover first what types of activities the interviewee enjoys in general, as we saw in our discussion of the "wellness triad" from Chapter 6. Questions such as the following may be fruitful for setting up such an exploration:

a. "What kinds of things do you like to do when you're away from work?"
b. "In the past, have you generally enjoyed your work?"
c. "Do you have any types of hobbies or sports you enjoy?"
d. "Do you enjoy reading or watching TV?"
e. "Do you like surfing the web, looking at YouTube or online gaming or shopping?"
f. "How much time do you spend on social media like Facebook or Twitter?"
g. "In the past, have you enjoyed socializing?"

Often I will spend considerable time exploring these interests further, because they can provide important insights to the clinician about the person's viewpoints and psychological integration, as seen, for instance, in the following:

> **Clin.:** Do you enjoy reading or listening to music?
>
> **Pt.:** I used to enjoy reading quite a bit … sort of odd stuff … (tiny smile) … like St. Augustine, Thomas Aquinas, and other theological books.
>
> **Clin.:** Sounds like pretty heavy reading?
>
> **Pt.:** Yeah, it is. But I used to enjoy it. (pause) … I used to be fairly religious … used to be (said with a trailing off of the voice).

From this dialogue it appears that religious themes may be important issues for this patient, perhaps contributing to his depressive anxiety or perhaps offering potential resources for healing. This questioning has not only laid the groundwork for the exploration of possible anhedonia, but it has also served the dual function of gathering pertinent intrapsychic material about the spiritual wing of the patient's matrix, while further engaging the patient. At this point one may continue the search for anhedonia with questions referring to the groundwork laid above.

a. "Over the past several weeks have you felt like doing these activities?"
b. "Do you find it as enjoyable to do these things as you used to or has there been a change?"
c. "Have you been feeling interested in your hobbies over the past several weeks?"

At times, interpersonal questions can uncover anhedonic complaints, as evidenced by the following:

> **Clin.:** You mentioned your grandchildren. Do you have a good time when you're around them now?
>
> **Pt.:** (sigh) Sort of … Don't get me wrong, I love my grandchildren, but I just can't seem to enjoy anything anymore, even them.

Uncovering the Neurovegetative Symptoms of Depression

What Are the Neurovegetative Symptoms of Depression?

Mr. Evans appears to be suffering from many of the neurovegetative symptoms of depression. Although it is difficult to find a standard definition of neurovegetative symptoms, I view them as symptoms suggesting that basic regulatory physiology has been disturbed. With such a definition in mind, in addition to anhedonia, the neurovegetative symptoms can be listed as follows: change in appetite, change in weight, sleep disturbance, change in energy, change in libido, altered concentration, and retarded or agitated motor activity. Although not always labeled as neurovegetative symptoms, other common physiologic correlates of depression exist including constipation, dry mouth, and cold extremities.

The neurovegetative symptoms are classic hallmarks of a major depressive disorder, fulfilling many of the symptoms in Criterion A for this disorder in the DSM-5. If they are not elicited spontaneously, they should always be actively sought. When done properly, such questioning powerfully engages the interviewee. It shows the interviewee two reassuring characteristics: (1) that the interviewer is interested in the individual as a person whose depression affects every aspect of his or her life, and (2) that the interviewer is knowledgeable, as witnessed by the fact that the questions seem right on the mark.

Tips for Exploring Early Morning Awakening and Other Sleep Disturbances

Sleep disturbance warrants a thorough discussion. Part of the lore of psychiatry has been that people suffering from major depressions often display early morning awakening. The exact frequency of this phenomenon is not entirely clear, although there is good evidence that both feeling worse in the morning and early morning awakening are frequently present in depressive episodes. As we shall see later, in one type of severe depression, melancholic depression, both of these symptoms are quite common and quite severe.

However, in my experience, early morning awakening of a milder, yet still disturbing nature, is common in major depressive disorders of even a mild to moderate severity. The symptom of early morning awakening often has a distinctive phenomenology.

It is not just that patients awaken earlier than they would like. It is that patients feel *as if they are abruptly awakened by* a steady stream of unpleasant worries. They find it extremely hard to shake these frets. Once one fret is gone, a new one appears. The worries are often accompanied by a growing feeling that the prospective problems of the day are insurmountable. It is very difficult to fall back to sleep, despite staying in bed. One of my patients, a physician, elegantly captured the pain as follows:

> *It's literally one worry after another. Frankly, the sensation is almost more like fear than worry. You just know you can't cope with everything you're supposed to do that day. It's simply overwhelming (patient tears up). You just lay there and toss and turn. You absolutely do not want to get up, because then you know that you have to start the day. On the other hand, you're miserable lying there in the bed (he pauses). What a horrible feeling, what a mess. I wouldn't wish it on anyone. And, you know, the really funny thing about it is that it usually gets better as the morning goes on once I get up. I don't know why I just don't make myself get out of the bed because there is no way I'm going to get back to sleep.*

I have found the following questions to be useful in spotting early morning awakening:

"Do you find yourself sort of jolted out of your sleep in the mornings by worries and frets, and you can't get back to sleep?"

"Do you find yourself waking up earlier than you want to and your mind is filled with worries and you just dread getting up, you just don't feel you can face the day?"

Another curious, but logical, aspect of early morning awakening is the patient's frequent puzzlement that when they went to sleep they were feeling better. It feels as if the worries somehow worsened during their sleep.

Other aspects of the patient's sleep cycle are worthy of careful exploration for a variety of reasons. Thorough questioning conveys to the patient that the interviewer is sensitively interested in the day-to-day disturbances of the patient's life caused by the depression. Furthermore, sleep disturbances can also provide early clues to other diagnostic possibilities. For instance, sleep continuity disturbances (e.g., waking up during the night) are common not only in depression, but also in psychosis, drug and alcohol abuse, and in the elderly. Difficulty falling asleep can also be seen in a variety of disturbances, including depression, mania, anxiety disorders, substance use disorders, adjustment disorders, and various psychotic processes.

Besides decreased sleep, one should also search for evidence of increased sleep or a tendency for daytime sleeping. A reversed diurnal pattern of sleep, whereby the patient sleeps during the day and remains awake at night, can be seen in entities such as depression, bipolar disorder, and schizophrenia. By eliciting a detailed sleep history, one may also stumble upon an unsuspected primary sleep disturbance such as sleep apnea, narcolepsy, or nocturnal myoclonus.

Sensitively Asking Patients About Libido

With regard to anhedonia, mention should also be made concerning the investigation of libido. At times interviewers feel shy about asking about libido. Seldom should this present a problem in engaging a patient if approached appropriately. In the first place, the topic should be broached smoothly while in a natural context. For example, if the clinician has been discussing the neurovegetative symptoms at length one might ask:

"It sounds like your depression has really upset your system. Do you think it has also affected your sexual drive?"

Alternatively, if the patient has been talking at length about the disruption of a romantic relationship by depressive symptoms one might query:

"From what you are saying, it sounds as if your depression has been causing a lot of tension between you and your husband. Do you think it has also affected your sexual relationship?"

I would like to add several points about questions concerning libido. I have found many patients relieved to know that decreased libido is a common feature of depression. Consequently, after asking about libido, I might add, "I ask about sexual drive because basic drives such as appetite and sexual desire are commonly decreased by depression." To such a statement, patients sometimes respond with sentiments such as "Thank God. I thought my loss of desire was just another one of my failures."

Another important issue is the tone of voice. If interviewers ask their questions matter-of-factly, without hesitation, it greatly decreases the risk that the patient will feel put off. In a different light, if the patient does react unusually strongly, then one may have incidentally learned something about the patient's views on sex, their body, or on what is proper for them to disclose. Such information is grist for the mill in later sessions.

As a final note, some people confuse sexual drive with actual intercourse. It sometimes helps to clarify this issue with remarks such as "By sexual drive, I mean your interest in having sex, not whether you are actually having it or not." If this point is not clarified, a patient who is not dating or in an intimate relationship may quickly state that libido is absent, "since I'm not seeing anyone," when in actuality a strong libido may be present.

Gracefully Weaving the Neurovegetative Symptoms Into the Interview

Questions dealing with the neurovegetative symptoms should seldom be asked in a checklist fashion with statements such as, "I need to ask a few questions now," or "Let me just go over a few things here." Instead, as we saw demonstrated in Video Module 2.1 and will view again in Video Module 9.1, they should be imperceptibly woven into the fabric of the conversation with appropriately spaced empathic statements – what we referred to in Chapter 4 as a "blended expansion" – as shown below:

Pt.: I don't know how to keep coping with all this strain, what with my hours at work decreasing and now my wife on my back.

Clin.: You're going through some tough times (empathic statement). Is this affecting your sleep at all?

Pt.: Oh my God, yes. I can't sleep at all.

Clin.: Tell me more about it.

Pt.: I'm waking up a couple of times a night. I just toss and turn thinking about Janet and whether she'll leave me. I don't know why she stays, except I think she needs the money.

Clin.: Sounds miserable (empathic statement). How many times do you think you actually wake up?

Pt.: Maybe two or three, it's pretty bad. Sometimes I have a hard time getting back to sleep. I feel horrible in the morning, not rested at all.

Clin.: Roughly what time are you waking up in the morning?

Pt.: Around 5:00 A.M.

Clin.: Do you wake up naturally or are you sort of jolted out of your sleep by worries?

Pt.: Oh no, I feel horrible. I can't get back to sleep no matter how hard I try. I just lay there worrying. It ruins the whole rest of my day.

Clin.: What do you worry about?

Pt.: Oh, basically the job. My boss is really fed up with me. And he probably has a right to be. I suppose that's why he cut my hours. (pauses) … I guess I'm worried he's going to fire me. And then I worry about my marriage, my kids, money, you name it.

Clin.: That's a lot of worries. (said gently)

Pt.: It is. (patient smiles sheepishly) Trust me. It is.

Clin.: It sounds like the mornings are really a rough time for you. Are you having any problems falling asleep too?

Pt.: Not really, and I never really have. Oh, maybe a little bit years ago, but not much even now, just a little.

Clin.: Roughly how long does it take you to fall asleep?

Pt.: Maybe 10, 20 minutes.

Clin.: Well, it sounds like your sleep has been pretty disturbed. I'm wondering whether all the loss of sleep has affected your energy at all?

> **Pt.:** None. Everything is an effort. Just getting up is an effort. Trying to cut the grass is like trying to swim the English Channel. I have no energy, no desire to do anything.
>
> **Clin.:** What about your golf or your Kindle, you said you liked to read a lot?
>
> **Pt.:** Sometimes I get a little satisfaction, but I really just don't enjoy them anymore. I haven't golfed in 4 weeks, and I used to golf three times a week. When I was a young man, I golfed five times a week. I haven't picked up my Kindle in months.
>
> **Clin.:** That must be an upsetting feeling, not wanting to do anything. (empathic exploration)
>
> **Pt.:** Yes it is (pause) … everybody just thinks I'm lazy … who knows. (through his empathic exploration the interviewer has uncovered a pocket of guilt)
>
> **Clin.:** It's not uncommon for people with depression to lose their interest in things, it's not that you're lazy. It's really quite common in depression. (interviewer adeptly assuages the patient's guilt) Sometimes it even affects their appetite. Have you noticed any change in your appetite?
>
> **Pt.:** As a matter of fact, food doesn't taste very good. I only eat two meals a day, and sometimes I don't even eat at all.
>
> **Clin.:** Have you lost any weight?
>
> **Pt.:** A little, I think.
>
> **Clin.:** Are your clothes getting too big or loose?
>
> **Pt.:** Actually, they are. I probably lost at least 10 lbs.
>
> **Clin.:** Over how long a time did it take to lose that weight?
>
> **Pt.:** Oh, about 2 months.
>
> **Clin.:** So your appetite has decreased, your energy is low, and your interest in things has decreased. What about your concentration? [and so on]

In summary, anhedonia and the other neurovegetative symptoms are critical areas to explore when considering any mood syndrome such as a major depressive disorder or persistent depressive disorder (dysthymia). Furthermore, by asking such questions, one can gain a vivid picture of what depression feels like for the interviewee. To the interviewee, the interviewer will appear to be one step closer to understanding.

The Concept of Melancholia

When we look back at the presentation of Mr. Evans, his anhedonia and neurovegetative symptoms appear to be particularly severe. Indeed, he fits a dimensional specifier in the DSM-5 called "with melancholic features."[7] Melancholia is a particularly severe variant of depression that is more frequently seen in an older population. In order to fulfill the criteria for melancholia the patient *must* be experiencing a loss of pleasure in all, or almost all, activities and/or doesn't feel much better, even temporarily, when something good happens, as was reflected by the comment of Mr. Evans' wife that, "Nothing cheers him up. Lord knows, I try. But nothing."

In addition, to warrant the specifier "melancholic" the patient must also have at least three out of six of the specific symptoms described below, the first of which relates to a distinctively unpleasant type of depressed mood. This phenomenologically distinct mood is often experienced as a profound sense of despondency, often to the point of despair.

Sometimes it presents slightly differently, primarily being characterized by either a marked moroseness or a so-called "empty mood."

This "empty mood" consists of an overwhelming sense of no connection with life. Patients have described this to me as if they have "no mood," or make statements such as, "I care about nothing." It is as if the person were an abandoned house, empty of dreams, activity, or light. It can be quite difficult to get the attention of a person experiencing these periods of empty mood. During the interview, you may find the patient looking listlessly ahead or downward, almost as if you were not in the room. In many respects, to the patient, you are not.

The other five criteria symptoms for a melancholic depression include a depression that is worse in the morning, severe early morning awakening (at least 2 hours before usual awakening), marked psychomotor agitation or retardation, significant anorexia or weight loss, and excessive or inappropriate guilt. As mentioned earlier, the tendency for the depression to be decidedly worse in the morning and the presence of a severe form of early morning awakening often go hand-in-hand.

Anxiety: Another Important Dimensional Specifier

Although in older diagnostic systems, anxiety symptoms and depressive symptoms were viewed almost as separate types of phenomena that clustered into two distinct categories of disorder – mood disorders and anxiety disorders – it has become apparent that there is much overlap. Indeed, from a phenomenological viewpoint it could be argued that some so-called depressive symptoms, such as motor agitation and early morning awakening, are experienced by patients as more of an anxious than depressive process. In any case, many people with depression experience anxiety and vice versa.

Whenever one explores depression, it is particularly important, in my opinion, to carefully screen for anxiety. As Jan Fawcett has repeatedly shown in his research, and explicitly warned in his writings, the presence of intense anxiety in depressive states should alert the clinician to the potential for suicide.[8-10] Moreover, patients who are experiencing prolonged and/or intense anxiety coupled with impulsivity – as might appear when manic qualities are also a part of the depressive soup, or as seen in a mixed bipolar disorder – can be particularly prone to suicide. Fawcett emphasizes that the presence of actual panic attacks can significantly raise the risk of suicide.

Once again, the dimensional quality of the DSM-5 gently nudges clinicians to attend to important aspects of clinical care, in this case, the risk of suicide and the role of anxiety in its manifestation in patients presenting with a primary mood disorder. In the DSM-5, the clinician's rating of the dimensional factor of anxiety in a depressed patient (from mild to severe) is not merely a diagnostic nicety; it is a sensitive probe towards a better estimate of suicide risk.

The Role of Substance Abuse in the Differential Diagnoses of Depression

The information from the first 30 minutes of Mr. Evans' interview highlights another important issue. He relates that he hopes to open a bar with his fiancée. Further questioning revealed that Mr. Evans had had moderate problems with drinking in the past, including evidence of both dependence and significant social dysfunction. He has not been drinking for over 1 year. Drinking, drug abuse, and depression often go hand-in-hand. Drinking itself can actually be an organic cause of depression. A variety of pieces of research have indicated strong associations linking alcohol misuse with both depressive and anxious symptoms and disorders.[11]

In most cases, these depressive symptoms clear after detoxification. But depressive symptoms can continue up to 2 months after detoxification, with sleep disturbances lasting as long as 6 months. Consequently, from an assessment perspective, when heavy drinking is reported in an initial interview, the validity of the diagnosis of a major depressive disorder is somewhat suspect and may best be viewed as a tentative diagnosis or a rule-out diagnosis. Many clinicians would wait to see if the depressive symptoms remained robust and present for some weeks after detoxification and sustained abstinence, before considering the diagnosis of depression confirmed. In actuality, depressive symptoms triggered by the alcohol abuse can actually remain for many months after detoxification.

As opposed to being caused by the drinking, the depression may precede the drinking or coincide. In a sense, these patients may be self-medicating with either alcohol or drugs as opposed to antidepressants. A true major depression is more likely if there is clear-cut evidence of depressive symptoms before the onset of sustained drinking. In any case, no survey of depressive symptoms is complete until a thorough drug and alcohol history has been taken, both of current and past use.

Important Data Points When Taking a Past Psychiatric History

Mr. Evans' case underscores another important point. Past psychiatric history may be very valuable. In particular, the following material should be actively elicited:

a. Any past psychiatric diagnoses (if the patient is depressed, carefully search for a past history of depression, mania, or hypomania).
b. Previous hospitalizations (names and dates of hospitalizations).
c. Previous outpatient treatment (including names of mental health professionals).
d. Previous medications (names, dosages, and length of time on medications). I also often ask if the patient liked the drugs, or if he or she experienced side effects.
e. Previous psychotherapy (name of clinician and when). I often ask the patient's opinion of the psychotherapy, as well as a brief description of what he or she did in therapy.
f. Any history of electroconvulsive therapy (ECT).
g. Current psychotherapies (current medications will be elicited in the medical history).
h. Past use of alternative medicine interventions (St. John's wort, acupuncture, meditation) and light therapy.
i. Periods of time when the patient feels that he or she could have benefited from mental health care but did not seek it.

As we have noted before, time limits are tough in contemporary clinical practice. You will often not be able to cover all of these past history points in the initial interview.

Instead, as time permits, the clinician will cover those that seem most important to this particular patient's history. Any past history that is missed can easily be garnered in the next interview or by the clinician to whom the patient is being referred as an outpatient or to inpatient staff.

Mr. Evans has provided an excellent gateway for understanding many of the elements involved in making a differential diagnosis where a major depressive disorder is present. He presents with many of the classic symptoms of a major depressive disorder, indeed, with melancholic features.

In our next chapter we will explore in even more detail the complex phenomenology of depression. We will see how an understanding of this phenomenology will lead us to an array of sophisticated interviewing techniques for uncovering depression and engaging those depressed patients and their families.

But we are not quite done with Mr. Evans, for our diagnostic impression is about to be challenged. If we stop here, it seems that we are at risk of falling into a common and easily sprung diagnostic trap. At this point, let us look at some further, revealing dialogue with Mr. Evans.

Clin.:	Mr. Evans, you've been explaining how very depressed you feel. I'm wondering if there has been a time in your life, even in high school or college or as a young man, or any time for that matter, when you felt just the opposite?
Pt.:	I'm not sure I know what you mean.
Clin.:	Well, has there ever been several days or even weeks when you felt really super energized, didn't feel a need for sleep, and just felt ready to take on the world. It might have even happened right after you were feeling depressed and might have seemed puzzling to you?
Pt.:	(very faint smile) Hmm, yeah, I had some problems once, I was really on the go.
Clin.:	Tell me a little about that time.
Pt.:	I was working real hard and suddenly it all became so easy, at least I thought it was easy. It was when I first had become a police officer. I was really excited about my career. I was really jacked up. It seemed like I just didn't need sleep. I went for days with only a couple of hours of sleep. I was like the Energizer Bunny.
Clin.:	Did you start to speak rapidly or did any of your friends remark that you were talking too fast?
Pt.:	Yeah. The other officers began calling me motor-mouth. At first I thought that was kinda funny. (pauses) … God, it all seems so foreign to me now. I'd give my right arm for one-tenth of that energy right now.
Clin.:	Certainly it would be nice for you to have some of that energy now, but do you think that you might have had too much energy back then?
Pt.:	Oh yeah, things got crazy back then.
Clin.:	How do you mean?
Pt.:	Well I didn't really know what I was doing. I couldn't get anything done well. Oh, I started plenty of stuff, but I didn't finish anything.
Clin.:	Did you start to do anything you were embarrassed about, like spending too much money or giving your money away?

> **Pt.:** Oh yeah, yeah. I did. I wanted to help everybody. I wanted to help the prisoners. That's why I tried to let a couple of them go (pause) … and that's when the Chief called me in and told me I needed a rest, and they put me in a hospital.
>
> **Clin.:** So things got so upsetting you needed a hospital?
>
> **Pt.:** Oh yeah.
>
> **Clin.:** What hospital was that?
>
> **Pt.:** St. Anthony's. It was a tolerable place.
>
> **Clin.:** Have you ever had any other episodes like that one?
>
> **Pt.:** Yeah, one other time but just for a couple of days. I didn't think anything of it.

Spotting Bipolar I Disorder: Traps and Nuances

The above dialogue strongly suggests that Mr. Evans is not suffering from merely an episode of major depressive disorder. Indeed, he is probably best viewed as having bipolar I disorder in a depressed phase. In the United States, patients have been reported as having a 12-month prevalence rate of bipolar I disorder of about 0.6%,[12] with a lifetime risk of dying by suicide at least 15 times that of the general population.[13]

This patient illustrates one of the easiest traps to fall into when interviewing a severely depressed patient. As both the interviewer and the interviewee become empathically absorbed by the depressive symptoms, contextual clues suggesting mania do not appear. Without such clues, the interviewer may forget to ask about current or past manic behavior. The depressed patient may be too preoccupied with depressive thought content, as was the case with Mr. Evans, to spontaneously bring up a manic history unless prompted to do so. Consequently, one should always inquire about manic symptoms with every patient. The DSM-5 criteria for mania and hypomania are as follows.[14]

DSM-5 DIAGNOSTIC CRITERIA FOR MANIA AND HYPOMANIA
MANIC EPISODE

A. A distinct period of abnormally and persistently elevated, expansive, or irritable mood, and abnormally and persistently increased goal-directed activity or energy, lasting at least 1 week and present most of the day, nearly every day (or any duration if hospitalization is necessary).

B. During the period of mood disturbance and increased energy or activity, three (or more) of the following symptoms have persisted (four if the mood is only irritable) are present to a significant degree and represent a noticeable change from usual behavior:

1. Inflated self-esteem or grandiosity.
2. Decreased need for sleep (e.g., feels rested after only 3 hours of sleep).
3. More talkative than usual or pressure to keep talking.
4. Flight of ideas or subjective experience that thoughts are racing.
5. Distractibility (i.e., attention too easily drawn to unimportant or irrelevant external stimuli) as reported or observed.
6. Increase in goal-directed activity (either socially, at work or school, or sexually) or psychomotor agitation (i.e., purposeless non-goal-directed activity).
7. Excessive involvement in pleasurable activities that have a high potential for painful consequences (e.g., engaging in unrestrained buying sprees, sexual indiscretions, or foolish business investments).

MANIC EPISODE—Cont'd

C. The mood disturbance is sufficiently severe to cause marked impairment in social or occupational functioning or to necessitate hospitalization to prevent harm to self or others, or there are psychotic features.

D. The episode is not attributable to the physiological effects of a substance (e.g., a drug of abuse, a medication, other treatment) or to another medical condition.

Note: A full manic episode that emerges during antidepressant treatment (e.g., medication, electroconvulsive therapy) but persists at a fully syndromal level beyond the physiological effect of that treatment is sufficient evidence for a manic episode and, therefore, a bipolar I diagnosis.

Note: Criteria A–D constitute a manic episode. At least one lifetime manic episode is required for the diagnosis of bipolar I disorder.

HYPOMANIC EPISODE

A. A distinct period of abnormality and persistently elevated, expansive, or irritable mood and abnormally and persistently increased activity or energy, lasting at least 4 consecutive days and present most of the day, nearly every day.

B. During the period of mood disturbance and increased energy and activity, three (or more) of the following symptoms (four if the mood is only irritable) have persisted, represent a noticeable change from usual behavior, and have been present to a significant degree:

1. Inflated self-esteem or grandiosity.
2. Decreased need for sleep (e.g., feels rested after only 3 hours of sleep).
3. More talkative than usual or pressure to keep talking.
4. Flight of ideas or subjective experience that thoughts are racing.
5. Distractibility (i.e., attention too easily drawn to unimportant or irrelevant external stimuli) as reported or observed.
6. Increase in goal-directed activity (either socially, at work or school, or sexually) or psychomotor agitation.
7. Excessive involvement in pleasurable activities that have a high potential for painful consequences (e.g., engaging in unrestrained buying sprees, sexual indiscretions, or foolish business investments).

C. The episode is associated with an unequivocal change in functioning that is uncharacteristic of the individual when not symptomatic.

D. The disturbance in mood and the change in functioning are observable by others.

E. The episode is not severe enough to cause marked impairment in social or occupational functioning or to necessitate hospitalization. If there are psychotic features, the episode is, by definition, manic.

F. The episode is not attributable to the physiological effects of a substance (e.g., a drug of abuse, a medication, other treatment) or to another medical condition.

Note: A full hypomanic episode that emerges during antidepressant treatment (e.g., medication, electroconvulsive therapy) but persists at a fully syndromal level beyond the physiological effect of that treatment is sufficient evidence for a hypomanic episode diagnosis. However, caution is indicated so that one or two symptoms (particularly increased irritability, edginess, or agitation following antidepressant use) are not taken as sufficient for diagnosis of a hypomanic episode, nor necessarily indicative of a bipolar diathesis.

Note: Criteria A–F constitute a hypomanic episode. Hypomanic episodes are common in bipolar I disorder but are not required for the diagnosis of bipolar I disorder.

Bipolar I Disorder

Over the years, several different types of bipolar disorder have been delineated. The classic form of bipolar disorder, which Mr. Evans would prove to be suffering from, is now called "type I" in the DSM-5[15] and consists of one or more major depressive episodes with at least one full-blown manic episode at some point in the history *or* a patient who presents *solely* with a single episode of mania (such patients generally will subsequently show depressive episodes, and a lifetime course consisting only of manic episodes is a relative rarity).

In bipolar I disorder, the mean age of onset for the first manic, hypomanic, or depressive episode is around 18 years of age. But earlier-aged adolescents (and some children) may show manic symptoms.[16] Mania can first appear after age 50 as well. (Late-appearing manias should alert the clinician to hunt for disease states related to structural damage to the brain, as with frontal lobe tumors or degenerative processes such as neurocognitive disorders [NCDs] that happen to impact more on behavior, personality, and language – as opposed to the memory deficits that hallmark the more classic presentation of NCDs such as dementias.) Manic episodes tend to come on fairly abruptly, usually over the course of days and can be quite startling and "unexplainable" to both the patient and family members.

I have found, though, that if the patient and family members are questioned carefully, they often describe early warning signs, sometimes unique to a specific patient, of impending mania. These signs may appear over the course of weeks. These early warning signs, if present, can prove to be invaluable in preventing relapse.

I remember a family interview in which I asked everybody in the room if they could think of anything else that warned them that their dad was heading for a manic break. There was a pause. One of the older sons piped up, "Oh yeah," shaking his head from side to side with an almost resigned sense of the inevitable, saying, "That hat with the little Swiss feather. It's a fedora, and, Dad," turning towards his dad, "when you pull that damn hat out of the closet, I book tickets for a quick vacation, because you're gonna be a wild man within 2 weeks." The entire family burst into laughter, including the patient. The "positive fedora sign" would prove to be an invaluable early harbinger of an impending manic episode with Dad.

Manic episodes tend to last for several weeks to several months, although some patients may tend to show significant partial symptoms between episodes. Compared to depressive episodes, they tend to be of shorter duration and, as was the case with onset, they tend to end more abruptly. Roughly 60% of manic episodes immediately precede a major depressive episode.[17] Many patients will show a characteristic style to these switches that can serve as a "fingerprint," helping the patient, family members, and clinicians to better predict upcoming episodes and hopefully prevent them.

Classic Euphoric Mania

In the prototypic manic episode, the patient seems to exhibit the opposite symptom picture from depression, with an elated (euphoric) mood, a grandiose sense of skill and mission, extremely high energy, and little need for sleep (often sleeping only a couple of hours per night and sometimes going for days with next to no sleep). Manic patients are also often hypersexual as well. Indeed, in a euphoric mania the patient's presentation almost seems to resemble a carbon opposite of the neurovegetative symptoms found in withdrawn depression.

Manic patients often exhibit striking changes in speech. They generally demonstrate a fast, pressured, and loud speech, throughout which they often crack jokes and speak on a plethora of barely related topics (thus appearing easily distracted). The term "flight of ideas" – seen as one of the manic criteria in the DSM-5 – refers to a style of speech originating from these manic tendencies. In flight of ideas, the speech is greatly speeded up (as are the patient's thought processes) and *although a logical connection between thoughts is generally maintained*, the connection is at times tenuous. The flow of the speech abruptly shifts from topic to topic, not infrequently triggered by external stimuli, plays on words, or humor.[18] In severe manifestations, the associations are so weak and so fast that the patient's language may appear to be disorganized and incoherent.

When I was writing this section on mania, I had one of the most remarkable synchronous events of my life. In a strange way it would prove to be of immediate value to us in our discussion of mania. I often write in the library of a local college and was stepping out of a study room for a break. At the time of the break, I was trying to decide what patient I wanted to describe in the chapter to illustrate a euphoric mania.

As I opened the door, I was abruptly confronted by a man who had his hand raised as if he was about to knock on the door. He appeared to be in his late 50s, with a rather wildly arranged patch of grey hair sprouting from his balding head. Without my saying anything, he immediately proclaimed, "I just did 15,000 jumping jacks in 30 minutes. It's a world record. I'm heading for Ripley's." Needless to say, I found this greeting a bit odd. But, things were about to get a good deal odder.

As I stepped into the hallway, I saw that Mr. Matthews, as we shall call him, looked a bit winded and was dressed in worn clothes inadequate for the wintry weather. I saw before me a man who was jubilantly pleasant and spoke with great speed and excitement about his recent exploits, of which there were many.

He stood uncomfortably close to me, and as I would gently step away to increase our interpersonal distance, he followed, maintaining his inappropriate closeness. In addition, he had an intense affect with very direct and unyielding eye contact. I must admit that despite the uncomfortableness of our interpersonal spacing, he was rather fun to engage, not unlike encountering Santa Claus on speed.

He gestured with enthusiasm as he commented, "You know, I walked around the Grand Canyon backwards." At which point he proceeded to do his best imitation of a Michael Jackson moonwalk. He quickly added, "I can do a hundred backhand push-ups in a row, want to see?" Before I could say no, he was on the ground doing a perfect set of six backhanded push-ups (I might add, a physical feat that is quite hard to do at any age).

An unwary student stumbled upon us, who Mr. Matthews immediately engaged with; "Hey, you know me, everybody knows me, I give talks at schools all over the country, a greatly admired athlete with college students, right? Frank Lloyd Wright, get it? I build buildings, the best in the business. Watch me as I fall into the waters. Get it? Right?" Mr. Matthews smiled and began laughing. At which point the student dully nodded yes and glanced anxiously at me. For those unfamiliar with Frank Lloyd Wright, he was a highly innovative architect, who happened to build a residence in Western Pennsylvania called "Falling Waters." One cannot find a much better example of a flight of ideas.

Mr. Matthews was demonstrating a classic euphoric manic presentation. His presentation highlights several points not delineated as DSM-5 diagnostic criteria *per se*, but they are subtle phenomenological symptoms and behaviors frequently seen in euphoric manias.

People experiencing a euphoric mania often show disruptions in the acceptable nonverbal rules for conversation, ranging from proxemic to paralanguage abnormalities. They frequently create a profound (and uncomfortable) increase in the sensation of immediacy (see Chapter 8, page 286) caused by their invasion of personal space. This uncomfortable immediacy sensation is exacerbated by the loudness of their voices and the directness of their eye contact. It is sometimes further accentuated by an unpleasant body odor, for during a manic fury, bathing quickly drops to a low rank on the patient's daily "to do" list.

As the above exchange involving Mr. Matthews demonstrates, patients coping with euphoric mania sometimes assume a false familiarity, abruptly engaging bystanders in conversation in which they assume the bystander already possesses information as if they had previously conversed. They often also display what I like to call a "demonstration propensity," as was aptly displayed by Mr. Matthews with both his moonwalking abilities and his ability to perform backhanded push-ups.

With someone whose mania is as advanced as Mr. Matthews, it is easy to spot a mania. But with much earlier manias, these same propensities may show themselves in muted forms that, if recognized by a savvy clinician, can lead to the early detection of a hypomanic or manic episode with resulting interventions that can prevent a tremendous amount of pain. Early intervention with mania can dramatically decrease its impact and ferocity, and may also lessen the number of medications and the sizes of the doses required to reverse the mania.

Before leaving the topic of spotting a euphoric mania, I want to mention a point that at first can appear to be paradoxical. All is not necessarily "rosy" inside the mind of a person displaying a euphoric mania. Besides showing an irritability that can also be seen in depressed patients, those experiencing a euphoric mania often display a peculiarity of affect called "affective lability." A patient experiencing affective lability can move from laughter to tears remarkably easily and sometimes back again in a matter of moments. In addition, euphoric manic patients can become remarkably impulsive, a characteristic of mania that often results in a darker side to the manic break (far from euphoric in nature), including substance abuse, car wrecks, and both violence and suicide.

It is this violent unpredictability that I most want to emphasize to the reader. It is important to realize that even in so-called "euphoric" manias, elements of anger and irritability may lie just below the surface. A state of euphoric mania, as described above with Mr. Matthews, can transform quickly into an angry and hostile state, sometimes prompted by the patient responding to limit setting or an attempt to structure the interview itself. Indeed, when I tried to re-direct Mr. Matthews, saying "Why don't you and I move downstairs to the lobby," he turned on me angrily, snapping "Don't push me buddy. I'm talking to this student right now." He then smiled and continued rambling away to the student.

Especially in an emergency department or on an inpatient unit, be on the alert when interviewing patients with a "happy mania." Be particularly on-guard if the patient is pacing and seems intent on getting his or her way. I have seen such patients turn hostile, and even violent, in a matter of seconds. We will also soon see that manias are often not purely "euphoric," but can come in all forms of mixtures and disguises. But first, Mr. Matthews brings to light another common aspect of manic presentations.

Psychotic Process in Mania

Mr. Matthews also raises one final point regarding bipolar disorder, albeit an important one. His grandiose statements appeared to be delusional in nature. If I had performed a clinical interview pressing him on his insight, I suspect I would have found that they were truly delusional in nature. About 60% of patients with bipolar disorder will show some psychotic symptoms, such as delusions or hallucinations, over their lifetime.

As illustrated by Mr. Matthews, most manic delusions consist of mood-congruent themes such as religious destinies ("I am the Christ") or special powers (as with 15,000 jumping jacks in 30 minutes). The term "mood-congruent" means that the patient's delusional or hallucinatory content seems to fit their immediate mood in a logical sense. Thus mood-congruent delusions in a depressed patient tend to be of a depressed nature (such as guilty concerns, death, self-loathing, etc.). Mood-congruent psychotic process during a manic episode suggests themes of grandiosity, remarkable powers, identifying as an extraordinary historical or religious figure (such as the Christ or Allah). In contrast, when patients have mood-incongruent psychotic process, the hallucinations and delusions do not fit the mood or are unrelated to the patient's mood state, and are possibly bizarre or paranoid in nature.

Mendelson nicely summarizes bipolar psychotic process, adding that about 30 to 40% of manic patients will have mood-incongruent delusions such as being controlled by others. Interestingly, about 25% of patients with bipolar disorder will experience psychotic process during their depressions, a fact often missed by clinicians. This rate is more than four times more frequent than the rate of psychotic process in unipolar depression.[19]

Other psychotic processes, such as auditory hallucinations, are common, especially in mania. Although relatively infrequent, patients have been known to self-mutilate (enucleate their eyes, mutilate their genitalia) or even kill themselves or others in response to command hallucinations during a manic episode. We will study how to effectively uncover such dangerous ideation in our chapters on psychosis. At this point let us return to Mr. Evans.

The Importance of Family Members and Collaborative Sources When Delineating Mania

A subsequent telephone interview with Mr. Evans' quite elderly mother revealed that he had demonstrated many of these classic features in his manic episode, which, in reality, occurred more than 30 years ago. He had been working, as he said, on a police force, but in a very small rural town in Pennsylvania. Over the course of several days he began talking very rapidly. His patrol partner became progressively worried about him, as he regaled him with news of his latest project. He was writing a three-book series on "How Police Officers Need to Be Nicer to People." He had not bathed for over a week and also reported that sleep was for "lower forms of life."

His mother related that both at home and in the police station he was talking constantly and was a veritable one-man comic monologue. His mother commented dryly, "He thought he was hysterically funny. He wasn't." When asked about hypomanic episodes in the past she commented, "I am very proud of him and he has done some wonderful things as a police officer over his life, helped a lot of people; but he was always my most unique child. I used to call him, my little nutball." She also mentioned that when he experienced his one actual manic episode, he had seemed to have problems thinking straight. When asked what this meant, she described him as having problems concentrating and remembering things.

There is one other detail from the interview with Mr. Evans' mother that provides an important lesson for any clinician. At one point she commented, "Did he tell you that he pulled a knife on his dad during that manic break. It's something we didn't tell the police department about." Here was a salient point that Mr. Evans had not shared with me during the interview, nor was his fiancée aware of it.

This telephone interview with Mr. Evans' mother highlights several important clinical points. People will often downplay past episodes of mania. I believe it is natural to do so. Mr. Evans had gone on to have an outstanding career in the police force. Being in an extremely small town, the police chief eventually decided to overlook Mr. Evans' brief manic interlude, eventually allowing him back on the force. It would have been uncomfortable for Mr. Evans, during our interview, to think back on the embarrassing behaviors that were present during his manic episode, especially any violent behaviors. On a conscious level, the behaviors caused by a manic process are often embarrassing (or guilt producing) for patients. To protect the patient from such memories, on an unconscious level, defense mechanisms such as rationalization, repression, and denial may bury the details of a manic episode deep into the unconscious of the patient. Consequently, it is common for past manic episodes to be "sealed over."

In the light of this, it is often important, if one uncovers a hint of history suggesting some hypomanic or manic symptoms in an initial assessment, to interview family members and other collaborative sources that might provide a more accurate picture of the severity of the manic symptoms, as was the case with Mr. Evans' mother. Also keep in mind that both patients and family members often do not spontaneously report hypomanic episodes unless the interviewer specifically asks about them, for the hypomanic symptoms seem so inconsequential compared to the manic or depressed symptoms.

Cognitive Deficits in Mania

Comments by Mr. Evans' mom on his "problems thinking straight" remind us that there is considerable evidence that patients with manias, as well as with depressions, may have specific cognitive deficits not caused simply because they are "wound-up" and having difficulty with attention. The manic process may actually cause cognitive dysfunction.[20–22]

This cognitive dysfunction may persist even when the patients are euthymic (a term indicating normal mood where there is no evidence of depression or mania).[23,24]

If manic patients become seriously sleep deprived, as well as dehydrated and physically exhausted by a manic overdrive that may stretch for weeks, they can present with a delirium accompanied by all of the cognitive dysfunction typical of a delirious state. On very rare occasions, serious cognitive dysfunction and frank confusion can occur as a typical part of a person's manic presentation. I have seen this only one time in my career. It was with a college student with extremely rapid cycling (multiple switches per day). In this patient, both his girlfriend and his parents related that in the hour before his manic episodes, he would sometimes appear slightly confused or cognitively impaired. For instance, one time he seemed confused about how to drive home and was manic half an hour later. In such instances it is important to rule out a seizure disorder, such as partial complex seizures, that could mimic such a presentation, although this patient proved to be seizure free and responded well to lithium.

Differential Diagnosis on Mr. Evans and Summary of Key Interviewing Tips

With regard to Mr. Evans, a summary of his diagnostic formulation seems in order. There was no evidence of a personality disorder upon further interviewing. Concerning any physical disorders, Mr. Evans complained of chronic and painful osteoarthritis in his knees.

Although there is no multiaxial system in the DSM-5, it is a diagnostic system that strongly urges the interviewer to always explore for personality dysfunction and the presence of medical conditions. Consequently, as I mentioned earlier in the book, I find it useful to indicate the presence or absence of these disorders, almost as if Axis II and Axis III from the DSM-IV-TR still existed. By doing so, I remind myself of the importance of always searching for personality dysfunction and for the presence of medical disorders with every patient. This documentation in the electronic health record (EHR) also indicates to future readers of the EHR whether or not the interviewer carefully looked for these disorders. If one carefully looked for a personality disorder and found none, if one does not document this fact clearly in the EHR, as in "none found," the reader of the document will have no idea if the previous clinician even looked for personality dysfunction.

Mr. Evans' formulation might appear as follows:

General Psychiatric Disorders:

Bipolar I disorder, major depressive episode (with melancholia)

Alcohol use disorder (in remission)

Personality Disorders:

None found

Medical Disorders:

Chronic osteoarthritis

Before leaving the discussion of Mr. Evans, some key differential diagnostic points are worth reiterating.

1. A major depressive episode may present without the reporting of a depressed mood. Instead the patient will be experiencing a markedly diminished interest in pleasure in all, or almost all, activities most of the day, nearly every day (anhedonia).
2. Early morning awakening has quite distinctive qualities that can help the interviewer spot it, while simultaneously engaging the patient more effectively. Severe early morning awakening is common in melancholic depressions.
3. Neurovegetative symptoms should be artfully woven into the fabric of the interview via blended expansions and should not be used in a checklist fashion.
4. Alcohol and drug abuse are commonly associated with depression. What may appear as a major depressive episode may actually be primarily related to alcohol or street drugs.
5. When patients present with depression, especially a severe episode, it is easy for the interviewer to forget to ask about manic or hypomanic symptoms, yet it is imperative to do so.
6. Past manic and hypomanic episodes may not be spontaneously reported and should always be elicited.
7. It is both natural and common for patients to "seal over" past manic symptoms because they are embarrassed by them or unconscious defense mechanisms have hidden them. In such instances, family members may provide more accurate information.
8. Do not be lulled by the pleasant interactions of a person with a euphoric mania. People experiencing the euphoria of mania can quickly become irritated and angry, at which point the interviewer should be on the lookout for potential violence.

Clinical Presentation #2: Danny Ramirez

Danny is an 18-year-old high school senior, a second generation Latino, whose dad is the principal of the local middle school. Danny has always been an excellent student and is active in community service. Of his many accomplishments, he is proudest of his being part of an environmental group that helped to revitalize a park area for the inner city, a project that received note in the official record of the House of Representatives in his home state. Throughout his life he has always enjoyed people and has been fascinated by various aspects of life, from a boyhood crush on Shakira to computer programming as an adolescent (although he still thinks Shakira is hot). At 8 years old, he developed severe OCD. His mother commented, "He's always been a really intense kid, I just wish he didn't take things so seriously." For many years he experienced what were believed to be reactive depressive symptoms in relation to the great difficulties caused by his OCD. But in high school, the depressive symptoms became much more striking. His angst became so great that his therapist became concerned about suicide. He cried frequently, reported problems concentrating and getting to sleep. Appetite was mildly decreased and mood reported as, "I'm always depressed. Life is shit." In addition, he was very irritable and bitterly angry at the world. His personality became much "darker" throughout high school, with three episodes of superficially cutting his wrists. Despite a very good relationship with his parents, he could become hostile and dramatic with them. One time when asked about having just scratched his wrists by his parents, Danny startled his parents by yelling loudly and angrily, "I just wanted to see my blood, I'm in so much pain!" The above information has just been elicited by a psychiatric consultant at the request of Danny's therapist (who feels he should be started on an antidepressant).

Discussion of Danny Ramirez

Bipolar I Disorder, Mixed Presentation

History Repeats Itself: An Evolving Diagnosis

Before discussing Danny's presentation, it is useful to review, from a historical perspective, a type of bipolar disorder we have not yet encountered – a mixed bipolar presentation. Historically, it is interesting to note that according to the DSM-IV-TR, to meet the criteria for a mixed bipolar disorder a patient needed to exhibit, for at least a week's duration, the *required* diagnostic criteria for both a mania and a depression *simultaneously*.

The first time I encountered this phenomenon, I was stunned by its apparent oddness. The patient, an X-ray technician, was in his mid-30s. He had a scraggly beard and a pair of wild eyes. He could barely sit still. He kept leaning forward as if about ready to bolt from his chair. His speech was extremely rapid and pressured with a tangential quality, suggesting mania. Yet the content of his speech was markedly depressive, with guilty ruminations, self-derogatory exclamations, and suicidal ideation. Within a split second his eyes would fill with tears, but just as quickly his face would transform into laughter. Such incongruities of behavior, affect, and thought content should alert the interviewer to a possible mixed state. According to the DSM-IV-TR, during a mixed presentation individuals often experience rapidly alternating moods (sadness, irritability, euphoria). Such patients can also experience agitation, irritability, anger, insomnia and appetite dysregulation, and may show psychotic and/or suicidal thinking.[25]

All of these traits are, indeed, characteristic of mixed bipolar states. But the DSM-IV-TR had a major problem with regard to its criteria requirements for a mixed bipolar disorder: It was the fact that its supposedly "prototypic picture" or "common presentation" of a mixed bipolar disorder was neither prototypic nor common. Although patients certainly can present with episodes in which they simultaneously demonstrate the criteria meeting both a depressive episode and a manic episode, in my entire career, I have only ever seen one patient who met the criteria for *both simultaneously* – our X-ray technician, above.

However, partial mixed states, in which patients show mixtures of depressive and manic symptoms in varying numbers and combinations, appear to be relatively common presentations.[26-30] Indeed, Goodwin and Redfield, in a recent edition of their classic text on bipolar disorder, state that research data suggests that, "… using broader criteria for mixed states, incorporating the clinical concept of dysphoric mania and perhaps also agitated depression, in patients with bipolar disorder, would result in more than 50% of episodes in bipolar disorder being diagnosed as mixed states."[31]

In this regard, the ubiquitous nature of mixed bipolar states suggests that the depiction of depression and mania as being polar opposites may not be as clear-cut as was once thought. Indeed, mania and depression may not represent opposite categorical entities. Instead, they may be better conceptualized as being part of a continuum.

The concept of mixed bipolar states receives support not only from recent research findings, but also from a most curious source – the past. In fact, it is probably inaccurate to state that modern psychiatry is discovering mixed bipolar states. In actuality, modern psychiatry, as suggested by Goodwin and Redfield, as well as others, is more accurately described as re-discovering the concept of mixed bipolar states.

In the late 1800s and early 1900s, these states were well defined by European psychiatrists, who were interested in both phenomenology and descriptive psychopathology. Emil Kraepelin, one of the greatest of the descriptive psychiatrists, devoted an entire chapter to mixed bipolar states in his *Lectures on Clinical Psychiatry*,[32] and he talks of "depressive or anxious mania" and "excited depressions" in his book *Manic-Depressive Insanity and Paranoia*.[33] Indeed, in 1899, Kraepelin viewed mixed states as the most common type of presentation of bipolar illness and carefully delineated six distinctive mixed states.[34] And Kraepelin was far from alone.

The great Eugen Bleuler, who for 25 years was a professor at the University of Zurich and Director of the famed Cantonial Hospital at Burghölzli, found that mixed states can present as unique, stable, and particularly destructive conditions.[35] His observations on the tendency of mixed bipolar states to have more severe presentations has been proven to be remarkably on the mark by more recent research. As early as 1882, Wilhelm Griesinger, writing from the University of Berlin, described a specific mixed state – "melancholia with destructive tendencies" – that, as we shall soon see, seems to capture the very essence of what is now sometimes called a dysphoric mania.[36]

The concept of mixed bipolar states is not merely a fascinating novelty of modern research or a quaint finding of distant phenomenological inquiry, it has major implications for contemporary intervention and healing. Patients that are showing a mixed bipolar presentation, who are quite depressed but also have several manic symptoms (but not enough to meet the criteria for a *full* mania – as would have been necessary for the diagnosis of a mixed bipolar disorder in the DSM-IV-TR system), are in my opinion fairly common. In the DSM-IV-TR, their bipolarity would often have been unrecognized, and they would have been misdiagnosed as having agitated depressions.

Consequently, I suspect that in the past several decades, many of these patients who might have benefited from mood stabilizers (such as lithium or Depakote) did not receive them. Moreover, many of them may have worsened when given antidepressants (as this can sometimes unleash manic symptoms, as we shall discuss later in this chapter), some with devastating results. It was up to the DSM-5 contributors to change the fashion in which clinicians conceptualized bipolar process so that these errors in treatment could be avoided. It was the concept of dimensionality that once again proved to be the key.

A Practical Solution From the DSM-5

In contrast to the DSM-IV-TR, the DSM-5 does not make it necessary to meet the criteria for both a mania and a depressive episode simultaneously in order to make the diagnosis of a mixed bipolar disorder. Keeping in mind recent research findings, as well as recognizing the value of historical descriptive psychopathology, the designers of the DSM-5 have created a system that allows one to more accurately describe and recognize people coping with mixed bipolar states. You will notice in the following DSM-5 descriptions that once a patient has met the criteria for either a depressive episode or a mania, he or she only needs three criteria of the opposite state in order to be viewed as having a mixed state. This flexibility is much more in tune with the reality of mixed presentations, hopefully allowing clinicians to make better treatment decisions.[37]

DSM-5 DIAGNOSTIC CRITERIA FOR MANIC OR HYPOMANIC EPISODE, WITH MIXED FEATURES

A. Full criteria are met for a manic episode or hypomanic episode, and at least three of the following symptoms are present during the majority of days of the current or most recent episode of mania or hypomania:

1. Prominent dysphoria or depressed mood as indicated by either subjective report (e.g., feels sad or empty) or observation made by others (e.g., appears tearful).

2. Diminished interest or pleasure in all, or almost all, activities (as indicated by either subjective account or observation made by others).

3. Psychomotor retardation nearly every day (observable by others; not merely subjective feelings of being slowed down).

4. Fatigue or loss of energy.

5. Feelings of worthlessness or excessive or inappropriate guilt (not merely self-reproach or guilt about being sick).

6. Recurrent thoughts of death (not just fear of dying), recurrent suicidal ideation without a specific plan, or a suicide attempt or a specific plan for committing suicide.

B. Mixed symptoms are observable by others and represent a change from the person's usual behavior.

C. For individuals whose symptoms meet full episode criteria for both mania and depression simultaneously, the diagnosis should be manic episode, with mixed features, due to the marked impairment and clinical severity of full mania.

D. The mixed symptoms are not attributable to the physiological effects of a substance (e.g., a drug of abuse, a medication, other treatment).

Reprinted with permission from the *Diagnostic and Statistical Manual of Mental Disorders, Fifth Edition*, (Copyright ©2013). American Psychiatric Association. All Rights Reserved.

DSM-5 DIAGNOSTIC CRITERIA FOR DEPRESSIVE EPISODE, WITH MIXED FEATURES

A. Full criteria are met for a major depressive episode, and at least three of the following manic/hypomanic symptoms are present during the majority of days of the current or most recent episode of depression:

1. Elevated, expansive mood.

2. Inflated self-esteem or grandiosity.

Continued

DSM-5 DIAGNOSTIC CRITERIA FOR DEPRESSIVE EPISODE, WITH MIXED FEATURES—Cont'd

3. More talkative than usual or pressure to keep talking.
4. Flight of ideas or subjective experience that thoughts are racing.
5. Increase in energy or goal-directed activity (either socially, at work or school, or sexually).
6. Increased or excessive involvement in activities that have a high potential for painful consequences (e.g., engaging in unrestrained buying sprees, sexual indiscretions, or foolish business investments).
7. Decreased need for sleep (feeling rested despite sleeping less than usual; to be contrasted with insomnia).

B. Mixed symptoms are observable by others and represent a change from the person's usual behavior.
C. For individuals whose symptoms meet full episode criteria for both mania and depression simultaneously, the diagnosis should be manic episode, with mixed features.
D. The mixed symptoms are not attributable to the physiological effects of a substance (e.g., a drug of abuse, a medication, or other treatment).

Note: Mixed features associated with a major depressive episode have been found to be a significant risk factor for the development of bipolar I or bipolar II disorder. As a result, it is clinically useful to note the presence of this specifier for treatment planning and monitoring of response to treatment.

Note that when making these diagnoses, the DSM-5 also allows you to add the dimension of anxiety as a specifier. I believe this added dimensional flexibility of the DSM-5 is important, for many mixed bipolar states, in my opinion, also have significant anxiety components. Using the specifiers for mixed states and anxious distress, clinicians can often paint a more valid picture of the patient's unique combination of symptoms when experiencing mixed bipolar process. There are as many types of mixed bipolar states as there are combinations of these depressive, manic, and anxious symptoms. Armed with a diagnostic system (the DSM-5) that allows one to recognize the unique qualities of each person's experience of bipolarity, we can now take a more careful look at Danny's presentation.

"Dysphoric Mania": One Type of Mixed Bipolar Disorder
Differentiating a Dysphoric Mania From an Agitated Depression

Danny's presentation is instructive for several reasons. As diagnostic systems such as the DSM-5 evolve and are implemented, it is hoped that the improved degree of understanding provided by the dimensional qualities of the system may allow us to uncover new categories of illness that can be more quickly spotted. In a paradoxical sense, dimensional systems sometimes help to ferret out hidden categorical entities. Danny may well represent one of these advances.

For years there has been debate as to whether or not one of the mixed bipolar states may be common enough (and demonstrate enough consistency of symptom pattern) to warrant a separate sub-category within the diagnosis of mixed bipolar disorder, in a similar sense that we now can specify some major depressive disorders as being "melancholic" in nature. As noted previously, early phenomenologists seemed to be aware of a style of mania that seemed to be in contrast to "euphoric mania." This type of mixed state seems to fit fairly closely to what in today's literature is sometimes referred to as a "dysphoric mania."

The issue remains debated. I personally agree with authors such as Strakowski and colleagues that one must be careful in creating new categories until appropriate research has been undertaken to show their validity, reliability, and usefulness.[38] But it is my hope that the dimensional advances of the DSM-5 will allow us to eventually clarify the issue. Danny may very well represent this particular type of mixed bipolar state.

Dysphoric mania is a state that I believe will eventually prove to have validity as a specifier, and I also believe it has potentially major therapeutic implications when uncovered during an interview. It is worth spending some time understanding its nuances and its implications for clinical interviewing.

If you will recall, Danny was 18 years old. He was presenting with a severe depression that was of concern to his therapist because of the risk of suicide. The therapist, who was quite skilled and had been seeing Danny for his depression and his OCD for several years, was hoping that Danny might be prescribed an antidepressant. The therapist felt that Danny had been given an adequate trial of psychotherapy (with a good therapeutic alliance) but it had not resulted in adequate relief. Indeed, the depression was intensifying and serious suicidal ideation was being expressed. Danny's therapist had commented to the consultant that, "Danny's pain is palpable when he is in my office. In fact, it's so intense it scares me. This kid is really hurting. I am worried he will kill himself." You will also recall that Danny had become somewhat dramatic in his behaviors, with several instances of self-cutting and comments to his parents like, "I just wanted to see my own blood!"

With a patient like Danny, who is clearly seriously depressed, one diagnosis that can be confused with a mixed bipolar state, such as a dysphoric mania, is an agitated depression (people with agitated depressions often report their thoughts to be racing and show marked pacing and irritability). Off the bat, one factor that helps with this differentiation is the simple fact that agitated depressions are more common in the elderly and significantly less common in adolescents and young adults.

Moreover, I believe that future phenomenological research will show that there are subtle, yet significant, differences in how the depression feels to patients experiencing a dysphoric manic state in contrast to patients experiencing an agitated depression. Agitated depressions often manifest with a striking overlay of anxiety and fretting. Whether the patient is worrying about mundane concerns, such as finances, business affairs or illnesses (common in the agitated depressions of the elderly), or more unusual material bordering upon, or moving into, the psychotic realm, as with delusional fears of disease and death, many people with agitated depressions appear to be overwhelmed by their worries. The result is an unpleasant sensation of *helplessness*. Consequently they often appear to be lost in a wave of agitated disorganization, almost paralyzed by their fears.

Patients experiencing dysphoric manias also have a high degree of anxiety. But, in contrast to people experiencing an agitated depression, I have found that individuals with dysphoric manias do not tend to feel, or look, as overwhelmed or helpless. Instead, they often report a sense of being driven to do something, almost anything, to fix their problems. Rather than presenting as helpless, they appear driven to action. *Curiously, they are overwhelmed, not by their anxieties, but by their need to take action on their anxieties.* I find this to be a distinctive sensation in manias, including mixed states such as dysphoric manias. Careful interviewing will uncover that it is reflected both in an intensity to the patient's affect and in the intensity with which the patient describes his or her *need* to act. It is one of the reasons that manic patients can quickly turn angry if they perceive that their needs are being thwarted by a clinician, even over something as apparently unimportant as the need to have a smoke.

As we will see with Danny, this compelling drive to act sometimes feels foreign to the patient (as if an unfamiliar part of themselves is pushing them to act). This manic sense of being driven by their urges can also be reflected in the suicidal ideation of these patients. For example, Danny commented later in his interview, "I don't really want to kill myself, but sometimes I almost feel like I have to, like something inside me is pushing me to do it." This sense of being driven to act on urges, from gambling and frantic buying to suicide and violence towards others, is typical of manic states including mixed states such as dysphoric manias; and I have personally found it to be atypical of agitated depressions.

If a clinician suspects the presence of a dysphoric mania, the following three questions can be of use in no particular order:

1. "Do you have any ideas of how to solve your problems?" (Although a patient with a dysphoric mania may not have decided upon the solution, they often have quite specific ideas for a possible plan or plans of action. People coping with agitated depressions often appear befuddled and/or irritated by this question.)
2. "Do you feel like you need to do something about this problem and you need to do something now?"
3. "Are you feeling sort of driven to do something to solve this problem, almost like you're going to need to do something about it even if you don't feel it's smart to do so?"

I have chosen Danny as our illustration of a specific type of presentation for a mixed bipolar state (dysphoric mania), because I feel that dysphoric manias are frequently missed in late adolescents and young adults, where they appear to be more common. In my opinion, missing this diagnosis can result in great and unnecessary pain. The question is: why are they so easily missed?

One of the reasons these dysphoric manias are misdiagnosed as agitated depressions is that some clinicians are unfamiliar with mixed presentations, an unfamiliarity re-enforced by the use of the DSM-IV-TR (which had an extremely narrow view of mixed bipolar states, as discussed earlier). Moreover, the intensity and vocalization by the patients of their depressive pain, as we will see below, is extremely striking. The patients will often spontaneously make comments to the clinician such as, "I'm extremely depressed. I'm depressed all the time. I hate life." Because the pain of their depression is so palpable, it is easy for the clinician to think of nothing but depression as a diagnostic possibility.

Another reason that these states can be easily missed is the fact that most of the classic manic symptoms may not be present, and those that are present tend to be of the dysphoric type, as opposed to the more classic picture of a manic patient appearing euphoric and grandiose. Danny's presentation reflects this potentially confusing picture. It is a camouflage of a sort, in which the mania fades into the depressive overlay, and it can lead even an experienced clinician to miss the presence of a mixed bipolar state. Let's see it at play with Danny.

Danny was experiencing his thoughts as being intensely speeded up at times and pressured, as is typical with a mania; but, curiously, according to both his therapist and his parents, Danny only infrequently showed rapid or pressured speech and it was of a mild nature. Phenomenologically, I have found that patients with dysphoric manias tend to find their internal pressure of thought (often filled with disturbing and dark images) to be unpleasant. Indeed, they often feel an intense desire to get away from it somehow. In contrast, I have found people experiencing an euphoric mania to frequently find their accelerated thinking to be exciting and creative. They feel no need to stop it and often make comments such as, "My thinking has never been so clear!"

Danny also did not move particularly quickly, nor was he prone to pacing (both of which, if present, might prompt a clinician to look for mania). He showed no flight of ideas, distractibility, excessive involvement in pleasurable activities (although he had a mild hypersexuality), or inflated self-esteem or grandiosity (as we saw in the euphoric mania exhibited by Mr. Matthews regarding his moonwalk around the Grand Canyon). Indeed, Danny was pessimistic of his future prospects.

He also reported a mild, but significant, tendency to stay up later than normal for him. At its most extreme, his parents once saw him doing pull-ups outside on a tree limb because he lacked a pull-up bar in the house. Not particularly odd until one hears the fact that it was being done at midnight! Thus Danny showed evidence of manic overdrive but he did not show the progressive tendency to stay up later and later, as is commonly seen in classic manias. At no point did he show any euphoria or increased happiness. The question is, Are there symptoms that could tip-off an interviewer to look for a mixed bipolar disorder in a patient who presents primarily complaining of severe depressive angst as was the case with Danny?

Three Practical Tips for Spotting a Dysphoric Mania. Let's take a look at three phenomenological factors that might prompt a clinician to more aggressively search for a dysphoric mania despite a depressive camouflage: (1) the prominent presence of anger, (2) the intensity of the patient's depressive angst, and (3) a discordance between the severity of patient's angst and the relative mildness of the patient's neurovegetative symptoms.

Regarding our first tip, one thing that the consulting psychiatrist noted quickly from the history, supported by both Danny and his parents, was the striking amount of anger Danny was experiencing. It was broad-based in nature, ranging from feelings of betrayal with friends to contempt for the world at large in response to current events. He had always socialized well with people and had maintained good friendships, but throughout high school his friendships, both male and female, were intense affairs with stormy moments. He had always been extremely conscientious (an "A" student, with great conduct) and had experienced a good relationship with his parents, sharing many of his thoughts and pains. As with his attitude towards his friends, his attitude towards his parents had become dismissive and contentious. The intensity of the anger felt during a dysphoric mania can be quite frightening and, indeed, these patients can be prone to both planned and impulsive violence.

The following questions may be of help here:

1. "Tell me a little bit more about your anger and who you are angry at?"
2. "How often in a day do you feel irritated or angered by the things people do?" (During a dysphoric manic episode, patients often feel irritated or angry for much of the day, with this angry overtone *being more prominent to them than their depressive feelings*.)
3. "Do you think the world is fair?" (They can look aghast at how stupid this question is, for, to them, it is obvious that the world is not fair and you may hear a diatribe making this point.)

There is one other aspect of the anger that patients with dysphoric manias experience to which I would like to draw your attention. For a moment, let us return to the historically rich clinical literature of descriptive psychiatry and phenomenology. In this regard, the words of Wilhelm Griesinger, written in 1882, can provide insights that remain remarkably useful for us in our everyday clinical work over 130 years later.[39] Griesinger, in describing a condition that he called "melancholia with destructive tendencies" – which today I think we would diagnose as a dysphoric mania – elegantly captures the patient's brooding anger, which can be pregnant with violence towards self or others:

> *In melancholia this emotional state of uneasiness, of anxiety, and especially of mental suffering, give rise to certain impulses … which always assume a negative, gloomy, hostile and destructive character. The negative ideas and feelings … may be directed either against the individual himself, against other persons, or finally against inanimate objects.*

When further describing the emergence of the patient's anger and hostility, I believe Griesinger captures a particularly useful phenomenological quality that characterizes the anger experienced by patients during a dysphoric mania:

> *In such cases we often see developed a feeling of bitter animosity towards the world, which becomes to such individuals perfectly hateful, gloomy, and fearful; and there frequently arise the impulses to commit these indeterminate acts, by which the individual thinks to repay the world, in some splendid crime, for all these griefs and imaginary evils, as well as all those painful impressions, the cause of which he is ever seeking, not in himself, but in the outer world.*

I believe that Griesinger is describing the type of rage that can explode behaviorally into violence towards loved ones or mass shootings in a Colorado movie theater or on a college campus. Note well that the *predominant* focus of the patient with a dysphoric mania on thoughts *directed towards the outer world* (as well as a desire to interact with that outer world) is, in my opinion, generally different to patients suffering from an agitated unipolar depression. *Although there can definitely be anger and intermittent focus on the outer world in unipolar depression, typically the principal focus is more consistently inwards upon oneself,* upon topics such as one's inadequacies, feeling overwhelmed, feeling guilt, somatic preoccupations, and withdrawal from the harshness of the world, even when feeling agitated.

This distinction, which can be readily apparent by merely recognizing the amount of time your patient spends talking angrily about specific people, the culture at large, and various "wrongs in the world," can be a useful indicator that the interviewer is sitting with an adolescent or young adult experiencing a dysphoric mania not an agitated depression. Such was the case with Danny, where the angry darkness of his worldview revealed itself in the consultant's interview, and was verified as being "really striking" by Danny's therapist. "This kid is a great kid. I've known him for several years, but something is really wrong here. I mean really wrong." At one point, Danny told the interviewer, "The world's a horrible place. It disgusts me. There's no reason for anyone to really go on living is there?"

With a patient like Danny, it can be productive to explore the patient's predilections on the web as well as his or her fantasies, for the patient's dark preoccupations often will reveal themselves. Questions such as the following may be of use:

1. "What types websites do you like to go to?" (Be on the lookout for websites focused upon anger at the culture, violence, and suicide.)
2. "How often do you have images of violence?"
3. "Do you ever picture yourself doing something violent?"

If psychosis ensues, the risk of danger to self and others suggests that an increased search for dangerous ideation is in order. Psychotic self-mutilation as a freestanding phenomenon, or in response to command hallucinations, can occur. Fortunately, at this point, Danny did not show thoughts of violence or evidence of psychotic process despite his dark musings.

Let us now move to our second tip for spotting a dysphoric mania – the intensity of the patient's depressive angst. If you will recall, Danny's psychotherapist had commented to the consultant, "Danny's pain is palpable when he is in my office. In fact, it's so intense it scares me. This kid is really hurting. I am worried he will kill himself." I have found that with people experiencing mixed bipolar states that fit the mold of a dysphoric mania, the intensity of the manic process seems to be translated into a particularly severe angst that possesses an almost bitter tone to it.

Note well that this intensely painful brooding angst presents as a *persistent* mood state, not solely as an intermittent rage response triggered by interpersonal affronts – this latter trait being commonly seen in people coping with borderline personality disorders (as we will see in Chapters 14 and 15). Patients with dysphoric manias may have an interpersonal reactivity as seen in some personality disorders, but it tends to be imbedded within this persistently dark mood. The intensity of the angst of these patients can increase their suicidal potential significantly. Coupled with the impulsivity of the underlying manic drive, the risk of suicide, in my opinion, can be high.

Let us wrap up our three tips on spotting dysphoric manias by looking at an often-missed third clue that a dysphoric mania may be present. I have found that the severity of the patient's reported psychological pain is frequently not matched by the severity of their neurovegetative symptoms. One would imagine that a person whose depression was causing this amount of angst (often accompanied by suicidal ideation) would also demonstrate equally severe neurovegetative symptoms. As we see with Danny, this is not always the case. His neurovegetative symptoms, although problematic, are not striking in nature. His appetite is mildly impaired. Energy and concentration were reported as fine, and there was a relatively mild difficulty falling asleep and no early morning awakening.

I suspect that the classic neurovegetative symptoms as seen in a unipolar depression are being overturned by manic energies and drives. Keep an eye out for such a discordance between the severity of a patient's depressive angst and the severity of their neurovegetative symptoms. I believe that it often points towards the fact that a patient is not just depressed. They may have a mixed bipolar state, specifically, a dysphoric mania.

Interestingly, some evidence exists that the depressions seen in bipolar disorder, in a general sense, may have a tendency to show some features not typical of classic unipolar depression. One study showed that bipolar depressions had an increased tendency to show atypical depressive symptoms, including mood reactivity (think of Danny's stormy relationships), overeating, oversleeping, and excessive fatigue.[40] In younger patients there is also a tendency for a higher percentage of "mixed" presentations, as we have been describing,[41] as well as an increase in depressive psychotic features.[42] There is considerable evidence that people experiencing mixed bipolar disorders have a significantly higher rate of suicide.[43-45]

It is time to wrap up our discussion of dysphoric manias. As phenomenological and empirical research unfolds using the now available dimensional qualities of the DSM-5, my hunch is that the sub-category of "dysphoric mania" will prove to be both valid and reliable. The term also has very high "descriptive essence" (the words capture the core of the syndrome effectively). I believe its therapeutic usefulness is high, and that these dimensional/phenomenological characteristics should be aggressively sought by clinicians, even if a specific category does not emerge as a unique diagnostic entity. Evidence suggests that patients who are experiencing a dysphoric mania frequently respond well to mood stabilizers. Many will respond poorly to antidepressants alone, and in some cases antidepressants will unleash the underlying manic rage even further.

Historical Tip-Offs That Raise the Suspicion of Mixed Bipolar States in General

Although we have been focusing upon a possible specific subtype of mixed bipolar disorder – dysphoric mania – it is important to remember that patients may experience many different types of mixed processes, including those in which euphoric symptoms are common. Whatever the type of mixed presentation, there are two historical factors that may also point towards a mixed bipolar process in a patient who presents with depression.

Look carefully at the patient's family history. It may have both bipolar I and bipolar II disorders (which we will be exploring presently), sometimes in surprising numbers. Patients with mixed bipolar disorder may also be more likely to show a positive family history for depression, anxiety disorders, and alcohol and substance disorders. Danny's family history was loaded with depression, alcohol dependence, and anxiety disorders. His paternal grandfather was adopted and nothing was known of the paternal family history from that point. (It could have been filled with bipolar disorder, but no one knows.)

The second historical factor that may raise suspicions of the presence of a mixed bipolar state is the discovery, when taking a psychiatric history, of other bipolar processes earlier in the patient's life, such as bipolar II disorder and substance/medication-induced bipolar and related disorder. Both of these can also present as mixed states. These disorders are so important that they deserve a closer examination. Before we do this, however, there is one differential diagnostic error that we should make sure we are not making.

Over-Diagnosing Bipolar Disorder: A Serious Diagnostic Error

Thus far, we have examined the importance of not missing bipolar process (which can be seen across age groups from childhood throughout adolescence and adulthood). We have particularly focused upon mixed states (including dysphoric manias), which can be easily missed. The consequences of missing these bipolar states are potentially serious.

There is a flip side to this coin, the consequences of which are also serious: it is the mislabeling of patients, especially children, adolescents, and young adults, as having bipolar disorder when they do not. The result of this misdiagnosis by clinicians is patients being placed on mood stabilizers, and sometimes antipsychotics, in the absence of symptoms for which these medications are helpful. Consequently, these patients are taking medications that can be of no value, yet have potentially serious side effects. This problem is so important that the DSM-5 has attempted to minimize its occurrence by addressing it directly. Let's see how.

The problem manifests when young patients display marked behavioral problems involving angry outbursts and disruptive behaviors. Such problems may manifest at home, at school, during recreational time, or all three. In truth, some of these adolescents may be experiencing normal responses to severe stresses such as bullying or violence at home. Many are dealing with disorders such as attention-deficit/hyperactivity disorder (ADHD) or an oppositional defiant disorder. Others may be dealing with a depressive equivalent.

The term "depressive equivalent" was coined to acknowledge a well known observation that children and adolescents, possibly as a result of differences in maturation of the brain when compared to adults, sometimes display depression less through depressed mood and classic neurovegetative symptoms and more through anger and disruptive outbursts. In any case, whether the behaviors are normal responses to stress, examples of ADHD or oppositional defiant disorder or a depressive equivalent, these patients should not be diagnosed as having bipolar disorder and, consequently, be exposed to medications they do not need and that may prove to be harmful.

In direct response to this problem, the DSM-5 created a category of mood disorder that can help clinicians to spot children and adolescents who are displaying angry outbursts as part of a depressive equivalent. This mood disturbance is called "disruptive mood dysregulation disorder."[46] The interested reader should learn about the details and presentation of this disorder in the DSM-5. Although this book is not a textbook concerning child and adolescent disorders, suffice it to say that disruptive mood dysregulation disorder cannot be made if the phenomenological criteria for a manic or hypomanic episode are present *or* if the disruptive behavior occurs only during an episode of major depressive disorder.

It is hoped that this new category will decrease the likelihood that clinicians will misdiagnose children and adolescents as having bipolar disorder when they don't, for the term bipolar disorder is explicitly reserved in the DSM-5 for episodic presentations of bipolar symptoms. As we have seen, an understanding of the phenomenology of depression, mania, and mixed bipolar disorder, together with the birth of this new diagnostic category, should allow clinicians, in my opinion, to more easily make this differential diagnosis. By reducing the rate at which children and adolescents are misdiagnosed as having bipolar disorder, the DSM-5 will have done a great service by preventing the unnecessary use of inappropriate medications.

Bipolar II Disorder

According to DSM-5 criteria, a diagnosis of bipolar II disorder is met when a patient has one or more depressive episodes with at least one hypomanic episode. Some authors refer to this spectrum of disorders (including hypomanic variations of substance/medication-induced bipolar disorder, described below) as "soft bipolarity" and argue, rightly so, that spotting these disorders has major implications for treatment.[47] Bipolar II disorder is surprisingly common, with a lifetime prevalence rate of 1 to 2%. In patients suffering with recurrent major depressive disorder, it has been estimated that 25 to 50% have features of hypomania.[48]

DSM-5 criteria specify that hypomania presents as bursts of low-grade manic-like symptoms *that last for at least four consecutive days.*[49] The patient may experience an inflated sense of self-importance or increased energy with less need to sleep; and/or the patient may feel more talkative and unusually social (perhaps having an increased sex drive as well). The patient's thoughts may seem to be racing, and there may be a significant increase in his or her irritability. These changes will be distinctly noticeable to those who know the patient well.

What separates these hypomanic symptoms from manic symptoms is not their characteristics, it is their disruptive severity and their duration. In hypomania, the "manic" symptoms are not severe enough to cause marked impairment in social or occupational functioning, nor are they severe enough to necessitate a hospitalization. In addition, the presence of any psychotic process rules out hypomania and requires a diagnosis of mania. Moreover, in true mania the symptoms must be present for at least a week.

Sometimes patients feel pretty good during milder hypomanic periods and relate to their interviewers that they are more productive, witty, and creative, which is sometimes true. Indeed, if we could all be programmed to have a consistent very low-grade hypomania without the irritability, the world might be a better place. It would certainly be a happier one.

However, the problem is that these episodes are often more disruptive and unpleasant than they are valuable. During the hypomanic episodes, patients often report feeling scattered, unproductive, and bothered by an unsettling sensation that "I am just not myself." They may be more likely to do things impulsively (e.g., initiate inappropriate drinking binges or regretted sexual liaisons). Because such episodes are an indication of an underlying instability of mood regulation in the brain, they can frequently transform into a depressed mood, which is sometimes severe. Unfortunately, a significant percentage of these patients go on to develop a full-blown bipolar I disorder.

As we saw with mixed bipolar disorder, this diagnosis is evolving. Daniel Smith argued convincingly, in my opinion, that the DSM-IV-TR diagnosis was too rigid, for many patients have hypomanic episodes lasting only 1 or 2 days, as opposed to the 4 days demanded by the DSM-IV-TR.[50] I feel that I have seen hypomanic bursts appear multiple times in a single day in some patients. It is interesting to note that the ICD-10, when describing rapid cycling in bipolar disorder, recognizes that mood shifts may occur in the course of a single day or two. I believe that the new dimensional qualities of the DSM-5 will eventually result in research that clarifies the frequency with which both manic and hypomanic bursts can occur (although keep in mind that currently the DSM-5 demands a minimum of 4 days of relatively consistent symptoms to be present in order to make the diagnosis of hypomania).

In addition to the more typical euphoric manic symptoms typical of the DSM-5 criteria for hypomania, keep an eye out for the presence of consistent dysphoric symptoms, for I have seen hypomanic bursts that consist primarily or solely of the dysphoric qualities of a mania. Look out for bursts of the following dysphoric symptoms: a preoccupation with violent and dark images; agitation; difficulty falling asleep; irritability; anger; an unpleasant racing of thoughts; a destructive impulsivity to gamble, drink, attempt suicide or violence; and an unpleasant sense of psychological angst and darkness.

With any person who presents with depression, it is important to look for episodes of hypomania suggestive of bipolar II disorder. The use of a mood stabilizer in these patients can sometimes significantly improve the quality of their lives. Although not proven, there is speculation that the addition of a mood stabilizer, such as lithium, in those patients who would have naturally evolved into having bipolar I disorder, might prevent them from experiencing this potentially catastrophic evolution. In addition, antidepressants used alone are commonly considered to be counter-indicated in these patients, for they may unleash further hypomanic bursts and/or a full-blown manic episode.

In my opinion, the diagnosis of bipolar II disorder is frequently missed. Every clinician should be on the lookout for it. As we have seen, it is a diagnosis that can be uncovered rather easily in the initial interview if the clinician asks questions that address it. If made, it is a diagnosis that can transform, and perhaps even save, a patient's life. Let's take a look at two screening questions that might help us to spot hypomania. Once again, from a clinical standpoint, I aggressively search for hypomanic bursts that may occur more briefly than appearing for 4 solid days as required by the current DSM-5 criteria.

After exploring depression with a patient, I find the following question to be a nice one for uncovering euphoric hypomanic episodes:

"Do you have periods of time, even just for hours or a couple of days or weeks, where you suddenly and unexpectedly feel unusually happy, super-energized, ready to 'take on the world' *and you can't explain why, it feels almost odd to you?*"

This screening question covers several of the more common symptoms when experiencing a euphoric hypomanic episode. It is made even more effective (and less likely to yield false positives) by the phrasing, "… and you can't explain why, it feels almost odd to you?" This part of the question stems from a sophisticated understanding of the people beneath the diagnoses of hypomania. It acknowledges a common response of these patients towards their symptoms (not just the presence of the symptom). This phenomenological understanding can help us to avoid mislabeling someone as having a hypomania when, in reality, they are experiencing normal feelings of "being on top of things" or "having a great day."

Many, although not all, people who are truly experiencing hypomanic symptoms are genuinely puzzled by their own mood shifts. The puzzlement is particularly acute if they have been feeling depressed and then suddenly and unexpectedly feel hypomanic, without any positive change in their environment or the interpersonal wing of their matrix that could explain it. If a patient admits to hypomanic symptoms, and to puzzlement in reaction to their presence, it increases the likelihood that the symptoms are valid and problematic enough to warrant the diagnosis of hypomania.

After asking the above question, the interviewer can use the question below as a follow-up screening for dysphoric hypomanic episodes:

"Do you have periods of time, even just for hours or a couple of days or weeks, where you suddenly, and unexpectedly, find your thoughts really speeded up on you, in an unpleasant rush that you feel you really can't control, and your thoughts are sort of angry and life just seems darker *and you can't explain why you suddenly feel so bad, the dark shift in mood feels almost odd to you?*"

Substance/Medication-Induced Bipolar and Related Disorder

As just mentioned, some patients only develop hypomanic or manic symptoms when given an antidepressant. It is important to realize that medications other than antidepressants (or other psychotropic medications) have been shown to occasionally unleash manic-like symptoms and/or suicidal ideation and/or violent ideation. Although definitive research is ongoing, offending agents *may* include amantadine (used to treat Parkinson's disease), isotretinoin (used to treat severe acne), varenicline (used to stop smoking), and steroids (used to treat a variety of illnesses and as an adjunctive agent by athletes and body builders). As one would expect, a variety of street drugs can induce bipolar process including stimulants, phencyclidine (PCP), and bath salts.[51] In addition, complementary and alternative medicines (such as St. John's wort), ECT, and light therapy can also trigger hypomanic or manic symptoms. In the DSM-5, one would record these diagnoses as "Substance/Medication-Induced Bipolar and Related Disorder with manic features" (noting what substance or treatment triggered the mania). In clinical and research literature, this syndrome has often been referred to in the past as bipolar type III disorder.

Shortly after the offending medication or intervention (antidepressant, St. John's wort, light therapy) is removed, most patients lose all manic or hypomanic symptoms and return to their baseline moods. However, if the hypomanic or manic symptoms still persist 1 month after the suspected triggering agent has been discontinued, then the diagnosis is switched to bipolar I disorder or bipolar II disorder.

As one follows the progress of patients who have met the criteria for substance/medication-induced bipolar and related disorder over the ensuing years, a small percentage will go on to develop bipolar type II disorder. Some of these will subsequently develop bipolar I disorder. A very small percentage will skip bipolar II disorder and directly develop bipolar I disorder. It is unclear whether the releasing agent simply speeded up a disease progression that would have unfolded at a later date without any use of an antidepressant or other agent, or whether, in some instances, it triggered a bipolar process in someone who would not otherwise have developed these disorders. In either case, it is likely, in my opinion, that the patient was genetically predisposed to bipolar process.

Either situation is a disturbing one. Consequently, I feel it is critical to aggressively hunt for hypomanic process and a family history of bipolar process in all patients presenting with depression before starting any antidepressant agent. When patients report current hypomanic symptoms or relate a history suggesting hypomanic process in the past, if clinically feasible, some clinicians prefer the use of psychotherapy alone. If it fails, then such clinicians might consider adding an antidepressant after the patient has been prophylactically loaded with a mood stabilizer such as lithium or Depakote. It is interesting to note that even one of the mood stabilizers, lamotrigine (which has antidepressant effects), has been documented to trigger or exacerbate suicidal ideation.[52]

Varying therapeutic approaches and debate as to how to best proceed with a depressed patient reporting a past history of hypomania go far beyond the scope of this book. I urge readers to seek out the appropriate literature on these complicated situations. Nevertheless, it is safe to say in a book on clinical interviewing that one should question for hypomanic or manic symptoms, past or present, with all patients presenting with depressed symptoms. Their presence can have major implications on how to proceed therapeutically and in a safe fashion.

We now come full cycle, back to Danny Ramirez. When the consultant asked the parents the following question, "With Danny's history of OCD early in his childhood and his repeated problems with depression, I would think he's been tried on numerous antidepressants. How has that gone for him? Have they helped at all?" Before he was even done with the question, the parent's glanced over at each other, shook their heads, and said, "Oh God."

At the age of 8, Danny's OCD erupted with a vengeance. (Note that there appears to be an even higher rate of OCD and other serious anxiety disorders in patients with bipolar disorder when compared to unipolar depressions, which already have a high frequency of co-morbidity with anxiety disorders.) Because of the severity of Danny's pain, an antidepressant was started, hoping that he would also eventually respond to cognitive–behavioral therapy (CBT). The antidepressant provided quick and remarkable help, with a 90% remission within 3 weeks, much to Danny's relief.

But within 5–6 weeks, Danny developed agitation, sleep problems, and "an attitude." Up until the use of the antidepressant, Danny had been the type of a kid who has a big superego, is pleasant with adults and siblings, receives excellent grades, and demonstrates great deportment at school. About 2 months after initiating antidepressant therapy, Danny began to talk back to his parents. He became highly oppositional, requiring multiple time-outs throughout the day. He had numerous angry outbursts, with several out-of-character episodes of screaming and swearing at his parents. The change in behavior was topped off by a bizarre incident of pulling out a kitchen knife and threatening to kill the family dog, a dog that Danny that had always loved. His parents told the consultant, "It was really amazing. It was like he had a totally different personality. It was sort of like he was Sybil or something."

He was promptly pulled off the antidepressant. All oppositional behavioral problems disappeared within 2 weeks; unfortunately, so did the relief from his OCD. His OCD returned with a crippling vengeance. Danny did not engage well in his CBT, despite really liking his therapist. Consequently, over the next 2 years various attempts were made to use different antidepressants at very low doses. Every single attempt resulted in dysphoric manic symptoms, highlighted by one frightening brief episode of paranoid psychosis. In short, Danny was a textbook illustration of person who, in the DSM-5 system, we would diagnose as having a history of a substance/medication-induced bipolar and related disorder.

Recognizing Suicidal Ideation Unleashed During Partial Manic Responses to a Medication

During episodes when dysphoric manic symptoms are partially or fully unleashed by medications or other treatment modalities, some patients can develop thoughts of self-mutilation and/or suicide (violent ideation has also been reported). Whether you are functioning as a consultant who is performing a one-time initial interview, engaged in ongoing psychotherapy with a patient who has been placed on an antidepressant by a prescribing colleague, or you yourself have prescribed the medication, several features of the patient's suicidal ideation, in my opinion, suggest that it may be related to an unleashing phenomenon (as opposed to the natural development of suicidal ideation in a patient whose depression is worsening).

Be suspicious that a worsening of your patient's depression is *not* the cause of the patient's emerging suicidal ideation when: (1) the suicidal ideation is unexpected and inconsistent with the patient's past suicidal ideation; (2) the patient reports the ideation as feeling very different from past suicidal ideation; (3) the ideation has a peculiar feeling of intensity and impulsiveness that has never been present before, and the ideation appears to be erupting with other co-existing phenomena characteristic of a dysphoric mania, such as agitation (ranging from pacing to a striking increase in nervous displacement activities such as finger picking, hair twirling, and foot twitching), angry outbursts, racing thoughts experienced as unpleasant, marked problems falling asleep, and intense psychological angst.

One of my psychotherapy patients, in her late 20s, provides an excellent illustration of this process. She had been doing reasonably well, but had had only a partial response to her antidepressant at a fairly high dose. I increased her antidepressant to an even higher dose to see if we could get a more robust response. Within about 10 days, although no new stresses had occurred in her life, she developed an acutely agitated state with extreme irritability, very low stress tolerance, and tearful episodes with mood lability. She reported, "I've been screaming at my kids and husband. It's like I'm a different person. It's so strange. I don't know what to do. I just don't know what to do." To her surprise she had also developed suicidal ideation of an intensity and quality that had frightened her. She stressed repeatedly in our session, "You have to understand, I don't want to die."

She reported that the morning of the day I saw her she had become particularly wound-up. While in her bathroom, she suddenly had the urge to electrocute herself by thrusting her hair dryer into the bathtub. She had never had such thoughts before. She reported feeling compelled by it, although in her heart she didn't want to die. It scared her, and she aggressively threw the hair dryer into the bedroom. When I asked whether the suicidal ideation felt the same as in the past, she quickly responded, "No. This was very different. It just came on so abruptly. It was very intense. And it felt different than anything I've ever felt before. It really frightened me."

Keep in mind that only 10 days earlier she had been doing fairly well (with about a 60% remission in her symptoms and no agitation or suicidal ideation whatsoever). Her last suicidal ideation, overdosing, had occurred over 8 years ago and was mild in nature. In my office, she appeared distraught and cried intermittently with her feet twitching rapidly whenever she crossed her legs. In short, she was "beside herself." Within 2 days of markedly decreasing the antidepressant, she felt "almost back to normal," with no suicidal ideation. By the fifth day she was fine. Her suicidal ideation never returned.

Cyclothymic Disorder and Rapid Cycling

Let me wrap up by describing two final diagnostic considerations that Danny's presentation brings to mind, for they may have potential ramifications for treatment in other patients. In a cyclothymic disorder, as defined by the DSM-5, over a 2-year timeframe an adult patient will experience intermittent and frequent bouts of low-grade depression and hypomania, neither of which reaches the proportions of a full-grade depressive episode or manic episode. During this 2-year timeframe, any combination of the depressive or hypomanic symptoms must be present for at least 50% of the time and no period of time in excess of 2 months can be symptom free.[53] Although clearly less disruptive than true bipolar disorder, cyclothymic disorder is painful, problematic, and puzzling to those people experiencing it. There is also a 15 to 50% chance that a person with cyclothymic disorder will eventually develop bipolar I disorder or bipolar II disorder.[54] If the clinician discovers cyclothymic disorder, he or she might be able to change a patient's life in a very positive fashion by prescribing a mood-stabilizing agent, as well as utilizing psychotherapy.

It should also be noted that the specifier "rapid cycling" can be added to either a diagnosis of bipolar I disorder or bipolar II disorder. To apply this specifier, the patient must have shown four or more mood episodes, in any combination, within 12 months. Whether these episodes are depressive, manic, or hypomanic, they must be demarcated by either a full period of remission between episodes or by an *immediate* switch into an episode of opposite polarity.[55] Rapid cycling characterizes roughly 10 to 20% of people presenting with bipolar disorder. Interestingly, bipolar disorder in general is fairly equally distributed between the sexes, whereas rapid cycling bipolar disorder is more common in women. On a practical level, the presence of rapid cycling can be associated with a poorer prognosis, and it often requires more complicated combinations of medications to achieve sustained remission.

Differential Diagnosis on Danny Ramirez and Summary of Key Interviewing Tips

The consultant that was seeing Danny at age 18 felt that Danny had been currently mis-diagnosed as having a major depression. He felt that Danny's symptoms were better characterized as a mixed bipolar disorder with dysphoric features. He also felt antidepressants were counter-indicated (unless used after a sound trial of a mood stabilizer first). He recommended the initiation of lithium.

His expectation was that the dysphoric characteristics of Danny's condition would improve markedly, including a disappearance of the angry, acting-out behaviors that could be mistaken for budding personality dysfunction, such as screaming "I just wanted to see my blood." He predicted that some true depressive symptoms would remain. He recommended that these be addressed by continued psychotherapy, hopefully without a need to add an antidepressant. He also felt that once the dysphoric manic symptoms were relieved by lithium, the psychotherapy would progress much more effectively (a healing matrix effect as described in Chapter 7).

The consultant also felt that if untreated with a mood stabilizer, Danny ran a high risk of developing severe manic symptoms, including psychotic process. His predictions proved to be right on the mark.

A brief trial of lithium was undertaken with excellent results. But Danny felt he did not have a bipolar disorder. Unfortunately, several subsequent psychiatrists concurred, telling his parents that Danny most likely had a personality disorder. Lithium fell by the wayside.

During his third year at college, as predicted by the original consultant, Danny experienced a ferocious psychotic manic episode, replete with command hallucinations to enucleate his eyes and a bevy of demonic delusions. At that time, he was diagnosed as having bipolar I disorder, mixed (with dysphoric manic symptoms). It required over 5 months to bring the mania into remission. Fortunately, because of the outstanding care he subsequently received and his own sophisticated understanding of how to effectively utilize his medications, 4 years after his manic episode Danny remained symptom free. He had completed college, become fully employed and had found a steady girlfriend.

Let us return to our original consultant's interview to see how Danny's differential diagnosis would be formulated today using DSM-5 criteria. It also serves as a refreshing reminder of how a well-trained clinician, in a single 50-minute interview, may arrive at a more valid, useful, and accurate diagnosis than clinicians who have seen the patient on a regular basis.

Danny's original presentation is consistent with a dysphoric mania. He clearly is reporting a severe depressive mood that has resulted in a marked decrease in his functioning both at home and at school, as well as interpersonally (the severity of his dysfunction would immediately eliminate hypomania as a diagnosis). It is persistent in nature, and severe enough, to generate significant suicidal ideation and intent. It has many of the identifying characteristics of a dysphoric mania including: an overlay of anger and hostility, a deep angst highlighted by a dark and gloomy worldview, and a surprising discordance between his relatively mild neurovegetative symptoms and the intensity of his depressive angst. He is plagued with racing thoughts, agitated anxiety, dark and foreboding images, problems falling asleep because of agitation, and an intense desire to do something to release his pain (including several episodes of self-cutting). All of this symptomatology is highlighted by a well-documented history in childhood of several medication-induced hypomanic and manic episodes (one of which included psychotic process).

Truth be told, it's tough to easily fit Danny's presentation into the DSM-5 system as it now stands for two reasons. (1) The DSM-5, despite its innovative dimensionality, in my opinion, still maintains a too restrictive criteria set for the diagnosis of a mixed bipolar disorder. In order to make this diagnosis, the patient *must fulfill the criteria* for either a major depressive episode or a manic episode – Danny does neither, yet he clearly is afflicted with a major mood disorder. (2) The DSM-5 tends to emphasize euphoric manic symptoms and lists few dysphoric manic symptoms in its criteria for mania or hypomania.

For such situations, the DSM-5 has a reasonable solution, although, in my opinion, it lacks descriptive essence. In any case, you could probably use the diagnosis of other speci-fied bipolar and related disorder. Of course, after his future psychotic episode in college, the DSM-5 diagnosis would have become bipolar I disorder, manic (mixed episode with depressed and anxious symptoms) with mood-incongruent psychotic features.

During his consultation, after collaboratively interviewing Danny's parents and having already spoken with Danny's therapist, no evidence of marked personality dysfunction was present. Indeed, Danny had been viewed as a pleasant and high-functioning indi-vidual, although a bit rigid and intense. Concerning medical issues, Danny had been evaluated medically on several occasions and deemed to be physically fit. Because of the severity of his symptoms, the consultant was recommending a more aggressive work-up, perhaps including a computed tomography (CT) scan and electroencephalogram (EEG). In any case Danny's differential diagnosis at the end of the consultant's initial interview would be as follows if we were using DSM-5 criteria:

General Psychiatric Disorders:

Other specified bipolar and related disorder ("dysphoric mania"; patient does not meet criteria for either a major depressive disorder or a manic episode)

Obsessive–compulsive disorder (with good insight)

Rule out bipolar and related disorder due to another medical condition

Personality Disorders:

None

Medical Disorders:

Rule out medical causes of bipolar disorder such as tumors, epilepsy

I believe that future research – made possible by the added dimensionality of the DSM-5 – will eventually substantiate the importance of dysphoric manic symptoms as well as their common appearance in mixed bipolar states. Indeed, it is my personal belief that future revisions of the DSM-5 may very well include a set of specifiers for dysphoric mania exactly as it has a set of specifiers for a melancholic depressive disorder.

Such an addition will serve to remind clinicians to look for this specific symptom cluster, the presence of which can significantly impact treatment planning. In addition, the term *bipolar I disorder (mixed, dysphoric mania)* captures the descriptive essence of Danny's complex and painful inner world distinctly and with a minimum of words.

Let us review the wealth of diagnostic interviewing points that Danny's presentation illustrates:

1. Some patients present with a curious mix of depressed symptoms and manic symptoms simultaneously (or that are cycling so fast that they appear to be merged).

2. Mixed presentations may be more common in late adolescents and young adults, where they are easily misdiagnosed as major depressions with irritability and/or agitation.

3. Mixed states, especially in this younger age group, may present primarily with dysphoric manic symptoms including: an intensely depressive angst, racing thoughts experienced as distinctly unpleasant, irritability, anger, a dark moodiness, stormy relationships, impulses for self-cutting and other self-damaging behaviors, suicidal ideation or violent ideation, and feeling intensely driven to get relief from their dark and racing thoughts and/or to "right" what is wrong with the world or the people in their world.

4. In the initial interview (as well as within ongoing sessions), be sure to monitor the potential for violent behaviors such as self-cutting, suicide, and violence towards others.

5. Three symptom characteristics may point towards the presence of a dysphoric mania in a patient complaining of depression: (1) persistent anger as a major presenting symptom, (2) intense psychological angst, and (3) intensity of a patient's psychological angst being markedly more intense than their neurovegetative symptoms.

6. Two historical markers can also suggest the possibility that a patient is suffering from a classic bipolar disorder (*or perhaps from one of the other types of mixed bipolar states*): (1) a positive family history for bipolar I disorder, bipolar II disorder, substance/medication-induced bipolar disorder, or cyclothymic disorder, (2) the patient has a personal past psychiatric history of bipolar II disorder, substance/medication-induced bipolar disorder, or a cyclothymic disorder.

7. Patients experiencing dysphoric manias may have a predilection to develop psychotic process.

8. The patient's dysphoric manic symptoms (especially angry outbursts, dark moodiness, stormy relationships, impulsive self-cutting and suicidal ideation and behaviors) can be easily mislabeled as evidence of personality dysfunction, resulting in an inappropriate personality diagnosis such as borderline personality disorder.

9. If you see behavioral characteristics suggesting diagnoses such as borderline personality disorder and histrionic personality disorder, be sure to carefully interview for evidence of mixed bipolar disorders of a dysphoric nature.

10. Be on the lookout for the opposite error (diagnosing patients with borderline personality disorder as having bipolar disorder, although some patients may have both).

11. Also be on the lookout for the similar error of misdiagnosing a child or adolescent with hyperactive ADHD, oppositional disorder, or a conduct disorder as having bipolar disorder. Keep in mind the diagnosis of disruptive mood dysregulation disorder.

12. Bipolar II disorder is diagnosed when the patient has at least one major depressive episode with one or more hypomanic episodes (with none of the hypomanic episodes reaching the full criteria for a manic episode).

13. Substance/medication-induced bipolar disorder is diagnosed when a patient *only* has hypomanic or manic episodes while taking a traditional medication (such as an antidepressant), a complementary alternative medicine (such as St. John's wort), or other non-pharmacologic interventions such as light therapy or ECT.

14. *Before starting any patient on an antidepressant agent*, carefully search for the following during the interview: (1) current symptoms or signs of hypomania (remember that hypomanic symptoms may be subtle and under-reported unless directly asked about), (2) a history of past hypomanic or manic symptoms, and (3) a family history of bipolar process, including relatives with hypomanic histories (often untreated, with families viewing them as "just sort of nutty" or as having a "motor mouth").

15. Medication/treatment-induced hypomanic or manic episodes can include impulsive suicidal ideation/behaviors or violent ideation/behaviors.

16. Suicidal thoughts and impulses triggered by a partial or full mania being unleashed by a medication or street drug may have different phenomenological characteristics than the typical suicidal ideation experienced by the patient during his or her previous or current depressive episodes. Such phenomenological differences may help the interviewer to distinguish suicidal ideation caused by the patient's underlying depression as opposed to suicidal ideation caused by a manic burst triggered by a medication or street drug.

17. Listen carefully to family members' opinions on symptoms, responses to medications, and diagnostic impressions. They can be invaluable.

Clinical Presentation #3: Mr. Whitstone

Mr. Whitstone was admitted to a general hospital for evaluation of bizarre behavior described by his family as paranoid. He is a distinguished-appearing 62-year-old White man who has been a prominent businessman. At the time of the interview, he is refusing all hospital care, including intravenous lines and medication. The interviewer has been called in as an emergency consultant. During the interview Mr. Whitstone appears guarded, thoroughly grilling the interviewer about his training and his purpose. Outside of his suspiciousness, Mr. Whitstone is cooperative. During the first 10 minutes of the interview he appears tense, complaining, "I'm really having trouble with my thinking. I can't concentrate anymore. But they don't understand." When asked whether he feels depressed, he answers, "No, I don't feel particularly depressed." He reports problems with appetite and sleep. But of all his concerns, he is most upset about his business company, since he feels "Someone in the company, and I'm not quite sure who, is out to get me. I'm pretty sure my life is in danger." He has not returned to work since his triple bypass heart surgery in January, 6 months earlier. He is alert and oriented times three with a stable level of consciousness. Three members of his family are at his bedside when the interviewer first enters the room.

Discussion of Mr. Whitstone

Patient Hesitancies to Admit to Depression and How to Transform Them

Mr. Whitstone had had heart surgery 6 months earlier. Currently he was refusing all medical help. One of the curious facets of Mr. Whitstone's presentation remains the fact that when asked directly about depression he stated, "No, I don't feel particularly depressed." Further questioning suggested differently. Since his bypass surgery in January, he had been experiencing many neurovegetative symptoms of depression, including difficulty falling asleep, sleep continuity disturbance, loss of appetite, weight loss, poor concentration, and anhedonia. Collaborative information from his wife and children pointed towards depression. They felt that he appeared withdrawn, sad, and not himself. Mr. Whitstone appeared to be depressed, and yet he denied it. Such a denial of depression is common. Donald Klein estimates that approximately 30% of people fulfilling the criteria of major depression will deny being depressed.[56]

When first asking about depression I have found the following series of questions to be useful in determining whether depressed mood may be present:

a. "How would you describe your mood over the past several weeks?"
b. "Tell me a little bit about how you've been feeling recently."
c. "Would you say that you've been feeling depressed?"

If the patient denies depression, the interviewer can switch to a different word than "depressed," which, for whatever reason, the patient may identify with more, such as:

a. "Have you been feeling sad at all?"
b. "Have you been feeling unhappy?"

It is not uncommon for a person suffering from depression to deny depression while admitting to sadness. Another useful question for uncovering depressed mood remains, "When was the last time you felt like crying?" The phrasing of this question automatically conveys that the interviewer feels it is both common and acceptable to cry, and is an example of one of our validity techniques (gentle assumption) from Chapter 5. Certain patients, especially males, feel hesitant to admit tearfulness. This question helps to skirt this resistance by asking only when they felt like crying. Such sensitive phrasing allows the self-conscious patient many avenues for saving face. The direct question, "Have you been crying?" may yield false negatives, since it does not offer any avenues for the patient except denial or admission of tearfulness.

Finally, if the patient denies both depression and sadness (Mr. Whitstone actually vigorously denied both), the following questions may unearth material suggesting depressed mood:

a. "Have you been feeling yourself recently?" or
b. "Have you been feeling up to par over the past several weeks?"

Cross-Cultural Issues in Recognizing Depression

Throughout the book we have emphasized the importance of understanding cultural and ethnic considerations during the initial interview. Such issues remain important in differential diagnosis as well. Sometimes cross-cultural differences can be the cause for missing the presence of a major depressive episode, for depression may be experienced or labeled differently depending upon the patient's culture.

For instance, in the Latino/a population, depression is likely to be associated with "bad nerves," and clinicians may be able to more effectively elicit depressive symptoms with questions such as, "When you are really stressed, do you sometimes experience 'nervios' or trouble with your nerves?" In addition, as seen with many cultures, in the Latino/a culture there can be a tendency to experience depression via somatic complaints such as headaches (sometimes called "brain aches"). Indeed, the syndrome of nervios encompasses a broad range of symptoms besides classic depressive symptoms including, trembling, tingling sensations, and mareos (dizziness with occasional vertigo-like qualities). Thus nervios can span a variety of DSM-5 diagnoses from depression and anxiety disorders to dissociative disorders and even psychosis.[57] In any case, the term "nervios" is an excellent gateway for uncovering depression and depressive equivalents in the Latino/a culture.

It is also worth noting that the rapid onset of "ataque de nervios" can meet the criteria for a panic attack, which demonstrate a considerable co-morbidity with major depressive disorders as described in the DSM-5. It is important for interviewers to realize that the symptoms of a panic attack may vary from culture to culture, even in cultures/ethnic groups that are stereotypically viewed as being loosely related cultural/ethnic entities such as Latino/a, Hispanic, Dominicano, Cuban, etc. (all of which may have distinctive differences in cultural heritage, customs, and beliefs, as well as being composed of various races and racial mixtures).

For instance, ataques de nervios in Puerto Rican and Dominican patients may be characterized by the appearance of abrupt trembling, uncontrollable crying and/or screaming, aggressive or suicidal behavior, and depersonalization/derealization symptoms.[58] An interviewer unaware of these common cultural manifestations of a panic attack in these patients may mislabel a Puerto Rican or Dominican patient – who is simply having a typical panic attack of the variety seen in their cultural matrix – as being histrionic or troubled by aggressive propensities.

In a metaphorical sense, this somatic tendency sometimes carries over into the label chosen for depression, as seen in Middle Eastern cultures where a depressive episode might be described as having "problems of the heart." In the Hopi nation the same episode would be described as being heartbroken. In Chinese and Asian cultures, a patient may be more comfortable complaining of being weak, tired, or feeling "imbalanced."[59]

As was the case with Danny, Mr. Whitstone's presentation also emphasizes the critical importance of sources of information other than the patient. A hallmark of shrewd interviewers remains the ability to know when their interview was inadequate. In the case of Mr. Whitstone, both his wife and other family members felt that he had been pervasively depressed for at least 2 months.

Problems With Concentration and Cognitive Functioning in Depression

When questioned whether he had been feeling up to par recently, Mr. Whitstone pensively yet openly discussed his concerns over inadequacy and his fears about his thinking:

> **Clin.:** In what ways haven't you felt yourself?
>
> **Pt.:** My concentration is shot. It's been very upsetting, let me tell you. I'm a fairly intelligent man, I've gone far. But about a month ago, I called my secretary to dictate a memo. I had to hang up, because I couldn't do it. (Mr. Whitstone was dismally moving his head from side to side.) It took me 2 days to write that memo (pause). I could normally do it in 20 minutes.

Other useful questions concerning cognitive processes include:

a. "Have you noticed if your thinking appears to have speeded up [hypomania, mania, mixed bipolar states, agitated depression] or slowed down [melancholic or withdrawn depression]?"
b. "Are you finding it more difficult to make decisions recently?"
c. "Do you find yourself feeling frustrated when you are trying to make a decision?"
d. "Does it ever seem like your thoughts are getting disconnected or confused?"
e. "Has it been difficult for you to hold a train of thought?"
f. "Are you finding it difficult to read or to follow people as they talk?"

We will examine the important role of the cognitive exam in further delineating the extent of a patient's cognitive dysfunction as well as its role in uncovering dementias masquerading as depressions and depressions masquerading as dementias (pseudodementia), in more detail later.

Spotting Atypical Depression

With Mr. Whitstone we have seen that a seriously depressed person may not always complain of depression. Another cause for diagnostic confusion is the presence of an atypical depression. Not all people with depressions present with classic neurovegetative symptoms, and in such cases the DSM-5 allows one to specify that the depression is "atypical" in nature.

I place the word atypical in quotes because these depressions are hardly atypical in nature. Estimates in both community and clinical settings indicate that 15.7 to 36.6% of depressions meet the criteria for atypical depression. As we saw earlier, these atypical features are seen even more frequently (in up to 50%) with bipolar type II depression and in dysthymia.[60] Some features, such as mood reactivity, also remind one of the "depressive" states seen in mixed bipolar process, and, indeed, atypical depressions are more common in bipolar I disorder, especially mixed presentations.

Spotting atypical depressions has distinct clinical implications. Their presence cues the clinician to thoroughly hunt for evidence of bipolar process, which, if present, may caution against the use of antidepressants without first covering the patient with a mood stabilizer or perhaps indicate only a psychotherapeutic intervention if possible. Even if hypomanic symptoms are not present, it reminds both the clinician and the patient to be particularly on the lookout for an unexpected unleashing of manic symptoms once an antidepressant is instituted, in which case the antidepressant can be promptly discontinued, hopefully before major manic symptoms have been precipitated. In addition, there is evidence that if a patient solely has an atypical depression (without bipolar process), and the patient's depression is not responding to medications such as selective serotonin reuptake inhibitors or tricyclics, they might preferentially respond to monoamine oxidase inhibitors[61] and/or cognitive psychotherapy.

So what do these atypical depressions look like? In the DSM-5, in order to be viewed as having an atypical depression, the patient must first meet the criteria for a major depressive disorder while simultaneously presenting with a phenomenon known as "mood reactivity." In addition, the patient must demonstrate two out of four secondary symptoms.

Let us first look at the concept of mood reactivity. In a classic depression, the patient's depressive symptoms, although somewhat fluctuating in intensity over time, are *persistently present over time* and don't respond much to environmental triggers. Thus, when anhedonia is present, a classically depressed patient will *not* suddenly respond with an uplift in mood and/or interest when an otherwise enjoyable activity for that patient presents itself (e.g., the chance to see a favorite movie) or respond positively and with animation to a compliment from a friend or employer. In contrast, patients with mood reactivity have the capacity to feel at least 50% better and can even become transiently euthymic (experience normal mood) when encountering positive events.[62,63] It has been noted that some of these patients can maintain a good mood for hours, or longer, if the positive re-enforcer continues (e.g., a weekend getaway with a new romantic interest).[64] It should be noted that some authors feel, and perhaps this will be reflected in future diagnostic systems, that the symptom of mood reactivity is not always present in atypical depressions and should not be viewed as necessary for making the diagnosis.[65]

In the DSM-5, once the patient demonstrates mood reactivity, in order to be viewed as having an atypical depression, two of the following four symptoms must be present: (1) significant weight gain or increase in appetite, (2) hypersomnia, (3) leaden paralysis, and (4) a long-standing pattern of interpersonal rejection sensitivity that results in significant social or occupational impairment. Of these symptoms, rejection sensitivity seems to be the most common, as seen in a study of 332 patients of whom 71% reported rejection sensitivity, 47% hyperphagia, 47% leaden paralysis, and 35% oversleeping.[66]

Let us look at these symptoms in more detail. Rejection sensitivity is unique among them, for it represents a personality trait, *which is lifelong in nature and is seen both during the depression and between episodes of the depression.* It can be exacerbated during the depressive episodes themselves. This diagnostic marker is one of the rare instances in the DSM-5 where a non-personality disorder includes a stable personality trait as one of its criteria. It is not surprising then to see that patients with atypical depressions have a higher rate of personality disorders such as histrionic, borderline, and narcissistic disorders.

The rejection sensitivity displays itself as an unpredictable and rapid negative response to both hostile and non-hostile interpersonal comments and/or interactions. Patients with atypical depressions tend to "take things in the wrong way" whether responding to conversation, comments in a chat room, a text message, or a tweet. Rejection, hurt, embarrassment, and anger may occur in response to relatively innocuous comments or behaviors. The result is a backlog of employment problems, broken friendships, stormy romances, and sometimes a maladaptive seeking of drugs and alcohol for solace. One can imagine that this entire array of behaviors can be further fueled by the patient's mood reactivity. *It is important to remember that not all patients with atypical depressions have rejection sensitivity.*

In addition, people with atypical depressions frequently find that during an episode of depression they find themselves with an increased appetite and/or a significant weight gain over the course of the episode. Note that this increase in appetite contrasts rather sharply with the more typical decrease in appetite found in more classic major depressive episodes.

Hypersomnia is sometimes present, including feelings of needing to sleep during the day and being just too tired to work, although the patient may feel suddenly more perky if pleasant activities are available (a type of energy reactivity akin to mood reactivity). To meet the criteria, the patient must show either a total of 10 hours of sleep per day (including nighttime sleep and daytime naps) or at least 2 hours more of sleep per day than the patient shows normally when not depressed.[67]

Perhaps the oddest of the symptoms is the sensation of "leaden paralysis." The term, in my opinion, is a poor one for it has nothing to do with feelings that a limb is paralyzed. Instead it refers to an unpleasant feeling of heaviness in the arms or legs (I have found it to be more common in the legs), creating the "leaden" sensation of the symptom's name. I find that patients may describe their legs as feeling weak, rubbery, or "just not right." Patients sometimes report being frightened by the sensation in a medical sense. Indeed, if present, it is important to make sure, especially in older patients, that this sensation is not being misattributed to depression when it is, in actuality, a symptom of peripheral arterial disease.

In closing our discussion on atypical depression, one should be aware that both classic depressions and atypical depressions may also show a tendency, especially in a primary care clinic, to present with pain or other somatic complaints. In such patients, if the interviewer vigorously pursues classic neurovegetative symptoms or looks for symptoms of an atypical depression, he or she will often uncover one lurking below the surface.

Many mental health providers will find themselves, at some point in their careers, working in a primary care setting, where it is important not to miss such depressions as well as other disorders that present with pain or somatization. During the course of a single year, about 10–12% of all adults in the United States will present to a primary care clinician during a timeframe in which they are suffering from a major psychiatric disorder. Disturbingly, more than 50% of these individuals will have two or more psychiatric disorders.[68]

In addition, roughly 50% of all people who die by suicide have been seen by a primary care clinician within 1 month of the suicide, *with 1 in 5 of these patients having seen a primary care clinician within 1 week of their suicide.*[69] It is not an exaggeration to say that the use of the types of skilled interviewing techniques that we will study and see demonstrated on video in our chapter on suicide assessment (Chapter 17) may represent one of the major hopes for lowering the suicide rate in the United States and internationally.

Psychotic Process in Depression

In our discussions of Mr. Evans and Danny, we noted that psychotic process is a relatively common phenomenon in bipolar disorder, especially during manic and mixed states, but also in the depressed phase of the disorder. Mr. Whitstone serves to remind us that psychosis can arise in unipolar depression as well, especially in agitated major depressions and in the elderly. As discussed earlier, the DSM-5 refers to such psychotic material as either mood-congruent or mood-incongruent. In a unipolar depression, the mood-congruent material frequently concerns itself with depressive ideation or themes of decay that would seem to be natural in a depressed individual. According to the DSM-5, such themes include personal inadequacy, guilt, disease, poverty, nihilism, or deserved punishment. Mood-incongruent delusions or hallucinations do not revolve about the above themes. They are more bizarre or peculiar and include phenomena such as paranoid delusions, demon possession, thought insertion, delusions of control, and other themes not necessarily related to depressive ideation. Mr. Whitstone's paranoia would fulfill the criteria for mood-incongruent psychotic features.

Ruling Out Non-Psychiatric Biological Causes of Depression

Finally, I have saved perhaps the most important point for last. When confronted with a mood disorder presentation, one should always "think organic." Further investigation revealed that Mr. Whitstone had qualities suggestive of delirium, including auditory hallucinations, rapid fluctuations in affect, and a few periods of a fluctuating level of consciousness according to the nursing notes. Besides the standard clues hinting at an organic state, Mr. Whitstone's history was suggestive of an organic etiology for several reasons: (1) He had not seemed normal since his bypass surgery; (2) he had been on anticoagulants, raising the possibility of emboli (blood clots) having been previously dislodged from his heart and passed to his brain or of a hemorrhage in his brain related to his anticoagulants; and (3) he was significantly dehydrated.

In relation to organic precipitants of depression, it is important to stress the need for asking questions about both over-the-counter medications and prescription medications. A brief list of medications that commonly affect mood includes cimetidine, propranolol, methyldopa, reserpine, amantadine, steroids, birth control pills, and opiates. Even thiazide diuretics can cause depression by altering electrolyte balance.[70] Be on the lookout for depressions triggered by the use of prescribed synthetic opioids, such as OxyContin and Percocet. The abuse of these drugs is of epidemic proportions in the United States. They are currently one of the leading causes of death/suicide by overdose.

When considering an organic cause of depression besides medications and intracranial disease, one should keep in mind extracranial diseases such as hypothyroidism, hyperparathyroidism, lupus, hepatitis, and carcinoma. Pancreatic carcinoma is notorious for initially presenting with depressive complaints. Looked at more systematically, Anderson[71] has separated the organic causes of depression into six categories, including:

1. Drugs and poisons
2. Metabolic and endocrine disturbances
3. Infectious diseases
4. Degenerative diseases such as multiple sclerosis
5. Neoplasm
6. Miscellaneous conditions such as chronic pyelonephritis or Meniere's disease

It is well beyond the scope of this chapter to discuss a thorough differential of the organic causes of depression, but I heartily urge the reader to review this material.

Naturally, even the best clinician will sometimes miss organic causes of depression despite a search for them. This failure is to be expected. But in the last analysis, there is no excuse for not having thought of looking for an organic cause of depression. In particular, one situation presents itself in which I unfortunately find it very easy to forget about possible organic factors.

This situation arises when the patient presents complaining of a significant life stress such as unemployment, housing problems, divorce, or a death in the family. In such instances it is easy to assume psychological causality, but this assumption can be patently misleading. Simply because a person has ample reason to be depressed does not mean that his or her depression does not also have a concurrent organic cause. Quite to the contrary, physical and psychological disabilities often go hand-in-hand. For instance, Schmale has reported a high incidence of separation events preceding the onset of medical illnesses.[72]

The clinician should think holistically, checking for both psychological and physiologic roots of depression. One can often be fooled by what appears obvious. On the one hand, apparent adjustment reactions may be hiding something more ominous biologically. On the other hand, the obvious endogenous depression may actually be triggered or sustained by some not-so-obvious psychological factor or family dynamic.

Differential Diagnosis on Mr. Whitstone and Summary of Key Interviewing Tips

In closing the discussion of Mr. Whitstone, let me diagnostically summarize his situation at the end of the initial interview.

General Psychiatric Disorders:

Psychotic disorder due to another medical condition, condition unknown (provisional diagnosis)

Rule out delirium

Rule out major depressive disorder (with mood-incongruent psychotic features, paranoid delusions)

Personality Disorders:

Possible paranoid or compulsive traits (derived from data elicited from the family)

Medical Disorders:

Significant dehydration

Status post-bypass cardiac surgery

Rule out embolism to brain or hemorrhage

By way of follow up, a rigorous organic evaluation, including delirium/dementia chemistry screen, EEG, CT scan of head, lumbar puncture, and echocardiogram (checking for clots in the heart which could have embolized to the brain) revealed no abnormalities. Moreover, once Mr. Whitstone was rehydrated he continued to be symptomatic. Apparently he was most likely suffering from a major depressive disorder with mood-incongruent psychotic features, although there may have been some brief periods of mild delirium, possibly secondary to dehydration, as well.

At this point I would like to summarize the major issues underscored by Mr. Whitstone's interview:

1. People suffering from depression often deny that they are depressed.
2. Specific questions should be asked in an effort to uncover dysphoric mood not readily described by the patient.
3. Become familiar with varying presentations of depressive disorders across cultures. (Also keep in mind that patients may vary on how likely they are to share depressive symptoms related to the degree of stigmatization associated with depression within their culture.)
4. Atypical depression often presents with mood reactivity accompanied by symptoms such as increased appetite, hypersomnia, "leadenness" of the limbs, and rejection sensitivity.
5. Outside information from family and significant others may be needed to delineate the diagnosis.
6. Even mood-incongruent psychotic features such as paranoia or thought insertion can occur during severe depressive episodes.

7. It is imperative to ask questions and to order appropriate lab work that can help to rule out possible organic causes of depression.

Clinical Presentation #4: Ms. Wilkins

Ms. Wilkins enters the outpatient office with hesitant steps. Her patterned blue dress is faded and wrinkled. She is a 26-year-old White single woman who reports, "I feel horrible. I am so very depressed. Last night I was thinking of maybe (pause, tearfulness) … killing myself." She reports numerous neurovegetative symptoms of depression such as sleep disturbance, decreased energy, decreased libido, and increased appetite. She reports, "I've been depressed for years." She truly appears very sad. As the interview proceeds, the interviewer feels a deepening desire to help as well as an increasing concern. There is also an angry quality to Ms. Wilkins as she relates, "My best friend is really a bitch. I can't believe I trusted her." Ms. Wilkins denies concrete suicidal or homicidal ideation at the time of the interview, stating, "I'm feeling in control now." She wishes to have both medication and psychotherapy.

Discussion of Ms. Wilkins

Despite her sad affect, further questioning revealed some intriguing differences when comparing Ms. Wilkins with our three previous individuals:

> Pt.: I'm really feeling horrible. My whole world is collapsing. I don't know who to trust.
>
> Clin.: How long have you been feeling this way?
>
> Pt.: Years, for years. I can't think of a time when my life went smoothly. It's all a big mess.
>
> Clin.: When you say "for years" do you mean your depression never lifts?
>
> Pt.: Well, not really, I mean, I have my good days. Even a bad apple has its good parts … so … sometimes I feel fine.
>
> Clin.: When looking back over the past several weeks, did you have some of those good days?
>
> Pt.: Oh, I actually had a couple of good days last week, right before the big blow-up with Janet, but I knew Janet would blow it.
>
> Clin.: Tell me how you felt on those days.
>
> Pt.: Fine. In fact, I was having a great day on Friday until Janet had to open her big fat mouth.
>
> Clin.: You say you've been feeling depressed for years, but it sounds like your mood changes a lot. Have you ever had a period of at least 2 weeks where for the entire 2 weeks you felt down and depressed?
>
> Pt.: That's a little hard to answer. I haven't felt that way for a long time … back home though, yeah, back home I was about 19, I was depressed for almost 4 months straight.
>
> Clin.: Tell me more about it.

The Need to Determine the Persistence of Depressive Symptoms and How to Do It

From this dialogue it becomes apparent that Ms. Wilkins is probably not currently experiencing a sustained depressive episode. She would later describe a history of intermittent, low-grade depressive symptoms for many years, meeting the criteria for having a persistent depressive disorder (dysthymia, refer to page 345 for DSM-5 criteria). Without a sustained alteration in mood or marked anhedonia lasting for 2 weeks, she will not fulfill criteria for a major depressive disorder. On the other hand, she appears to have undergone a 4-month major depression in her teens. Further interviewing revealed that this episode was accompanied by persistent neurovegetative symptoms. She currently notes some *fluctuating* neurovegetative symptoms, including some difficulty falling asleep, increased appetite, and low energy. From her history she appears to have had a major depression at age 19, which is currently in remission. This previous depression had responded to paroxetine successfully.

The above dialogue emphasizes two points: (1) A detailed history of the present disorder should be carefully elicited. In this exploration, the interviewer pays particular attention to both the time course and the duration of the symptoms. The foundation of a good diagnostic interview remains a good history of the presenting disorder. (2) One should rigorously evaluate whether the depressive symptoms are sustained or whether they fluctuate towards normal. Many people whose depressed feelings come and go will describe their symptoms as unrelenting unless questioned carefully, perhaps related to the fact that depressive feelings often tend to be experienced as intolerable, thus overshadowing the moments of normal mood. *The DSM-5 criteria, for a major depressive episode, require that the depressive symptoms need to have each been present nearly every day for a period of at least 2 weeks.* Consequently, if the interviewer uncovers a significant fluctuation of symptoms, then he or she must look elsewhere than a major depressive disorder for a diagnosis.

Incidentally, I have found that statements such as, "I've been depressed for years," are, curiously enough, often indications that a classic major depressive disorder is not present. When questioned in more detail, such people often do not describe a sustained depression. Instead, they relate histories of depressive symptoms that fluctuate in response to environmental rewards or pleasures, as is commonly seen in some personality disorders, with a dysthymic disorder, in substance abuse, and in some atypical depressions. The following questions may be of value concerning the exploration of mood fluctuation:

a. "Do you find that your mood can shift during a single day?"
b. "Would you describe yourself as a moody person?"
c. "When you are feeling down, do you ever find that a friend or 'something to do' can perk you up quickly?"

If the patient answers "yes," then the interviewer, using behavioral incidents, asks the person to describe some examples of such experiences. Another very useful question for determining whether a depression is persistent or not is:

"Some people tell me that, when they are depressed, their symptoms stay with them day after day. Others tell me that their symptoms come and go almost like a roller-coaster. Where on that continuum would you place yourself?"

As mentioned earlier, the lack of sustained depressive symptoms suggests other diagnoses such as dysthymia, cyclothymic disorder, certain personality disorders, or drug abuse or atypical depressions.

Red Herrings: Disorders That Mimic Major Depressions

In contrast to Danny, Ms. Wilkins presents the opposite diagnostic trap – misdiagnosing a patient who actually has a personality disorder as solely having a major depressive disorder. Missing a personality disorder, especially severe disorders such as borderline personality disorder, can have major ramifications for a patient including: missed opportunities to use effective psychotherapies (such as dialectical behavioral therapy), inappropriate triage to inexperienced clinicians, the development of dangerous dependencies on the therapist, exposure to unnecessary medications, and lack of appropriate attention to suicide potential.

Upon further interviewing during her initial assessment, Ms. Wilkins described a long history of angry outbursts (e.g., throwing a hammer through a window), severe loneliness, intense feelings of boredom and emptiness, confusion over homosexual versus heterosexual relationships, and a series of overdoses. She also described a lengthy history of self-cutting her wrists and of burning her fingertips. These non-lethal self-injurious behaviors could occur in the middle of a series of days when she was feeling good, the behaviors occurring abruptly after a perceived interpersonal stress.

Later in the interview, Ms. Wilkins would provide further information suggesting that her problematic behaviors were long-standing, persistent, and not caused by substances or other disorders such as mania. She denied any history of bipolar process in her family and she had no history of unleashed manic symptoms upon use of antidepressants. She met the criteria for a diagnosis of borderline personality disorder. In addition, the interviewer sensitively uncovered a history of sexual abuse as a child, a situation that we shall see in our chapter on personality disorders is not uncommon with people presenting with a borderline personality disorder.

Her presentation emphasizes the following simple but easily forgotten principle: No matter how severely depressed a person looks, the diagnosis is not always that of a major depressive disorder. In fact, when it comes to looking severely upset, individuals with borderline personality disorder have a knack for such a dramatic presentation. With this in mind, when the interviewee complains of sadness or depression, the following diagnoses should be considered in addition to a major depression or a bipolar disorder:

a. Persistent depressive disorder (dysthymia)
b. Cyclothymic disorder
c. Borderline personality disorder
d. Other personality disorders such as the histrionic personality, narcissistic personality, avoidant personality, dependent personality, or obsessive–compulsive personality
e. Alcohol or drug abuse
f. Adjustment disorders with depressed mood
g. Medical etiologies of depression such as hypothyroidism
h. V-codes such as marital problems or housing and economic problems (*normal* depressive responses to situational stresses)

Far from being a complete differential, this list represents the common entities that are often misdiagnosed as major depressive episodes. In contrast to a major depressive episode, these entities tend to show significant fluctuation in both mood and symptomatology. To mislabel these disorders as a major depressive disorder can lead to serious errors in triage or medication prescription, as mentioned earlier. To further illustrate the point, it could be a fatal mistake to prematurely prescribe antidepressants for Ms. Wilkins, subsequent to having mistakenly diagnosed her as having a major depressive disorder. Indeed, Ms. Wilkin's psychiatric trail is littered with empty bottles signifying her suicidal gestures by overdosing.

Tips for Delineating an Accurate History of the Presenting Disorder

Delineating the history of the presenting disorder and determining the consistency of the symptoms are not tasks as easily accomplished as one might think. The process is greatly complicated by a variety of factors, including: (1) patient difficulties with memory, (2) unconscious distortion of the facts by the patient, (3) conscious or histrionic distortions by the patient, and (4) misunderstandings by the patient of the questions asked. These problems are compounded when the clinician becomes lost in the facts and has no general approach to eliciting the history of the presenting disorder.

Consequently, it is worth spending some time examining some approaches to gathering a valid history of the present disorder for the classic psychiatric diagnoses unrelated to personality dysfunction. This history can be broken down into three contiguous phases: the early phase, the mid-phase, and the recent phase of the disorder (the 2 months directly preceding the interview). All three phases are important, but because of the time constraints facing the intake clinician, an emphasis should be placed, in my opinion, on the early phase and the recent phase.

The early phase may provide critical diagnostic information, because it allows the clinician to see the natural unfolding of the pathologic process. A patient may present with striking hallucinations while also reporting depressive feelings. If the patient has a major depression, then the early phase will generally demonstrate the appearance of marked depressed symptoms first, followed by psychotic symptoms. However, as we shall see in Chapter 11 on the differential diagnosis of psychotic disorders, the patient with schizophrenia (although the patient may have mild prodromal depressive symptoms) will generally demonstrate psychotic symptoms and agitation first, with more severe depressive symptoms appearing later. Unless the clinician asks the patient or collaborative sources such as parents and other family members for this information, it can easily remain buried in the history. It is also during the history of the early phase that the interviewer has the opportunity to hear about the symptoms of the disorder without the distorting impact of medications.

A careful delineation of the recent history is an absolute necessity, because it provides the information needed to determine the patient's immediate level of functioning and the present diagnostic reality of the patient. As noted above, this immediate diagnostic picture can be confusing if the patient is currently taking medications, because the patient's symptom picture may be incomplete, since partial remission may be present. As obvious as this point may seem, it is surprisingly easy in a busy clinic setting to be trapped into thinking that a patient is *not* experiencing a major depressive episode when, in actuality, it is hiding beneath the facade created by partial treatment. In such circumstances, it is important to explore the symptom picture at the time directly preceding the use of medications.

With the understanding that it may be valuable to emphasize the early phase and the recent phase, two rather different approaches can be utilized when eliciting the history of the presenting disorder. Both are effective. Clinicians must determine which seems best suited to their style and the needs of the specific patient.

In the first technique, as the patient discusses the history of the presenting disorder, an effort is made to quickly direct the patient to the early phase of the illness. The history is then taken chronologically from past to present, with less emphasis upon the middle phase. Stressors and responses to stressors are frequently elicited as the history naturally unfolds. The strength of this approach is the detailed and well-ordered history that results. The weakness is the fact that because patient histories are frequently both complex, and fascinating, the clinician can easily spend too much time on the early and middle phase, coming away with a hazier picture of the immediate problems and current presentation.

A brief piece of dialogue will demonstrate two important features concerning the delineation of the onset of the disorder.

> **Clin.:** When did this depression first begin for you?
>
> **Pt.:** Uh … a couple weeks after Thanksgiving … yeah, after Thanksgiving everything began to fall apart.
>
> **Clin.:** Think carefully, in the months before Thanksgiving were you feeling totally normal or were you already feeling not quite yourself? (time-related anchor question)
>
> **Pt.:** Huh … actually I had been feeling somewhat depressed shortly after Patty, my daughter, went away to college.
>
> **Clin.:** What were the first symptoms you noticed?
>
> **Pt.:** I felt tearful at times and unusually tired … yes, yes, I remember being struck at how little I wanted to get out of bed in the morning. But I'm not really certain when that feeling began … no, now that I think of it, that might have happened much later, I'm just not certain (looking frustrated).
>
> **Clin.:** It's hard to remember details like this and you're doing an excellent job. Let's focus upon Thanksgiving. Did you have a hard time getting out of bed then?
>
> **Pt.:** Oh yes, that I do remember. I didn't want to clean the house either or even cook the turkey.
>
> **Clin.:** What was your appetite like over Thanksgiving?
>
> **Pt.:** Very poor.

As illustrated in the preceding dialogue, when first asked to date the onset of their disorder, patients frequently give an inaccurately late date, because it is easiest to remember when they began to feel really bad, usually a point several weeks or months after the onset of the illness. Consequently, they should be gently pushed by asking a second time, as shown in the example. Another useful method of increasing the validity of the data, as illustrated in the above dialogue, is to use a validity technique we described in Chapter 5 called the "time-related anchor question," delineated by Danny Carlat. Time-related anchor questions prime the memory of the patient by using specific holidays or personal events that can function as a trigger for increasing memory production.[73]

The second approach for eliciting the history of the present disorder consists of focusing the patient upon the recent and current phase of the illness first. The clinician then skips to the early phase and delineates the remainder of the history chronologically, with less emphasis upon the middle phase. This method provides the clinician with a sound understanding of current symptoms, stresses, and level of functioning, ensuring that these critical areas do not get short shrift because of time constraints. Patients also frequently like talking about recent symptoms first. Generally, this method also provides the early generation of a good diagnostic differential, which can help guide the subsequent questioning concerning the earlier phases of the history of the presenting disorder.

When delineating the recent history, it is often useful to frame the time period with comments such as, "Let's look for a moment at just the last 2 weeks. All of the following questions deal only with the last 2 weeks. During that time how has your energy been?" Because the patient has been coping with large amounts of psychological pain and confusion, even with the above framing, it is easy for that person to eventually begin discussing earlier symptoms without letting the clinician know that this is the case. Consequently, it is useful to remind the patient several times of the timeframe with statements such as, "Once again, just looking at the past 2 weeks, what has your sleep been like?"

Let us now return to the presentation of Ms. Wilkins, because her history provides several more practical interviewing points.

Ruling Out Peripartum Depressions, Grief, Adjustment Disorders, and V-Codes

Pay particular attention to mood disturbances in the months directly after a patient has given birth. The tremendous hormonal shifts associated with pregnancy, birthing, and breastfeeding can trigger mood disturbances. Ms. Wilkins was neither pregnant nor postpartum, effectively ruling out this diagnosis.

Sometimes women who develop postpartum mood disorders may have had significant mood disturbances during the pregnancy itself. It is also important to note that a true postpartum depression is strikingly more severe than the normal moodiness (postpartum blues) seen in many women following birth. Postpartum depressive episodes can evolve into bipolar disorders and mixed states, including psychotic process, as we shall discuss in Chapter 11. It is important in these postpartum psychotic states to ask questions that can sort out whether there may exist some danger to the newborn (as with a belief the child is demon possessed or the patient is experiencing command hallucinations to hurt the child). Whether the depressive episode begins prepartum or postpartum, in the DSM-5 these major depressive disorders are indicated by adding the specifier "with peripartum onset."[74]

With further questioning, Ms. Wilkins denied the recent death of any close friends or family. This point is mentioned because her initial symptoms would have been consistent with an uncomplicated bereavement. In addition to the natural depressive responses accompanying grief, it is not uncommon for a full major depressive episode to occur during the acute phase of grief. If it does – or if the patient demonstrates severe depressive symptoms not typical of his or her culture – one should consider adding the diagnosis of major depressive disorder.[75]

On the other hand, if the bereavement lasts too long a time and/or begins to persistently intensify over the months following the death, then the diagnosis of a major depressive disorder should be made instead of an uncomplicated bereavement. Also clinicians can use their phenomenological understanding to help differentiate normal grief from the development of a pathologic depressive episode.

In normal grief, the depressive symptoms are less persistent and consistent than in a major depressive episode. Indeed, in normal grief it is common to see wave-like "pangs of grief" as the person is reminded of the deceased. In a similar fashion, in normal grief the neurovegetative symptoms may not be as severe or persistent in nature. Guilty cognitions are more commonly seen in true major depressive episodes when they assume a generalized feeling of being inadequate, worthless, or weak. In contrast, if guilty ruminations appear in normal grief, they tend to be specific towards letting down the deceased, as with not visiting enough, not getting a chance to say good-bye, or not telling the deceased how much he or she was loved.

An uncomplicated bereavement is one of the many "V-codes" in the DSM-5 system (close to a hundred such codes are enumerated). A V-code is a situation or life stressor that the clinician feels is playing a significant part in the person's current difficulties and warrants attention from the clinician. *It is important to remember that V-codes are not mental disorders.* V-codes are, in essence, reminders to subsequent clinicians of various aspects of the person's matrix where intervention may be valuable. They can include factors such as current marital problems, spouse or partner abuse, problems at work, financial or housing problems, as well as quite specific situations such as deployment to a war zone for a soldier or the spouse of a soldier.[76]

The diagnosis of adjustment disorder specified with depressed mood describes those occurrences in which there is a clear-cut psychosocial stressor within 3 months of the depression. These disorders are viewed as exceeding normal response by either the distress being markedly out of proportion to the experienced stressor and/or there is significant impairment in social, occupational, or other areas of functioning. But even if there is a clear-cut stressor within the specified timeframe, if the criteria for a major depressive episode are fulfilled, then the diagnosis of adjustment disorder is no longer applicable and should be dropped, and the diagnosis of major depressive disorder should be made. Note that adjustment disorders can be classified with various specifiers, such as depressed mood, anxiety, conduct disturbance, or admixture of such symptoms.[77]

Differential Diagnosis on Ms. Wilkins and Summary of Key Interviewing Tips

Note that Ms. Wilkins seems to clearly have had a true major depressive episode about 8 years earlier, which raises the possibility that she could, theoretically, be currently starting into a second or recurrent episode, although her symptoms are not yet persistent enough to meet such a disorder. In addition, she reports some phenomena, such as mood reactivity, interpersonal rejection sensitivity, and an increased appetite, that are consistent with an atypical depression (a type of depression seen with some regularity in people fitting the criteria for a borderline personality disorder and some other personality diagnoses). Ms. Wilkins diagnostic summary, after her initial interview, would be as follows:

General Psychiatric Disorders:

Persistent depressive disorder (dysthymia)

Personal past history of childhood sexual abuse (one of the V-Codes, included in the differential diagnosis to ensure that appropriate attention is given to this factor in treatment)

Rule out major depressive disorder, recurrent

Rule out major depressive disorder, recurrent, with atypical features

Personality Disorders:

Borderline personality (principal diagnosis)

Medical Disorders:

None

Notice that if a personality disorder is the main presenting problem (often becoming the focus of care) or the reason for a hospital admission, it can be useful to identify it as the "principal diagnosis."

By way of summary, Ms. Wilkins' presentation illustrates the following points:

1. A careful history of the presenting disorder is the foundation of the diagnostic component of an initial interview.
2. The duration of the depressive mood should be thoroughly discussed. To fulfill a major depressive disorder it must last at least 2 weeks in length with little fluctuation in symptoms.
3. Many other diagnoses may present with depression. In particular, one should be careful to check for a borderline personality disorder, dysthymia, drug or alcohol abuse, an adjustment disorder, or a V-code.
4. The clinician should develop a well thought-out approach to the history of the presenting disorder. Otherwise, it is easy to become lost in the database.
5. Patients frequently date the onset of their illness later than it was in reality. Once a date is given, ask the patient to carefully consider whether he or she had felt completely normal in the month or two before that date.
6. One can prime the patient's memory by referring to holidays or to special events in the patient's life (the use of a time-related anchor question).
7. When gathering the recent history, it is useful to frame the time period for the patient and intermittently remind him or her of the timeframe being discussed.
8. Uncomplicated bereavement (a V-code) may simultaneously fulfill the criteria for a major depressive episode. If this occurs, the process is still labeled an uncomplicated bereavement and the diagnosis of a major depression is added as a concurrent disorder.

Clinical Presentation #5: Mr. Collier

Mr. Collier and his wife presented at the psychiatric emergency room. Mr. Collier is a 26-year-old White man who is casually but nicely dressed. He has dark brown hair and a strong jaw. His voice is rich with a vigorous, almost aggressive, tone. He answers quickly with authority. While he interacts with his wife, the interviewer finds it easy to picture Mr. Collier giving his wife "the third degree." Mr. Collier complains bitterly of severe depression "ever since I was a teenager." He continues, "I remind myself of my father." He reports a tendency to sleep during the day and frequently feels tired. On the other hand, he reports that his energy can be pretty good if he has something to do that he likes doing. Along these lines, he reports a robust appetite and sex drive. In fact, he reports that, "I still enjoy life a fair amount. I love getting out with my buddies and there is nothing better than Super Bowl Sunday!" He complains of intermittently "feeling sort of worthless and lazy." He is definitely upset that he has been sharp with his kids. A day before their emergency room visit he slapped his 5-year-old daughter, Jackie, on the face. This incident frightened him and prompted the emergency room visit. He occasionally has fleeting suicidal ideation, remarking, "If I had to, I guess I'd jump in front of a car or bus … you know, to make sure my wife gets the insurance." He denies current suicidal ideation. He states, "I'm the problem here. Help me and you'll help my family."

Discussion of Mr. Collier

In some respects, Mr. Collier's interview sounds reminiscent of Ms. Wilkins' presentation. Further questioning revealed that, like Ms. Wilkins, his mood tends to fluctuate. He would not meet the criteria for a major depressive disorder for he has not had a recent period of pervasively depressed mood lasting for 2 weeks or more. He denies any manic or hypomanic symptoms other than chronic irritability.

Questions pertaining to the history of his present disorder revealed that he had felt intermittently depressed for over 10 years. He had had no periods of good mood lasting consistently longer than a month or two. Mr. Collier did not relate further symptoms consistent with a borderline personality or any other personality disorder, although he displayed, and his wife supported, that he had some mildly narcissistic traits. The above information, once again, suggests a diagnosis of dysthymia, a relatively common psychiatric syndrome. There is substantial research evidence that dysthymia can respond well to antidepressant medication, as well as psychotherapy, suggesting both modalities as a potential tool for intervention.[78]

Dysthymia (also called persistent depressive disorder – see DSM-5 criteria on page 345) often presents, as it did with Mr. Collier, with a low-grade depressive mood (and two or more common depressive symptoms) being present most days over a minimum of a 2-year timespan. If the patient, at any point, meets the criteria for a major depressive disorder, it is added as a concurrent diagnosis.

Techniques for Eliciting a Family History

Mr. Collier's comment that "I remind myself of my father," warrants further follow-up. This statement may be the first indication that mood disorders run in his family. Research has shown genetic predispositions for many psychiatric disorders are common, ranging from severe processes such as psychotic depression and bipolar disorder to much milder processes such as dysthymia.

For instance, the heritability of bipolar disorder has been estimated to be about 60% to 80% in genetic studies of the concordance of the disorder in monozygotic (same egg) twins.[79] In a similar fashion, patients with major depressive disorders show a higher prevalence of relatives with major depressive disorders and depressive personalities. Other studies have suggested some genetic correlation between mood disorders and alcoholism. For instance, in a well-known study – the Collaborative Study on the Genetics of Alcoholism (COGA) – Nurnberger and associates found that alcoholism and depression do, indeed, tend to run in families, with evidence that some of this concurrence may be related to genetic factors.[80]

An accurate family history can help patients in several ways. Sometimes, the presence of a specific disorder in the family history (such as bipolar disorder) can alert the clinician to more carefully hunt for similar symptoms in the patient that might have been overlooked in the earlier interviewing. The presence of processes such as psychosis or a strong history of suicide in the family may prompt the interviewer to seek more careful follow-up or recommend hospitalization to the patient (if one is "on the fence" as to whether or not hospitalization might be useful for observation or more intensive treatment). In addition, if one uncovers the same psychiatric disorders in family members as with the patient, it is useful to ask, "Do you know if your dad (or whomever is being discussed) responded well to any medications?" Excellent response in a family member can be an indicator that the patient may have a positive response to that specific medication. Finally, as we have already seen, the presence of bipolar process in family members (or the unleashing of a manic process after the use of an antidepressant in a family member) should alert us to be careful with the use of antidepressants in the patient.

Difficulties in Taking a Family History and How to Transform Them

Despite its importance, elaborating a valid family history in the first 50 minutes is no easy task. A variety of variables can get in the way, including: (1) the patient's lack of information about his family history; (2) the patient's decreased concentration and other cognitive impairments decreasing the accuracy of his statements; (3) the patient's protection of other family members; (4) the patient's culture disapproves of sharing information on psychiatric disorders; and (5) the interviewer's ineffective exploration of the patient's family history. This last variable is the only one over which we have direct control.

Frequently, vague questions such as "Does anyone in your family have a mental illness?" can often lead to blanket negatives. The interviewee may have no idea that the interviewer is including blood relatives such as aunts, uncles, or cousins in such a question. Along the same lines, the interviewee may have no idea that the interviewer is including alcoholism as a mental disorder. To anticipate these problems, it may be of value to help the patient understand the reason for obtaining a family history. Such an approach also "focuses" patients, increasing their willingness to jog their memories. Just one of many lead-ins is illustrated below with a patient we shall call Carl:

> Clin.: Carl, you mentioned earlier that you sometimes remind yourself of your father. In what ways is this true?
>
> Pt.: Hmm … Well, my father often seemed upset to me as a kid. He got irritable and would yell at us, all of us, even Annie, the baby. He just seemed troubled.
>
> Clin.: Do you think he was depressed?
>
> Pt.: Yeah, I do.
>
> Clin.: Had he ever received help from a therapist or psychiatrist?
>
> Pt.: Oh, no! He would never do that. He didn't believe in that sort of thing; even so, I think he needed help.
>
> Clin.: While we are talking about your father's depression, I would like to touch upon other family members. Sometimes we can gain clues from psychiatric problems in relatives that may give us better ideas of how to help you.

Following such an introduction to the topic, the clinician can proceed to discuss each member of Carl's nuclear family, inquiring specifically about drinking, schizophrenia, and other affective disorders. With regard to more distant family members, it is important to state whom you are interested in.

> Clin.: The rest of these questions concern any of your blood relatives, including grandparents, aunts, uncles, and cousins. Have any of your father's blood relatives had depression or schizophrenia? (repeat these questions later for the other side of the family)
>
> Pt.: Well, I'm not really sure. I had an aunt who was sort of crazy.
>
> Clin.: How do you mean?
>
> Pt.: They put her away for a while because she had a nervous breakdown.

The preceding exchange illustrates several points. First, one needs to be careful with technical words like "schizophrenia" or "bipolar disorder." Many patients do not know what these terms mean and will consequently deny their presence. A brief definition may help clarify the issue. Second, it can be of use to ask the question, "Has anybody in your family been hospitalized or institutionalized for a mental disorder?" People may remember a concrete hospitalization concerning a distant relative much easier than a nebulous process like depression. Third, terms such as "bad nerves" or "nervous breakdown" are common labels for serious disorders such as schizophrenia, bipolar disorder, or an agitated depression. Such terms warrant further inquiry.

Another important question is simple and to the point, "Has anybody in your family ever tried to kill themselves or actually did kill themselves?" Surprisingly, after having denied any serious psychiatric illnesses in their family, interviewees will suddenly recall a suicide following this question.

This phenomenon parallels the finding that subsequent interviewing will often reveal positive family history that went undetected in the initial interview. In a similar way, it is remarkable how interviewing family members of the patient regarding a history of familial mental disorders pulls forth some surprises. If possible, questioning family members, in addition to the patient, about mental illness and suicide in the family tree is a good habit to cultivate.

Cross-Cultural Sensitivity When Taking a Family History

As one would expect, cross-cultural differences can impact on the eliciting of a family history of psychiatric disorders. Generally speaking, there is a hesitancy in all cultures to relay personal information about psychiatric disorders in family members. In some cultures, this hesitancy is particularly strong. As an example, individuals from Asian cultures may experience relatively extreme stigmatization concerning mental illness. To admit to mental illness in oneself or one's family members may, essentially, be a cultural taboo. In this regard, clinicians may need to be sensitive and employ subtlety in the phrasing of potentially disengaging questions about the presence of mental illness in family members.

When asking about past family psychiatric history with an Asian patient, it can be of use to avoid asking direct questions such as, "Does anyone in your family have a mental illness?" or "Anyone in your family with psychiatric problems?" Michael Cheng[81] suggests that with Asians and Asian Americans it is sometimes best to proceed with questions that cue directly off the symptoms of the patient himself or herself, focusing more upon phenomenology or stress, such as:

1. "Has anyone in your family ever had similar difficulties as yourself?"
2. "Has anyone in your family had mood problems like the ones you've been having?"
3. "Has anyone been feeling anxious like you've been feeling?"
4. "Has anyone in your family been particularly stressed, like you've been recently?" (If the answer is yes, the clinician can ask whether the family member has been having similar symptoms.)

Even the term "nervous breakdown" may sound less stigmatizing to an Asian American than "psychiatric illness." If there appears to be confusion over the less direct questions above, one can ask, "Has anyone in your family, perhaps related to stress, had a nervous breakdown?" These questions are often of use with almost any patient who is particularly afraid of stigmatization, no matter what his or her cultural background.

Another potential problem arises if the interviewer is unaware that a particular culture may use a different word than "depression" for a depressive equivalent. We saw this problem earlier with the word "nervios" often being used instead of depression (or other psychiatric disorders). Consequently, when inquiring about a psychiatric family history with a Latino/a patient (or his or her family members), it can be useful to ask, "Have there been any of your family members who, when very stressed, developed nervios?" It should also be kept in mind that many cultures will express depressive equivalents with somatic symptoms, particularly true in Asian and Hispanic cultures. It is also quite striking in some refugee populations.[82]

A final impediment to uncovering a valid family history occurs when the interviewer is unaware that there are specific major mental disorders unique to the patient's culture that are not present in the culture of the interviewer, as we shall examine in Chapter 12. Obviously, when taking a family history, the interviewer may need to ask directly about such culture-specific disorders in order to hear about them. A subtle variation occurs when a similar disorder exists to a DSM-5 disorder, but it might not be viewed as being "psychiatric" in nature in the patient's culture, hence not shared with the interviewer when questioning about a family history of psychiatric disorders.

A nice example of this process can be found when interviewing a patient or refugee from Vietnam. In Vietnamese culture, there is a syndrome called *trung gio*.[83] The syndrome has many of the symptoms of a panic attack as defined in the DSM-5. Interestingly, these attacks are viewed as being literally caused by the wind. Anticipation of such attacks on a windy day can even result in what might be called agoraphobic tendencies in the DSM-5. Our point, regarding family history, is that such attacks might not be conveyed by the patient as being present because they are not necessarily viewed as being a mental disorder. Instead, they are viewed as being caused by the movements of the wind. In hunting for a family history of panic disorder with a Vietnamese patient, after asking directly about panic attacks, the interviewer might add, "Have any of your family members tended to have problems with *trung gio* and feel very frightened and upset when they go out in the wind?"

Family History as a Reflection of Family Dynamics

Before leaving the issue of family history, I would like to add one final point. The family history may provide more information than just that relating to genetic inheritance of mental illnesses. The tone of voice and the manner in which the patient talks about family members may provide subtle clues concerning family relations themselves. At times, it pays to take a brief excursion into interpersonal and dynamic issues during this part of the interview, as illustrated below.

> **Clin.:** Do you feel your brother had problems with depression or drugs?
>
> **Pt.:** Him (said with an astonished and sarcastic tone)! No. He's lily white. He's never had any problems.
>
> **Clin.:** You sound almost surprised by my question.
>
> **Pt.:** Oh, it's just that he has always been everybody's favorite.
>
> **Clin.:** How have you noticed that?
>
> **Pt.:** He always made better grades. Report card day was a real pain in the ass for me. I used to …

In this example, "family history" has taken on a richer meaning.

Differential Diagnosis on Mr. Collier and Summary of Key Interviewing Tips

Before looking at Mr. Collier's diagnostic summary, three points should be made. First, with regard to medical problems, Mr. Collier related having bronchitis secondary to smoking. Second, on an interpersonal level, further interviewing indicated significant marital distress. Couples therapy was recommended. This disruption on the intimate wing of Mr. Collier's matrix would prove to be a core issue with regard to Mr. Collier's depression. Third, the physical slapping of his child demanded much more careful inquiry during the initial interview. Both parents related this action as a one-time incident. Mr. Collier's diagnostic summary is as follows:

General Psychiatric Disorders:

Persistent depressive disorder (dysthymia)

(with early onset and moderately severe)

Relationship distress with spouse or intimate other (V-code)

Encounter for mental health services for perpetrator of parental child abuse (V-code)

Personality Disorders:

No disorder but may have narcissistic traits

Medical Disorders:

Chronic bronchitis secondary to smoking

Note that when using the V-code regarding child abuse, it is critical that you explain in detail in the body of your EHR the exact abuse and your estimate of its severity. This V-code can have powerful legal ramifications. In this case, after extensive interviewing, if the clinician believed in the truthfulness of the reporting by Mr. Collier and his wife, he would state that the physical abuse appeared to be limited to one example of slapping. A wise interviewer would return to this topic in later sessions to see if more abuse was relayed upon further engagement with Mr. and Mrs. Collier.

Also, after completing this initial interview, I would also advise that the clinician should consult with a superior to determine whether an interview with the child was indicated. During this consultation, a decision could be made as to whether any further requirements existed for reporting to appropriate protective agencies (various states may have differing laws and regulations governing such reporting of potential abuse).

In conclusion Mr. Collier's presentation emphasizes several points:

1. Individuals with persistent depressive disorder (dysthymia) commonly experience psychological symptoms of depression as well as some neurovegetative symptoms, but neither their psychological symptoms nor their neurovegetative symptoms persist in a sustained manner for over 2 weeks, unless a major depressive disorder is concurrently present. Also note that if a major depressive disorder does not go into a full remission within 2 years, the diagnosis of a persistent depressive disorder should be added.

2. The depressive symptoms of a dysthymia can often rapidly shift towards normal if there is something "fun" to do, similar to the mood reactivity seen in atypical depressions.

3. A detailed family history should be an integral component of all comprehensive initial assessments.

4. Blanket questions such as "Does anybody in your family have a mental illness?" will often yield false negatives.

5. Patients may not view alcohol dependence or drug dependence as mental illnesses, and you should clearly mention them specifically.

6. Some patients will need you to explain potentially confusing terms, such as schizophrenia or bipolar disorder in everyday language, or they will simply deny their presence in the family history.
7. Consider carefully cross-cultural differences when taking a family history.
8. A family history occasionally provides a nice take-off point for exploring family dynamics.

The above five case discussions are not intended to be an exhaustive review of the diagnostic subtleties associated with mood disorders. Instead, I have attempted to present a sound, and hopefully exciting, introduction to the process of differential diagnosis during an initial interview. My goal has been to show some of the practical interviewing strategies and techniques for arriving at a DSM-5 diagnosis, while simultaneously showing how an accurate uncovering of these diagnoses can have profoundly useful ramifications for our patients' healing.

I believe it is an opportune time for us to look at some video material. In Video Module 9.1 below, I will demonstrate the expansion of the diagnosis of a major depressive disorder exactly as described in this chapter. In addition, as mentioned earlier, the interviewing principles delineated in this chapter on mood disorders are equally applicable to most of the major psychiatric disorders. Thus they can serve as models from which you can generalize to the expansion of these other disorders.

Consequently, in our *optional* second video, Video Module 9.2, I thought it might be fun for the interested reader to have a chance to see both didactic material and subsequent interviewing demonstrations in which I illustrate expansions on three disorders that you will commonly encounter in your clinical practice: panic disorder, generalized anxiety disorder, and adult attention-deficit disorder. Our optional second video package allows us to look at didactics and interview segments that cannot be covered in our book due to space limitations. It's a bonus of sorts. I hope you find this additional material to be both useful and enjoyable.

VIDEO MODULE 9.1

Title: Sensitively Uncovering the Symptoms of Major Depressive Disorder

Contents: Contains both expanded didactics and annotated interview excerpts demonstrating the diagnostic expansion of a major depressive episode.
Important note to the reader: After viewing Video Module 9.1, you can proceed directly with the text below OR you may view optional Video Module 9.2.

VIDEO MODULE 9.2

Title: Sensitively Exploring the Diagnostic Criteria for Other Psychiatric Disorders such as Panic Disorder, Generalized Anxiety Disorder, and Adult Attention-Deficit Disorder

Contents: This video module contains three sequentially unfolding learning segments. Each segment contains didactic material and an interview demonstration of how to effectively expand the diagnostic region of the three disorders indicated in the title of the module.

In our next chapter, we will move past the art of differential diagnosis and begin to explore how depressive symptoms are uniquely experienced by our patients and those who love them. We will see how depression impacts and resonates throughout the matrix of each patient who enters our offices. From the perspective of person-centered interviewing, the art of differential diagnosis is always performed hand-in-hand with the art of understanding the person beneath the diagnosis. We will now turn our attention to this equally important second art.

REFERENCES

1. Blake W. *Songs of innocence and of experience*. Franklin Center, PA: Franklin Library; 1980. [Original publication, 1794] p. 86.
2. American Psychiatric Association. *Diagnostic and statistical manual of mental disorders*. 5th ed, DSM-5. Washington, DC: American Psychiatric Association Publishing; 2013. p. 160–1.
3. *DSM-5*. 2013. p. 168–9.
4. Carlat DJ. *The psychiatric interview*. 3rd ed. Philadelphia, PA: Lippincott Williams & Wilkins; 2012. p. 122.
5. *DSM-5*. 2013. p. 165.
6. American Psychiatric Association. *Diagnostic and statistical manual of mental disorders, DSM-IV-TR*. Washington, DC: American Psychiatric Publishing; 2000. p. 371.
7. *DSM-5*. 2013. p. 185.
8. Fawcett J. Suicide and anxiety in DSM-5. *Depress Anxiety* 2013;30(10):898–901.
9. Fawcett J. Depressive disorders. In: Simon RI, Hales RE, editors. *The American psychiatric publishing textbook of suicide assessment and management*. 2nd ed. Washington, DC: American Psychiatric Publishing; 2012. p. 109–21.
10. Fawcett J, Clark DC, Busch KA. Assessing and treating the patient at risk for suicide. *Psych Annals* 1993;23:245–55.
11. Gratzer D, Levitan RD, Sheldon T, et al. Lifetime rates of alcoholism in adults with anxiety, depression, or co-morbid depression/anxiety: a community survey of Ontario. *J Affect Disord* 2004;79(1–3):209–15.
12. *DSM-5*. 2013. p. 130.
13. *DSM-5*. 2013. p. 131.
14. *DSM-5*. 2013. p. 124–5.
15. *DSM-5*. 2013. p. 123.
16. *DSM-5*. 2013. p. 130.
17. *DSM-5*. 2013. p. 130.
18. Sims A. *Symptoms in the mind: an introduction to descriptive psychopathology*. 2nd ed. London: W. B. Saunders Company, Ltd.; 1996. p. 137.
19. Mendelson D, Goes FS. A 34-year-old mother with religious delusions, filicidal thoughts. *Psych Annals* 2011;41(7):359–62.
20. Martínez-Arán A, Vieta E, Reinares M, et al. Cognitive function across manic or hypomanic, depressed, and euthymic states in bipolar disorder. *Am J Psychiatry* 2004;161(2):262–70.
21. Murphy FC, Rubinsztein JS, Michael A, et al. Decision-making cognition in mania and depression. *Psychol Med* 2001;31(4):679–93.
22. Stefanopoulou E, Manoharon A, Landau S, et al. Cognitive functioning in patients with affective disorders and schizophrenia: A meta-analysis. *Int Rev Psychiatry* 2009;21(4):336–56.
23. Bora E, Yucel M, Pantelis C. Cognitive endophenotypes of bipolar disorder: A meta-analysis of neuropsychological deficits in euthymic patients and their first-degree relatives. *J Affect Disord* 2009;113(1–2):1–20.
24. Deckersbach T, McMurrich S, Ogutha J, et al. Characteristics of non-verbal memory impairment in bipolar disorder: the role of encoding strategies. *Psychol Med* 2004;34(5):823–32.
25. American Psychiatric Association. *Diagnostic and statistical manual of mental disorders*. 4th ed, Text Revision (DSM-IV-TR). Washington, DC: American Psychiatric Association Publishing; 2000. p. 362.
26. Goodwin FK, Jamison KR. *Manic-depressive illness: bipolar disorders and recurrent depression*. Oxford: Oxford University Press; 2007. p. 96–8.
27. Frye MA. Diagnostic dilemmas and clinical correlates of mixed states in bipolar disorder. *J Clin Psychiatry* 2008;69(5):e13.
28. Akiskal HS. Searching for behavioral indicators of bipolar disorder II in patients with major depressive episodes: the "red sign", the "rule of three" and other biographic signs of temperamental extravagance, activation, and hypomania. *J Affect Disord* 2005;84:279–90.
29. McElroy SL, Keck PE Jr, Pope HG Jr, et al. Clinical and research implications of the diagnosis of dysphoric or mixed mania or hypomania. *Am J Psychiatry* 1992;149(12):1633–44.

30. Himmelhoch JM, Mulla D, Neil JF, et al. Incidence and significance of mixed affective states in a bipolar population. *Arch Gen Psychiatry* 1976;**33**(9):1062–6.
31. Goodwin FK, Jamison KR, 2007, p. 96–8.
32. Kraepelin E. *Lectures on clinical psychiatry*. 2nd ed. Birmingham, AL: Classics of Psychiatry and Behavioral Sciences Library, Division of Gryphon Editions, Inc.; 1988. p. 69–78 [Original work published 1904].
33. Kraepelin E. *Manic depressive insanity and paranoia*. Edinburgh, UK: E & S Livingstone; 1921.
34. Kraepelin E. *Psychiatry: a textbook for students and physicians*. Sixth ed. Translated by Helga Metoui. Canton, MA: Science History Publications; 1990. p. 8 [Original work published 1899].
35. Bleuler E. *Textbook of psychiatry*. Birmingham, AL: Classics of Psychiatry and Behavioral Sciences Library, Division of Gryphon Editions, Inc.; 1988. p. 479 [Original work published 1924].
36. Griesinger W. *Mental pathology and therapeutics*. Birmingham, AL: Classics of Psychiatry and Behavioral Science, Division of Gryphon Editions, Inc.; 1989. p. 176–9 [Original work published 1882].
37. *DSM-5*, 2013, p. 149–50.
38. Strakowski SM, Fleck DE, Maj M. Broadening the diagnosis of bipolar disorder: benefits vs. risks. *World Psychiatry* 2011;**10**(3):181–6.
39. Griesinger W. 1989, p. 176–91.
40. Forty L, Smith D, Jones L, et al. Clinical differences between bipolar and unipolar depression. *Br J Psychiatry* 2008;**192**(5):388–9.
41. Akiskal HS, Benazzi F. Family history validation of the bipolar nature of depressive mixed states. *J Affect Disord* 2003;**73**(1–2):113–22.
42. Mitchell PB, Wilhelm K, Parker G, et al. The clinical features of bipolar disorder: A comparison with matched major depressive disorder patients. *J Clin Psychiatry* 2001;**62**:212–16.
43. Goldberg JF, Garno JL, Leon AC, et al. Association of recurrent suicidal ideation with nonremission from acute mixed mania. *Am J Psychiatry* 1998;**155**:1753–5.
44. Dilsaver SC, Chen YW, Swann AC, et al. Suicidality in patients with pure and depressive mania. *Am J Psychiatry* 1994;**151**:1312–15.
45. Goldberg JF, Garno JL, Portera L, et al. Correlates of suicidal ideation in dysphoric mania. *J Affect Disord* 1999;**56**:75–81.
46. *DSM-5*. 2013. p. 156.
47. Smith DJ. How to recognize and treat bipolar II disorder. *Current Psychiatry* 2009;**8**(7):41–8.
48. Smith DJ. 2009, p. 41.
49. *DSM-5*. 2013. p. 1124–5.
50. Smith DJ. 2009. p. 42.
51. *DSM-5*. 2013. p. 144.
52. Vaks YK, Nandu B. A 34-year-old woman with depression, suicidal ideation. *Psychiatr Ann* 2011;**41**(7):367–9.
53. *DSM-5*. 2013. p. 139.
54. *DSM-5*. 2013. p. 140.
55. *DSM-5*. 2013. p. 150–1.
56. Klein D, Gittelman R, Quitkin F, Rifkin A. *Diagnosis and drug treatment of psychiatric disorders*. Baltimore: Williams & Wilkins; 1980. p. 226.
57. *DSM-5*. 2013. p. 835.
58. Lewis-Fernández R, Hinton DE, Laria AJ, et al. Culture and the anxiety disorders: recommendations for the DSM-5. *Depress Anxiety* 2009;**0**:1–18.
59. *DSM-IV-TR*. 2000. p. 353.
60. Cristancho MA, O'Reardon JP, Thase ME. Atypical depression in the 21st century: Diagnostic and treatment issues. *Psychiatric Times* 2011;**28**(1):42–6.
61. Cristancho, et al. 2011. p. 44–6.
62. *DSM-5*. 2013. p. 186.
63. Nierenberg AA, Alpert JE, Pava J, et al. Course and treatment of atypical depression. *J Clin Psychiatry* 1998;**59**(Suppl. 18):5–9.
64. *DSM-5*. 2013. p. 186.
65. Cristancho, et al. 2011. p. 43.
66. McGrath PJ, Stewart JW, Harrison WM. Predictive value of symptoms of atypical depression for differential drug treatment outcome. *J Clin Psychiatry* 1992;**12**:197–202.
67. *DSM-5*. 2000. p. 186.
68. Hirschfield RM. The comorbidity of major depression and anxiety disorders: recognition and management in primary care. *Prim Care Companion J Clin Psychiatry* 2001;**3**(6):244–54.
69. Ahmedani BK, Simon GE, Stewart C, et al. Health care contact in the year before suicide death. *J Gen Intern Med* 2014;**29**(6):870–7.
70. Bernstein JG. Medical psychiatric drug interaction. In: Hackett T, Cassam N, editors. *Massachusetts General Hospital handbook of general hospital psychiatry*. Saint Louis, MO: C.V. Mosby; 1978. p. 502.

71. Anderson WH. Depression. In: Lazarre A, editor. *Outpatient psychiatry: diagnosis and treatment.* Baltimore, MD: Williams & Wilkins; 1979. p. 259.
72. Akiskal H, McKinney W. Research in depression. In: Guggenheim F, Nadelson C, editors. *Major psychiatric disorders, overview and selected readings.* New York, NY: Elsevier Science Publishing Co.; 1982. p. 77.
73. Carlat D. 2012. p. 30–1.
74. *DSM-5.* 2013. p. 186–7.
75. *DSM-5.* 2013. p. 161.
76. *DSM-5.* 2013. p. 715–27.
77. *DSM-5.* 2013. p. 286–9.
78. Stein DJ, Kupfer DJ, Schatzburg AF. *The American psychiatric publishing textbook of mood disorders.* Arlington, VA: American Psychiatric Publishing, Inc. (APPI); 2005.
79. Kerner B. Genetics of bipolar disorder. *Appl Clin Genet* 2014;7:33–42.
80. Nurnberger J, Foroud T, Flury L, et al. Is there a genetic relationship between alcoholism and depression? *Alcohol Res Health* 2002;26(3):233–44.
81. Cheng MKS. *Asking Asian Americans about a family history of mental illness: some cross cultural tips.* Posted as the Interviewing Tip of the Month, #7, 2002 at the Training Institute for Suicide Assessment and Clinical Interviewing (TISA) website, <http://www.suicideassessment.com/tips/archives.php?action=prod&id=7> [accessed September 2015].
82. Chaplin SL. Somatization. In: Tseng W-S, Jon Stretlzer J, editors. *Culture & psychopathology.* New York, NY: Brunner/Mazel, Inc.; 1997. p. 767–86.
83. Lewis-Fernández R, et al. 2009. p. 6.

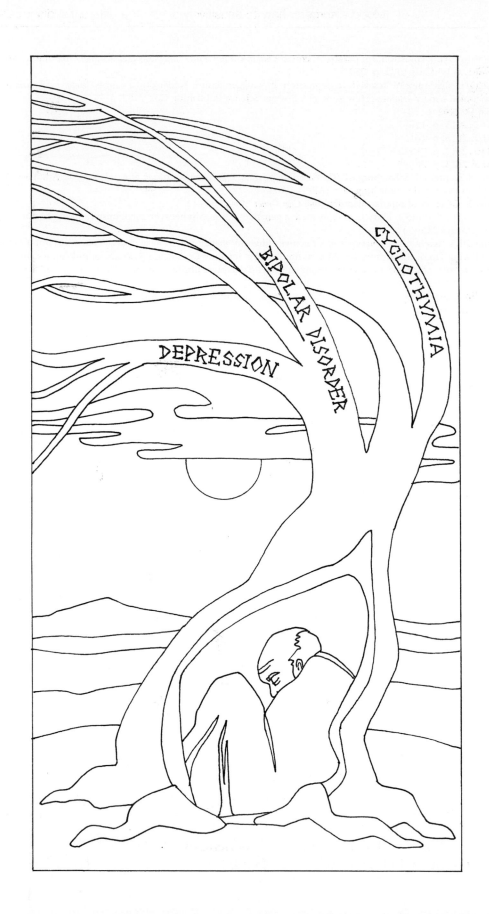

CHAPTER 10

Interviewing Techniques for Understanding the Person Beneath the Mood Disorder

When the low heavy sky weighs like a lid
Upon the spirit aching for the light,
And all the wide horizon's line is hid
By a black day sadder than any night; ...
When like grim prison bars stretch down the thin,
Straight, rigid pillars of the endless rain,
And the dumb throngs of infamous spiders spin
Their meshes in the cavern of the brain, ...

Charles Baudelaire
Spleen[1]

INTRODUCTION

In this chapter, we will search for a more sophisticated understanding of how a mood disorder is experienced by a patient in each wing of the patient's matrix as first described in Chapter 7 on treatment planning. For the sake of conciseness we will collapse the matrix into the following five wings: biological, psychological, dyadic, familial/societal, and worldview (as reflected in the patient's spirituality and framework for meaning). We will begin with the very smallest system of interaction – biological – and move outwards through progressively larger systems. We will see how these disorders create damage, and trigger core pains, throughout the wings of the patient's matrix from biological and psychological disruptions to the damage done to the patient's family, friends, workplace, spirituality, and worldview.

Because there is no time to explore all of the mood disorders, we will focus, specifically, upon the symptoms of depression, using depressive symptoms as a prototype through which we might better understand these damaging matrix effects in other mood disorders, indeed, in all psychiatric disorders. We will see how each depressive symptom is experienced uniquely by the person beneath the diagnosis, for every depression is a unique one.

I also believe that in order to effectively uncover psychiatric symptoms, it is critical to understand how patients experience these symptoms personally, in a phenomenological sense. As we shall soon see, this empathic familiarity on the part of the interviewer, if present, is quickly recognized by patients, resulting in a markedly more pronounced sense of safety. From the clinician's questioning, it becomes clear to the patient that this interviewer has seen these symptoms before, often many times, and respects their complexity and nuance.

The more an interviewer understands the concepts explored in this chapter, the more open the interviewer will be to the subtle clues suggesting depression in an initial encounter, thus decreasing the likelihood that a depressive state will be missed or its severity underestimated. Simultaneously, this understanding helps the clinician to better phrase his or her questions in a fashion that empathically resonates with the patient, enabling the patient to share the intimate details of their pain more readily, including suicidal ideation and the other harsh realities left in a depression's wake. From this understanding, interviewers enhance their sensitivity, their clinical acumen, and their ultimate engagement with patients. The interview is, at once, both more human and more clarifying.

At another level, our more sophisticated understanding of the human matrix will emphasize the sometimes-overlooked fact that interviewers – whether they want to or not – will, by their very presence, become a subsystem touched by the patient's depression. The interviewer will both affect and be affected by the depressive processes being explored. Awareness of this fact can lead to important insights in intervention. Blindness to this fact can lead to short-sighted conclusions and misplaced interventions. With these ideas in mind, our exploration begins. At its conclusion, hopefully we will have a truer understanding of what it is like to be at a place where:

> *… all the wide horizon's line is hid*
> *By a black day sadder than any night.*

THE PAIN BENEATH DEPRESSION

Fields of Interaction

The Biological Wing of the Matrix

As one enters the room occupied by a person experiencing depression, the physiologic ravages of the process are often disturbingly apparent. In a severely depressed person the initial glance may reveal unkempt hair, ragged or mismatched clothes, dirty nails, untied shoes, and a vacant look to the eyes. More striking may be the slowness of movement and the person's lack of responsiveness. It may take a few seconds or longer for the depressed person to acknowledge the interviewer, if such acknowledgment occurs at all. In a similar manner, more subtle decrements in responsiveness may be the first clues of a milder depressive state. Thus, the interview begins with the first look, before any words are uttered.

The slowness of movement probably parallels the disquieting sensation of heaviness often reported by depressed people. Depression, as Baudelaire suggested with his line, "When the low heavy sky weighs like a lid …", often feels like a heavy shawl weighing down upon the patient's shoulders. As noted in the last chapter, the arms and limbs of the patient may feel weighted down, a sensation called "leaden paralysis" in the DSM-5. This abnormal sensation may be related to the powerfully intense sense of inertia that can accompany depression. It becomes distressing for the depressed person to initiate movement; it seems so much easier to simply rest. A young woman with a depressive disorder vividly describes this phenomenon:

> It is so strange. Depression is exhausting in a physical sense. You know, most people have chores they have to do just to keep their lives going. And if the chores are waiting for you, and you sit there and look at them, they just seem overwhelming. And I could easily sit for 2 hours in a chair just looking at some clothes I left on the bedroom floor and not be able to motivate myself to pick them up. My body just feels heavy, as if it wouldn't want to respond unless I absolutely forced it to … Hmm … You know it is actually almost as if your brain lost half of its ability to control your body in the sense that even making a decision to pick something up required so much energy that you don't want to make it. You feel like it couldn't possibly be worth it. I just want to vegetate.

This sensitive excerpt brings up another important point with the opening comment, "It is so strange." Depressed patients, at times, present a peculiar dichotomy in the manner in which they cognitively and affectively experience their profound condition. On a cognitive level, they often feel they are the root of their problem, their speech becoming an entangled web of self-recrimination and belittlement. They cognitively experience their depression as being actively caused by their own flaws. Simultaneously, they emotionally experience the depression as coming on them or over them from an outside source. In a sense, they feel invaded and violated. They feel they are the passive recipients of a phenomenon that they do not understand or control. This incipient "loss of control" presents a terrifying threat to their sense of ideal self. Jaspers, with a single word, captures the pith of this process when he describes depressed patients as experiencing a physical and emotional "ossification."[2]

At present, the etiologic meaning of such radical changes in movement and body perception in the patient's biological wing remains unclear. Such changes may represent a variety of damaging *inter*-wing matrix effects: psychological defenses to withdraw the patient from painful external circumstances, social indicators that the person needs help, cultural attempts to withdraw a malfunctioning person from a potentially dangerous environment, or spiritual angst revealing itself as the need to withdraw from a meaningless world. Or they may be caused by a direct *intra*-wing matrix effect being the direct results of a primary biochemical imbalance. Any combination of the preceding factors is possible. No matter what the etiology of these phenomena, they create frightening experiences for anyone suffering from a depression. In essence, even patients' bodies become strangers to them – one more step toward their intense sense of isolation.

The other neurovegetative symptoms also represent an array of biological markers of depression. Baseline energy withers. Appetite and libido dry up as if parched by the intensity of the process. These feelings of altered functioning can become immensely disturbing to patients, sometimes being perceived as further evidence of their personal failure. With these phenomena in mind, questions such as the following may add depth to the interview:

a. "What has your body felt like to you recently?"
b. "What does it feel like to you to have lost your energy and drive?"
c. "You mention that you have lost your energy, your appetite, and your ability to sleep. How have all these changes made you feel about yourself?"

As well as allowing patients the chance to ventilate, these questions emphasize that the interviewer is interested in them as unique people whose depression they alone can explain.

Before leaving the biological field, I would like to briefly describe some of the biologic ramifications of an agitated depression. Here too there exists a peculiar dichotomy, as described by an elderly male patient in response to a question about losing energy, "I don't know exactly what you mean, but yeah, I've got energy all over the place, driving me constantly, but no, I don't have any sustained energy to do anything." The result in an agitated depression is often an inability to begin tasks, the patient being disabled by the frenzy of his or her own agitation.

Note the difference between the disorganized energy seen in an agitated depressive episode when compared to the organized energy frequently seen in a patient experiencing a dysphoric mania as described in the last chapter. Although the patient with a dysphoric mania may not successfully complete many tasks, they are compelled to try them and initially may approach them with a remarkably well-organized drive. As opposed to the almost frantic inertia seen in a patient suffering from an agitated depression, a patient with a dysphoric mania may develop and initiate surprisingly intricate and well-developed plans of action with regards to self-harm, suicide, and violence to others.

Returning to depression, in an agitated depressive state there exists a nagging need to move. The energy is unbridled and disobedient. Consequently, the body tends to assume an incessant display of "bad nerves." Hands wring each other in a frenzy of confusion. Fingers pick at the body or pluck the clothes. Sitting becomes an act of will power. From deep inside the legs there erupts a need to move. Pacing becomes a necessary method of release as natural as breathing. Especially when the patient is experiencing a depressive episode marked by melancholia, this agitated state may appear worse in the morning. In the interview it can be revealing to ask, "What part of the day seems worse to you?" It is important to remind oneself that a relatively calm patient interviewed at 4:00 P.M. may have looked remarkably more agitated at 8:00 A.M. Depression nags the body with an intermittent voice.

The Psychological Wing of the Matrix

Depression has a calling card. This calling card consists of a distinct set of changes that occur within the mind of those experiencing the depression. Not all depressed people experience these feelings, but many do in one combination or another. Four broad areas are touched by depression and will be the focus of this discussion: (1) perception of the world, (2) cognitive processes, (3) thought content, and (4) psychodynamic defenses. An understanding of the above processes can increase the ability of the interviewer to recognize the subtle clues of depression and can increase empathic abilities, as well.

1. Depressive Changes in How the World Is Perceived

Concerning the perception of the world, depression alters both the sense of time and the size of the world actively engaged. In a person experiencing a severe major depressive episode, the concept of current or future change frequently appears conspicuously absent. A mantle of flatness suffocates spontaneity. Moment-by-moment existence seems void of any chance of alteration. Without this feeling of possible change, time passes arrogantly slowly. In a literal sense, time passes painfully.

Such a state of psychic monotony can have a curious effect on the interviewee's perception of the future. In effect, if change does not exist, then the future is essentially meaningless. All days are merely replicas. Our sense of the future is partially dependent upon our sense that the future may be different. To the depressed interviewee, the future is draped in a radically bland light. This perception may be one reason why depressed people often appear unmotivated. Without a perceived future why should they attempt change? This phenomenon has been described by the phenomenologist Eugene Minkowski as a "blocking of the future."[3]

The second alteration in world perception does not involve time. It revolves about space. The "active world" of the depressed person undergoes a profound alteration. By "active world" I refer to that part of a person's environment that he or she remains interested in engaging. In depression, the active world shrinks. The patient's sense of space gradually vanishes creating a "cataract of the mind." This shrinking of the active world can powerfully short circuit environmental reinforcement and reward. The depressed person becomes a behavioral isolate. The woman quoted before elegantly depicts this process.

> I'm so focused inward … When I feel depressed it is such a great pain, and I am paying so much attention to it trying to control it, that I walk down the street and really don't see much at all … I screen out other people because I don't want to interact with others … I probably miss a lot. Even in the sense that I can walk down the street where I work and there can be roses blooming. And if I am really depressed, I don't even see them. And I love roses. Whereas, if I am feeling better, even despite the smell of the buses running around, I will still smell the roses. And I will admire them …

It can come as quite a shock to the interviewer to realize that the interviewer may not be a feature of the interviewee's active world. To engage such patients, the clinician needs to enter their world as best as possible. Consequently, the interview with a severely depressed patient may require a change in style. At times, the clinician must be more active while also accepting, with patience, the interviewee's difficulty in responding.

The Window Shade Response

In an even more striking example of the patient's need to consciously shut out the world, there is a specific sensation that sometimes plays a role in the shrinking of the patient's world. To me, the phenomenon appears to be fairly unique to withdrawn depressive states, and it is not reported by patients with agitated depressions or anxiety disorders. I have found it to be a surprisingly reliable marker of the presence of a moderate to severe depressive episode.

It is a phenomenon perhaps related to the well-documented tendency of depressed patients to withdraw to their beds for much of the day. When patients seek out their beds, if they sleep, it is a fitful sleep at best. In point of fact, I find that they are seldom returning to their beds primarily to sleep. Instead, they are returning to their beds because they can shut their eyes while in their beds, for it is the natural place in our culture where it is acceptable to shut one's eyes. With the closing of their eyes, they have effectively shut out the stresses of their world. The result is a desperately needed and immediate sense of relief. Sometimes severely depressed patients will actually draw their bed sheets over their head, an action often paralleled beforehand by the pulling down of the window shades so as to darken the room and further isolate themselves from the outside world.

And here we can see the connection with the uniquely depressive phenomenon that I hinted at above. Specifically, patients coping with depression not infrequently feel a need to shut their eyes, even while standing or walking about. It is as if the depressed patient is escaping the world by pulling down the ultimate window shade – their own eyes. Sometimes this need to shut the eyes is almost overpowering.

This "window shade response" was poignantly described by a particularly articulate lawyer, who first introduced me to the phenomenon. I have since found it to be common in moderate to severely depressed patients. He described it as follows. Note that he too, as with the patient above, emphasizes the "overwhelming" sensation experienced when depressed:

Sometimes the world is so overwhelming to me. It is mind-boggling how overwhelming the simplest of things is … I don't want to see or talk to anyone. It is almost painful, and yet it sounds so silly. I'll tell you another thing that is really interesting, it's almost weird. When I'm depressed, I will find myself almost compelled to shut my eyes.

It is so odd. It is not a desire to rest or sleep, it's not sleepiness. I just want to shut everything out. As soon as I shut my eyes, I feel some relief. And I just don't want to open them and face the world again … It really feels like I'm driven to do it, because the relief feels so good … It can come over me, and that's exactly what it feels like, like the urge to shut my eyes is somehow coming over me, almost against my will, almost any time when I'm really depressed.

During this last depression, I forced myself to keep up with my morning walks before work, which I'm really proud I did. It was tough to do, but I'm glad I did it. But here's the strange thing. I'd be walking on the old dirt road up behind my house through a beautiful woodland and I would feel compelled to close my eyes while I was walking. And I did! I would do it for several paces intermittently. I didn't even want to see the woods around me. I didn't want to see anything. It's hard to believe that several hours later, I'd be in court trying to do my best for my client. If they only knew what I looked like just 3 hours earlier.

To uncover the "window shade response" I have found the following question to be useful:

"When you're really depressed, do you sometimes have an intense desire to just shut your eyes? It seems almost odd to you how strongly you want to shut your eyes, to just shut the world out?"

I think you will find the presence of the window shade response to be a surprisingly reliable marker of a moderate to severe depressive state in the interviewee. As I noted above, in my experience, it does not appear to be present in patients experiencing a pure anxiety disorder such as a generalized anxiety disorder or obsessive–compulsive disorder. In addition, it is very engaging to inquire about the phenomenon, for depressed patients are often surprised that you are familiar with the sensation.

2. Cognitive Changes Caused by Depression

Changes in the Flow of Thought and Ideational Caging

A second broad area of alteration concerns changes in the cognitive processes of the depressed person. In a melancholic depression, the thought process slows, as if the stream of thought were frozen by an unexpected drop in temperature. In contrast, in an agitated depression thought races, as if the same stream had sustained a turbulent boil. In both cases, the thought process becomes disjointed. Concentration becomes annoyingly elusive.

Besides these alterations in the speed and flow of thought, depression creates an ideational caging. The term "caging" suggests that the mind becomes trapped within a small network of limiting themes. Such depressive rumination can lock the depressed person into worries about the past, the present, or the future. Once within the cage, the depressed patient has great difficulty attending to new and perhaps therapeutic influences. In the interview, caging may demonstrate itself as a frustrating tendency for the patient to return to a specific topic. Or, alternatively, the patient may repeatedly ask the same question, despite the interviewer's reasonable reassurances.

Such caging can seriously block an interview. One method of trying to circumvent it consists of attempting to acknowledge it while simultaneously refocusing the patient, as illustrated below. This strategy may look familiar, for it is one of the strategies that we examined in Chapter 3 for effectively transforming "wandering interviews." In this interview, the clinician had done an excellent and sensitive job of providing the patient a chance to ventilate and describe her financial concerns. When an effort was made to learn more about her depressive symptoms, the patient would not move on.

> **Clin.:** Mrs. Jones, can you tell me a little bit about the effect of all these troubles on your sleep?
>
> **Pt.:** Sleep, can't sleep … (pause) can't sleep because of the bills. I just know we won't be able to pay the bills. Oh God, my children, we'll be ruined.
>
> **Clin.:** No question about it, the money situation needs to be addressed. I'm also trying to figure out more about your depression too, it's also a big problem for you right now. It might be even making it harder to fix the money situation. The reason I'm trying to learn more about your sleep is that it will help me to understand more about your depression and what type of medications might help you the most, that's why I'm asking you about it. For instance, how long has it been taking you to fall asleep?
>
> **Pt.:** I don't know, all I think about are the bills. I know that somehow I'm to blame. What will we do? What will we do! Somebody has got to help.
>
> **Clin.:** Mrs. Jones, I know it can be really hard to not talk about your financial concerns, and we'll spend a lot more time doing so later; but, you know, in order to help you, I think I need to learn more about what your depression has done to you and what it feels like to you. To help us stay focused, I'm going to ask you some important questions, and if we get sidetracked I will pull us back to the question. It will help us figure out which of your symptoms we can help you with as fast as possible. Once again think carefully, how long is it taking you to fall asleep? (the preceding is said with a calm but firmer tone)
>
> **Pt.:** It's bad, real bad, maybe 2 or 3 hours; I just can't fall asleep. My nerves are shot.
>
> **Clin.:** Can you stay asleep or do you keep waking up?
>
> **Pt.:** Stay asleep! I wish. God knows. I can't ever get a good night's sleep. Ever. Ever.

With proper timing, such an intervention may open a cage. At other times, the caging of the patient will not yield despite the interviewer's best intentions.

Cognitive Distortions as Conceptualized by Aaron Beck

Aaron Beck, one of the founders of cognitive psychotherapy, has delineated many specific cognitive impairments in depression. Beck has pointed out that depressed patients may over-generalize, with statements such as "Everything has fallen apart" or "No one cares about me." They can exaggerate, in essence creating the proverbial mountain out of a molehill with a statement such as, "My boss Mr. Henry looked angry. He's dissatisfied with me. I'm sure it is only a matter of time until I'm fired."

They also have a tendency to ignore the positive. For instance, a businesswoman confused me with the following statement, which illustrates this principle: "It's the best Christmas season we've ever had. We're really selling books all over the place. But I set myself a remarkably high quota. If we don't meet it, I will have failed miserably as a manager."

Beck has also described a trio of distortions – the cognitive triad – that frequently appears in depression: (1) negative view of the world, (2) negative concept of the self, and (3) a negative appraisal of the future.[4]

First Distortion in Beck's Triad: Negative View of the World

This negative view of the world is partially generated by the tendency of the depressed patient to continually validate his or her depression. The patient speaks as if he or she had placed a negative filter over his or her eyes, as witnessed by the following taped comments:

When I'm really depressed every negative, every unpleasant thing that I could possibly think of that might be happening to another person like someone being hit by a car or someone getting cancer or a dog being injured will trigger personal fear and worry that the world is bad. And so the depression has no justification to ever lift because everything about life is horrible. It's all just proof that depression is reality just looking itself in the face …

Second Distortion in Beck's Triad: Negative Self-Concept

With regard to negative self-concept, the tendency to assume self-blame may be a major contributing factor. I do not think I have ever seen this quality as strikingly portrayed as in *The Bob Newhart Show*, a show whose re-runs are still quite popular with mental health professionals. In this show, Newhart plays a psychologist with a client named Mr. Herd who epitomizes the self-blamer. A typical exchange might be as follows:

Dr. Newhart: (after entering the office) I can't believe it, I left my wallet at home.

Mr. Herd: I did it … You were worried about me and forgot your wallet over me … I'm sorry, I'm really sorry. I won't let it happen again.

Although funny in the Newhart show, the process of self-blame stands as a vicious cognitive trap. In a sense, it may represent a milder variant of the much more ominous symptom known as delusional guilt.

Third Distortion in Beck's Triad: Negative View of the Future

Another jarring twist in cognitive process comes to mind at this point. Depressed patients sometimes exhibit a trait that I prefer to call "an immunity to logic," which can be very frustrating to the family, therapist, or initial interviewer. Facts are simply irrelevant. This immunity to logic, which is just one example of the processes that can lead to a negative view of the future, was brilliantly depicted by Minkowski, while at the same time illustrating the blocking of the future mentioned earlier. Minkowski spent several months living with a man experiencing a psychotic depression. The following excerpt refers to Minkowski's vain efforts to convince his apartment-mate that he would not be horribly mutilated and subsequently executed:

From the first day of my life with the patient, my attention was drawn to the following point. When I arrived, he stated that his execution would certainly take place that night; in his terror, unable to sleep, he also kept me awake all that night. I comforted myself with the thought that, come the morning, he would see that all his fears had been in vain. However, the same scene was repeated the next day and the next, until after 3 or 4 days I had given up hope, whereas his attitude had not budged one iota. What had happened?

It was simply that I, as a normal human being, had rapidly drawn from the observed facts my conclusions about the future. He, on the other hand, had let the same facts go by him, totally unable to draw any profit from them for relating himself to the same future. I now knew that he would continue to go on, day after day, swearing that he was to be tortured to death that night, and so he did, giving no thought to the present or the past. Our thinking is essentially empirical; we are interested in facts only in so far as we can use them as basis for planning the future. This carry-over from past and present into the future was completely lacking in him; he did not show the slightest tendency to generalize or to arrive at any empirical rules.[5]

Although this is a description of a psychotically depressed man, a similar, albeit milder, process commonly accompanies non-psychotic depression.

All of these disturbances in cognitive process may be encountered by the initial interviewer. By training themselves to listen for such abnormalities, interviewers may increase their ability to detect depression. For instance, people with atypical depressions, or somatic presentations of depression, may initially betray their underlying depression by the use of such pathologic processes. Of course, the presence of such processes in a less severely disturbed patient may also alert the interviewer to the possible use of cognitive psychotherapy as a future treatment modality. At this juncture, I would like to turn attention to the third major psychological area affected by depression, thought content itself.

3. Alterations in Thought Content Found in Depression

The distinction between cognitive process and cognitive content is sometimes a blurred one, but I would like to focus briefly on four content themes: loneliness, self-loathing, helplessness, and hopelessness. These factors blend with one another, reinforcing their mutual perpetuation.

Depressive Loneliness

The loneliness of the depressed person can become practically insurmountable. As shown earlier, processes such as caging and the shrinking of the active world separate the depressed patient from friends, family, and even the clinician. Their loneliness reaches such an intensity that it may begin to assume a qualitative difference from the more common loneliness encountered in daily living. Put differently, they are not only lonely – they feel that they *are* alone.

The loneliness assumes an irrefutable realization that they are isolated, somehow cut off permanently from others. Such isolation does indeed diminish social reinforcement and therapeutic intervention. Thomas Joiner has emphasized that acutely suicidal patients may feel intense loneliness even when surrounded by caring loved ones. Indeed, the existence of loved ones is sometimes cruelly twisted by depressive process into a guilt-ridden sense that one is a burden to others, a cognition further increasing the draw towards suicide in depression as seen below.[6,7]

Depressive Guilt and Self-Loathing

Combined with this alienation from others, depressed patients may also experience a profound alienation from, and hatred of, themselves, accompanied by intense guilt.

Such a self-loathing only intensifies their feeling of loneliness, because they are repulsed by their own company. To the guilt-laden patient, it seems as if he or she lacks any real existence or purpose at all except for his or her pain. As described above, these feelings can shift imperceptibly into the potentially lethal thought that "I am truly a burden to those I love." It is a thought that Joiner feels can be one of the most reliable of interpersonal harbingers of a suicide attempt. Sometimes guilt-laden thoughts may emerge in the interview in a more oblique fashion as in, "Don't bother with me. Talk with someone you can help." The initial interviewer needs to probe beneath such comments, hunting for the more dangerous logic that "others would be better off if I were dead."

Carlat suggests the following types of questions for helping patients share even subtle feelings of guilt[8]:

"Have you felt especially critical of yourself lately?"
"Do you feel that you are essentially a good person, or do you have doubts?"

Depressive Helplessness

From their social isolation and their repugnance toward themselves, feelings of helplessness emerge naturally. This profound sense of helplessness can contribute to the inertia that effectively prevents therapeutic encounters. Phrased succinctly, depressed patients wonder "Why bother?" The interviewer can easily estimate the role of this factor by simply asking, "Have you been feeling helpless?" A more sophisticated gauge may emerge with the question, "At this time, what kinds of ways of getting help do you see for yourself?" A blank negative or dismal shake of the head in response to this question should alert the interviewer to the potential seriousness of the depression.

Depressive Hopelessness

Finally, all of the above depressive themes may lead to hopelessness. Beck has demonstrated that hopelessness represents a more specific and sensitive predictor of suicide potential than depressive mood itself.[9] As such, the interviewer can begin to measure the degree of hopelessness with an indirect question, such as "What do you see for yourself in the future?" and/or follow up more directly with, "Are you feeling hopeless?"

4. Psychodynamic Defenses and Their Role in Depression

I have found the discussion by MacKinnon, Michels, and Buckley in the 2nd edition of their book, *The Psychiatric Interview in Clinical Practice*,[10] to be particularly illuminating in this area. I shall summarize some of their points, focusing on those defenses that can most easily confuse the interviewer.

As we noted earlier in our discussion of Mr. Whitstone in Chapter 9, some people have trouble admitting depression into their cognitive awareness. They tend to verbally deny depression. In fact, they may be truly unaware that they are depressed. Such an ironic state may be the result of psychodynamic defenses such as denial and repression. Despite these defenses, careful questioning will often uncover the depression by eliciting neurovegetative symptoms or evidence of depressive cognitive functioning such as caging or generalization. Other common defenses include isolation and rationalization. The patient may isolate all his or her depressive rumination onto one symptom complex. The patient may simultaneously deny depression, as illustrated by "I've got no real problems other than the fact that I can't sleep at night and I've got daily headaches."

The patient's anger can provide the interviewer with the first glimpse of the depressive phenomenon. Analytic theorists such as Abraham and Freud have stressed the idea that depression may represent anger turned inward.[11] This anger may originate from a variety of situations, including perceived abandonment, rejection, frustration, direct or indirect attacks on oneself, or feelings of betrayal or injustice.

In line with this thinking, anger often pierces the sadness of the person experiencing an agitated depression. Thus a patient who quickly verbally attacks the interviewer may be betraying his or her depression to that very same interviewer. I have even been surprised to see anger unexpectedly shooting through the apathy of the supposed "melancholic depression," as evidenced by vicious diatribes against past doctors or relatives. As we have already seen, anger also routinely disrupts the existence of people displaying borderline personality disorders, dysthymia, atypical depressions, and mixed bipolar states.

Anger and depression can form a damaging, self-enhancing feedback loop, as follows. The patient lashes out at a close friend. From this angry display, the patient develops guilt for having such inappropriate feelings. This guilt triggers further depression. As the depression deepens, the patient becomes increasingly irritable. Soon enough, the patient lashes out again, thus completing and fueling the cycle.

A third confusing clinical picture resulting from psychodynamic defenses involves the defense of projection, with resultant paranoia. MacKinnon emphasizes that depression and paranoia may alternate with each other. The person's intense self-incrimination can become too painful. Deflection of this pain occurs through projection. Instead of hating himself or herself, the person finds that "other people hate me," or "others want to punish me." This last statement sometimes demonstrates the projection of suicidal ideation outwards. The need to consider paranoia as a defense against depression dramatically demonstrates itself in the following vignette provided by one of my colleagues.

Apparently he had consulted on a patient who presented as psychotically paranoid in a medical hospital. This patient denied all suicidal ideation; furthermore, he related few neurovegetative symptoms. Transfer to the psychiatric hospital was recommended in the morning. The patient was checked throughout the night but was not placed on a one-to-one observation. During a period of non-surveillance, the patient quickly and efficiently hanged himself. Little more need be said.

A final dynamic mechanism that can easily fool the interviewer exhibits itself in the process of pseudo-hypomanic defenses against depression. One needs to be wary of anybody who appears "too happy" while describing numerous unsettling stressors. If watched carefully, the surprisingly buoyant person may betray sadness by a minute quivering of the chin or a hesitancy to the voice. At these moments, a quiet statement such as, "You know, as you are talking you seem sort of sad to me" may open a floodgate of tears.

The Dyadic Wing of the Matrix

When two people interact, a dyadic system is born. Depression often first shows itself through its impact on the flow of communication and affection within this dyadic system. In this sense, depression exists as an interpersonal phenomenon, seldom, if ever, restricted to the world of a single individual. Perhaps the following description by a patient will illustrate the power of depression to alter the interpersonal field:

> It makes it harder to interact with people. It decreases your motivation for talking … first of all because you are so acutely aware of how depressed you are that you are convinced that other people are going to recognize it immediately, and it is very embarrassing to think that. So it makes you feel as if any interaction with other people will make you feel as if you will need to put on a front. It requires a lot of energy to do that. And that makes you very tired. It is sort of a circular motion … you see how much energy it will take to relate so you avoid doing it. I have even noticed that if I enter a store or see a Burger King and I want coffee I tend to speak softer and not really smile like I normally do. When I am depressed I want to limit the interaction as much as possible so I don't smile and I don't really look at them. I just want to get it over with and get away …

This excerpt illustrates several subtle facets of interpersonal disruption. At one level, the depressed person feels withdrawn and consequently attempts to decrease interaction. This decrease in interaction robs the depressed person of the chance to gain positive reinforcement from others, as mentioned earlier. But, perhaps more importantly, depression decreases the quality of the remaining interactions. The decreased smiling, the decreased spontaneity, and the curtness of interaction displayed by the patient can be perceived by others as coolness or aloofness. Once perceived in this manner, people may treat the depressed person with increased reserve. For instance, an employee behind the counter at a fast food chain may snap at the person, thus further creating a hostile environment. This generates a self-fulfilling prophecy in which the patient creates a hostile world, a world lacking rewards for interactions with others.

This destructive cycle can be one of the forerunners of the learned helplessness sometimes seen in depression and postulated by Seligman as an etiology of depression.[12] Seligman discovered that if you experimentally expose an animal, such as a dog, to inescapable aversive stimuli, the dog will eventually stop attempting escape. The animal appears to give up. It does not attempt to find new ways of coping. Once this learned helplessness has occurred, exploration ceases. With the cessation of exploration, the chance for new learning and positive reinforcement vanishes. In a sense, the helplessness has ensured its own survival. A very similar process may occur in humans, perhaps made even more damaging by the uncanny ability of the human to cognitively reframe such interactions into self-derogatory beliefs such as, "Obviously, nobody likes me," or "I don't even know why I bother."

The interviewer can search for evidence of interpersonal dysfunction and learned helplessness with questions such as the following:

a. "Do you find yourself going out as frequently as you used to?"
b. "Tell me what it is like for you when you are around people at work?"
c. "When you talk with people what kinds of feelings do you have, like if you meet a friend on the street?"
d. "How do people seem to be treating you?"
e. "Do you find yourself easily irritated or 'flying off the handle' recently?"
f. "Does it require much energy to be around people such as your friends?"
g. "Are you spending the same amount of time on social media?"

The Impact of the Patient's Depression on the Interviewer

At this point one of the more fascinating elements of interviewing presents itself. I am referring to the fact that not only are the friends and family of the patient affected by the patient's depression, but also the interviewer cannot escape the process. It benefits clinicians to periodically look within themselves at their own emotional responses. In the first place, such intuitive responses may be the tip-off that one has encountered a depression or a depressive equivalent. In the second place, negative feelings generated in the interviewer can seriously damage engagement. The interviewer may inadvertently distance the interviewee by tone of voice or nonverbal cue. Put differently, the interviewer needs to adjust to the needs of the patient in a continuous, adaptive creativity. To accomplish this process, interviewers must be aware of the impact of patients on themselves and vice versa.

There exist several emotions commonly felt by interviewers besides generally acknowledged reactions such as sympathy, empathy, or a desire to help. For instance, the depressed patient's slowness of movement and speech, caging, and hesitancy to answer questions can create a sense of frustration in the interviewer. Questions may have to be asked repeatedly. Answers may be vague. The interview may loom as a long and tedious process. Such feelings of frustration may be useful indicators that the clinician should be on the lookout diagnostically for a major depressive episode while being wary of countertransference.

In a similar fashion, the patient's depressive manner of interaction may create anger in the interviewer as well as frustration. At times, interviewers may subsequently feel guilt because they suddenly catch themselves being "non-caring." This resultant guilt may provide the initial clue to a diagnosis of depression. This guilt also provides the interviewer with a vivid, experiential glimpse into the world of family members and friends who interact with a depressed patient on a daily basis. Occasionally, the first suggestion that one has encountered an atypical depression may be a growing sense of unexpected sadness within the interviewer.

A final feeling that an interviewer may experience while interviewing a depressed patient arises from both the withdrawal of the patient and the shrinking of the patient's active world. In short, as the patient introverts, the interviewer may feel ineffectual or out of touch. Such feelings are to be expected. They do not necessarily suggest that the interview is going poorly.

The preceding interactions emphasize the need for interviewers to adjust both their pace and their expectations. The interview with the depressed patient requires both a calm and a calming style. Indeed, any suggestions of haste or irritation may be interpreted in a highly disengaging fashion by the depressed patient. A frustrated interviewer may be perceived as, "Just like everyone else, you find me irritating." Such an interaction hardly sets an ideal platform for a therapeutic alliance.

How a Clinician's Behaviors Can Submerge a Depression From View

So far I have been describing the impact of the patient on the therapist, generating feelings such as sadness, annoyance, or guilt. Flipping the coin, one finds that the therapist can unwittingly affect the patient's presentation. With regard to depression, this phenomenon occurs most frequently with atypical depression, dysthymia (persistent depressive disorder), and in depressions accompanying a personality disorder.

People with these disorders are often highly responsive to their immediate surroundings. A patient with dysthymia or with a histrionic personality can sometimes be cheered up deceptively rapidly if the patient feels that someone is showing an interest, an example of the "mood reactivity" described in Chapter 9. Therefore, an overly warm or extroverted interviewer can unknowingly shift the patient's affect. To such an interviewer, the presentation of the patient may not seem very sad or depressed. Such an initial impression might mislead the interviewer into downplaying the significance of the depressive complaints.

It should also be remembered that "happy people" are often very annoying to depressed people, being perceived as incapable of understanding how miserable they feel. The interviewer best approaches the patient from the calming middle ground of gentle warmth and interested listening.

Effectively Addressing Tearfulness

While interviewing depressed patients, the clinician will undoubtedly encounter tearful patients. The first time a patient cries in an interview, it is generally comforting to allow the patient to cry for a brief period. If the patient is on the brink of tears, statements such as, "You seem sad right now," or as MacKinnon and Michels[13] suggest, "Are you trying not to cry?" may be very helpful. Said with a soft tone, they will offer the patient a chance to ventilate, thus decreasing a sense of discomfort. Many patients feel embarrassed or vulnerable at such moments. I generally address this unstated issue with a statement such as, "It's all right to cry. We all cry at times. It's our body's way of telling us we are hurting; (after a brief pause) maybe you can tell me a little more about what is hurting you."

After allowing the patient some time to ventilate, I generally will ask, "Would you like a tissue?" while simultaneously offering one in my outstretched hand. Such an interaction has many metacommunications. The clinician is conveying an acceptance of crying as a normal aspect of sadness. Simultaneously, respect is given to the patient's current needs. Rather than just giving the patient a tissue, the clinician asks if one is needed. By the process of asking, the clinician conveys confidence that the patient is still in control, fully capable of making decisions.

During the tearfulness and as it subsides, the interviewer has an ideal chance to learn about the core pains of the patient. Tearfulness tends to decrease the use of defenses. At such a point, pertinent and startling information may emerge. If the clinician had prevented the tearfulness by cutting it off abruptly or by changing topics, then valuable information might have been lost.

Of course, at times, one might find a patient whose uncontrollable crying prevents progress. To further the interview, statements said reassuringly but firmly such as the following may be effective, "Mr. Jones this is obviously very upsetting and would be to anybody. Take a moment to collect yourself. It's important for us to talk more about what is bothering you."

But, generally speaking, interviewers tend to prematurely shut down crying, perhaps because it is disturbing to feel another person's pain. Another emotion may also contribute to this premature shut-down, for the patient's tearfulness can make the interviewer feel awkwardly helpless. On a deeper level, it remains important for interviewers to understand their spontaneous feelings when someone cries. In this regard, part of the interviewer's basic training should be a search for answers to questions such as the following:

a.   What do I feel when someone cries?
b.   Do I ever perceive crying people as weak or ineffectual?
c.   How often do I cry and how do I feel about myself when I do?
d.   Have I ever seen my parents, family, or friends cry, and how did I feel then?

By exploring such questions, the interviewer decreases the risk that countertransference issues will adversely affect the ability to deal with a crying patient. In the last analysis, many a powerful therapeutic alliance has been forged by a clinician's calming and mature response to a patient's first tears.

The Familial and Societal Wing of the Matrix

In an immediately practical sense, it is important to interview family members, for they may provide invaluable information regarding the patient's history. Sometimes patients may be so withdrawn or their cognitive abilities so impaired that they have trouble providing reliable information. In this situation, family members may provide valid information regarding the patient's symptoms and the situational and interpersonal circumstances that may be triggering or impacting upon the patient's depression.

Additionally, family members are potentially illuminating sources for collaborative treatment planning, as well providers of information on what interventions have been either useful, damaging, or unproductive in past care. To not invite family input or to ignore it once given is not only foolish, but it will often antagonize the family members (and rightly so), who are living with the patient and who must cope with the patient's symptoms on a daily basis once leaving the interviewer's office.

On a more complex level, sometimes depression seems to possess a life of its own, independent of the person labeled as depressed. It is within the family that this phenomenon comes most vividly to mind. To understand a patient's depression in an initial interview fully, one must understand its contextual role in the family and within the culture that is shaping that family.

Family interaction may be the primary root of the depression, as in a hateful sibling rivalry or incest. At other times, the depression may have its roots in a biochemical process yet damaging matrix effects will reverberate throughout the family. A case in point would be a spouse laid off from work secondary to a severe endogenous depression. Surely, all members of the family will feel the pains of this depressive process, almost as if the biochemical imbalance were in their own neurochemistry. Finally, family pathology may feed a depression already caused by another wing of the patient's matrix, such as the biochemical or psychological system. For instance, an abusive spouse may re-enforce a depressed patient's guilt by making denigrating comments such as, "You're letting everybody down, especially the kids, you're truly worthless."

Cultural biases can also impact on how a depression reverberates throughout the members of a family. In Asian cultures, a family member's depression may be viewed as a bad reflection upon the entire family, in which case added shame and guilt may fall upon the patient struggling with the depression. Such cross-cultural influences may also make it harder for a clinician, when interviewing an Asian American, to hear the truth about a patient's degree of disability from family members for there may be covert cultural pressures to keep this quiet.

An Illustration of the Insidious Impact of Depression on a Family

I will accent this topic by describing an interview that I supervised in person. The interviewer was talking with the identified patient, whom I shall refer to as Mrs. Ella Thomas. The husband and son of Mrs. Thomas were also present in the same room. Mrs. Thomas was a gray-haired woman with angry eyes that seemed resentful of all 70 of her years. She fidgeted and cried throughout the interview. At times she would suddenly change topics, whining out such statements to her husband as, "You've got to help me, Leonard! I can't go on. The pain! The pain!" She complained about the hospital and warned that, "I had better get my sleeping pills or I'll leave."

As the interview proceeded, an atmosphere of increasing tension pervaded the room. Her husband had refused to have a chair brought for himself. Consequently, he stood throughout the interview, stationed reservedly behind his wife. As the interview progressed, he tightly rolled his lips upon each other, while his arms closed over his chest. Mrs. Thomas' son sat down, his body turned sideways to his mother. He occasionally tossed a glance at her when his eyes were not staring at his shoes or the floor. Later in the interview, with an angry tone plucking each word, the son challenged the clinician, "Why can't she have those meds?" I felt a growing sense of discomfort inside me. The poor interviewer was nervously breaking eye contact with Mrs. Thomas, while he sheepishly performed a mental status.

I can safely say that no one in that room was comfortable. That room represented a classic reflection of the impact of depression on a family system and even on the hospital system itself. Diagnostically, Mrs. Thomas had an agitated major depressive disorder. In reality, this entire family was experiencing a depressive episode. But it did not stop at the boundary of her age-spotted skin. Depression is often reflected in the actions and words of family members. Her husband and son demonstrated the frustration and anger often generated in those who love the patient. These people experience a sense of helplessness, fearing that nothing will change, despite their best efforts. Not personally experiencing the patient's anhedonia and loss of energy, they cannot understand why the patient does not help himself or herself. They also find their own daily activities continuously interrupted by the complaints and actions of the depressed person. If the initial interviewer has the opportunity to meet family members, sometimes their statements and nonverbal messages may be the first clue that depression is the diagnosis.

Addressing the Pain of Family Members

The interviewer should keep in mind that family members who are desperately trying to help their loved one may need support themselves. The problem is not "just Ella's problem." Our mission includes helping to relieve the pain of family members as they deal with the devastation that depression has brought to their worlds. Occasionally, secondary to such frustration, family members will develop a major depressive episode of their own. In a sense, like a virus, the depression will have replicated itself. If one senses that an accompanying family member appears to be depressed, it can be comforting and rewarding to interview them alone briefly, to see how they are coping. I find that the following question, asked gently, can be a powerful doorway into the family member's pain:

"I can see that you are providing great support for your mother during her depression but I'm wondering who is providing you with support?"

I have seen family members burst into tears following such a question as they simply answer, "No one."

Occasionally, you will need to inquire about suicidal thought in a family member. It is not uncommon to help family members to connect with appropriate mental health follow-up for themselves if necessary.

In the last analysis, it is difficult to over-estimate the pain generated in family members by watching their loved one suffer. The angst of seeing a child or spouse suffer from a mental disorder while feeling helpless to relieve his or her pain is, quite frankly, beyond words. I can vouch for this pain, for I have felt it myself.

One of our greatest gifts as clinicians is to take the time to help relieve the suffering of those family members who love the patients for whom we are providing care for illnesses ranging from depression to bipolar disorder and schizophrenia. In this regard, be sure to checkout the wonderful article, "Practical Interview Strategies for Building an Alliance with the Families of Patients Who have Severe Mental illness" by Murray-Swank,[14] (complete article available in Appendix IV).

Uncovering Potentially Damaging Family Impacts on the Patient

As illustrated above, the pent-up frustration and anger of family members may be expressed not only towards the patient but also towards the interviewer. Unfortunately, as described earlier in the section on dyadic process, the negative feelings generated by Mrs. Thomas may backfire upon her, creating a hostile environment even within the hospital.

From a very different perspective, depressions sometimes play a curious role in a family, for the family system may in some way need Mrs. Thomas' depression as a stabilizing force, as theorists such as Bowen or Minuchin have discussed.[15] Family members with low self-esteem may find a boost in self-worth as they embrace the role of a caretaker "who is the only person who is really helping Mom." Or an adult child who always felt "put-down" by a parent might find it exhilarating to be one-up on that parent and in charge of care. At an unconscious level, these family members "may not want Mom to get better," potentially undercutting treatment recommendations made in the closing phase of the interview. All of these points emphasize the need for the interviewer to carefully explore the family dynamics in order to understand the depression.

Within the individual interview, family tensions may be spontaneously brought up by the patient. At other times, questioning may be needed to illuminate the issues. Questions such as the following represent some good jumping off points:

a. "Who in your family seems to understand your depression and who doesn't?"
b. "Who in your family are you concerned about right now?" (The answer may uncover a family member who is having trouble coping with the patient's depressive state.)
c. "How do you think your family members view your depression?"
d. "What kinds of suggestions have your family members been making to you about how to feel better?"
e. "Have you been feeling any pressure from anyone in your family to get better?"
f. "Has anyone in your family told you that you 'just need to pick yourself up by the bootstraps'?"
g. "Has anyone in your family said something to you like, 'I'm sick of you being depressed all the time.'"
h. "What kind of pressures has your spouse been coping with recently?"
i. "Do you think your spouse views you as a problem?"

Questions such as the above must be asked in sensitive fashion with the clinician always being aware of their impact on the patient. When used effectively, they will often yield valuable information about the "psychodynamics" of the family. They may elicit interpersonal tensions between specific family members, where more direct questioning might have elicited denial.

For instance, when answering the question about pressures on the spouse, the patient may relate feelings of guilt for being a burden, feelings of anger towards the spouse for perceived neglect, disgust at the spouse's over-attention to work or other family members, or he or she may seem detached and uninterested in the spouse. From such a question, one may also learn valuable information about situational stressors in the family system as well.

The Impact of Depression on Societal and Cultural Systems

Larger systems other than the family may experience damaging matrix effects from the patient's depression. On a direct level, impact of the depression will be seen in systems such as the job environment, church groups, social organizations, and social media such as Facebook, Instagram, and Twitter, where the patient's participation may plummet.

From a different perspective, such systems may act as major stressors triggering the depression in the first place. Conversely, they may act as important supports, helping to buffer the patient from their depression. Society itself can be an integral system involved in depression. Careful questioning might reveal that the husband of Mrs. Thomas had been forced to retire secondary to economic layoffs. Or perhaps her family had recently relocated because of increasing taxes in their former state. Likewise, the hospitalization of patients such as Mrs. Thomas may ultimately affect the Medicaid and Medicare systems or the Affordable Care Act. The societal cost in treating depression, and in lost productivity in the workplace, is estimated in the billions of dollars per year, a striking example of a damaging matrix effect.

Cultural Impacts on the Patient's Depression

In the same sense that depression impacts on the patient's family and cultures, cultures impact on how depressions are perceived and the degree with which they are stigmatized. Indeed, if a patient's culture strongly disparages depression, and perhaps suicidal thinking as well, the culture can strikingly increase depressive guilt and shame. Here we see a stigmatizing viewpoint, housed within the cultural wing of the patient, causing inter-wing damage on the patient's psychological response to his or her own depressive symptoms. We have already seen how cultural stigma might limit the accuracy of information provided by family members by compelling them to downplay the severity of the their loved one's symptoms.

If one is unfamiliar with the cultural beliefs of an interviewee regarding depression, the interviewer should not be hesitant to ask about them. The very act of asking can help the patient to share serious depressive symptoms, perhaps even suicidal ideation more readily. It does not matter if one is a Muslim clinician trained in Pakistan who is interviewing a Christian White American or vice versa, questions such as the following can be useful:

1. "You know, I'm not entirely certain how depression is viewed in the West. Back in the States, do people tend to talk about depression openly or do they hush it up?"
2. "I'm curious about how your family and friends view depression?"
3. "Help me to get a better understanding of how Christianity views suicide, for instance is it viewed as a sin and could one get to heaven if one had killed oneself?"

The answers to such questions can be quite revealing. They may prove to be the gateway to an engaging and potentially life-saving discussion. No matter how you mark it, cultures shape depressive episodes. Conversely, depression leaves its mark throughout all the interlocking wings of the patient's matrix. The sensitive interviewer understands these inter-relationships and attempts to make a reconnaissance of each system during the initial and subsequent interviews. Through this diligent search, the puzzle of depression may become clearer and avenues of therapeutic intervention more apparent. As we've just seen in our review of the cultural ramifications of depression, spirituality itself can partially shape depression. It is time to explore this impact in more detail.

The Wing of the Matrix Encompassing Worldview and Spirituality

As we have emphasized repeatedly throughout our book, one should attempt to understand how patients view their symptoms, their problems, their life, and their beliefs. Such views represent the patient's worldview or framework for meaning as described in Chapter 7.

In an initial interview, one will seldom have the time to explore this framework in depth as it relates to the patient's depression, but even a few minutes of discussion may provide clues for engagement or for future therapeutic discussion. Such questioning may also further foster an understanding of the person beneath the depression, as well as providing hints as to possible causes of the patient's depression. Failure to have evolved a framework for meaning or a sudden breakdown in a pre-existing framework can function as triggers or perpetuators of the patient's depression, representing an existential crisis.

To investigate these areas of existential framework, several regions of information may be of value. At times, demographic questions concerning religious background may act as springboards for further inquiry. Significant information may present itself following questions such as, "What role does religion play, if any, in your life?" If asked with a nonjudgmental tone, I have found that people generally respond naturally and specifically. Very quickly, the interviewer will register the role of religious doubt or ambivalence in the current crisis. In Chapter 20 devoted to advanced strategies for exploring cross-cultural issues and diversity, we will examine in detail various interviewing techniques for exploring religious beliefs and spiritual perspectives, which play such a pivotal role in the cultural matrix of our patients and ourselves.

Religion/spirituality is not the only axis upon which a framework for meaning is built. Other areas include family, job, community, charities, patriotism, and subcultures such as those associated with sports and hip hop music. Ignorance of these factors can result in markedly disrupted engagement. Moreover, as we saw earlier in Chapters 6 and 7, these systems can have a very powerful influence on whether the patient will follow up with treatment recommendations. Consequently, it remains critical for the initial interviewer to understand these factors, as illustrated below:

Clin.: What kinds of things do you like to do in your spare time?

Pt.: When I felt better, I used to love to sing.

Clin.: Oh … (with an increased interest in tone of voice) What kinds of music did you like to sing?

Pt.: All types, but I really loved gospel music. What a beautiful way to bring God to people … I think if you put all of your trust in God, He will help you. Man is not the answer. Man provides artificial answers.

Clin.: Have you been praying recently in an attempt to gain some guidance?

> **Pt.:** Yes I have. Every day. It helps, but I wonder if maybe I ask for too much. Perhaps I am to blame.

This vignette provides a wealth of information for the clinician. In the first place, religion obviously plays a major role in this person's life. The interviewer may want to further examine the possible therapeutic supports that religion could provide, such as meetings with a pastoral counselor, minister, or choral church activities. However, it is possible that religion may be feeding some guilty ruminations that are part of the depressive process itself. Perhaps even more important, the clinician has some clues concerning where engagement could go wrong. In particular, the patient's statement, "Man is not the answer. Man provides artificial answers," serves as an alert to the clinician. Specifically, the patient may find treatment modalities such as psychotherapy or medication as clearly "artificial answers." Premature reference in the interview to such treatments could easily rupture engagement. The clinician will need to proceed cautiously, trying to gently find out what this particular patient wants in the way of help.

It is beyond the scope of this chapter to discuss the numerous ramifications that the search for meaning may play in depression. I refer the reader to authors such as Frankl,[16] Yalom,[17] Josephson and Peteet,[18,19] and Cloninger,[20] who address these issues in the detail they deserve. In closing, I am reminded of another example in which understanding the patient's framework for meaning helped in the initial interview of a patient with depressive complaints. I had been asked to see this patient as a psychiatric consultant on a medical ward.

Mr. Kulp (as I shall refer to him) was a 55-year-old man with alcoholism suffering from moderately severe Parkinson's disease (a progressive form of muscular rigidity). He had been admitted with suicidal ideation following a drunken spree. He had many stressors, not the least of which was a markedly battered self-image created by the stiffening of his body from his Parkinson's disease. Mr. Kulp had always prided himself on being an energetic breadwinner for his family. He viewed himself as a tough Marine.

This latter affiliation surfaced when I asked him if he liked to read. He mentioned that he loved to read, pointing to his books. When I asked if I could see them, he enthusiastically showed them to me. All of them concerned Marines and various war heroes, which led to a discussion of his former Marine days, including his boot camp experiences. At the time, I did not know exactly what to make of this information. Later its usefulness would become apparent.

By way of understatement, Mr. Kulp did not respond positively to my recommendations that he needed to enter a local alcohol rehabilitation center. As the discussion proceeded, I felt that he would decide against entering the program. He balked, stating that it would be too big of a time commitment and too tough. At which point I made a comment to the effect, "Well Mr. Kulp, I guess you're right. It's a tough commitment, but not your first. It's sort of like boot camp was a tough commitment. But you needed boot camp. It made a good soldier of you. Maybe you and your family need this program." This statement appeared to affect Mr. Kulp. He eventually decided to enter the rehabilitation program. Perhaps he would have entered anyway, but the understanding of his framework for meaning certainly seemed to help. Suddenly the rehabilitation program was not viewed as a foreign entity; it was akin to his familiar and respected boot camp. Mr. Kulp had been given a chance to be a soldier again.

REFERENCES

1. Baudelaire C. *The flowers of evil*. Franklin Center, PA: The Franklin Library; 1977. p. 123.
2. Jaspers K. Symptom complexes of abnormal affective states. In: *General psychopathology*. Manchester, UK: Manchester University Press; 1963. p. 598 [Original work published 1923].
3. Minkowski E. Findings in a case of 'schizophrenic' depression. In: May R, editor. *Existence*. New York, NY: A Touchstone Book; 1958. p. 133.
4. Beck AT. *Cognitive therapy and the emotional disorders*. New York, NY: The American Library; 1976. p. 105.
5. Minkowski E. 1958. p. 132.
6. Joiner T. *Why people die by suicide*. Cambridge, MA: Harvard University Press; 2005.
7. Joiner TE, Van Orden KA, Witte TK, Rudd MD. *The interpersonal theory of suicide: guidance for working with suicidal clients*. Washington, DC: American Psychological Association; 2009. p. 57.
8. Carlat D. *The psychiatric interview*. 3rd ed. Philadelphia, PA: Wolters Kluwer/Lippincott Williams & Wilkins; 2012. p. 168.
9. Beck AT, Kovacs M, Weissman A. Hopelessness and suicidal behavior. *JAMA* 1975;**234**:1146–9.
10. MacKinnon RA, Michels R, Buckley PJ. *The psychiatric interview in clinical practice*. 2nd ed. Washington, DC: American Psychiatric Publishing, Inc.; 2006. p. 229–80.
11. Akiskal H, McKinney W. Research in depression. In: Guggenheim F, Nadelson C, editors. *Major psychiatric disorders: overview and selected readings*. New York, NY: Elsevier Science Publishing Co., 1982. p. 73.
12. Akiskal H, McKinney W. 1982. p. 74.
13. MacKinnon RA, Michels R, Buckley JR. 2006. p. 256.
14. Murray-Swank A, Dixon LB, Stewart B. Practical strategies for building an alliance with the families of patients who have severe mental illness. *Psychiatr Clin North Am* 2007;**30**(2):167–80.
15. Gurman AS, Kniskern DP, editors. *Handbook of family therapy*. New York, NY: Brunner/Mazel Publisher; 1981.
16. Frankl VW. *The doctor and the soul*. New York, NY: Vintage Books; 1973.
17. Yalom I. *Existential psychotherapy*. New York, NY: Basic Books; 1980.
18. Josephson AM, Peteet JR. *Handbook of spirituality and worldview in clinical practice*. Washington, DC: American Psychiatric Publishing, Inc.; 2004.
19. Peteet JR. Putting suffering into perspective: implications of the patient's worldview. *J Psychother Pract Res* 2001;**10**:187–92.
20. Cloninger CR. *Feeling good: the science of well-being*. Oxford, UK: Oxford University Press; 2004.

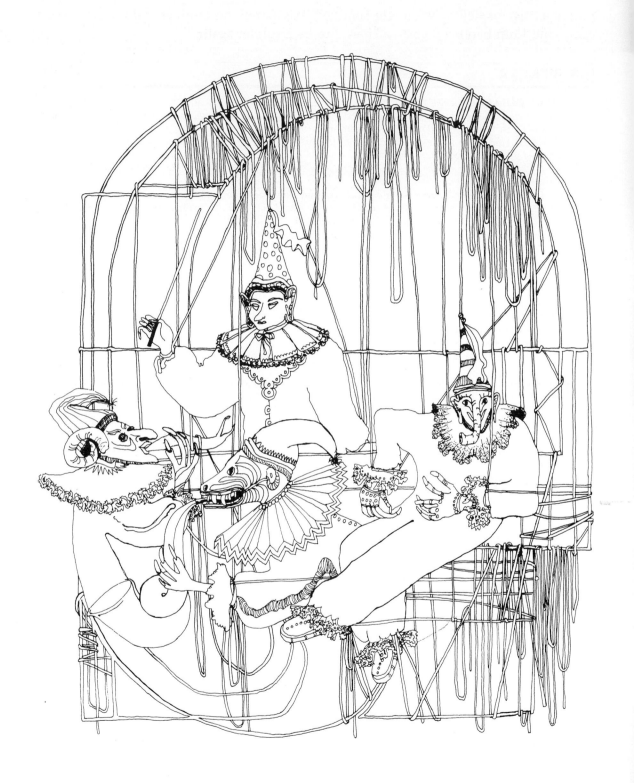

CHAPTER 11

Psychotic Disorders: How to Sensitively Arrive at a Differential Diagnosis

And then a Plank in Reason, broke,
And I dropped down, and down –
and hit a World, at every plunge,
And finished knowing – then – …

Emily Dickinson

INTRODUCTION

One wonders what the world is like when a plank in reason splinters, as Emily Dickinson describes the slip into psychotic process. The more we, as clinicians, can develop a feeling for this world, the easier it is to uncover subtle psychotic states. As intuitive understanding increases, it also becomes easier to understand the needs of the patient, an understanding that leads directly into a more compassionate, person-centered interview.

To begin our exploration, we will turn to Gérard De Nerval, a poet of extreme talent, who had the misfortune of falling through a plank in reason sometime during the middle of the Victorian Era. De Nerval was a gifted Symbolist poet, who was also a world traveler and a man deeply interested in philosophy. He was blessed with a child-like awe of nature. In 1841 he experienced his first psychotic break. Some 14 years later, psychotic process would lead him on a cold winter night to an iron gate bordering an alley near the Boulevard St-Michel. There, the following morning, he was found hanging from a railing with his neck fatally embraced by an apron string.[1]

On the morning after his suicide, fragments of a work entitled *Le Rêve et la Vie* were found in his pocket. It is this piece that provides us with our first glimpse into the world of psychosis:

First of all I imagined that the persons collected in the garden (of the madhouse) all had some influence on the stars, and that the one who always walked round and round in a circle regulated the course of the sun. An old man, who was brought there at certain hours of the day, and who made knots as he consulted his watch, seemed to me to be charged with the notation of the course of the hours …

I attributed a mystical signification to the conversations of the warders and of my companions. It seemed to me that they were the representatives for all the races of the earth, and that we had undertaken between us to re-arrange the course of the stars, and to give a wider development to the system. An error, in my opinion, had crept into the general combination of numbers, and thence came all the ills of humanity. …

I seemed to myself a hero living under the very eyes of the gods; everything in nature assumed new aspects, and secret voices came to me from the plants, the trees, animals, the meanest insects, to warn and to encourage me. The words of my companions had mysterious messages, the sense of which I alone understood.[2]

In some respects, it is De Nerval's last statement that provides one of the most telling clues as to the nature of psychotic process. As psychotic process becomes more intense, the patient's world becomes progressively more unique to the patient, receding further from the experience of the world as witnessed by others. In this sense, psychosis can be defined in simple terms as a breakdown of perceptual, cognitive, or rationalizing functions of the mind to the point that the individual experiences reality very differently than other people within the same culture.

De Nerval's world became filled with a maelstrom of curious and disturbing sensations. His words sensitively depict a variety of classic symptoms of psychosis, including delusions, ideas of reference, and hallucinations. It also demonstrates the fact that some aspects of psychotic process may be exciting and even beautiful. But – and this is an important "but" – psychosis is almost invariably ultimately accompanied by an intensely painful collection of fears. The patient senses impending catastrophe. For instance, De Nerval states, "An error, in my opinion, had crept into the general combination of numbers, and thence came all the ills of humanity." Such paranoid perception can create a tremendous sense of urgency and responsibility in those experiencing psychotic process. Perhaps for De Nerval, it was the realization that he could not correct this heinous error in the universe that led him to believe that his life should be ended because he had failed both God and humanity.

There are many aspects of psychotic process that, to my mind, demarcate it from the innovative workings of eccentric and/or creative men and women, whose thought is clearly at variance with the worldview of most people but is not a psychotic process. Creative thinking may bear a resemblance to psychotic process, but it is not identical to it. We shall see that it is not so much the content of the psychotic thinking that is pathologic, but more the way in which the thinking occurs that marks the process as psychotic.

THE DIFFERENTIAL DIAGNOSIS OF PSYCHOTIC STATES

Now that we have arrived at a working definition of psychosis, an important point needs to be emphasized. The word "psychosis" is not a diagnosis. Psychosis is a syndrome that can result from any number of psychiatric disorders delineated in the DSM-5. As we have already seen, mood disorders such as major depressive disorder and bipolar disorder can present with psychotic symptoms. It is never enough to simply state that the patient appears to be psychotic, because one must proceed to determine what diagnostic entity is causing the psychotic process. With some disorders such as schizophrenia and psychotic bipolar disorder, timely recognition can lead to early intervention, lower doses of antipsychotic medications, and an untold reduction in the patient's severity and duration of suffering. Other disorders that can sometimes feature psychosis such as deliria and central nervous system infections, can prove to be acutely life threatening, requiring immediate diagnostic recognition. In this chapter we will look at the interviewing techniques and strategies that will allow us to spot these diagnostic distinctions in a sensitive, rapid, and accurate fashion.

To accomplish this task, we will look at seven clinical vignettes that illustrate the diversity of possible disorders that can present with psychotic symptoms. Once again, the emphasis will be upon a discussion of both the symptoms experienced by the patients and the practical interviewing techniques that allow us to more sensitively and effectively uncover these symptoms. In the process we will explore the interface between interviewing and the delicate art of differential diagnosis.

Before proceeding with this clinical material, it may be of value to review the DSM-5 criteria for schizophrenia, because schizophrenia may very well represent the classic example of a psychotic illness. One of the main goals in the approach to any psychotic patient remains the determination of whether or not schizophrenia is present. To this end the DSM-5 criteria are as follows[3]:

DSM-5 DIAGNOSTIC CRITERIA FOR SCHIZOPHRENIA
SCHIZOPHRENIA
DIAGNOSTIC CRITERIA 295.90 (F20.9)

A. Two (or more) of the following, each present for a significant portion of time during a 1-month period (or less if successfully treated). At least one of these must be (1), (2), or (3):
   1. Delusions.
   2. Hallucinations.
   3. Disorganized speech (e.g., frequent derailment or incoherence).
   4. Grossly disorganized or catatonic behavior.
   5. Negative symptoms (i.e., diminished emotional expression or avolition).
B. For a significant portion of the time since the onset of the disturbance, level of functioning in one or more major areas, such as work, interpersonal relations, or self-care, is markedly below the level achieved prior to the onset (or when the onset is in childhood or adolescence, there is failure to achieve expected level of interpersonal, academic, or occupational functioning).
C. Continuous signs of the disturbance persist for at least 6 months. This 6-month period must include at least 1 month of symptoms (or less if successfully treated) that meet Criterion A (i.e., active-phase symptoms) and may include periods of prodromal or residual symptoms. During these prodromal or residual periods, the signs of the disturbance may be manifested by only negative symptoms or by two or more symptoms listed in Criterion A present in an attenuated form (e.g., odd beliefs, unusual perceptual experiences).

D. Schizoaffective disorder and depressive or bipolar disorder with psychotic features have been ruled out because either (1) no major depressive or manic episodes have occurred concurrently with the active-phase symptoms, or (2) if mood episodes have occurred during active-phase symptoms, they have been present for a minority of the total duration of the active and residual periods of the illness.

E. The disturbance is not attributable to the physiological effects of a substance (e.g., a drug of abuse, a medication) or another medical condition.

F. If there is a history of autism spectrum disorder or a communication disorder of childhood onset, the additional diagnosis of schizophrenia is made only if prominent delusions or hallucinations, in addition to the other required symptoms of schizophrenia, are also present for at least 1 month (or less if successfully treated).

Specify if:

    The following course specifiers are only to be used after a 1-year duration of the disorder and if they are not in contradiction to the diagnostic course criteria.

    First episode, currently in acute episode: first manifestation of the disorder meeting the defining diagnostic symptom and time criteria. An *acute episode* is a time period in which the symptom criteria are fulfilled.

    First episode, currently in partial remission: *Partial remission* is a period of time during which an improvement after a previous episode is maintained and in which the defining criteria of the disorder are only partially fulfilled.

    First episode, currently in remission: *Full remission* is a period of time after a previous episode during which no disorder-specific symptoms are present.

    Multiple episodes, currently in acute episode: *multiple episodes* may be determined after a minimum of two episodes (i.e., after a first episode, a remission, and a minimum of one relapse).

    Multiple episodes, currently in partial remission.

    Multiple episodes, currently in full remission.

    Continuous: Symptoms fulfilling the diagnostic symptom criteria of the disorder are remaining for the majority of the illness course, with subthreshold symptom periods being very brief relative to the overall course.

    Unspecified.

Specify if:

    With catatonia (refer to the criteria for catatonia associated with another mental disorder, pp. 119–120, for definition).

    Coding note: Use additional code 293.89 (F06.1) catatonia associated with schizophrenia to indicate the presence of the comorbid catatonia.

Specify current severity:

    Severity is rated by a quantitative assessment of the primary symptoms of psychosis including delusions, hallucinations, disorganized speech, abnormal psychomotor behavior, and negative symptoms. Each of these symptoms may be rated for its current severity (most severe in the last 7 days) on a 5-point scale ranging from 0 (not present) to 4 (present and severe). (See Clinician-Rated Dimensions of Psychosis Symptom Severity in the chapter "Assessment Measures").

Note: Diagnosis of schizophrenia can be made without using this severity specifier.

It should be noted that there also exists a diagnosis, schizophreniform disorder, that is applied when a patient meets Criterion A of schizophrenia (as well as having ruled out depressive disorder with psychosis, bipolar disorder, and schizoaffective disorder) but the symptoms do not last for 6 months nor necessarily result in a marked decline in functioning. In the schizophreniform disorder, the symptoms (including prodromal, active, and residual phases) must last at least 1 month but less than 6 months. Many patients who have received this diagnosis provisionally will eventually receive the diagnosis of schizophrenia if their symptoms last longer than 6 months and significant impairment in functioning begins to appear.

For psychotic presentations of an even shorter duration, the DSM-5 delineates the diagnosis of brief psychotic disorder. This diagnosis is used when the patient has one (or more) of the following symptoms, with at least one of the symptoms being in the first three listed: (1) delusions, (2) hallucinations, (3) disorganized speech, and (4) grossly disorganized or catatonic behavior. The timeframe is at least 1 day but less than 1 month, with the patient eventually having a full return to his or her previous level of functioning. If the psychotic episode is triggered by a specific stressor, this stressor should be specified. Such psychotic episodes are often called brief reactive psychoses in the clinical literature.

To begin our discussion, let us meet some people who have had the misfortune of falling through a plank in reason. As with Chapter 9, where we examined the differential diagnosis of mood disorders, it is assumed, for the sake of discussion, that the following clinical material was obtained during an initial assessment interview unless otherwise noted.

Clinical Presentations and Discussions

Clinical Presentation #1: Mr. Williams

Mr. Williams presents to the emergency department (ED) accompanied by three police officers. His behavior has not put the officers in particularly good moods. As one officer states, "This guy is wacko. Every once in a while he tries to bolt, as if something was after him." The officer has no idea what the "thing" is that appears so disturbing to Mr. Williams. In the interview, Mr. Williams presents as a 33-year-old male who initially appears relatively calm despite the beads of perspiration on his forehead. He is just finishing supper from his dinner tray and is neatly wiping his mouth with a napkin. His pants are torn and soiled; obviously, they are not strangers to the harshness of street life. He appears oriented to person, place, and time. As he begins to talk, he becomes more animated, displaying tangential speech with occasional glimpses of derailment (also known as a loosening of associations in the clinical literature). He also appears to be increasingly more distracted as evidenced by his having trouble focusing on the interviewer's questions. He denies any recent drinking or drug use, but his story is vague, concerned primarily with the appearance of some creature that has been following him. Suddenly, in the middle of the interview, his eyes widen as he stares down at his feet. He cannot attend to the interview because his attention is riveted to the floor. He begins kicking at some invisible object and angrily looks at the clinician, yelling, "Get rid of that thing!"

Discussion of Mr. Williams

Phenomenology of Visual Hallucinations and Illusions: Their Diagnostic Implications

While with the police, Mr. Williams had appeared to be responding to visual hallucinations, a process that reappeared during the interview itself. And here is the first clue to the diagnostic entity causing his immediate psychosis: The presence of visual hallucinations should alert the clinician to the possibility that a general medical condition may be causing the disorder. Schizophrenia can cause visual hallucinations but auditory hallucinations are significantly more frequent. However, general medical causes of psychosis (e.g., substance abuse and withdrawal, endocrine disorders, infections, toxins, and seizures) frequently present with extremely vivid visual hallucinations, with or without auditory hallucinations.

Fish has suggested that the quality of the visual hallucination may tend to vary depending on whether schizophrenia or a general medical process is present,[4] but no specific characteristics clearly differentiate them. Nevertheless, some characteristics seem to be more common in each category and may provide clues to etiology.

Visual hallucinations in patients whose psychosis is caused by a general medical condition, as seen with delirium, tend to vary from the classic psychoses by preferentially occurring at night, by being briefer in duration, and by being more frequently perceived as moving. They may also have little personal significance to the patient. For example, a patient with schizophrenia may hallucinate about a recently deceased relative, whereas the delirious patient may see snakes.[5]

With patients for whom the psychosis is caused by drugs or other general medical conditions, the hallucinations may appear more frequently and more vividly when the patient is in a darkened room or has his or her eyes shut. This is not the case with people with schizophrenia, who tend to see their hallucinations with eyes open or who experience little difference whether the eyes are open or closed.[6,7] In this sense, it is of value to ask patients, "When you see your hallucinations, what happens if you close your eyes?" With a hospitalized patient it is of value to check with the nursing staff concerning whether the patient is hallucinating more at night.

With people suffering from schizophrenia, visual hallucinations seldom occur by themselves. They usually present with auditory hallucinations or hallucinations from some other sensory modality.[8] Also of interest to the interviewer is the fact that schizophrenic hallucinations are frequently superimposed on an otherwise normal-appearing environment or may even appear with the surrounding environment absent. In hallucinogenic drug-induced psychoses, the entire environment frequently seems distorted with numerous illusions and hallucinations.[9] In a similar vein, the visual hallucinations of schizophrenia tend to appear suddenly, without preceding visual illusions or less formed visual hallucinations; whereas visual hallucinations caused by a general medical condition, as seen in delirium, tend to have a prodrome of visual illusions, simple geometric figures, and alterations of color, size, shape, and movement.[9]

Patients with schizophrenia tend to see concrete things such as faces, body parts, or complete figures, as opposed to geometric patterns or poorly formed images. On the other hand, once patients whose psychosis is caused by a general medical condition begin seeing concrete images, it has been my experience that the images frequently appear extremely real to the patients. The delirious patient may look on with terror, pointing towards the hallucination, eyeing it warily, or moving away from it as it appears to approach. Occasionally the patient's affective response may be pleasurable, as experienced with hallucinations of miniature people, so-called Lilliputian hallucinations, sometimes seen in the early stages of delirium tremens (DTs) and other medically related states.[10]

In Mr. William's case, the interviewer asked him if he could point more closely to the creature in question. Mr. Williams hesitantly obliged by cautiously moving his hand towards the open space in front of his feet. Abruptly he halted, "I ain't getting no closer!" It became even more apparent that the hallucination was vivid and quite realistic. At times, these types of hallucinations can create a peculiar sensation in the interviewer, because the actions of the patient, like the movements of a mime, create the feeling that one ought to be seeing something.

Sometimes the terms "hallucination" and "illusion" are confused. Mr. Williams presents with a true hallucination, for with hallucinations the perceptual image arises from an open space and is not triggered by an environmental stimulus. Whatever Mr. Williams is seeing, he is seeing it in the open space in front of his feet, not triggered by any object in the room itself. In contrast, with an illusion, the image is triggered by some actual object or stimulus. For instance, one patient vividly described watching the face of a man standing beside him on the bus. He saw the man's face begin to twist in a grotesque fashion and saw his eyeballs shatter and begin to bleed. This experience represents a visual illusion and also emphasizes that such illusions may be as striking and terrifying as true hallucinations.

Recognizing Psychotic Process Induced by Alcohol Withdrawal

We have seen that the appearance of vivid visual hallucinations ought to arouse suspicion that an organic agent may be at work. Mr. Williams presents with one of the more typical organic causes of psychosis that the initial interviewer must constantly keep in mind – abuse and withdrawal from alcohol, street drugs, or medications. It is important to realize that there exist two different manners in which drugs may precipitate a psychosis: by acute intoxication or by withdrawal. First, let us look at the issue of withdrawal, because Mr. Williams is suffering from a substance withdrawal delirium caused by an abrupt discontinuation of his drinking. Such a delirium is traditionally called delirium tremens – DTs.

It is beyond the scope of this book to provide a thorough review of drug abuse, and the reader should study this topic elsewhere in detail. However, there are some basic facts with which all assessment clinicians should be familiar, for psychoses triggered by substance abuse can be life threatening in nature, whether presenting in a clinical environment where they are encountered frequently (emergency department, inpatient unit, community mental health center) or one where they are seen much less often, yet, nevertheless, can present (college counseling center or private practitioner's office). They are also one of the most common causes of psychotic process. All initial interviewers need to be familiar with their symptomatic presentation and physical signs.

With regard to withdrawal states, alcohol and sedative/hypnotic drugs are the most likely to cause psychotic features. They are also the most likely to result in death if not recognized and treated. Withdrawal from these drugs is significantly more dangerous than withdrawal from drugs such as heroin or amphetamines. Some estimates of the mortality rate of patients with definite DTs from alcohol, who have been hospitalized, have been as high as 15%, although with good management this number should be markedly lower.[11]

As people begin to withdraw from alcohol and sedative hypnotics, they generally move from mild symptoms of withdrawal towards progressively more severe states such as DTs. As withdrawal occurs, patients frequently experience sleep disturbances, nausea, anxiety, over-alertness, tremulousness, and a peculiar intensification of their sensory modalities. Delirium tremens, itself, often persists about 5 to 10 days, with 62% of episodes resolving in 5 days or less.[12]

Even if patients such as Mr. Williams deny recent alcohol abuse, they may willingly admit to withdrawal symptoms if asked matter-of-factly and without the suggestion that they have "a personal problem." In this regard, questions such as the following may be useful:

a. "Since you stopped drinking, have you been noticing any problems with your sleep, because many people use alcohol to help with their sleep and without it, they have problems falling asleep?"
b. "Have you been feeling edgy over the past couple of days, you know, just can't seem to relax?"
c. "Over the past couple of days, have you been feeling sick in your stomach?"
d. "Recently, have you found yourself to be more edgy, you know, being startled by noises or upset by people moving or talking loudly near you?"

To develop DTs, the patient must have used alcohol heavily for a long period of time, minimally imbibing 4 to 5 pints of wine, or 7 to 8 pints of beer, or 1 pint of "hard" liquor every day for several months. It does not typically occur under the age of 30, although it clearly can, and it usually requires consistent use of large amounts of alcohol for several years,[13] most often appearing after a decade or so of abuse. This chronic use of alcohol sets up a complex set of compensatory physiologic changes in autonomic body regulation. When the alcohol is abruptly stopped, these compensatory changes go unchecked, resulting in such abnormalities as increased pulse, increased temperature, normal or elevated blood pressure, rapid breathing, muscle twitching, and sweating. As the syndrome becomes more serious, the patient may become so tremulous that walking appears to be difficult.[14]

While interviewing the psychotic patient, the clinician should do a quick survey to see if any of these physiologic signs of withdrawal are present. With Mr. Williams, he was noted to appear sweaty. The clinician also knew that his pulse rate was elevated at 100, with a mild increase in temperature. This emphasizes an important point. *In general, a patient presenting with an acute psychosis should have his or her vital signs taken before the clinical interview, thus alerting the clinician that an acute organic process may be at work.*

Mr. Williams proceeded to become more agitated, claiming that some kind of bug was crawling on him and that some "wires are running around on the floor. They're shocking the hell out of me, man!" It is not uncommon for people with DTs to hallucinate about small animals, and sometimes large objects such as trains or the proverbial pink elephant. Tactile hallucinations or illusions such as mice or lice crawling on the skin also occur, as seen with Mr. Williams.[14]

The clinician astutely cut this interview short, proceeding rapidly with a physical examination and appropriate medical management, which raises another important point. These patients need prompt medical attention. If one is not a physician, then one must immediately arrange to have such a patient seen by one. An appointment for "later in the day or tomorrow" is inadequate and potentially dangerous.

Before leaving the topic of DTs, a few more points are worth mentioning. Seizures ("rum fits") sometimes precede DTs, usually occurring during the first 2 days after the cessation of drinking. More than one in three patients who have withdrawal seizures will go on to develop DTs. DTs usually begin 24 to 72 hours after the cessation of drinking but can appear much later, even as long as 7 or more days later.[14] While performing an initial assessment on a psychotic patient in the hospital, a few issues are worth considering.

During their hospital stay, some patients may have a temporary alcohol or drug source, such as a friend, who eventually stops bringing them drugs. In these cases, DTs may not appear until much longer into the patient's hospitalization. Keep in mind that even patients with a higher income may purposely lie about alcohol consumption and may consequently develop withdrawal problems only as the hospitalization proceeds. Curiously, surgery may delay the appearance of DTs as well. *All these facts considered, clinicians should be alert to the possibility of drug withdrawal in any patient who develops a psychosis at any time during a hospital stay, especially if the patient's vital signs are abnormally elevated.*

Recognizing Psychotic Process Induced by Street Drugs

Violently psychotic patients, frequently brought in by the police, serve as a bridge to the next topic, patients who are acutely intoxicated by a psychosis-producing agent. The list of offending agents is extensive and includes common agents such as methamphetamine, lysergic acid diethylamide (LSD) and other hallucinogens, marijuana, cocaine, crack, and phencyclidine (PCP). For a concise and practical discussion, the reader is referred to specialized texts, such as Goldfrank's classic article on PCP and outstanding general textbooks such as the recent work of Fischer and Harrison.[15,16]

By way of example, I will briefly describe some of the more typical aspects of a patient intoxicated on PCP, a drug originally developed in the 1950s as an anesthetic-analgesic agent. These patients frequently present as markedly psychotic, although they can present without any psychotic features. In addition, they can be extremely violent. In this regard, any violent patient should alert the clinician to the possibility of PCP abuse. Even at low doses this drug can produce the "three As" of PCP use: analgesia, amnesia, and ataxia (problems with gait). The analgesia can result in self-mutilatory behaviors such as eye gouging. If use of PCP is even remotely suspected, the initial interviewer should have safety officers informed and immediately available during the interview.

On a behavioral level, the psychotic features of these patients may be quite bizarre, such as running naked in public or crawling around on all fours like an animal. They may develop paranoia, disorientation, auditory hallucinations, and visual hallucinations.

The physical examination may provide important clues, such as the various types of nystagmus (abnormal eye jerks) and hypertension, reported as occurring in 57% of these patients.[17] These patients generally show miosis (smaller than normal pupils) but may also present with mydriasis (larger than normal pupils), especially if they also ingested an anticholinergic agent. Increased muscle tone and increased salivation are also common. Rather than presenting as agitated, these patients may present lethargically or in a coma if they have ingested high doses of the drug.

At the time of writing this chapter, a new, still-legal drug was hitting the streets. It can create psychotic states similar to PCP, but is more common than PCP. It is known as "bath salts" and, in actuality, is not a single agent but is often a concoction of chemicals that are sought for their psychedelic effect. Unfortunately, wildly psychotic states can result – ranging from public nudity to extreme violence. One rare, but particularly bizarre, behavior associated with bath salts has been cannibalism, as seen in a young man under the influence of bath salts, who was found naked, eating the flesh off of a homeless man's face on a street in Miami. Another newer class of drugs that can also trigger psychotic states has been the synthetic cannabinoids, referred to by various street names including "spice."

One cannot leave the topic of street-drug induced psychosis without addressing methamphetamine in more detail. The rise of illicit meth labs has been striking – so commonplace, in fact, that it has been the subject of a popular television series; *Breaking Bad* is based on the exploits of a former high school teacher turned master of meth production. Chronic use of methamphetamine can create a psychotic state that appears remarkably like paranoid schizophrenia or a mixed bipolar disorder such as a dysphoric mania with psychosis. The two most common psychiatric symptoms with meth use are persecutory delusions and auditory hallucinations.[18] Even when patients stop the use of the drug, psychotic symptoms can persist.[19,20] Other persistent symptoms, despite continued abstinence, can include cognitive impairment, social instability, and an increase in lifetime suicide attempts.[21] For the initial interviewer, any patient presenting in an agitated state (often accompanied by severe problems sleeping), anger, paranoia, and auditory hallucinations should be considered as a potential methamphetamine user with appropriate drug screens ordered, even when street drug use is adamantly denied.

Returning in a more general sense to psychosis as precipitated by drugs, a few more points are worth noting. The rapid appearance of a full-blown psychosis in a matter of hours should make the clinician very suspicious of a drug-induced psychosis, as might be seen with LSD, PCP, or bath salts. Processes such as schizophrenia tend to develop more slowly over days, weeks, or months. Some patients may not know that they have been given a drug; it may have been slipped to them or sprinkled on a joint. In this regard, it is always worthwhile checking with friends who may know more about the actual circumstances surrounding the drug ingestion. One should always be on the lookout for two possibilities when faced with drug-intoxicated, psychotic patients:

1. Is the patient actually under the influence of more than one street drug?
2. Is it possibly a medication rather than a street drug that is precipitating the psychosis in this patient?

Recognizing Medication-Induced Psychosis

I am reminded of a young woman with a chronic history of paranoid schizophrenia. She had been doing very well in the hospital and was consequently sent home on a pass. Within a few hours of returning from her pass, she began to appear agitated and reported feeling apprehensive. In another 30 minutes she became grossly psychotic and reported that small dragons were chasing her. Indeed, she was seen racing down the hall as if pursued by a bevy of such monsters. The physical examination revealed dilated and poorly responsive pupils, a dry mouth, and an elevated pulse. It was discovered that she had taken "a few extra" Cogentin (benztropine mesylate) tablets while at her apartment. Cogentin is a prescribed anticholinergic agent that helps to alleviate some of the side effects of antipsychotic medications such as a Parkinsonian syndrome.

If taken in excess, these anticholinergic agents can quickly precipitate a delirium, as was the case with this patient. Elderly patients appear to be particularly susceptible to such anticholinergic deliria. It is therefore important to inquire about both prescription and non-prescription medications. Keep in mind that specific medications may have a mild anticholinergic effect, but when given together these medications may have an additive effect strong enough to precipitate a delirium, especially in the elderly.

Classes of medications that may have anticholinergic properties include some over-the-counter hypnotics and "cold medicines," certain antidepressants, some antipsychotics, certain antiparkinsonian medications, some medications for peptic ulcer disease, and even antihistamines.[22] The clinician must always carefully elicit a medication history from both the patient and the patient's family.

At the time of the writing of this third edition, the class of medications known as the semisynthetic opioids, such as oxycodone and OxyContin (its time-released preparation), as well as hydrocodone (Vicodin, Hycodan and, in combination with acetaminophen, Percocet) have achieved an epidemic prevalence in the United States. They have also led to a striking increase in the subsequent use of heroin and a sharp rise in heroin overdoses and deaths. OxyContin (because of the particularly high concentration of oxycodone in each tablet for it is a time-released medication) has become a major drug of abuse. Some of the common street names for oxycodone are: ox, oxy, kicker, cotton, hillbilly heroin, 40 and 80. I mention them here for a specific reason. In general, these substances are not highly associated with the production of acute psychotic symptoms,[23] but because of this recent upsurge in their use, clinicians should keep them in mind as etiologic agents when patients are presenting with psychotic features and substance use is suspected.

These medications at high doses have been reported to cause vivid and terrifying visual hallucinations. If a patient presents with vivid visual hallucinations in a clinic or emergency department setting, abuse of these agents should be considered. Also, be on the lookout for these agents as the cause of psychotic process, including vivid visual hallucinations, in any post-operative or pain patient. Sometimes with post-operative patients, the hallucinations do not appear for days after the patient's discharge from the hospital, until after they have returned home, much to the shock of both the patient and his or her family members. These psychotic presentations often have accompanying agitation and intense anxiety.

In concluding our discussion of medication-induced psychosis, the clinician should also keep in mind one other broad category of agents that could precipitate a medication-induced psychosis, namely, herbs and other natural agents. A naturally occurring source of anticholinergic agents is a family of plants known as the Solanaceae. Such an innocuous sounding name actually houses a variety of not so innocuous plants, including *Atropa belladonna* (commonly called deadly nightshade), jimsonweed, mandrake, and henbane.[24] Historically, ointments and potions made from such agents may have resulted in the psychotic states that, at least partially, functioned as the source of the wild phenomena reported by the witches of the Middle Ages, such as flying through the night sky to a Sabbat. In the present, it remains important to consider the ingestion of herbs and other "natural foods" while evaluating an unexplained acute onset of psychosis.

Effectively Interviewing and Collaborating With Law Enforcement Officers

Thus far, the material gained from the actual interview with Mr. Williams has been the focus of discussion. However, in addition, one of the most important interviews to perform when a patient is brought to the emergency department by the police is with the officers, and there is an art to this process. The first trick is training oneself to take the time to perform this interview. Both the police and the clinician are frequently harried, but nevertheless this interview can provide invaluable information.

In particular, one wants to establish the following: (1) What were the circumstances in which the patient was found? (2) Is the patient a known alcohol or drug abuser? (3) Do the officers know the patient's family and has the family been contacted? (4) Did the patient appear disoriented or demonstrate any signs of psychosis? (5) Has the patient appeared drowsy or been unconscious? and (6) Has the patient been in a fight involving a possible head blow?

Actively psychotic patients, especially paranoid patients, can be surprisingly violent, especially if they perceive, from a paranoid perspective, that they are fighting for their lives. I believe it is important initially to inquire as to whether an officer may have been injured while bringing the patient under control. This inquiry is both medically important and builds sound collaborative relationships among law enforcement officers and emergency department staff.

As with any type of professional, a particular police officer may be talented or not so talented in their work. In this regard, officers vary on their understanding and effective handling of psychiatric patients. Since the last edition of this book, law enforcement agencies, coupled with concerned patients, family members, and mental health professionals, have developed several outstanding programs for training law enforcement officers to be particularly effective and compassionate with patients coping with mental illness. I believe all initial interviewers should be aware of such efforts and tap them, if possible, in building healthy collaborative relationships with police departments, whether the interviewer works in an emergency department, on a crisis team, or at a college counseling center. Two such innovative programs are the Crisis Intervention Team Memphis Model – CIT – (http://cit.memphis.edu/) and the Connecticut Alliance to Benefit Law Enforcement – CABLE – (www.cableweb.org).

Considering the difficulties of subduing a person experiencing an agitated psychotic process, it is expedient to discover how the patient was subdued, including whether or not a Taser was used. The clinician should also determine whether an officer delivered a head blow, either justly or unjustly. Uncovering a history of a physical confrontation can help alert the clinician to the possibility of a subdural hematoma or an intracranial bleed as the source of the psychosis, especially in older patients who have been struck. It may also help the clinician understand and perhaps decrease the patient's fear that more violence may follow.

A sensitive interviewer approaches these topics in a manner that places the officers at ease. It is important to remember that most officers resort to violence only when absolutely necessary. Angry countertransference feelings directed towards the police can only get in the way of gaining valid information from them. The following type of approach may be useful:

Clin.: It really looks like you had your hands full tonight.

Police: You can say that again, this guy's really out of it. It took three of us to get him down.

Clin.: Yeah, he's wound up, maybe he's on something. Listen, did any of your officers get hurt? We'd be glad to take a look at them and check them over.

Police: No, don't worry about it, thanks anyway.

Clin.: By the way, did you need to Taser him to calm him or wrestle him down?

Police: Didn't need to Taser him, but like I said, it took three of us to wrestle him down. I think he was hallucinating and must have felt we were after him or something.

Clin.: When you were wrestling him down, did he accidentally get struck on the head?

Police: No, can't say that he did.

Clin.: The reason I ask is that if he got a blow on the head we need to make sure he didn't get a small fracture or something like that?

Police: Hmmm … Well, you might want to take a look, this guy was really wild; someone might have used a baton on him or he could have smacked his head on the ground. I'm not sure. It all happened really fast. He was out of control.

Clin.: Okay, thanks a lot for all your help. We'll take a look at him. I hope the rest of your night goes better than this. Sounds like you guys did a great job. Thanks for bringing him in.

This matter-of-fact type of exchange tends to yield accurate answers while unobtrusively reminding the officers of the dangers of a head blow.

Differential Diagnosis on Mr. Williams and Summary of Key Interviewing Tips

The interview with the police revealed that Mr. Williams had a long history of alcohol use (severe), although he did not appear intoxicated at that point in time. They also thought that he had a history of "stuffing his face with any drug he could get his hands on." Further interviewing with Mr. Williams revealed that he had a history of DTs. The physical examination and lab work revealed no other probable cause for the psychotic presentation. He was felt to be in the early stages of DTs and was begun on Valium (diazepam). In a matter of several hours he calmed down, and all psychotic symptoms vanished. His case would be summarized as follows:

General Psychiatric Disorders:

Substance withdrawal delirium (alcohol)

Alcohol use disorder (severe)

Rule out unknown substance use disorder

Personality Disorders:

Deferred

Medical Disorders:

Rule out a variety of alcohol-related diseases such as hepatitis, gastritis, and pancreatitis

As we leave the discussion of Mr. Williams, several key points are worth summarizing.

1. Visual hallucinations, especially if they appear to be particularly vivid and real to the patient, are frequently seen in psychoses caused by physiologic insults to the brain, including street drugs, medications, and medical disease.
2. Despite the fact that such physiologic psychoses may tend to have some features that distinguish them from entities such as schizophrenia, all psychoses can present in a similar fashion. Consequently, any patient presenting for the first time with psychotic features should be promptly medically evaluated.
3. One of the most frequent physiologic causes of psychotic symptoms is the use of street drugs or alcohol.
4. Withdrawal from alcohol in heavy drinkers may lead to an alcohol withdrawal delirium (commonly called DTs). DTs can be fatal if not treated promptly.
5. The onset of a marked psychosis in a matter of hours in a previously normal individual is strongly suggestive of a drug-related etiology.
6. Both over-the-counter and prescription medications may cause psychotic states, especially in the elderly. Anticholinergic medications are notorious for precipitating deliria.
7. Although not a common presentation, be on the lookout for psychotic process, especially visual hallucinations, triggered by the use and/or abuse of medications containing oxycodone or hydrocodone.
8. If police bring in the patient, the officers should be questioned thoroughly, for they may have pivotal information regarding differential diagnosis.
9. Any patient who presents violently should be thoroughly evaluated for evidence of psychotic process and the possible use of drugs such as PCP or newer "legal" drugs such as bath salts, synthetic cannabis, and other designer drugs.

Clinical Presentation #2: Mr. Walker

Mr. Walker is a 20-year-old male. He is thin and his hospital gown tends to hang forlornly on his gaunt frame. Beneath his black hair a rather handsome face sits quietly darkening with a day's worth of beard. He has been admitted to an inpatient unit after having been referred by a college counseling center, who had seen the student shortly after his return from Christmas break. One of the unit's social workers is performing an initial intake. As the interviewer enters the room, Mr. Walker acknowledges him with a slight nod of his head. His speech is soft and mildly slowed. He appears almost shy. As he speaks, there is barely a hint of facial expression, his voice painted gray by a conspicuous lack of highlights. All seems bland. Mr. Walker proceeds to describe a chaotic situation at home. He is being avidly pursued by three filthy women who enter his house at night. They attempt to force sex on him. When asked if he knows who these women are, he nods, stating that one is "that devil Miss Brown." He proceeds to describe a recent party he attended, where sex games were played. He relates that he had been tricked into going. As he entered the kitchen three men tied him to a chair and stripped him. When asked what happened, he pauses and proceeds to say, "They violated my anus." As he says these words a slight smile steals across his face. It had been verified that no such rape had occurred. His speech is without any evidence of derailment (loosening of associations), tangential thought, thought blocking, or illogical thought. He is alert and well oriented. Both he and his family deny that he has used any street drugs. His family says he has been acting oddly for almost a year, making vague accusations about a Miss Brown even during the summer. During the interview the clinician feels uncomfortable and somewhat frightened.

Discussion of Mr. Walker

Spotting Disturbances of Affect as Seen in Schizophrenia

One of the first things to note about Mr. Walker is the peculiar blandness that he demonstrates when describing brutal scenes of sexual abuse. This blandness represents an important diagnostic clue, because Mr. Walker is suffering from schizophrenia.

Affect refers to a patient's manner of expressing emotion and spontaneity through facial expressions. Criterion A-5 from the DSM-5 includes "diminished emotional expression," a concept that is traditionally described as a reduction in affect. Diminished affect is viewed as one of the negative symptoms of schizophrenia, a cluster of symptoms we will explore in detail shortly. Abnormalities in affect can be seen in other psychotic states, but it is particularly common in schizophrenia. At present, let's turn our attention to the changes in affect typical of schizophrenia.

A useful interviewing habit consists of asking oneself if the patient seems to be appropriately disturbed while describing traumatic incidents. In the case of Mr. Walker, as he related his rape, there was little display of fear, anxiety, or anger. His affect changed very little. When present in a mild degree, this type of affect is usually called "restricted." If present to a moderate degree, this type of unresponsive affect is usually called "blunted." If the patient demonstrates essentially no change in affect, it is usually referred to as a "flat" affect. Mr. Walker also nicely demonstrates the concept of an inappropriate affect. Rape victims do not generally smile as they describe their assaults. This peculiar combination of flattened affect and inappropriate affect is not infrequent in schizophrenia. It is one of the qualities that can create an unsettling emotional response in a clinician, as it did in this case.

An important point to remember concerning reduced affects is the ironic and sometimes confusing fact that some antipsychotic medications frequently also cause a blunting of affect as a side effect. The wary clinician must keep this point in mind, because a patient inappropriately labeled as having schizophrenia by a previous clinician may present with a blunted or flat affect related to current medication. This blunted affect may be misinterpreted by the new clinician as further "proof" that the patient has schizophrenia, resulting in a perpetuation of the first diagnostic error.

Diagnostic Significance of the Presence of Delusions: Delineating Schizophrenia From Delusional Disorders

Perhaps even more striking than Mr. Walker's blunted affect is the fact that he is clearly delusional. The appearance of delusions of any kind should alert the clinician to the possibility of schizophrenia. A delusion is a false belief that is firmly held by a patient but is not believed by others in the patient's general culture. When firmly entrenched, a patient will persist in his or her delusional belief despite incontrovertible evidence that it is false. Over the course of time, patients may vary on the intensity of their belief, a process I like to call having greater or lesser distance (insight) from their delusional belief. When a patient has gained considerable distance from a delusion, the patient will be able to see that the belief may very well be untrue. If this perspective is maintained, one can say that the patient is no longer delusional but is now experiencing an overvalued idea.

The delusions of schizophrenia are frequently bizarre in the sense that they are patently absurd and have no possible factual basis. The patient may feel that alien or demonic forces are controlling his or her body or that thoughts are being inserted or withdrawn from his or her body. Other delusions tend to be concerned with magical, grandiose, or intensely hyper-religious themes. For example, a patient may believe that God wants the patient to cut off a finger and sprinkle the blood over the earth in order to bring flowers into bloom. When schizophrenia is highlighted by paranoia, the patient may present with delusions of persecution or jealousy, as did Mr. Walker. Such delusions, although clearly not true, may not be bizarre in nature.

But this point raises an important diagnostic issue, for how does one separate schizophrenia from a different DSM-5 diagnosis called a delusional disorder? The distinction is actually somewhat easier to make than one might assume if one keeps the following guidance in mind.

In schizophrenia the delusions are only part of the pathologic process. Other aspects of psychotic process are present in addition to the delusion itself. Specifically, in schizophrenia, if delusions are present, the patient's delusions are accompanied by one of the following: some type of hallucinatory process, evidence of disorganized thought, grossly disorganized or catatonic behavior, or the presence of "negative symptoms" such as the affective flattening seen with Mr. Walker. Problems with the formation of thought may manifest as incoherence or as a marked loosening of associations (referred to as "derailment" in the DSM-5). In addition, patients with true schizophrenia will invariably demonstrate a significant decrease in social and/or occupational functioning over time.

In contrast, patients with delusional disorders tend to demonstrate *only* delusions, although they can show infrequent hallucinations. If present, these infrequent hallucinations are always tied directly into the patient's delusional system (as with a patient with a paranoid delusion about his neighbor complaining of occasionally hearing his neighbor yelling, "I'll get you someday, watch your back, watch your back," or a patient deluded that he is infested with parasites may have tactile hallucinations within his abdomen). Also in contrast to schizophrenia, patients with delusional disorders tend to show surprisingly good baseline functioning at home and at work, as well as demonstrating a reasonably normal and appropriately reactive affect. We will look at the phenomenology of delusions and delusional disorders in more detail later in this chapter.

Keep in mind that not all patients with schizophrenia have delusions.

Negative (Deficit) Symptoms of Schizophrenia

An important advance in the DSM-IV system that was continued in the DSM-5 was the addition of the term "negative symptoms" and a recognition of their importance in the amount of pain they cause patients. Historically, in the DSM-III, much emphasis was placed upon those symptoms that people with schizophrenia show that most people do not experience, such as hallucinations and delusions. These "extra" phenomena are now called "positive symptoms," indicating that they are an unwanted "excess."

We are now aware that schizophrenia also afflicts brain structures in such a way that the person *loses* certain normal functions. These lost functions are referred to as "negative symptoms" or "deficit symptoms," the latter being the term that I prefer. Such symptoms include decreased affect, as described above, alogia (decreased speech production and interest in speaking), avolition (decreased drive and ability to sustain interest), anhedonia (loss of interest in pleasurable activities), and asociality (reduced interpersonal interactions).[25] Some clinicians also view anergia (loss of energy) as a deficit symptom.

Empirically, Rado summarized the research findings on the impact of the "deficit syndrome," a term referring to patients afflicted with a predominance of negative symptoms.[26] During the first episode of schizophrenia, negative symptoms appear in patients somewhere between 50 and 90% of the time. The deficit syndrome is associated with more severe cognitive disorganization, as well as poorer insight into the illness. Patients with significant amounts of these deficit symptoms tend to have poorer psychosocial, vocational, and recreational functioning. They also tend to experience higher levels of anxiety and a lower appraisal of competence, as well as a decrease in interpersonal skills. As we shall see later in this chapter, these deficit symptoms are frequently devastating to both functioning and self-esteem and are in some instances more disabling than positive psychotic symptoms such as hallucinations and delusions.

The Importance of Family Members in Uncovering Psychotic Process

Mr. Walker's presentation becomes even more clearly typical of schizophrenia following an interview with his mother.

Clin.:   What does your son do down in his room all day long?

Moth.:   That is what is so peculiar. He talks with her.

Clin.:   How do you mean?

Moth.:   He talks with this devil woman. I'll hear voices that sound like a woman's voice coming up out of the basement. It is really weird. Late at night I can hear him arguing with her, swearing at her, and sometimes it sounds like holy hell is breaking out down there. I'm terrified; I never go down there.

Clin.:   When he is with you, does it ever look like he is hearing voices?

Moth.:   Oh yes, he's always mumbling to himself like he's answering someone. But the strange thing is that he's not always like this. Sometimes he seems so calm and almost normal and other times he's in a frenzy. Just last night he came screaming up out of that basement with a butcher knife in his hand. He kept screaming at me that I'd better make them stop. I couldn't take it anymore so I brought him in.

From the above, it is apparent that Mr. Walker is hearing voices and clearly fulfills the criteria for schizophrenia. It also serves to stress the importance of carefully interviewing family members or other significant others. For whatever reasons, psychotic patients may withhold information critical to the diagnosis, and the family often gratefully provides the missing pieces.

Mr. Walker also illustrates the fluctuating nature of psychotic process. Even in schizophrenia, as we shall see later in the chapter, the severity of the psychotic process may vary substantially. Many an interviewer has been lulled into a belief that a patient is not psychotic during the interview. In such cases it is always wise to listen carefully to the family, because the interviewer may simply be catching the patient during a period of decreased psychotic process. Moreover, patients with psychotic process may not be too eager to tell the "shrink" that they are plagued by voices. Their more rational side warns them that such talk may provide a quick ticket into the hospital.

Differential Diagnosis Between Schizophrenia and Mood Disorders With Psychotic Features

Let us turn our attention to one of the exclusion criteria for schizophrenia as delineated by the DSM-5. Criterion D directly addresses the issue of affective symptoms. Several points are worth remembering here that can help us to differentiate between schizophrenia and mood (affective) disorders with psychotic features. In the preceding chapter we noted that a major depression or a bipolar disorder may eventually manifest with psychotic symptoms; thus these diagnoses are important to rule out when psychosis is suspected. The particular psychotic symptoms may be either mood-congruent or mood-incongruent. *It is important to note that in a major depressive disorder with psychotic features or a bipolar disorder with psychotic features, the psychotic symptoms generally appear a considerable time period after the onset of the mood disorder. It is almost as if the depressive or manic process builds to a crescendo that culminates with the blooming of psychotic process. In contrast, with schizophrenia, the psychotic process is usually an earlier part of the process, predating the most severe mood symptoms.*

Diagnostic mistakes can be made in either direction (mislabeling someone with schizophrenia as having a psychotic mood disorder and vice versa). Factors in such misdiagnoses can range from sloppy interviewing and/or a misunderstanding of the phenomenology of these disorders to the fact that some people present with confusing admixtures of psychotic and mood symptoms. In this regard, Guze reports that most people suffering from schizophrenia experience affective syndromes at some time during the course of their illness.[27] Moreover, anhedonia is frequently seen in schizophrenia, where it presents as one of the negative symptoms.[28] Such patients may be mistakenly diagnosed as having a mood disorder. In contrast, some patients are mislabeled as having schizophrenia when, in actuality, they have a bipolar disorder or major depression. This error is not a benign one, for such patients might benefit from lithium or antidepressants. American psychiatrists have tended to over-diagnose schizophrenia, while under-diagnosing bipolar disorder.[29]

Two points are worth emphasizing here that can help us with our differential diagnosis. First, family members and the records of other mental health professionals can be invaluable in gaining a clear history of which came first, the psychotic symptoms or the mood symptoms. *Second, it is always important when evaluating a patient who has had numerous psychotic breaks to return to the first break in an attempt to determine the role of depressive or manic symptoms in the chronology of the illness.*

The role of the timing of mood versus psychotic symptoms is particularly important in the differential between bipolar disorder (manic phase) and schizophrenia, for an agitated mania can look exactly like the psychotic presentation of a patient suffering with schizophrenia. Keep in mind that a patient can be manic without being psychotic. The mania itself is manifested by excessive energy, unstable mood, agitation, decreased need for sleep, pressured speech, and other classic manic symptoms. The mania does not become psychotic unless reality contact is disturbed, as manifested by the presence of delusions, hallucinations, or other psychotic symptoms such as grossly disorganized thought. It has been estimated that about 50 to 70% of manic patients display psychotic symptoms.[30]

As with depression, psychotic symptoms in mania tend to appear significantly later than the mood symptoms. This point once again helps to ease the difficulty of distinguishing between schizophrenia and mania with psychotic process. However, to make use of this difference, the interviewer must make a concerted effort to learn about the very first episode of the patient's illness.

Interestingly, there is mounting evidence that the clear-cut distinctions between schizophrenia and psychotic bipolar disorders, delineated above, may be somewhat misleading.

Let me explain more clearly what I mean. We have already seen in Chapter 9 that even *within the broad category* of mood disorders, diagnoses sometimes seem to overlap. For instance, within mood disorders, *especially with late adolescents and young adults* who present with angst ridden depressions (sometimes including psychotic features), the diagnosis of an agitated major depression is sometimes wrong. In reality, some of these patients are suffering from a type of mixed bipolar disorder called a dysphoric mania. In short, there may be more of a continuum within broad diagnostic categories, such as the mood disorders, than was formally thought. Specifically, the mood disorders of depressive disorder and bipolar disorder may be more related than has been traditionally recognized.

Extending this idea, then, is it possible that there may exist continua not just *within* a single broad diagnostic category like mood disorders but also *between* broad diagnostic categories themselves, for instance, between mood disorders and schizophrenia?

The answer appears to be evolving towards "yes." The clear-cut distinctions described above that can distinguish schizophrenia from psychotic mood disorders may prove to be most true for patients at each end of what, for want of a better term, we will call the schizo–bipolar continuum. In short, there may be many patients who have a relatively pure form of schizophrenia (psychotic symptoms appear early, followed by marginal mood disturbances relatively late in the process) and there may be patients with a relatively pure form of bipolar disorder (manic symptoms appear quite early, followed by psychotic symptoms relatively late in the disorder). But a significant cohort of patients seems to lie in-between these two diagnoses.

Schizoaffective Disorder and the Schizo–Bipolar Continuum

It is now apparent that we have stumbled upon a curious diagnostic dilemma. We have seen that in schizophrenia the psychotic symptoms usually predate marked mood symptoms. And in the mood disorders the psychotic symptoms generally appear later in the process, after the mood symptoms have been around for a while. But what diagnosis is appropriate when the psychotic symptoms appear at or near the same time as the affective symptoms? Indeed, even in patients with a relatively classic presentation of schizophrenia, one can find that during the prodrome of the illness, there may be many months of low-grade mood disruption, especially of a dysthymic nature.

The diagnosis that helps to fill this gap is "schizoaffective disorder," and it is defined in the DSM-5 as follows[31]:

DSM-5 DIAGNOSTIC CRITERIA FOR SCHIZOAFFECTIVE DISORDER

A. An interrupted period of illness during which there is a major mood episode (major depressive or manic) concurrent with Criterion A of schizophrenia.

Note: The major depressive episode must include Criterion A1: Depressed mood.

B. Delusions or hallucinations for 2 or more weeks in the absence of a major mood episode (depressive or manic) during the lifetime duration of the illness.

C. Symptoms that meet criteria for a major mood episode are present for the majority of the total duration of the active and residual portions of the illness.

D. The disturbance is not attributable to the effects of a substance (e.g., a drug of abuse, a medication) or another medical condition.

Specify whether:

    295.70 (F25.0) Bipolar type: This subtype applies if a manic episode is part of the presentation. Major depressive episodes may also occur.

DSM-5 DIAGNOSTIC CRITERIA FOR SCHIZOAFFECTIVE DISORDER—Cont'd

295.70 (F25.1) Depressive type: This subtype applies if only major depressive episodes are part of the presentation.

Specify if:

With catatonia (refer to the criteria for catatonia associated with another mental disorder, pp.119–120 for definition).

Coding note: Use additional code 293.89 (F06.1) catatonia associated with schizoaffective disorder to indicate the presence of the comorbid catatonia.

Specify if:

The following course specifiers are only to be used after a 1-year duration of the disorder and if they are not in contradiction to the diagnostic course criteria.

First episode, currently in acute episode: First manifestation of the disorder meeting the defining diagnostic symptom and time criteria. An *acute episode* is a time period in which the symptom criteria are fulfilled.

First episode, currently in partial remission: *Partial remission* is a time period during which an improvement after a previous episode is maintained and in which the defining criteria of the disorder are only partially fulfilled.

First episode, currently in full remission: *Full remission* is a period of time after a previous episode during which no disorder-specific symptoms are present.

Multiple episode, currently in acute episode: Multiple episodes may be determined after a minimum of two episodes (i.e., after a first episode, a remission and a minimum of one relapse).

Multiple episodes, currently in partial remission.

Multiple episodes, currently in full remission.

Continuous: Symptoms fulfilling the diagnostic symptom criteria of the disorder are remaining for the majority of the illness course, with subthreshold symptom periods being very brief relative to the overall course.

Unspecified

Specify current severity:

Severity is rated by a quantitative assessment of the primary symptoms of psychosis, including delusions, hallucinations, disorganized speech, abnormal psychomotor behavior, and negative symptoms. Each of these symptoms may be rated for its current severity (most severe in the last 7 days) on a 5-point scale ranging from 0 (not present) to 4 (present and severe). (See Clinician-Rated Dimensions of Psychosis Symptom Severity in the chapter "Assessment Measures.")

Note: Diagnosis of schizoaffective disorder can be made without using this severity specifier.

The vagueness of this definition certainly would be at home in the campaign speech of any presidential candidate. But then at this stage of current diagnostic knowledge, this degree of vagueness may be appropriate. The vagueness of the definition serves to remind us that categorical diagnostic entities are not necessarily real-life entities, but rather represent labels for the most commonly observed patterns of behaviors. In this regard, there has been growing recognition that traditional diagnostic "entities" such as schizophrenia, schizoaffective disorder, and psychotic bipolar disorder, may perhaps be better conceptualized as being on a dimensional continuum rather than being a set of distinct disease entities. Future versions of the DSM system may more accurately reflect this dimensional quality.

In the late 1970s, Tsuang pioneered the idea that the diagnosis of schizoaffective disorder represents a heterogeneous category with two probable subtypes, an affective subtype and a schizophrenic subtype. According to this theory, schizoaffective disorder is not likely to represent a genetically distinct category.[32] It appears that Tsuang was ahead of his time. More recent studies have indicated substantial genetic overlap between schizophrenia and psychotic bipolar disorder.[33,34]

In addition to genetic evidence, there is increasing data from cognitive, neurobiological, and epidemiological studies that there is significant overlap between schizophrenia and psychotic bipolar disorder.[35,36] Even in their prodromal states, there seems to be some overlap – for example, the appearance of subtle cognitive changes in both disorders during this phase.[37] A nice summary of how the concept of schizophrenia has been evolving over the past two centuries, up to and including the DSM-5, has been provided by Bruijnzeel and Tandon.[38] The net result of this exploration of the overlapping characteristics of schizophrenia, schizoaffective disorder, and bipolar disorder is the growing interest in conceptualizing a "psychosis spectrum" between schizophrenia and bipolar disorder, in which the schizoaffective states lie between the purer forms of the syndromes located at opposing poles of the spectrum.[39,40]

At the present moment, the bottom line with the differential diagnosis of schizoaffective disorder is that people with schizoaffective disorders have many of the striking psychotic processes seen in schizophrenia but also have persistent and significant mood disturbances. They seem to differ from people who have psychotic bipolar disorder or an agitated, psychotic depression in that people with schizoaffective disorder have periods when they are quite psychotic but their mood is fairly normal. This latter state is seldom seen with people suffering from a pure mood disorder, whose psychotic process tends to "rear its head" primarily during a marked disturbance in mood. People with schizoaffective disorders seem to differ from those with classic schizophrenia in having prolonged periods of time, both early and throughout the process, in which there are striking mood symptoms, frequently without accompanying psychotic symptoms. In the DSM-5, the diagnosis of schizoaffective disorder requires that the disturbance in mood continues for the majority of the duration of the disorder (as seen in Criterion C, above). If psychotic symptoms begin to appear without concurrent mood symptoms, then the diagnosis must be changed to schizophrenia.

These recent insights into the nature of schizoaffective disorder (including the concept of a schizo–bipolar spectrum) are not merely of academic interest – they have practical implications for initial interviewers and their patients, for diagnoses play a significant role in future treatment interventions. When an initial interviewer determines that a patient meets the criteria for schizophrenia, future clinicians may be less likely to consider the use of mood stabilizers such as lithium and Depakote.

In contrast, the diagnosis of schizoaffective disorder serves to remind clinicians that the patient may have an affective component to the illness, suggesting the use of such medications. If there is a bipolar quality to the schizoaffective disorder, it also alerts the clinician to be cautious in adding an antidepressant, for fear of exacerbating or unleashing an underlying manic process. The diagnosis may also have some prognostic importance, because some authors feel that schizoaffective disorders have a significantly better prognosis than schizophrenia.[41]

Differential Diagnosis on Mr. Walker and Summary of Key Interviewing Tips

No history suggestive of a personality disorder or a medical problem was found upon further interviewing with Mr. Walker. Apparently he had been displaying a downhill course for almost a year, thus fulfilling the time criteria for schizophrenia. His family reported that he had appeared intermittently depressed, but not strikingly so. They were not entirely clear about the time course of the interplay between depressive symptoms and the psychotic process, but they did not feel that Mr. Walker had been consistently depressed. They did not see evidence of a marked depression before the onset of his delusions, nor during the early months of the process. Once within the hospital, lab tests and other medical examinations would need to be ordered to rule out a general medical condition, such as chronic use of methamphetamine or hyperthyroidism, as the cause for his psychosis, but his history does not particularly suggest such an entity. Consequently, the working diagnostic formulation would probably look as follows:

General Psychiatric Disorders:

Schizophrenia

Rule out schizoaffective disorder

Personality Disorders:

None

Medical Disorders:

None

Before leaving the discussion of Mr. Walker, several key points are worth summarizing:

1. Aberrations in affect such as blunting, flattening, and inappropriate affect are frequently seen in schizophrenia.
2. Some antipsychotic medications can cause a blunted or flat affect. Consequently, when a patient is on an antipsychotic, it is difficult to determine whether the unusual affect is secondary to the medication or a psychopathologic process.
3. In order for a patient presenting with delusions to fulfill the criteria for schizophrenia, he or she must also demonstrate one of the following: hallucinations, disorganized speech, grossly disorganized or catatonic behavior, or the negative symptoms of schizophrenia (e.g., decreased affect, alogia, avolition, anhedonia, and asociality).
4. Psychotic process frequently fluctuates. The interviewer should keep in mind that the patient may not be strikingly psychotic during the interview itself.
5. Collateral interviews with family members may provide invaluable diagnostic information.
6. Recent evidence-based research is suggesting that there may be significant genetic, cognitive, epidemiologic, and phenomenological overlap between schizophrenia and psychotic bipolar disorder, suggesting a continuum between the two disorders.

7. If you are interviewing a patient who is clearly psychotic, before making the diagnosis of schizophrenia, carefully look for a history of mood symptoms that may suggest a schizoaffective disorder, a diagnosis that could have marked implications for psycho-pharmacologic interventions.
8. Also take a detailed family history, for the presence of many blood relatives who have experienced mood disorders may further hint that the patient lays somewhere on the mood end of the schizo–bipolar spectrum.

People coping with schizophrenia may move into partial or full remissions, conditions that may be indicated in the DSM-5 by adding specifiers such as "multiple episodes, currently in full remission" or "first episode, currently in partial remission." It is important to remember that patients with schizophrenia need not be psychotic continuously. The disorder itself can show fluctuations and may also be transformed with the use of antipsychotic medications.

Clinical Presentation #3: Ms. Hastings

Ms. Hastings walks into her first session at a private outpatient clinic run by a group of psychologists with a disgruntled look on her face. She is 57 years old and appears a bit bedraggled. The first words out of her mouth are, "Can you help me with my husband?" Her speech is fluent, without any evidence of derailment, illogical thought, or bizarre ideation. In fact, she is somewhat eloquent but clearly upset. When asked to elaborate, she responds with an indignant snort, "It's the divorce game, that's all!" She proceeds to relate an elaborate tale of infidelity on the part of her husband. At the present time, she says, he has hired a variety of men to harass her into a state of insanity. Her craziness will provide grounds for his sought-after divorce. The men are using "conventional spy tools," and she is beginning to feel that her own mother may be in on the plot. Her story is literally illustrated by a journal filled with drawings and time schedules she has compiled on the activities of her husband and "his goons next door." She denies hallucinations or a previous psychiatric history. She also denies most depressive symptoms except, "I'm edgy of course, wouldn't you be?"

Discussion of Ms. Hastings

Unlike Mr. Walker, Ms. Hastings does not present with a blunted or odd affect. On the contrary, she seems convincingly quite normal. Her affect is appropriately upset for someone believing that she is the object of foul play. She does not complain of any hallucinations, and subsequent interviewing revealed that she has none. There is no evidence of a formal thought disorder (i.e., problems with the formation of thoughts as seen with derailment or severely illogical thought) or the other psychotic symptoms frequently seen in schizophrenia. Furthermore, she has no evidence of any psychotic disorder before the age of 50.

Types of Delusional Disorders

The only psychopathology that Ms. Hastings displays is a concrete delusional system. As we noted earlier, such a delusional system alone cannot fulfill the criteria for schizophrenia unless the delusion is accompanied by at least one other Criterion A symptom (hallucinations, disorganized speech, grossly disorganized or catatonic behaviors, or negative symptoms). Instead, Ms. Hastings displays one of a curious collection of disorders referred to as delusional disorders. We briefly addressed the distinction between these disorders and schizophrenia when discussing Mr. Walker. It is now useful to explore their phenomenology and their implications for the interviewer in an initial interview. In the DSM-5, these disorders comprise seven types: persecutory type, jealous type, erotomanic type, somatic type, grandiose type, mixed type, and unspecified type. All seven of these disorders share the following criteria of a delusional disorder[42]:

DSM-5 DIAGNOSTIC CRITERIA FOR DELUSIONAL DISORDER (297.1 (F22))

A. The presence of one (or more) delusions with a duration of 1 month or longer.

B. Criterion A for schizophrenia has never been met.

Note: Hallucinations, if present, are not prominent and are related to the delusional theme (e.g., the sensation of being infested with insects associated with delusions of infestation).

C. Apart from the impact of the delusion(s) or its ramifications, functioning is not markedly impaired, and behavior is not obviously bizarre or odd.

D. If manic or major depressive episodes have occurred, these have been brief relative to the duration of the delusional periods.

E. The disturbance is not attributable to the physiological effects of a substance or another medical condition and is not better explained by another mental disorder, such as body dysmorphic disorder or obsessive–compulsive disorder.

Specify whether:

   Erotomanic type: This subtype applies when the central theme of the delusion is that another person is in love with the individual.

   Grandiose type: This subtype applies when the central theme of the delusion is the conviction of having some great (but unrecognized) talent or insight or having made some important discovery.

   Jealous type: This subtype applies when the central theme of the individual's delusion is that his or her spouse or lover is unfaithful.

   Persecutory type: This subtype applies when the central theme of the delusion involves the individual's belief that he or she is being conspired against, cheated, spied on, followed, poisoned or drugged, maliciously maligned, harassed, or obstructed in the pursuit of long-term goals.

   Somatic type: This subtype applies when the central theme of the delusion involves bodily functions or sensations.

   Mixed type: This subtype applies when no one delusional theme predominates.

   Unspecified type: This subtype applies when the dominant delusional belief cannot be clearly determined or is not described in the specific types (e.g., referential delusions without a prominent persecutory or grandiose component).

Specify if:

   With bizarre content: Delusions are deemed bizarre if they are clearly implausible, not understandable, and not derived from ordinary life experiences (e.g., an individual's belief that a stranger has removed his or her internal organs and replaced them with someone else's organs without leaving any wounds or scars).

Continued

DSM-5 DIAGNOSTIC CRITERIA FOR DELUSIONAL DISORDER (297.1 (F22))—Cont'd

Specify if:

The following course specifiers are only to be used after a 1-year duration of the disorder:

First episode, currently in acute episode: First manifestation of the disorder meeting the defining diagnostic symptom and time criteria. An *acute episode* is a time period in which the symptom criteria are fulfilled.

First episode, currently in partial remission: *Partial remission* is a time period during which an improvement after a previous episode is maintained and in which the defining criteria of the disorder are only partially fulfilled.

First episode, currently in full remission: *Full remission* is a period of time after a previous episode during which no disorder-specific symptoms are present.

Multiple episodes, currently in acute episode.

Multiple episodes, currently in partial remission.

Multiple episodes, currently in full remission.

Continuous: Symptoms fulfilling the diagnostic symptom criteria of the disorder are remaining for the majority of the illness course, with subthreshold symptom periods being very brief relative to the overall course.

Unspecified

Specify current severity:

Severity is rated by a quantitative assessment of the primary symptoms of psychosis, including delusions, hallucinations, disorganized speech, abnormal psychomotor behavior, and negative symptoms. Each of these symptoms may be rated for its current severity (most severe in the last 7 days) on a 5-point scale ranging from 0 (not present) to 4 (present and severe). (See Clinician-Rated Dimensions of Psychosis Symptom Severity in the chapter "Assessment Measures.")

Note: Diagnosis of delusional disorder can be made without using this severity specifier.

Ms. Hastings demonstrates many of the classic findings that you will encounter when interviewing a patient suffering from a typical delusional disorder. These patients frequently appear surprisingly normal. One would hardly suspect any psychopathology, until one uncovers the topics within the delusional system, at which point, these patients often describe elaborate ramifications and subplots that would gratify the needs of any soap opera buff. Their delusions are generally unshakeable. They simply do not believe that there is anything wrong with them, as evidenced by the fact that Ms. Hastings did not seek help for herself but for the problem she was having with her husband. In the long run, the striking inability of these patients to see that their beliefs are delusional can make these patients frustratingly resistant to therapy.

All of the following delusions can occur in other psychotic disorders, such as schizophrenia and deliria, but *when seen as the only sign of psychopathology*, they are viewed as the distinct diagnosis called delusional disorders in the DSM-5.

Arguably, the best-known type of delusional disorder is the persecutory (paranoid) type. Paranoid delusions consist of beliefs that a person, organization, or a bizarre entity (such as aliens or vampires) are trying to thwart the patient's goals, harm the patient psychologically, or physically harm or kill the patient and/or loved ones. The exact nature of the aggressor may vary from patient to patient and tends to be consistent with the patient's cultural matrix. The common manifestations and characteristics of paranoid delusions may change over time as cultures shift. Thus, in our wired age, it is reasonable to anticipate that more and more patients will complain of being monitored by the webcams in their computers or of being clandestinely tracked via their smart phones. (It should be remembered that both of these processes can, in reality, be accomplished by hackers.)

A different type of delusional disorder has been referred to as "the Othello syndrome," in which the patient becomes convinced that his or her spouse is having a sexual affair, referred to as the jealous type in the DSM-5.[43]

In erotomanic delusional disorders, sometimes referred to as Clérambault's syndrome, the patient comes to believe that a person has fallen madly in love with him or her. The patient may proceed to pursue the alleged lover across the country or into the bedroom.

Erotomanic delusions are potentially dangerous, for the patient may eventually grow intensely angry with the perceived lover, because of the person's repeated rejections. At times, this anger manifests itself as, "if I can't have this person, no one can." The result can be violent assaults or murder. The classic "Hollywood stalker" is usually a person suffering from an erotomanic delusional disorder.

Because of their potential dangerousness, erotomanic delusions are particularly important to spot in an initial assessment. To do so effectively, it is important to remember that the delusion is *not* that the patient loves the targeted other. The delusion is that the patient is firmly convinced that the other person is truly in love with the patient, no matter how frequently or vociferously the targeted person denies any feelings towards the patient. Consequently, psychotic denial doggedly creates a false and painful world for the patient, reflected by the patient using rationalizations such as, "She is denying that she loves me because she needs to maintain her marriage for her children," or "He is simply waiting for his wife to die from cancer so that he can marry me." Such denials and rationalizations can occur despite the targeted person angrily telling the patient to leave them alone or filing protective restraining orders.

I have found that the following types of questions are useful for teasing out the presence of a true erotomanic delusion as opposed to neurotic preoccupation and wishful thinking. The questions are asked in a sensitive fashion without any hint of an accusatory tone of voice:

1. "What type of evidence do you have that this person loves you?"
2. "What leads you to think that he (or she) loves you, when he has asked you to never contact him (or her) again?"
3. "How do you put it together that she loves you, if she has actually gone to court to get a restraining order against you."
4. "What do you think is stopping this person from openly admitting their love to you?"

When the answer to the last question is a spouse, partner, or love interest of the targeted person, the interviewer must keep in mind that the delusional patient could be considering murdering the person who is in the way of "true love." The patient may actually believe that he or she is doing a favor for the targeted love object by releasing them from an unwanted relationship, through murder, to be with their real love – the patient.

Another type of delusional disorder consists of an unshakeable belief that one has a serious medical illness, the so-called hypochondriacal paranoia or somatic type of delusional disorder. These patients differ from those suffering from simple hypochondriasis by the fact that the belief has reached a truly delusional proportion and is essentially unshakeable. These patients may also believe that a plot has evolved to hide the truth from them.

People coping with the somatic type of delusional disorder are generally concerned that there is something wrong with their *bodily functions or sensations*. For instance, they may present with the belief that they are emitting a foul odor, infected with a parasite, or perhaps that they are being infested by insects that are crawling on their skin at night. They may also feel that a specific body part is deformed or malfunctioning. In the literature, this disorder is often referred to as a monosymptomatic hypochondriacal psychosis. (Note that in the DSM-5, if a patient presents with a pathological preoccupation that there is something grossly wrong with the *appearance* of a specific body part, whether non-delusional or delusional, they will more likely meet the diagnosis of body dysmorphic disorder, which is a more common disorder than somatic delusional disorder. Body dysmorphic disorder is viewed in the DSM-5 as sitting within the obsessive–compulsive disorder spectrum.)

By way of example, one of our patients was convinced that "my muscles of mastication are disordered." He had carefully produced a beautifully drawn anatomic atlas illustrating the problems with his jaw. At the interview he just happened to bring along a human skull, which he used to demonstrate in a disturbingly convincing fashion his specific anatomic defects. Sometimes these patients proceed to develop schizophrenia.

The term "mixed subtype" applies when no single delusional theme predominates. Ms. Hastings seems to fit this mixed subtype, for both jealous and persecutory themes are strongly displayed. Unspecified type applies when the clinician cannot determine the underlying delusional belief or is convinced that the patient's belief is fairly unique and does not fall into one of the previous categories.

Brief mention should also be made of the shared psychotic disorder. In this relatively rare condition, sometimes poetically referred to as "folie à deux," two patients share the same delusion. One of the patients develops the delusion after the other patient has evidenced it for some time, and, in this sense, the other patient is said to be induced into a delusional system. Frequently one of the patients is a dominant and powerful personality while the second patient tends to be dependent and suggestible. The second patient's delusion may even crumble if not in the presence of the dominant figure.[44]

Paranoid Delusions: Techniques for Uncovering Potential Dangerousness

Persecutory delusions can be seen in delusional disorders, but in everyday practice they are much more commonly encountered as part of the psychotic process seen in disorders such as schizophrenia, bipolar disorder, psychotic depression, and substance-induced psychotic states. No matter where they appear, arguably the most important immediate task for the clinician is to determine if the patient intends to harm or kill the supposed persecutor as a means of proactive self-defense. With Ms. Hastings, it would be important to determine whether she intends harm to either her "cheating" husband or his "goons next door."

Robinson has developed two effective questions that can be of immediate value in addressing this potentially disengaging task in a sensitive fashion[45]:

1. "Do you feel a need to protect yourself against your husband?"
2. "Have you felt a need to possibly take action against your husband or harm him?"

In addition, Phil Resnick, a leading innovator in forensic psychiatry and risk assessment, has described an interview strategy that can shed some light on the likelihood of a patient pre-emptively attacking a supposed persecutor. I will borrow liberally from his writings in order to more effectively describe his interviewing strategy, which he appropriately calls, "confrontation with a paranoid persecutor."[46] It should be noted that paranoid psychotic patients are often suspicious of clinicians, especially if they are fearful of the consequences of openly sharing (involuntary commitment, police involvement). Thus, as Resnick emphasizes, rapport should be carefully established before initiating this approach.

As an example, we will use a patient who has described fears of being killed by the mafia to an initial interviewer. The interviewer might inquire, "Mr. Jones, if you were to see an individual walking toward you in an alley who was dressed like a mafia hit man and he had a bulge in his jacket, how would you respond?"

One patient might say that he would not do anything because the mafia has so much power that they could easily kill him if they chose to. A second patient might say that as soon as the "mafia hit man" came within range, he would take out his .357 Magnum and blow his head off. If these patients were asked simply whether they had any thoughts of killing anyone, both might honestly answer no. However, they have different thresholds for killing in misperceived self-defense. Such information can help the clinician decide as to whether hospitalization is indicated, as well as whether a potential victim should be warned of danger from the patient.

Let us see Resnick's strategy of "confrontation with a paranoid persecutor" illustrated with a reconstructed interview directly from his work[47]:

Clin.: Tell me what's troubling you?

Pt.: I know that my wife is poisoning me. She and our mail carrier are getting it on and they want me out of the way.

Clin.: How do you know that this is going on?

Pt.: My food has been tasting funny, so I know she is trying to poison me. The postman also looks at me with murder in his eyes.

Clin.: Do you have any other evidence?

Pt.: I can just tell by looking at her. She has also had less interest in having sex with me.

Clin.: Have you taken any steps to try to resolve this?

Pt.: I went to the police but my wife denied it and they say I have no real evidence. I started carrying a gun for protection.

Clin.:	What would you do if you were sitting on your porch and the mailman walked up to you and started to take something out of his mail bag?
Pt.:	I would have to shoot him in self-defense because I know he and my wife are getting impatient because I am not dying fast enough from the poison.

Delusions in the Elderly and Paraphrenia

Diagnostically, if a patient presents with a delusional disorder, it is critical to rule out a psychotic disorder due to another general medical condition. This is particularly true in patients who first develop delusional symptoms over the age of 40. There exist numerous medical illnesses that can present with delusions. Perhaps at the top of the list one should consider a brain tumor, because these tumors tend to occur in later adult life. Indeed, malignant gliomas tend to arise in middle age, while metastatic tumors from other parts of the body are more common in the elderly.[48] Other frequent general medical causes include medications, endocrine disorders, infections, and complex partial seizures (temporal lobe epilepsy).

Especially with the elderly, the interviewer should also consider dementia. Roughly 20% of patients with Alzheimer's disease demonstrate paranoid symptoms at some point. Paranoid delusions tend to occur later in the process with these patients, although suspiciousness may occur early on.[49]

The issue of paranoid symptoms raises a pertinent diagnostic point. Some elderly patients present with concrete paranoid delusions frequently accompanied by auditory hallucinations and some other features common in schizophrenia, almost as if these patients were presenting with a late-onset schizophrenia. This particular syndrome raises some problems for the DSM-5, because these patients could technically fulfill the criteria for schizophrenia, for it has no upper limit on age of onset. But it is unclear whether these psychoses, when first appearing in the elderly, are genetically or phenomenologically the same as true schizophrenia.

In the DSM-5, if the hallucinations are not prominent, one could probably use the diagnosis delusional disorder, persecutory type. With prominent hallucinations, the diagnosis of unspecified schizophrenia spectrum and other psychotic disorder could probably be used reluctantly, a syndrome that would have been called atypical psychosis in the DSM-IV-TR. I say "reluctantly" because such presentations are neither uncommon, atypical, nor unspecified, as these "grab-bag" diagnoses seem to suggest. One study revealed that at least 10% of patients who were admitted with psychotic features over the age of 60 presented as described above.

European psychiatry pioneered the study of these late-onset psychoses. In Europe, the syndrome is frequently called paraphrenia.[50,51] In the United States it is more often called late-onset schizophrenia.[52] However, both these terms are reserved for the first-time appearance of psychosis in older patients, *in instances where there is no mood disorder, delirium, or dementia.* Although some authors provide empirical evidence that the syndrome can appear commonly before the age of 50, and even below the age of 30,[53] most authors view paraphrenia as a disorder that manifests in the older patient. It can appear as an early variant, with onset between 40–60 years of age (in which case it tends to show many of the characteristics of a late-appearing schizophrenia) or as a late-appearing disorder, first manifesting after the age of 60 (a syndrome which appears to have significant differences in phenomenology from classic schizophrenia).

It is these differences in symptom presentation that warrant our attention as initial interviewers. With the graying of our populations, many clinicians will be working with the elderly, and late-onset psychosis will be ever more frequently encountered. I prefer calling this late-appearing psychosis "paraphrenia," for I am not convinced that it is merely a late-appearing form of schizophrenia.

Paraphrenia typically presents in late life with well-organized paranoid delusions. Grandiose, erotic, and somatic delusions can occur, but are much less frequent. Delusions are often accompanied by auditory hallucinations, thus demarcating them from paranoid delusional disorders (in which hallucinations are generally absent and, if present, are infrequent in number). Interestingly, in paraphrenia it is not uncommon for the patient to experience hallucinations in multiple sensory modalities including olfactory, tactile, visual, and gustatory.[54]

Before these overt psychotic symptoms appear, the patient may show prodromal symptoms for months or even years. These symptoms include suspiciousness, irritability, seclusiveness, and odd behavior. Unlike patients with schizophrenia, however, these patients, even when grossly psychotic, do not usually show problems with restricted, blunted, or inappropriate affect; nor do they demonstrate a formal thought disorder.[55] Unlike schizophrenia, these patients tend to show a good preservation of their personalities, fewer negative symptoms, and are less likely to show progressive deterioration than in classic schizophrenia. They also tend to respond reasonably well to antipsychotic medications. Paraphrenia is 6- to 10-fold more common in females than males.[56]

An unusual associated finding is the fact that about 15 to 40% of these patients have some degree of hearing loss. It has been suggested that a hearing loss may predispose the patient to misinterpret the conversation of others in such a way as to create paranoid ideation.

As compared to patients with delusional schizophrenia, where the persecutory delusions not uncommonly have a peculiar or unlikely quality (e.g., being pursued by aliens or watched by foreign spies), the persecutory delusions in paraphrenia tend to be more mundane and believable (e.g., a neighbor is trying to break into the patient's house or the grocery man is plotting to get the patient's social security checks).

One more peculiarity of paraphrenia is worth mentioning. A well-designed phenomenological study by Castle showed that over half of the patients with paraphrenia reported an odd belief called a "partition delusion."[57] In a partition delusion, a person is concerned that people, objects, gases, or some form of radiation is entering their homes, passing through the objectively impermeable walls. Perhaps this intense fear of home invasion is prompted by the fact that many of these patients live alone and are socially isolated.

In this regard, it should be kept in mind that delusions are often only shared with interviewers if interviewers ask directly about them specifically, a trait perhaps even more common in the elderly. Thus, partition delusions, because of their oddness, will often go hidden unless asked about directly, as with the following question framed as a normalization:

"Some of my patients tell me that they are afraid that something is being pushed into their houses, right through the walls and windows, like a gas, a poison, or even radiation. Do you have any worries like that?"

At times, the interviewer can deftly tie the question directly into a paranoid delusion that the patient has been sharing, in this instance about a neighbor with which the patient had formed a persecutory delusion:

"Do you feel that Mr. Roberts is trying to break into your house, or perhaps pass something dangerous into your house like a gas or a poison, or has figured out a way to look through your walls?"

Differential Diagnosis on Ms. Hastings and Summary of Key Interviewing Tips

For a moment, let us review the diagnostic issues associated with Ms. Hastings. In this particular interview, there was little time to explore for personality disorders, and the clinician would need to defer regarding personality dysfunction. She complained of peptic ulcer disease, chronic bronchitis, and the recent onset of a hacking cough associated with a long history of heavy smoking. With such a history of smoking, the issue of lung cancer is certainly worth considering. Her diagnostic formulation would appear as follows, if there proved to be no truth to her accusations concerning her husband's infidelity and murderous intentions:

General Psychiatric Disorder:

Delusional disorder (mixed; both jealous and persecutory types present as central themes)

Rule out psychotic disorder due to another medical condition

Personality Disorder:

Defer

Medical Disorders:

Peptic ulcer disease

Chronic bronchitis

Rule out lung carcinoma

Concerning medical disorders, as mentioned earlier, numerous entities should be ruled out; however, for the sake of conciseness, it is probably more practical to only list those diagnoses for which the initial interview has raised some specific suspicions, as with the cigarette smoking history suggesting lung cancer in the case of Ms. Hastings.

Let us review the major issues that surfaced with the case of Ms. Hastings.

1. The diagnosis of a delusional disorder can be classified into seven subtypes: persecutory, jealous, erotomanic, somatic, grandiose, mixed, and unspecified. (It should be noted that, at this time, it is not yet clear whether these sub-categories will prove to have any association with etiology or treatment response.)

2. Outside of the delusional content of their speech, people with delusional disorders frequently appear and behave quite normally (other than inappropriately pursuing and contacting the target of the delusional process).

3. If paranoid delusions are present, one must ascertain whether the patient may be intending to harm or kill the supposed persecutor (specific interviewing techniques and strategies, such as "confrontation with a paranoid persecutor," can be intentionally utilized to address this critical task).

4. In any patient diagnosed as having a delusional disorder, one should rule out a general medical cause (a brain tumor, etc.) of the delusional symptoms.

5. Paranoid symptoms are not uncommon with people suffering from primary degenerative diseases, such as a neurocognitive disorder due to Alzheimer's disease (Alzheimer's dementia).

6. Paraphrenia, although not currently recognized as a separate DSM-5 diagnosis, may well represent a specific syndrome in elderly patients. It is characterized by a delusional system that is associated with hallucinations first arising in the elderly.

Clinical Presentation #4: Ms. Fay

Ms. Fay is a 23-year-old divorced woman who is being seen in the outpatient clinic at a community mental health center for the second time in 2 weeks. She is casually dressed in jeans and a yellow blouse that tends to overshadow her curly, dull blonde hair. She has come alone to the clinic and relates, "I just had to talk to someone again. I'm a nervous wreck." Indeed, she appears decidedly nervous in that she wriggles uneasily in her chair while incessantly picking at her nails. It seems difficult for her to maintain eye contact. She states to the male clinician, "You make me nervous. These are hard questions." She relates that things are terrible at home, where she lives with her mother and her two children. She never gets a moment's rest and reports significant problems falling asleep, as well as a general inability to relax. Her speech is mildly pressured and characterized by an evasive style, which clearly frustrates the interviewer. She bluntly denies any delusions or hallucinations, but seems greatly concerned with an incident of sexual abuse from her distant past, which she prefers not to discuss at the moment. As the interviewer proceeds, she becomes intermittently more anxious and coyly giggles at times, perhaps out of nervousness. One senses that if she could burrow beneath her chair to escape scrutiny, she would most surely do so. At the time of her first evaluation, she was diagnosed as having a relatively severe generalized anxiety disorder.

Discussion of Ms. Fay

The Life Cycle of a Psychosis

As Ms. Fay had appeared at her previous clinic interview 2 weeks earlier, she currently presents with an overwhelming sense of anxiety, succinctly stated by Ms. Fay as, "I'm a nervous wreck." She flatly denies any overt signs of psychosis such as delusions or hallucinations. She does not demonstrate any marked evidence of a formal thought disorder such as a gross loosening of associations (derailment). She does not appear overtly psychotic; rather she seems consumed by her own anxiety.

It is this anxiety that warrants more careful exploration, because anxiety stands as one of the most frequent early signs of a developing psychosis. To further our understanding, it may be useful to review what could be called the "life cycle" of psychotic process.

There exist certain overt signs of psychotic process, one or more of which must be present for a clinician to view a patient as experiencing psychotic process. These "hard signs of psychosis" include the following: hallucinations, delusions, or evidence of a formal thought disorder (e.g., a moderate to severe loosening of associations or other problems in the formation of thought). In a strict diagnostic sense, unless at least one of these signs are present one does not call the patient psychotic by DSM-5 standards. In addition, in a clinical sense, the following symptoms represent hard signs of psychotic process: gross disorganization, gross disorientation, and bizarre behavior.

The conservative approach used by the recent DSM systems for using the term "psychosis" is, in my opinion, a wise one, because it eliminates the dangerous habit of loosely labeling people as psychotic. Such sloppy clinical work can lead to problems, such as the inappropriate use of the diagnosis "schizophrenia" when the diagnosis "schizotypal personality" is more appropriate. *In a similar vein, it is important to realize that the mere presence of one of the above hard signs does not necessarily indicate that a patient is psychotic.* For instance, as we shall see later, auditory and visual hallucinations are occasionally seen in people who are not psychotic and specific cultural nuances may determine whether or not a particular behavior or experience is psychotic in a pathologic fashion.

It is equally important to realize that in a clinical sense (pathologically experiencing the world in a strikingly different way than most people within his or her culture) as opposed to a strict diagnostic sense (meets the criteria for psychosis in the DSM-5), a patient can be psychotic without demonstrating these hard signs, especially in the earliest phases of a psychosis or when a psychotic process is fluctuating over time. We can arrive at a better understanding of this apparent paradox by examining how psychotic process naturally unfolds.

Most patients do not abruptly develop the hard signs of psychosis in the course of a day or two, as if the light switch of reason was suddenly snapped off. Instead, patients with classic psychotic disorders (such as schizophrenia, schizoaffective disorder, bipolar disorder, and major depressive disorder with psychotic features) generally move more slowly into the world of psychotic process.

An excellent example of this concept can be provided by looking at one possible mode of development of a single psychotic symptom such as a delusion. The phenomenologist Lopez-Ibor has discussed this specific process in detail[58] (Figure 11.1). In the following discussion we will follow his model with some minor adjustments.

Delusional Mood

In the beginning of a psychotic break, the patient frequently develops what Lopez-Ibor calls a "delusional mood." During this phase, the patient begins to feel that something is not quite right. There may be an intensification of perceptions such as sight and sound. In a sense, the world is almost clearer than before, because the environment appears

LIFE CYCLE OF A DELUSION

delusional mood ⟶ delusional perception ⟶ concrete delusion

Possible indicators of psychotic process

A) Soft signs

↓

Alerts clinician to the possible
presence of psychosis

↓

Can be caused by a variety
of non-psychotic processes

B) Hard signs

↓

Usually indicates active
psychotic process

Hard and soft signs of psychosis

Softs signs

Unusually intense affect

Angry or agitated affect

Glimpses of inappropriate affect

Guardedness or suspiciousness

Vagueness

Evidence of a very mild formal
thought disorder

Pre-occupation with an incident
from distant past

Expectation of familiarity from
interviewer

Inappropriate eye contact

Long latency before responding
or thought blocking

Hard signs

Delusions

Hallucinations

Moderate or severe formal
thought disorder

Gross disorientation

Bizarre mannerisms and
body language

Figure 11.1 Life cycle of a psychotic process.

more vivid. New details never before recognized take on new significance; they may never have even been noticed before. There frequently exists an unsettling feeling that something ominous may be about to happen, although at other times life may seem refreshingly vibrant. The following excerpt captures this peculiar state of affairs as described by a patient who had experienced delusional mood:

> *If I am to judge by my own experience, this "heightened state of reality" consists of a considerable number of related sensations, the net result of which is that the outer world makes a much more vivid and intense impression on me than usual. ... The first thing I note is the peculiar appearance of the lights. ... They are not exactly brighter, but deeper, more intense, perhaps a trifle more ruddy than usual. Certainly my sense of touch is heightened. ... My hearing appears to be more sensitive, and I am able to take in without disturbance or distraction many different sound impressions at the same time.*[59]

Delusional Perception

Eventually this process becomes more intense, developing a second phase, which is called "delusional perception," a term clarified by the phenomenologist Kurt Schneider. With delusional perception, the perception itself may be normal in a sensory way, but the patient's interpretation of the perception is clearly distorted. The anxiety of the patient begins to snowball as the patient becomes convinced that something is not right and that danger is present. *In this phase, not only is the environment noticed in a more intense fashion, but also the details of the environment are felt to be directly related to the patient.* The world becomes at once both highly personalized and terrifying. Ideas of reference occur. In a sense, patients feel that people are talking about them but do not yet know why.

> *Not knowing that I was ill, I made no attempt to understand what was happening, but felt that there was some overwhelming significance in all this, produced either by God or Satan. ... The walk of a stranger on the street could be a "sign" to me which I must interpret. Every face in the windows of a passing streetcar could be engraved on my mind, all of them concentrating on me and trying to pass me some sort of message.*[60]

At this point the patient may already be showing marked changes in daily functioning, avoiding this person or that person, meticulously checking on people's behaviors, re-reading comments on Facebook to hunt for a hidden personalized meaning, staying awake at night and ruminating endlessly. In a very real sense of the word, these patients are already psychotic, because their perception of reality is markedly different than the reality of those around them. No hard signs of psychosis in a diagnostic sense have appeared yet, but they are just around the corner.

The Emergence of Concrete Delusional Ideation

In the third phase, the phase of "delusional ideas," the slippery suspicions of the first two phases are transformed into concrete beliefs. Patients suddenly "know" what people are saying about them and why. The paranoid feelings become concrete delusions that are both more elaborate and entrenched. Here, indeed, the classic hard signs of psychosis flower. In a sense, as the phenomenologist Clérambault stated, the psychosis is already old when the delusions have begun. It is almost as if the delusion evolves as an answer to why the world has felt so ominous to the patient.

Soft Signs of Psychosis: How to Spot Hidden Psychotic Process

As mentioned earlier, psychotic process tends to fluctuate, and patients may move in and out of these various phases. In the early phases of an initial psychotic episode, or in the early phases of a psychosis emerging from a sound remission (as might happen when a psychosis "breaks through" medications), a patient could be having delusions one day but not the next, as they slip back and forth between non-delusional periods and periods of delusional perception, delusional mood, or frank delusional ideation. For these reasons, the initial interviewer needs to pay keen attention to any evidence that the patient may be in one of the less obvious phases of psychosis. If such soft signs of covert psychosis are present, then the interviewer more carefully explores for the harder signs. These soft signs of psychosis are frequently overlooked by clinicians, as was the case with Ms. Fay during her first visit to the evaluation center. Their phenomenology is worth examining in more detail.

In the first place it is important to emphasize that the presence of the "soft signs of psychosis" does not imply that the patient is necessarily psychotic. *In fact, usually the patient with soft signs is not psychotic. In most instances the soft signs are being caused by a non-psychotic process such as anxiety, an immature interpersonal style, or somewhat idiosyncratic interpersonal habits.* Their importance lies in the fact that their presence alerts the clinician that psychotic process *may* be present, and that the interviewer should thoroughly hunt for it.

For instance, a mild and infrequent loosening of associations, one of the soft signs, does not necessarily indicate that a patient is actively psychotic. People with schizotypal personalities may routinely demonstrate this finding, in which case it represents an ingrained personality style, not evidence of psychosis (see Figure 11.1). The vast majority of people who present with intense anger are not psychotic (many factors could be at play, ranging from being appropriately angry to characterologically angry or intoxicated), but the presence of intense anger in an initial interview, whether it occurs in an outpatient clinic or an emergency room, should alert the clinician to carefully search for psychotic process.

There exist a variety of soft signs that suggest a given interviewee may be experiencing psychotic processs, and that the interviewer should actively look for it, including the following: (1) mild or infrequent evidence of a formal thought disorder, such as a mild loosening of associations, infrequent bits of illogical thought, idiosyncratic speech, or mild to moderate tangential speech; (2) unusually intense affect; (3) angry or agitated affect; (4) infrequent glimpses of inappropriate affect; (5) guardedness or suspiciousness; (6) vagueness; (7) preoccupation with an incident from the distant past; (8) immediate discussion of personal details as if the interviewer already knew the patient well; (9) long latency before answering questions; (10) poor eye contact in a patient who does not appear depressed; and (11) inappropriate staring. The list could certainly be made longer, but the above signs serve as a good introduction.

Note that both verbal and nonverbal clues may suggest underlying psychotic process (see Figure 11.1). Interviewers must understand the cultural norms for nonverbal behaviors, such as eye contact, to make sure that the clinician is not misinterpreting a normal nonverbal behavior as a soft sign of potential psychotic process – yet another potentially damaging aspect of the kulturbrille effect.

When a clinician spots some of the soft signs of psychosis, he or she may want to expand the region of psychotic questioning in more detail, delicately probing for the hard signs of psychosis, such as evidence of delusions and hallucinations. The belief that psychotic patients will always spontaneously reveal their hallucinations and delusions is patently false. Frequently, one must ask for specific symptoms before they are proffered.

Helping Patients to Share Delusional Material

Tapping Intense Affect

If a patient appears unusually affectively charged or anxious about a particular topic, it is often rewarding to gently guide the patient into a further discussion of this topic by showing interest and asking clarifying questions. With this technique one structures the conversation very little. Instead, an attempt is made to unleash further affect, because as the patient becomes more and more emotionally involved, defenses may decrease, allowing more dramatic evidence of psychotic process to emerge. Eventually, as the patient senses a friendly ear, delusional material may be shared. It is not infrequent for interviewers to simply run-over these areas of intense affect, thus robbing themselves of a natural gate into the patient's psychotic world.

Tapping Odd Language, Illogical Thought, and Idiosyncratic Phrasing

Similarly, when a patient uses an illogical or idiosyncratic phrase, it is often wise to ask for further elaboration. It is paramount that this request for clarification sounds non-judgmental and carries a tone of true interest. As the patient proceeds to explain the ideas behind the reasoning, it is not infrequent for further and more substantial evidence of psychotic process to emerge. The psychotic patient essentially guides the interviewer into regions of questioning more likely to unearth substantial evidence of psychosis.

Indirect Techniques for Exploring Delusional Material

Robinson, both in his illuminating book and in his subsequent writing,[61,62] has delineated a basic strategy for helping patients to more accurately and comfortably share their delusional material. The keynote of Robinson's approach is to demonstrate a gentle, genuine, and respectful curiosity about the patient's beliefs. I don't believe I can explain it any better than Robinson, so we will let him speak for himself:

> *When patients mention something that could be of a delusional nature, respond with curiosity. An interested, conversational manner helps to elicit detailed information because patients who harbor delusions are generally so immersed in them that they occupy the majority of their thoughts. Your approach is three-fold: (1) grease the wheels so that the patient feels comfortable sharing information with you, (2) uncover the extent and logic*

of the delusional material; and (3) determine the degree to which the delusion has become entrenched in the patient's thoughts (i.e., determine how much insight is preserved or how much distance the patient has from the delusion).

Examples
1. *"I'm interested in what you just said, please tell me more." (greasing the wheels)*
2. *"How did this all start?" (greasing the wheels)*
3. *"What has happened so far?" (uncovering the extent and logic)*
4. *"Why would someone want to do this to you?" (uncovering the extent and logic)*
5. *"How do you know that this is the situation?" (determining distance)*
6. *"How do you account for what has taken place?" (determining distance)*

Illustrative Dialogue

Clin.: *Do you have thoughts that you focus on a lot of the time and feel strongly about? (looking for overvalued ideas or delusions)*

Pt.: *I don't understand what you mean.*

Clin.: *I'm asking about ideas that you have that perhaps those around you don't share or agree with, but you know to be true and are puzzled why others may not seem to be convinced, and might even argue with you about them.*

Pt.: *I have an infestation with a parasite and asked my family doctor to help me out. Initially she tried, but then seemed to give up and I couldn't understand why, so I've spent a lot of time looking for a non-prescription treatment.*

Clin.: *That's interesting. How did this start? (greasing the wheels)*

Pt.: *I stepped on a nail about 3 months ago and got an infection. As part of the treatment, I had to soak my foot a couple times a day. On one occasion, a spider fell into the tub, and you know how dirty those things are. Well, before I could get it out, the water got infected with parasites that the spider was carrying.*

Clin.: *What happened after that? (uncovering the extent and logic)*

Pt.: *Well, the parasites got into my foot because of the wound and then immediately spread throughout my body causing a variety of physical problems. I haven't been well since that very moment.*

Clin.: *How do you know that this is the cause of your physical problems? (determining distance)*

Pt.: *Internet research. But before I continue, I need to ask you something?*

Clin.: *What's that?*

Pt.: *Do you believe me?*

How to Respond When a Delusional Patient Asks, "Do You Believe Me?"

There is no single or "right" way to respond to such a question from a delusional patient. But, it is important to feel comfortable with various flexible ways of handling it, for it is not an uncommon question. The fashion in which the clinician responds can have critical ramifications for engagement, whether the question is asked in a clinic office, inpatient unit, or emergency department. Wherever it arises, it is important to appear comfortable when providing an answer. Robinson has some practical and effective approaches for handling this potentially awkward situation and once again, I believe it is best to simply let him speak for himself[63]:

A major concern of many patients when first sharing a delusion, as in an emergency room setting, is that they will be viewed as being seriously mentally ill. This fear is a natural one for a person experiencing a delusion, and to some degree, may even reflect that the patient has some distance from the delusional material. How the clinician handles this delicate moment may prove to be pivotal to the relationship and how much more material the patient will be willing to share. Clinicians do not want to be deceptive, yet we need to develop enough of an alliance with patients to hear more about their thoughts.

In such situations, you should continue to actively empathize with the patient to preserve rapport and facilitate the sharing of more information. In addition, tactfully avoid being the arbiter of reality and telling patients whether or not you agree with them (or whether or not you think they are right). Examples include statements such as:

1. *I'm keeping an open mind.*
2. *I can't decide without more information.*
3. *My job is to understand what your views are.*
4. *The story is an unusual one, so I really want to hear more before making a decision, tell me about … (Refer patient back into an affectively charged detail from the story.)*

There is seldom a situation in which a clinician would openly agree with a patient's delusional thoughts (e.g., saying something like, "Of course I believe you."). Such false endorsements can undermine a therapeutic alliance and also come back to haunt the clinician later in the interview when the patient asks the clinician to follow through on the endorsement with, "You'll call the police for me then?"

As with all principles there are exceptions in which the clinician may need to temporarily endorse a delusion, but these are very rare. Such a situation could arise when the clinician feels that the patient might become violent towards him or her if there is not immediate agreement with what the patient is saying.

In my own practice, I have found the fourth technique described by Robinson to be one of my favorites ("The story is an unusual one, so I really want to hear more before making a decision, tell me about …"). It conveys a respectful interest, yet communicates an open yet non-affirming stance. It often allows the clinician to quickly return to a sensitive uncovering of the extent and logic of the patient's delusion. Let's see a variation of it at work:

    Pt.:   Do you believe me?

  Clin.: Well, the story is undoubtedly an unusual one, so I really want to make sure I understand better what is going on before making a decision. Help me to understand exactly what problems the parasites are now causing in your body? (note the tie-in with a personally affectively charged topic for the patient, inviting spontaneous elaboration, which simultaneously moves the patient away from an insistence upon knowing whether or not the clinician believes the story at that exact moment)

Pt.:   Oh, they are all over the place (patient continues animatedly). They have entered my brain so I can't always think straight or concentrate, and I feel this very subtle moving in my head. I think it might be the parasites moving around.

Clin.:   That sounds very disturbing. (actively empathizing)

Pt.:   Oh yeah, oh yeah. It is. They have also moved into my feet, and I have a strange burning sensation in the bottoms of my feet, especially when I am walking.

Clin.:   What have you been doing to help yourself with the physical problems? (uncovering the extent and logic of the delusion)

This clinician has adeptly responded to the patient's inquiry and has effectively continued to explore the extent of actions the patient has taken regarding his delusion of infestation. Looking for the extent of action a patient takes on delusional material provides invaluable information regarding the patient's "distance" from the delusion (i.e., how much the patient believes or does not believe that the delusion is absolutely true). In some types of delusions it also provides critical information related to dangerousness to self or others. For instance, patients with delusions of infestation have been known to mutilate themselves by attempting to dig out the parasites, information that the clinician's last question is attempting to uncover.

Hallucinations and Other "Hard Signs of Psychosis" in the Normal Population

As mentioned earlier, the presence of hallucinations, and the other hard signs of psychosis, does *not* necessarily indicate that a person is psychotic. Some hallucinations are seen in people who are not psychotic. Mistaking such a hallucination as a marker of psychosis can lead to serious misdiagnoses such as schizophrenia or major depression with psychosis. Consequently, it is worth spending time exploring this area of potential misinterpretation carefully.

Auditory and Visual Hallucinations in the Normal Population

In the past decade, a variety of studies have helped us to better understand both the prevalence and phenomenology of non-psychotic auditory hallucinations.[64-75] Such research has provided evidence that "non-clinical individuals" report a lifetime prevalence rate of auditory hallucinations ranging 1–2% to 15–18% of the population,[76] although others have estimated the prevalence to be as high as 40% in people without psychiatric disorders.[77] The most common types of hallucinations that are not caused by a psychiatric disorder are hypnogogic hallucinations (experienced as one is falling asleep) and hypnopompic hallucinations (experienced as one is awakening).

Times of extreme stress and/or prolonged sleep deprivation can also trigger hallucinatory phenomena in otherwise normal individuals. This process is illustrated by the rather common appearance of both visual and auditory hallucinations in people who have lost a spouse. One study involving 300 widowed men and women found that nearly half had experienced hallucinations of their lost partner with visual hallucinations slightly outnumbering auditory hallucinations.[78] Older surviving spouses (ages 40 and over) were more likely to experience hallucinations, with some experiencing hallucinations of their spouse over the course of a decade or more without any evidence of psychosis.

With an older patient, keep in mind the rather curious, yet not uncommon, Charles Bonnet syndrome, in which central or ocular visual impairment (as can be seen with cataracts) produces visual hallucinations.[79] This syndrome is considered as being akin to the "phantom limb" phenomenon but occurring in the visual system. It has been estimated that 60% of elderly patients with a severe visual loss may experience one or more visual hallucinations. Note that the hallucinations in the Charles Bonnet syndrome are only visual in nature. They are usually both vivid and complex, often creating surprisingly convincing images of people or small animals. By way of illustration, a case was reported in which the patient began spreading birdseed in his room at a long-term care facility in order to feed the "birds" who were strutting about his room on a daily basis. This syndrome can be easily misdiagnosed as psychotic in nature, sometimes mistaken for an early delirium or part of a dementia in the elderly. If the eye defect can be corrected (as with cataract surgery) the hallucinations vanish.

Cultural Competence: Its Importance in Distinguishing True Psychotic Symptoms From Culturally Accepted Behaviors

Not only are hallucinations sometimes experienced in non-psychotic individuals, they are sometimes enjoyed and even sought. Historical figures of great stature, including Socrates, Descartes, and Julius Caesar, admitted to auditory hallucinations, as well as mystics such as Swedenborg and artists such as William Blake. In addition, auditory hallucinations have played an important role in specific spiritual disciplines in the past, such as the Greek oracles and the chief priests and sadhus of Egypt and India, both with and without the use of psychedelics or other psychoactive drugs.[80] For centuries, shamans have valued the hallucinations, whether drug-induced or not, that are experienced in their pathworking trance states, as they still do today. None of these experiences represent pathologic psychotic states.

Other "hard signs" of psychosis may not be indicative of psychosis in all situations. Some beliefs such as in witchcraft, ghosts, and extrasensory perceptions are quite acceptable in various cultures and should not be viewed as delusions *per se*. Indeed, the concepts of ghosts, channeling, and spells are common in American culture, with shelves devoted to their exegesis in New Age bookstores and a web teeming with countless New Age websites. Obviously these bookstore owners, webmasters, and their consumers are not delusional. Even processes such as a loosening of associations may be seen in culturally normal phenomena such as channeling and speaking in tongues.

Nor is the presence of disturbing hallucinations necessarily evidence of psychosis, although their disturbing nature greatly increases the likelihood that the hallucinations are psychotic in origin. Once again, a cultural familiarity is important.

For instance, in Taiwan, a woman who is coping with the naturally complex emotions arising following an abortion may experience the persistent crying of a child. From a

Taiwanese religious and cultural perspective, this crying is felt to represent the child's dismay that its reincarnation has been prevented. This crying, although an example of a hallucination and one that is disquieting, should not to be misconstrued as evidence of psychosis. Without an understanding of this cultural and religious phenomenon, the patient could easily be mislabeled as experiencing a brief psychotic break or a schizophreniform disorder.[81]

The Interface Between Cultural Phenomena and the Life Cycle of a Psychosis

We have come to a situation that we encountered earlier, in Chapter 6, but we are now better prepared to understand it. If you will recall we ended that chapter describing a young woman with schizophrenia whose mother was a Pentecostal minister. The patient was suffering from delusions of demon possession, accompanied by intense paranoia and auditory hallucinations, that would prove to be symptoms of an emerging schizophrenia. Here was an instance in which both the client's culture, and her mother, clearly believed in possession and exorcism (non-delusional beliefs in that culture), yet both the mother and the clinician were able to discern that this particular belief, in this particular patient, represented a psychotic state. Similarly, in reference to our Taiwanese example above, a woman 2 months post-abortion could be, by mere chance, simultaneously developing schizophrenia or might be developing a major depression with psychotic features triggered by the emotional trauma of the abortion. With such patients, how does one tell whether hallucinations or beliefs are simply cultural reflections or represent part of a pathologic process – psychosis?

With our understanding of the life cycle of a psychosis, we can now address this clinical dilemma with a new sophistication and with a clearer-cut interviewing strategy. When considering whether a hallucination or belief is psychotic in nature, as opposed to a non-pathologic culturally accepted phenomenon, try to determine whether the hallucination or belief is embedded within a psychotic cluster of phenomena, as might be seen with delusional mood or delusional perception. This psychotic matrix, although sometimes subtle, will tend to show itself *not* only while the patient is experiencing his or her hallucinations but also is likely to have been present before the hallucinations began and remains after the hallucinations have stopped.

More specifically, psychotic processes seen in disorders such as schizophrenia and bipolar disorder don't tend to materialize out of nowhere, nor do they then abruptly shut-off with the person immediately experiencing the world as totally normal. There is generally both a prodrome and a residuum that will be highlighted by some of the soft signs of psychosis. Another tip-off that one is seeing truly psychotic symptoms is that careful interviewing may uncover the presence of other hard signs of psychosis, not viewed as normal in that patient's culture.

Another phenomenon that may alert the astute clinician to the presence of true psychotic process (concerning an otherwise culturally acceptable belief) consists of the subtle twisting of the culturally held belief into a more vicious and denigrating psychotic variation. Scott describes a potential illustration of such a psychotic distortion. Among Bantu peoples, it is culturally acceptable to hear voices that provide instructions to carry out Bantu customs designed to allay guilt feelings that are shared by the entire tribe. With psychotic process, these voices may shift into a more accusatory tone in which the hearer of the voices is singled out as being worthy of guilt. Similarly, with the Bantu, the normal auditory hallucinations are often of a known person (e.g., a relative), whereas psychotic voices may emanate from unknown sources.[82]

You will recall in Chapter 6 that it was the patient's mother, a Pentecostal minister, who recognized that her daughter's experiences were not the typical experiences of members of her congregation, neither during possession nor following exorcism. Her daughter's hallucinations and delusional beliefs were part of an ongoing matrix of delusional mood and delusional perception of an insidious and destructive pattern.

Indeed, two other processes that tend to be seen with genuine psychotic processes, as opposed to culturally accepted normal experiences, are (1) the intensely disturbing quality of the phenomena, and (2) their tendency to disrupt normal functioning in an ongoing fashion. Nevertheless, the presence of hallucinations that seem pleasant at times does not rule out genuine psychotic disorders. Patients coping with schizophrenia occasionally experience pleasurable voices, and may even miss them when alleviated by antipsychotic medications.

Returning to our Taiwanese example, most women experiencing post-abortion depression and hallucinations of "their child" crying are not psychotic. But a specific patient experiencing this phenomenon who also relates weeks of feeling odd, describes persistent concerns that somebody or something is observing her, and also relates that she has been preoccupied with suspicious knocking sounds coming from her heater may actually be psychotic. In this case, the culturally accepted crying appears to be imbedded in an ongoing psychotic matrix. Indeed, the crying itself is probably being transformed by the psychotic process into a new psychotic symptom, for the crying of the infant is now being experienced with an intensity, meaning, and disruption that non-psychotic, post-abortion Taiwanese women do not experience. Given time, new hallucinations of voices berating her and delusions of demons may very well appear, providing conclusive evidence that she is experiencing psychotic process, not just a culturally accepted hallucination.

Back to Ms. Fay: An Illustration of How to Tap a Piece of Illogical Thought for Underlying Delusional Material

At this point we can return to Ms. Fay. A re-constructed excerpt of her interview proves to be particularly germane. In it we shall see some of the soft signs of psychosis; in particular, the interviewer will follow up on an isolated piece of illogical thought.

> **Clin.:** Tell me a little bit more about what your anxiety has been like.
>
> **Pt.:** (giggles inappropriately) That's very hard to say … I get uptight and I just don't know what to do with myself. I suppose it all has to do with self-image and all that stuff.
>
> **Clin.:** How do you mean? (greasing the wheels for psychotic process)
>
> **Pt.:** Sometimes when I'm alone I just get really frightened and … I don't know … well, I … I don't know if I'm coming or going. I guess I'm just too anxious to be a woman. I don't know what else to say. What else do you want me to talk about?
>
> **Clin.:** When you say that you are too anxious to be a woman, what exactly are you referring to? (tapping an odd use of language)

Pt.:   I get panicky, you know all goose flesh all over. I never know exactly when it is going to happen but it always does.

Clin.:   But how does that tie in with your being a woman? (looking for illogical thought)

Pt.:   It just does. Women have to do certain things and I'm unclear what exactly they are. It was all so much simpler years ago when my mother was growing up. But today what with short skirts and rock videos, it's all more confusing and there is a lot more responsibility out there, so I'm just too anxious to be a woman and I'm also too anxious to be a man, so there you have it!

The phrase "I'm just too anxious to be a woman," is a curious one. The patient did not appear cognizant of this fact and made no spontaneous attempt to explain herself. At this point the clinician wisely asked for further clarification. Her subsequent explanation was also vague, although one can surmise to what she was probably alluding. Her subsequent reply was also somewhat illogical, giving even further suspicion that a psychotic process is at hand.

Differential Diagnosis on Ms. Fay and Summary of Key Interviewing Tips

As the interview progressed she appeared to become more anxious, but she never displayed or related any hard signs of psychosis. Of course, during the interview she did display a variety of soft signs, including vagueness, guardedness, a few inappropriate giggles, some small bits of illogical thought, and the hint of a preoccupation with a distant past sexual event with her brother.

She described a variety of sustained symptoms of generalized anxiety, while denying any regularly occurring panic attacks. She also described periods of fleeting paranoia and magical thinking, but said she had always had such feelings "cause I grew up in a bad family." She denied any persistent symptoms of depression or mania. But she did describe episodes of angry outbursts and periods of being very moody. She was evasive when questioned about previous suicide gestures.

Ms. Fay represents an excellent example of a person who leaves the interviewer with the feeling that psychotic process is lurking beneath the clinical facade but cannot be clearly identified. Because of the presence of a large number of soft psychotic symptoms, the clinician would tend to arrange for both rapid and close follow-up care.

At the end of this interview her diagnostic conceptualization was as follows:

General Psychiatric Disorders:

Generalized anxiety disorder (provisional)

Rule out unspecified schizophrenia spectrum and other psychotic disorders

Personality Disorders:

Rule out schizotypal personality

Rule out borderline personality disorder

Medical Disorders:

None known

The diagnosis of unspecified schizophrenia spectrum and other psychotic disorders (atypical psychosis) was entertained because there were no strong indicators of a mood disorder and no clear-cut signs of schizophrenia or paranoid disorder, but the clinician was suspicious of some underlying psychotic process.

This suspicion proved to be well founded, because several weeks later Ms. Fay was admitted to the hospital with several striking paranoid delusions concerning her brother accompanied by many of the symptoms of mania. Apparently, the clinician had caught her at a time when, clinically speaking, she was actively psychotic (for she was already experiencing the world strikingly differently than others in her culture), but had not yet developed the hard signs of psychosis in a diagnostic sense. He had, in essence, seen her "before the storm erupted," during the phase of delusional mood or delusional perception. Or she may have actually already had delusional ideas that she was not yet ready to share. Figure 11.2 summarizes the inter-relationships between the stages of the life cycle of a psychosis and the appearance of soft and hard signs of psychotic process. It also re-emphasizes the point that psychotic phenomena tend to fluctuate.

Later interviews with Ms. Fay and with her family revealed a history of intermittent affective instability with both manic and depressed features. Her psychotic symptoms appeared early on in the process. It was unclear which appeared first, the affective symptoms or the psychotic symptoms. Consequently, her Axis I diagnosis was changed to: schizoaffective disorder, rule out bipolar disorder. Further observation and history would eventually determine whether she was experiencing a true bipolar disorder or not.

Fortunately, Ms. Fay eventually stabilized upon a combined treatment of lithium and Haldol (haloperidol). Even during periods of stability, she continued to appear very manipulative and quite dramatic. She also continued to have significant problems with anger and impulsive control. Her parents related these symptoms were life-long in nature, lending further support to the idea that Ms. Fay might also have some characterologic problems, such as histrionic or borderline traits or even a borderline personality disorder. Further interviewing of her personality traits, historically, would be necessary to determine the presence of personality psychopathology, as we shall see in Chapter 14 on personality dysfunction.

Ms. Fay serves as an intriguing example of the subtle signs of psychotic process and the need for the initial interviewer to constantly seek out the soft signs of psychosis. At times, such dedicated diligence, associated with prompt subsequent treatment, may help prevent the patient from suffering the full-blown wrath of a psychotic illness.

Before leaving her presentation, it is worth summarizing some of the major points it highlights.

1. A person may be psychotic in a clinical sense, without demonstrating the hard signs of psychosis in a diagnostic sense (such as delusions or hallucinations).
2. The so-called soft signs of psychosis should always alert the clinician to the possibility of a smoldering psychotic process.
3. In the life cycle of a psychosis, hard signs of psychosis generally do not erupt without a prodromal phase of psychosis in which the patient's experience of reality is clearly abnormal but only the soft signs of psychosis are apparent.

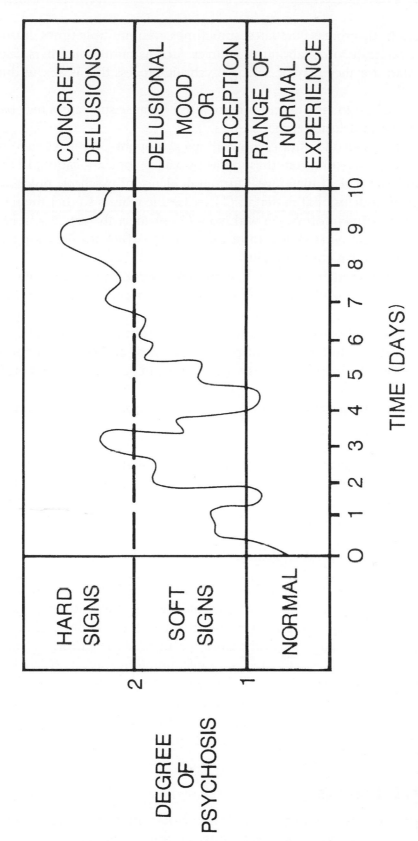

Figure 11.2 Evolution of a psychosis.

4. Because psychotic process fluctuates, sometimes even multiple times during a single day, listen carefully to collaborative sources such as family members, friends, and inpatient staff, for they may be seeing psychotic process that is absent during your interview.

5. Generally, it is best to tap areas of intense affect because such areas may be outward manifestations of delusional material.

6. If the patient uses an odd phrase, shows illogical thought, or utilizes an idiosyncratic phrase, it is often useful to tap these areas by asking for clarification. In the process of clarifying, the patient may reveal further evidence of psychotic process.

7. When exploring delusional material: (1) grease the wheels so that the patient feels comfortable sharing information with you, (2) uncover the extent and logic of the delusional material, and (3) determine the degree to which the delusion has become entrenched in the patient's thoughts.

8. Always consider whether an isolated, seemingly psychotic symptom may be viewed as normal in the patient's culture; if so, it may not represent a true marker of psychotic process.

9. Remember that an isolated, culturally acceptable hallucination or belief will not be embedded in an ongoing matrix of psychotic process and should *not* be accompanied by the soft signs of psychosis as might be seen in delusional mood or delusional perception.

10. A patient may have a severe psychotic illness, such as schizophrenia, and also have a personality disorder.

We can now leave the outpatient clinic at a community mental health center and return to an emergency room where Mr. Lawrence was brought in by the police and a crisis clinician. Mr. Lawrence was apparently suffering from an acute exacerbation of his chronic paranoid schizophrenia.

Clinical Presentation #5: Mr. Lawrence

Mr. Lawrence is a good-looking man about 30 years of age. Despite his good looks he is not particularly attractive at the moment, because he is in the midst of a rage. He was found in his apartment smashing a typewriter through the bedroom window. He had trashed the apartment, madly throwing white paint over his furniture. The landlord found him screaming. Mr. Lawrence has a long-standing history of schizophrenia with paranoid delusions. He has been violent at times in the past. Tonight he refuses hospitalization, and the crisis worker has to involuntarily commit him, because he apparently seems to be in the midst of yet another acute psychotic relapse. It took two policemen to bring Mr. Lawrence into the emergency room, and on the way in he managed to creatively coin a few new obscenities.

Discussion of Mr. Lawrence

At first Mr. Lawrence presented in an agitated and violent manner. At one point he threatened to beat one of the nurses, and subsequently tried to do so, eventually requiring restraints. It's possible that somehow the nurse had been incorporated into a delusion, although the patient denied the typical delusions he had demonstrated in the past.

I was "on-call" and was called to see if I would give permission to have Mr. Lawrence admitted to the inpatient unit to seclusion (secondary to his violence in the emergency department). I always prefer seeing any psychotic patient myself before proceeding with admission and told the ED staff that I was on my way.

By the time I had arrived on the scene I was surprised to find that Mr. Lawrence was lying calmly on a cart and appeared quite cooperative, but I attributed his calmness to the sedating effects of the haldol he had been given. He denied any hard signs of psychosis and also denied any recent suicidal gestures, although he commented that he had been thinking of killing himself several days earlier. Eventually we were able to remove the restraints, at which point Mr. Lawrence took a peculiar turn in his clinical course.

He related that he needed to go to the bathroom. As he walked towards the toilet he appeared to stagger a bit. Once he reached his destination, he looked about, as if he had been suddenly teleported into an unfamiliar space, and asked, "What am I doing in here?" When told that he had wanted to go to the bathroom, he appeared puzzled and denied ever making such a request.

As the interview proceeded Mr. Lawrence began to appear drowsy, which he attributed to being up all night and drinking heavily. He could only repeat three or four digits forwards, whereas he had been able to repeat seven forwards earlier. He also began grasping at some invisible objects near his feet.

If you think that Mr. Lawrence is beginning to sound similar to our first patient, Mr. Williams, who presented with DTs, it is because Mr. Lawrence is also suffering from a delirium (sometimes referred to as an acute confusional state in the literature). It was a delirium that would eventually threaten his life.

The interview was promptly stopped at this point. I relayed my concerns to the emergency room physician that I was suspicious that Mr. Lawrence had overdosed, despite his denial both to the crisis clinician, earlier, and to myself. An electrocardiogram (ECG) revealed some subtle abnormalities. Roughly 30 minutes later Mr. Lawrence stopped breathing. Fortunately, his life was saved through the effective use of an artificial respirator. Imagine, for a moment, what his fate might have been if he had been admitted to a seclusion room as initially requested by phone.

A Deadly Trap: Missing Deliria in Patients With Illnesses Such as Schizophrenia

In retrospect, the correct diagnosis was a tricyclic overdose leading to a paradoxic rage response. This rage was followed by a delirium. Mr. Lawrence's case provides a springboard into a discussion of several important points. In the first place, it is important to note that it was assumed initially, by the crisis clinician and the emergency room staff, that Mr. Lawrence was merely experiencing an exacerbation of his schizophrenia, because he had frequently presented with paranoia and violence in the past. This is one of the more dangerous clinical traps when dealing with a patient who has been labeled with a chronic psychotic process. It is both easy, and natural, to assume that the old etiologic agent is at work without vigorously searching for a new one.

A useful point to remember is that psychotic processes caused by a single etiology, such as schizophrenia, frequently present in a relatively similar fashion during each episode for a given individual. The soft signs, or early warning signs, are often similar from episode to episode, as are the subsequent hard signs. The psychotic process tends to present with an identifying fingerprint of sorts for each patient.

Consequently, in any patient for whom a new episode of psychosis appears distinctly different to previous episodes, the clinician should become suspicious that something new has been added to the picture etiologically. In the case of Mr. Lawrence, he usually presented with delusions and hallucinations. In this episode, neither symptom was present. This is an arena in which a patient's previous electronic health record (EHR) can be remarkably useful, providing a history of the patient's past episodes.

The second major point has been stated earlier but certainly warrants repeating. Any patient presenting with a delirium requires an immediate medical evaluation. Crisis clinicians are not infrequently faced with this clinical situation and they must constantly be on the lookout for it. It is critical for all initial evaluators to become adept at recognizing the clinical presentation of a delirium. With knowledge and common sense, it is not usually difficult to recognize; yet this diagnosis is frequently missed, often by physicians themselves.

We can begin our exploration of the presentation of a delirium by reviewing the DSM-5 criteria, which appear below (for information on the numerous specifiers, see the DSM-5 itself)[83]:

DSM-5 DIAGNOSTIC CRITERIA FOR DELIRIUM

A. A disturbance in attention (i.e., reduced ability to direct, focus, sustain, and shift attention) and awareness (reduced orientation to the environment).

B. The disturbance develops over a short period of time (usually hours to a few days), represents a change from baseline attention and awareness, and tends to fluctuate in severity during the course of the day.

C. An additional disturbance in cognition (e.g., memory deficit, disorientation, language, visuospatial ability, or perception).

D. The disturbances in Criteria A and C are not better explained by another preexisting, established, or evolving neurocognitive disorder and do not occur in the context of a severely reduced level of arousal, such as coma.

E. There is evidence from the history, physical examination, or laboratory findings that the disturbance is a direct physiological consequence of another medical condition, substance intoxication or withdrawal (i.e., due to a drug of abuse or to a medication), or exposure to a toxin, or is due to multiple etiologies.

Practical Tips for Spotting a Delirium: The Nature of the Beast

It is important to note that not all delirious patients are disoriented.[84,85] Generally these patients develop disorientation, but at times, especially in the early stages of the process, they may be completely oriented. In this sense, deliria can present in a variety of fashions, which is part of the reason they are sometimes misdiagnosed.

The following guidelines provide a practical platform for clinical assessment. In the first place, a delirium occurs when there exists a rather diffuse pathophysiologic dysfunction in the brain. Such a diffuse dysfunction will frequently show itself in one of two ways – a fluctuating level of consciousness or a marked problem with concentration and the ability to attend to the environment. These two processes should alert the clinician to the possibility of a delirium. Indeed, if either of these processes appears in a patient demonstrating the soft or hard signs of psychosis, then one should strongly consider a delirium work-up.

It therefore becomes critical to evaluate these two aspects during the initial interview of any psychotic patient. Unfortunately, it is easy to overlook their significance if the patient is agitated, as was the case with Mr. Lawrence. Let us begin with the evaluation of the level of consciousness.

People with a delirium tend to present in one of three ways: (1) hypoactive, (2) hyperactive, or (3) a mixed picture of the previous two states. In the hypoactive state, which represents the most common state, the patient may appear drowsy or may actually be hard to arouse. This type of "quiet delirium" is common in elderly patients. Their somnolent behavior does not bother anyone, and consequently their condition may be overlooked. In the hyperactive state the patient is "wired." The patient appears unusually responsive to any stimulation from the environment and tends to appear driven. This is sometimes accompanied by marked agitation or aggression. We saw this presentation earlier with Mr. Williams, the man suffering from DTs. Finally, patients may present with a mixture. One of the hallmarks of the delirious patient is the tendency for the level of consciousness to fluctuate. This fluctuation may be so extreme as to move the patient back and forth between hypoactive and hyperactive states. Mr. Lawrence first presented to the emergency room staff with a rage-like, hyperactive state and later presented to me in a drowsy, hypoactive state.

If one is actively looking for changes in the level of consciousness, they are not hard to spot. But in a busy clinical situation the trick is to be aware of their importance. A problem arises in the fact that patients tend to move in and out of delirious states relatively quickly. An alert nurse may note a brief episode of delirium that will simply not be present during clinical rounds the following morning. A frequent physician error is to assume that if the patient looks good on rounds, then "what's the fuss?" Unfortunately such a patient may be developing permanent brain damage during the periods of delirium. Consequently, this type of patient needs a medical work-up despite a good appearance during rounds.

This tendency for the delirious patient to demonstrate a fluctuating level of consciousness is paralleled by changes in the electroencephalogram (EEG).[86] In the hypoactive state, the EEG usually demonstrates a generalized diffuse slowing of the background activity. During the hyperactive state, fast activity is often seen. At times a normal EEG may be found.

With regard to determining whether or not the patient is having trouble concentrating and attending to the environment, the task becomes more difficult. The difficulty lies in the fact that subtle problems with attention and concentration may not be apparent unless tested. At times, the clinician may be able to determine that concentration is reasonably good, by noting the patient's ability to converse in a natural and intelligent fashion. At other times, as was the case with Mr. Lawrence, more formal testing is required, especially if the evaluator is truly suspicious of the presence of a delirium.

Four Cognitive Tests Useful for Recognizing a Subtle Delirium

Four tests come to mind, which as a battery will generally pick up any significant problems with concentration and the ability to attend to the environment. These four tests are: digit spans forwards and backwards, the vigilance test, constructions, and an examination of the patient's handwriting.

In the digit span test, one asks the patient to repeat a series of digits (starting with two digits and advancing to seven digits if the patient proceeds to answer correctly) to see if the patient can place incoming information into immediate memory storage and then quickly retrieve it. Deliria often disrupt this process.

It is important to ensure that one is testing the patient's immediate recall memory, as opposed to the patient's ability to simply repeat back a digit span without using memory. To ensure that memory recall is being tested, the clinician can say the following:

"I'm going to give you some numbers to remember. We will start with something easy, say two numbers, and then we will do longer strings of numbers. Watch me carefully as I say the number to make sure you got it. Then wait a moment. I will point to you. Do not repeat the number back to me until I point to you. This will help us to test your memory. Any questions? … Good, let's start: eight; five." (Pauses for several seconds, and then points to the patient.)

It is important to say the digits in a steady rhythm so as not to allow the patient to remember clumps of digits. Consistency in rhythm is particularly important when you are testing for seven-digit recall. If said like a telephone number, the patient may find them artificially easy to remember.

After testing seven digits forwards, the clinician can ask the patient to recall digits backwards, once again starting with two-digit recall. With the digit span test one should expect an average adult to be able to repeat about seven digits forwards and four to five digits backwards.

In the vigilance test, the clinician recites (for about 1–2 minutes) a string of letters randomly from the alphabet. The patient is asked to make a hand tap on the table every time the letter "A" is said. If the patient is experiencing problems attending to the environment, both errors of omission and commission will tend to occur, especially as you go deeper and deeper into the string of letters. A normal adult should make few if any errors in the vigilance test. As the series continues, some delirious patients will even forget what letter they are hunting for. I have found this test to be a surprisingly sensitive one for picking up problems in concentration as seen in subtly delirious states.

The patient may also be asked to make copies of constructions, such as a cross or a cube. Once again the delirious patient may find such a task difficult. Also note the time and the ease with which a patient performs constructions. Sometimes a patient can complete a construction such as a cube correctly, but it requires great time and concentration to do so. In an engineer or architect, such delays may actually indicate early cognitive dysfunction for they should be able to do a cube with great ease.

Finally, problems with writing (dysgraphia) are common and include spelling errors, clumsily drawn letters, reduplication of strokes in letters such as "M" or "N," and problems with alignment and linguistics.[87] The patient can be asked to write his or her name, a sentence or two of their own creation, and/or copy a sentence or two from a book or magazine. This test is significantly more telling if one can compare the patient's handwriting to a sample of his or her handwriting done prior to the behavioral symptoms. (Keep in mind that tests based upon the patient's writing are limited in use to patients who are literate and have been taught to use script, which is frequently not taught in grade schools due to the switch to computer keyboards, although deliria can also cause errors in printing). In Chapter 16, where we will focus our attention upon the mental status, I will be demonstrating the effective use of these four tests in Video Module 16.2.

These four tests represent an excellent quick screen for deficits in concentration, attending abilities, and immediate recall, but one may have difficulty using them with a hostile patient. Few hostile patients are eager to demonstrate their artistic abilities or play word games. When these tests are deemed to be inappropriate, one can learn a great deal by carefully observing the patient. The delirious patient may demonstrate difficulties in concentration, attending, and other cognitive problems through an inability to follow commands, a problem remembering questions, a tendency to appear overly sensitive to noises and other outside stimuli, or simply an appearance of confusion, as was the case with Mr. Lawrence in the bathroom. The trick is in remembering to look for these processes on a routine basis when encountering a psychotic patient.

Inouye has developed a systematic approach to spotting delirium called the Confusion Assessment Method (CAM) that many view as one of the best methods for diagnosing a delirial state, which requires only about 5 minutes to perform.[88] As one would expect from the above considerations, it focuses upon the patient's problems with both concentration and fluctuation in levels of consciousness. The CAM is not a structured test, but it brings a structured approach to delirial assessments. It focuses upon nine characteristics, symptoms, and behaviors: (1) acuteness of onset, (2) inattention, (3) disturbed thinking, (4) altered level of consciousness, (5) disorientation, (6) memory impairment, (7) perceptural disturbances, (8) psychomotor agitation, and (9) psychomotor retardation. We will not review its use in detail here, but the interested reader can find a manual for its use on the web.[89]

Thus far our focus has been on the two key characteristics of a delirium – problems with concentration/attending to the environment and fluctuations in the level of consciousness. It may be valuable now to review a few of the more common clinical characteristics.[90–92]

1. Hallucinations or illusions have been estimated to occur in 40 to 75% of delirious patients. Visual and auditory hallucinations are frequent, and the presence of visual hallucinations should always arouse suspicion of a delirious or organic state.

2. Rapidly changing delusions, especially of a paranoid nature, are common. These delusions tend to be of a much more fleeting and malleable nature than the delusions seen in schizophrenia or one of the delusional disorders.

3. Other problems with a formal thought disorder such as derailment or illogical thought may appear.

4. Short-term memory and orientation are frequently impaired.

5. Deliria tend to fluctuate. In particular, patients tend to be more disoriented and delirious at night, a process that has been referred to as "sundowning."

6. Deliria tend to emerge in a matter of hours or days, but this is not always the case. Insidious onsets can occur.

7. Although deliria are generally believed to be related to organic etiologies, it is believed that stress and psychological mechanisms can lead to a delirious presentation in some instances.

8. Affect is typically abnormal, with a high incidence of emotions such as fear and anxiety.

9. A characteristic phenomenon is the tendency for the patient to misidentify the unfamiliar as familiar. For instance, a nurse's aide may be identified as a brother or sister.

A variety of other odd behaviors have been reported during deliria, ranging from wandering aimlessly about the hospital to drinking copiously from the toilet. One particularly peculiar process has been reported in which the patient continues habitual behaviors in totally inappropriate places. For instance, in an "occupational delirium," patients perform behaviors in the hospital that are normally only done at their place of work. The term "carphology" has been coined for the behavior of picking at one's bedclothes, another abnormal behavior sometimes seen in deliria.

With regard to etiology, the list is extensive. In Table 11.1, a list of common causes is presented. It is beyond the scope of this book to elaborate on the medical differential and on the appropriate laboratory and physical examinations. The first and crucial step remains the uncovering of the delirium during the interview itself.

In a practical sense, interviewers must train themselves to rule out delirium any time a patient presents with a psychosis. Unless this active process of viewing delirium as a part of the differential becomes a clinical habit, one runs the risk of missing it. The patient is the one who pays for such an error, and the cost may be permanent brain damage or worse.

Differential Diagnosis on Mr. Lawrence and Summary of Key Interviewing Tips

At this point let us summarize the DSM-5 differential diagnosis on Mr. Lawrence:

General Psychiatric Disorders:

Medication-induced delirium (overdose on antidepressant)

Schizophrenia in remission

Table 11.1 Common Causes of Delirium

Metabolic

1. Hypoxia, hypercarbia, anemia
2. Electrolyte imbalance, hyperosmolarity
3. Hyperglycemia or hypoglycemia
4. Abnormal levels of magnesium or calcium
5. End-stage liver or kidney disease
6. Vitamin B_1 deficiency (Wernicke's encephalopathy secondary to a thiamine deficiency)
7. Endocrine disorders (hyperthyroidism or hypothyroidism, hyperparathyroidism, and adrenal disorders)

Infections

1. Systemic (e.g., pneumonia, septicemia, malaria, and typhoid)
2. Intracranial (e.g., meningitis, encephalitis)

Neurologic Disorders

1. Hypertensive crisis, stroke, subarachnoid hemorrhage, vasculitis
2. Seizures
3. Trauma

Drug Withdrawal

1. Alcohol hallucinosis, rum fits, delirium tremens
2. Other withdrawal states (e.g., from barbiturates, as well as acute intoxication with street drugs)

Intoxication

1. From agents such as digoxin, levodopa, anticholinergics, and street drugs

Post-operative Sequelae

1. Especially following cardiac surgery

Personality Disorders:

Deferred

Medical Disorders:

Respiratory arrest secondary to overdose

Major points worth reviewing include the following:

1. Psychoses such as those seen with schizophrenia or bipolar disorder often present in a similar fashion from episode to episode.
2. If a patient's psychotic presentation seems different than is typical from previous episodes, then the clinician should strongly consider the possibility of a new etiologic agent.
3. The presence of a delirium always warrants an aggressive medical evaluation and can easily be missed in chronic patients.
4. The clinician should always consciously look for evidence of a fluctuating level of consciousness or a significant problem with concentration and attending to the

environment in all psychotic patients; these two characteristics are tip-offs that a delirium may be present.

Clinical Presentation #6: Kate

The moment that one sees the look of concern on the faces of this young girl's parents, one feels that something is very wrong. Kate is 14 years old. She is slightly overweight. Her black hair drops in a tangle down her back. Her parents relate that they feel she is very depressed and that she has become more depressed over the past 2 months. Things had reached a crisis point when 5 days earlier Kate had thrown a slumber party. No one came. Since then she has been acting oddly, talking about "reality" and wandering about the house. The most bizarre incident occurred two nights ago, when Kate knocked at her parents' bedroom door at 2:00 A.M. When they opened the door, Kate stood topless, stating in a dull monotone that she felt a need to talk. At no time had Kate been delusional or heard voices. During a brief break in her interview, Kate left her examination area and was found wandering about in the clinical exam area of the ED peeking behind the curtains of the other examination areas. Kate's parents had taken her to two emergency rooms in the past week. At both places her parents were told that she was hysterical. Referrals were made for outpatient therapy.

Discussion of Kate

During the interview it was easy to see why hysterical traits had been reported. Kate seemed to be preoccupied, as if pulled into an autistic cocoon. At one point, she turned and while looking me squarely in the eyes she dramatically said, "Tell me Doctor, what is reality?" She denied hallucinations and delusions. Her speech was halting and was interspersed with inappropriate giggles. At times she displayed mild thought blocking and seemed distracted. She was completely oriented, demonstrated an alert and stable consciousness, and when cognitively tested, displayed no specific problems with concentration (other than a single error when doing reversed digits and one error on the vigilance test), attending to the environment, or other deficits.

Her numerous soft signs suggested that a psychotic process was present, and she was hospitalized. Her physical examination was normal in the emergency room without any neck stiffness nor complaints of headaches. We were somewhat suspicious of drug abuse, but it seemed unlikely from the history taken from the parents. By the time of admission, morning had almost broken, and I requested an immediate neurological consult to be placed upon arrival on the unit, for her presentation seemed difficult to explain, and I had concerns of a possible neurologic complication such as a central nervous system infection. The admission bloodwork and the results of the spinal tap performed hours later by the neurological consultant revealed a diagnosis of viral encephalitis. Approximately 1 week after her admission, Kate, unfortunately, lay dying in the intensive care unit.

Spotting Non-Delirial Psychoses Caused by Underlying Medical Conditions

Diagnostically speaking, Kate did not present with a delirium. Not all general medical causes of psychosis manifest as a delirium. While looking over the spectrum of general medical etiologies of psychotic process outlined in Table 11.2,[93] it is important to

Table 11.2 Organic Causes of Psychosis*

Space-Occupying Lesions of the CNS	Metabolic and Endocrine Disorders
Brain abscess (bacterial, fungal, tuberculosis, cysticercosis) Metastatic carcinoma Primary cerebral tumors Subdural hematoma	Adrenal disease (Addison's and Cushing's disease) Calcium-related disorders Diabetes mellitus Electrolyte imbalance Hepatic failure Homocystinuria Hypoglycemia and hyperglycemia Pituitary insufficiency Porphyria Thyroid disease (thyrotoxicosis and myxedema) Uremia
Cerebral Hypoxia	
Anemia Lowered cardiac output Pulmonary insufficiency Toxic (e.g., carbon monoxide)	
Neurologic Disorders	**Nutritional Deficiencies**
Alzheimer's disease Distant effects of carcinoma Huntington's chorea Normal pressure hydrocephalus Temporal lobe epilepsy Wilson's disease	B_{12} Niacin (pellagra) Thiamine (Wernicke–Korsakoff syndrome)
	Drugs, Medications, and Toxic Substances
Vascular Disorders	Alcohol (intoxication and withdrawal) Amphetamines Analgesics (e.g., pentazocine [Talwin], meperidine [Demerol])
Aneurysms Collagen vascular disease Hypertensive encephalopathy Intracranial hemorrhage Lacunar state	Anticholinergic agents Antiparkinsonian agents Barbiturates and other sedative-hypnotic agents (intoxication and withdrawal) Bromides and other heavy metals Carbon disulfide
Infections	Cocaine Corticosteroids
Brain abscess Encephalitis and postencephalitic states Malaria Meningitis (bacterial, fungal, tuberculosis) Subacute bacterial endocarditis Syphilis Toxoplasmosis Typhoid	Cycloserine (Seromycin) Digitalis (Crystodigin) Disulfiram (Antabuse) Hallucinogens Isoniazid L-Dopa (e.g., Larodopa) Marijuana Propranolol Reserpine (Serpasil and others)

CNS, Central nervous system.
*Adapted from Bassuk EF, Beck AW, editors. *Emergency psychiatry*. New York, NY: Plenum Press, 1984.

remember that a psychosis secondary to a general medical condition like encephalitis can present in a fashion suggestive of any classic psychosis, such as schizophrenia or bipolar disorder. Frequently, delirium is not a part of the picture. This point once again emphasizes the need to "think organic" when evaluating a patient presenting with the onset of psychotic symptoms.

More importantly, in the emergency room, and even in a clinic setting, one of the critical triage decisions involves ruling out a life-threatening cause of psychosis. The most common life-threatening illnesses that present with an acute psychosis include the following[94]:

1. Hypoglycemia
2. Hypertensive encephalopathy
3. Poor oxygenation (perhaps related to a heart attack, pulmonary embolus, anemia, or a hemorrhage)
4. Infections such as encephalitis or meningitis
5. Drugs, including medications, street drugs, withdrawal states, industrial toxins, and actual poisons
6. Intracranial trauma (including hemorrhage, actual trauma related to head injury, and other causes of increased intracranial pressure)
7. Wernicke's encephalopathy (not generally life threatening but should be viewed as a medical emergency, because if untreated, permanent brain damage can occur)

Other serious entities to consider in the differential diagnosis include hepatic failure, uremia, subacute bacterial endocarditis, and a chronic subdural hematoma. Autoimmune encephalitis is another important entity to keep in mind, for it can present with psychotic symptoms as well as other psychiatric features, including catatonia, anorexia/bulimia, obsessive–compulsive symptoms, anxiety, depression, and lethargy. These autoimmune encephalitides are often accompanied by problems with memory and cognition, and are frequently (*but not always*) followed by neurological deficits such as seizures, ataxia, parkinsonism and memory loss. In this collection of disorders, the immune system inadvertently attacks brain cells as it mounts a response to a pathologic agent such as seen in rheumatic fever caused by streptococcal infections or a cancer (paraneoplastic autoimmune encephalitis). Fortunately, this list does not represent a particularly extensive differential. If the clinician remembers to think of these entities, they are generally easy to rule out – but that is an important "if." In actuality, these entities are rare enough as causes of acute psychotic process that they are likely to be overlooked, unless clinicians train themselves to consistently consider them.

When to Refer for a Physical Exam and What to Do If You Can Perform One

A brief, well-directed physical examination will often uncover many of the life-threatening processes mentioned above, but not always as evidenced by Kate whose physical exam was normal. In fact, a patient presenting with the onset of new psychotic symptoms should seldom, if ever, leave an emergency room without a screening physical examination. If a new patient presents to a community mental health center, college counseling center, or a private practice with psychotic symptoms, every effort should be made to have the patient seen as quickly as possible, hopefully immediately after the mental health assessment.

The physical examination can be performed quickly and is geared towards uncovering evidence of a life-threatening dysfunction. To this end, it focuses on the following five areas: (1) vital signs, (2) autonomic system dysfunction, (3) heart and lung dysfunction, (4) neurologic dysfunction and head trauma, and (5) abnormalities of the eyes.

Abnormal vital signs should be retaken. If they remain abnormal, an etiology for the dysfunction should be sought. Keep in mind that the pulse may be naturally elevated in an agitated patient, but agitation alone seldom causes sustained pulses over 120 to 130.

Autonomic dysfunction is frequently present during a life-threatening illness. Agents such as the anticholinergic medications, mentioned earlier, frequently cause the patient to present with hyperthermia, blurred vision, dry skin, facial flushing, and delirium. The mnemonic "hot as a pepper, blind as a bat, dry as a bone, red as a beet, and mad as a hatter" has been used to describe this toxic state.

A note of caution should be added: the anticholinergic syndrome is often incomplete, or it may be hidden by other active agents such as opiates. For instance, Mr. Lawrence, who overdosed on Elavil, an antidepressant with many anticholinergic properties, presented with an increased pulse and a dry mouth, but his pupils were normal in size and reactive. His skin color was pale, not flushed as would be expected in a classic anticholinergic syndrome. Many contemporary psychiatric and non-psychiatric medications have anticholinergic properties.

This discussion also emphasizes the usefulness of looking at the patient's eyes. The clinician should look for abnormal size or responsiveness of the pupils, as well as asymmetry. Horizontal and vertical nystagmus should be sought. The eye grounds may reveal evidence of increased intracranial pressure.

Neurologically, one scans for evidence of focal weakness and changes in reflexes. Reflexes, including the suck reflex, snout reflex, palmomental reflex, and the Babinski sign, can be quickly screened. The clinician should check for signs of neck rigidity as well as for hemotympanum of the ears or other signs of a slight skull fracture.

Finally, the clinician should listen to the heart and lungs if an abnormality of the cardiovascular or respiratory system is suspected.

A screening physical examination as described earlier can quickly flush out a serious physical condition, sometimes even in the early stages. A common error in this regard is to admit an extremely agitated patient directly to a seclusion room and subsequently fail to perform a follow-up physical examination when the patient has calmed down. Once the patient has calmed, the physician, nurse clinician, or physician assistant should attempt a screening examination no matter how late it is at night. At times, when one is strongly suspicious of the presence of a serious illness, the patient may need to be physically restrained to allow for examination.

Differential Diagnosis on Kate and Summary of Key Interviewing Tips

At this point we can return to Kate in an effort to summarize her DSM-5 diagnosis. Note that although Kate does not present with delusions, hallucinations, or a formal thought disorder other than some mild thought blocking (the three classic hard signs of psychosis), she does present with one extremely odd behavior by history – appearing topless when knocking at her parents' bedroom door – and the somewhat odd behavior demonstrated in the emergency department – wandering about in the exam area. These odd behaviors should appropriately raise the clinician's suspicion of the presence of an underlying psychotic disorder in the differential diagnosis. In addition, the thought blocking she demonstrated during the interview itself is usually a sign of active psychotic process. Although Kate has some signs suggestive of delirium (possible episodes of confusion and mild cognitive deficits), she does not currently meet the criteria for delirium. At the time of her admission, before any lab work had returned, her differential may have looked as follows:

General Psychiatric Disorders:

Unspecified schizophrenia spectrum and other psychotic disorders (provisional)

Rule out:
1. Brief psychotic disorder
2. Psychotic disorder due to another medical condition
3. Unknown substance use disorder
4. Substance/medication-induced depressive disorder
5. Substance/medication-induced psychotic disorder
6. Major depressive disorder with psychotic features
7. Unspecified delirium

Personality Disorder:

Defer

Medical Disorders:

Rule out general medical causes of psychosis (such as infection, partial complex seizure disorder, etc.)

Before leaving the topic of Kate's presentation, it may be of value to summarize some key points.

1. A delirium is not the only way in which a medical illness may manifest as a psychosis. Diseases such as encephalitis can mimic processes such as schizophrenia.
2. The clinician should routinely consider the various life-threatening illnesses when evaluating a patient who is psychotic.
3. A screening physical examination should be performed on any patient presenting with psychotic features (as well as any appropriate lab work).
4. The absence of all the typical signs of the anticholinergic syndrome does not rule out this syndrome, because it may present with only some of the physical signs.

Let us now move on to our final case presentation. Ms. Flagstone represents an anomaly among our other cases: She is not acutely psychotic.

Clinical Presentation #7: Ms. Flagstone

Ms. Flagstone walks into the outpatient clinic at a community mental health center, dressed in a stylish fashion, with a cigarette in hand, waving it about like a baton of sorts, until she is politely asked to put it out by the receptionist. During the initial interview with her assigned outpatient therapist, her affect changes periodically as she relates a long-standing history of "just not going anywhere in my life." At times she is tearful but is able to quickly pull herself together. She is very dissatisfied with her poor relationships with men, despite her good looks and thick black hair. Her speech rate and volume are within normal limits. Although mildly tangential at times, she does not display any loosening of associations or thought blocking. She is well oriented and denies any history of delusions. When asked about hallucinations she denies any except for one episode 2 years earlier. She continues as follows:

> I've really never told anyone this story, but it has had a profound effect on me. At the time I was extremely upset. Everything was horrible in my life. Fortunately, I was not taking any drugs or else I might not have found God. I was in my kitchen doing the dishes when a sudden light filled the room. I just knew it was a message from God. He had come to bring me back to the His flock. From inside the light I heard the Angel Gabriel speak. He said, 'Janet, you are with child.' I knew this was a test from God and I showed strength by accepting the mission. He talked with me, and I convinced him of my great love of God. At that point the angel told me that all was well and that I was back with God, my father. A blinding light moved in and out of the room many times. The whole thing only lasted about 15 minutes, but my life has never been the same since.

This episode is the only time that she has ever heard a voice, and she denies that she has any special mission for God other than to be a good Christian.

Discussion of Ms. Flagstone

Upon further interviewing, the entire episode with the Angel Gabriel seemed to last roughly 15 to 30 minutes (no soft signs immediately before or after the experience); moreover, the voice of the angel was loud and distinct. At one point the voice of the angel actually conversed with the voice of God. Apparently, near the time of this episode, Ms. Flagstone had been fired from a job and had also been feeling "slightly paranoid near my co-workers."

She also related that she undergoes periods in which she feels, "not quite myself, as if I wasn't quite real." These episodes last only for about 10 minutes and occur during times of intense stress. She finds these episodes very disturbing. Further interviewing would reveal that Ms. Flagstone had never experienced ongoing psychotic process, yet how does one explain the voices and the episodes of depersonalization?

"Micropsychotic Episodes" Seen in People Coping With Personality Disorders

The answer lies in the fact that psychotic process is not limited to classic major psychiatric diagnoses such as schizophrenia, bipolar disorder, major depression, and delirium. A variety of personality disorders may present with "micropsychotic episodes." These episodes tend to last from minutes to hours. At times they may extend longer, but as soon as the episodes appear to be lasting a day or longer, one should immediately begin suspecting a more serious ongoing psychotic disorder. It is much more characteristic for these events to be short-lived, as demonstrated by Ms. Flagstone, who upon further interviewing seemed to fulfill many of the criteria for a histrionic personality disorder; however, this diagnosis is difficult to verify in a single hour and will require further interviewing.

Micropsychotic episodes, as experienced by people with personality disorders, are characteristically precipitated by stress, or they may be unleashed by drug abuse, or both. Processes such as fleeting paranoid ideation, depersonalization, and derealization are frequently experienced. If drug abuse or stress is frequent, then both the frequency and duration of the micropsychotic episodes may increase.

Diagnostically speaking, micropsychotic episodes are seen most frequently in the following three disorders: paranoid personality disorder, schizotypal personality disorder, and borderline personality disorder. Although seen much more rarely, micropsychotic episodes have been reported in patients dealing with histrionic and/or narcissistic process if the patients are under intense stress or their natural defense mechanisms are outstripped by the pressures of their daily life. For instance, a highly respected priest with a severe narcissistic personality disorder, who is discovered to be an active pedophile, may be at risk for micropsychotic process. The public humiliation may prove to be so intense as to overcome his protective narcissistic defenses. The result could be intermittent brief lapses of subtle paranoia.

Psychotic Processes With a Rapid Onset/Offset

In classic psychotic disorders, such as schizophrenia, schizoaffective disorder, bipolar disorder, and major depression with psychosis, we have seen that the hard signs of psychosis, such as hallucinations and delusions, tend to be imbedded within a psychotic matrix. These disorders usually have a prodromal phase lasting days, weeks, or even months, in which the soft signs of psychotic process appear first before the hard signs appear. We have seen that this phenomenological distinction may help an interviewer to distinguish between culturally accepted hallucinations and beliefs (that are not psychotic) and genuine psychotic process.

Some psychiatric disorders can create rapidly appearing and disappearing genuine psychotic process, as we just saw with Ms. Flagstone. There was no prodromal phase with soft signs of psychosis in the days preceding her micropsychotic episode. The episode also ended abruptly with an immediate return to her baseline functioning.

In psychotic states precipitated acutely by street drugs and medications, psychotic symptoms such as hallucinations can also occur very rapidly, in a matter of minutes to hours. The hallucinogens such as LSD, peyote, and other variants of mescaline, have striking effects in this respect. As with drugs impacting directly on brain functioning, other underlying neurologic disorders such as seizure disorders may also precipitate psychotic phenomena rapidly.

Also keep in mind that particularly intense flashbacks, as sometimes seen in post-traumatic stress disorder (PTSD), can essentially achieve psychotic proportions in which hallucinations and/or paranoia may erupt. It is fairly common for people experiencing intense flashbacks to experience auditory hallucinations of the voices and/or sounds that were present during the original trauma.

At other times, the PTSD patient will experience an atypical type of flashback in which the emotions experienced during the assault (such as extreme fear and/or anxiety) will appear during the flashbacks, occurring without a memory of the exact circumstances of the traumatic incident. Such episodes may be misinterpreted as being evidence of enduring psychotic or paranoid process if the clinician is unaware of such phenomena. I am reminded of a patient of mine who would sometimes, without warning, experience intense fears. Her fear was so great that she would sometimes arm herself with a gun and point it intermittently towards her front door. The episodes of fear would last for an hour or two. But there were no associated memories flashing through her mind during these atypical flashbacks, just fear and hypervigilance. Interestingly, these episodes were often triggered by the sound of a phone ringing. It was conjectured that perhaps she had been assaulted at a young age, with the memory still repressed, and that, during the assault, a phone had been left to ring unanswered in the background.

Differential Diagnosis on Ms. Flagstone and Summary of Key Interviewing Tips

With regard to Ms. Flagstone, her voices and depersonalization episodes probably warrant the label of micropsychotic episodes. They were always brought on by stress and appeared abruptly. Further interviewing revealed that they were not preceded by mood states suggestive of the soft signs of psychosis.

After the first interview, the differential on Ms. Flagstone looked something like the following:

General Psychiatric Disorders:

Defer (probably none; but because of her tangential speech and mood shifts, entities such as cyclothymic disorder or dysthymia could be kept in mind)

Personality Disorders:

Histrionic personality disorder (provisional, but more historical information needed before diagnosis can be made)

Rule out other specified personality disorder (mixed with histrionic, schizotypal, and borderline traits)

Medical Disorders:

Rule out partial complex seizures

Recognizing Psychotic Process Triggered by Seizure Disorders

The need to rule out a seizure diagnosis may surprise the reader, and rightly so, because I have not yet provided some pertinent information. Ms. Flagstone reported that she had become extremely interested in a variety of philosophical and religious issues. She had filled nearly 20 journals with her thoughts, none of which were psychotic. She also reported brief episodes of feeling very uncomfortable in her abdomen, a sensation that seemed to move upwards into her throat area. All of these phenomena could be components of partial complex seizures (formerly called temporal lobe epilepsy), including her periods of depersonalization and her mood shifts.

Epilepsy presenting with partial complex seizures is the "masquerader *par excellence.*" It can mimic essentially any psychiatric disturbance and is particularly good at presenting as a psychotic disturbance. A query should be made for partial complex seizures in any patient presenting with psychotic symptoms. Indeed, with our immediately previous patient, Kate, you will recall that a partial complex seizure disorder was also a part of the differential diagnosis, especially because of her episodes of odd behavior (such as distractedly walking about the back halls of the ED).

Psychotic symptoms may emerge during the seizure itself or between seizures (the period known as the interictal phase). The seizure activity sometimes begins with a phase known as the aura, in which patients may experience a variety of odd sensations, including fear and anxiety. Patients may feel that they are experiencing a given situation for a second time (known as *déjà vu*), or they may have the opposite feeling that nothing is familiar (known as *jamais vu*). The patient sensing strange and pungent odors may also be a predominant symptom. Peculiar abdominal feelings are very frequent. In some cases, these feelings are the only symptoms, and the patient is said to have "abdominal seizures."

As the seizure develops, the patient loses conscious awareness and usually displays various automatisms such as picking at himself or herself, wandering about, and displaying bizarre mannerisms or odd behaviors. To uncover such processes, a useful question remains, "Have you ever found yourself somewhere and you didn't know how you got there?" Two other pertinent questions are, "Have you ever had periods of losing consciousness?" and "Have your friends or family ever told you that they have seen you doing very odd things that you don't remember?"

Curiously, personality changes or psychotic-like activity may appear between partial complex seizures during interictal periods.[95] Ms. Flagstone reported some of the more common interictal phenomena seen in such presentations: preoccupation with religious or moral issues, a tendency to write copiously, decreased sexual drive, intense mystical experiences, a deepening and intensification of emotions, and what has been called interpersonal viscosity. This latter term refers to a tendency to want to keep talking and be near to people.

It is certainly not always possible to explore all these issues during the initial interview because of time constraints. However, in later sessions these questions should be rigorously pursued if suspicious of seizure activity. Collaborative interviews with family/friends can be particularly useful if one is suspicious of the presence of partial complex seizures. Family/friends may be quite puzzled by the behaviors of the patient (periods of confusion, aimless or bizarre behaviors) and the patient is completely unaware of them due to post-seizure amnesia.

It is an unfortunate error to label someone as having schizophrenia when the actual problem is a partial complex seizure disorder. Such a person would be robbed of the chance to benefit from a course of antiseizure medications, and would also be needlessly exposed to the potentially serious side effects of antipsychotics.

At this juncture, we are rapidly drawing to a close on our case discussions. It seems appropriate to summarize some of the points brought forward by the case of Ms. Flagstone.

1. Some personality disorders may present with psychotic symptoms, so-called micropsychotic episodes.
2. Micropsychotic episodes are most common in people coping with paranoid, schizotypal, or borderline personality disorders. They are less frequently seen in people with decompensating histrionic or narcissistic personality disorders during times of intense stress and/or substance use.
3. These micropsychotic episodes tend to extend from minutes to hours and are often triggered by stress or drugs. Paranoia, depersonalization, and derealization are common.
4. Partial complex epilepsy may present with psychotic symptoms both during seizures or between seizures.
5. Consequently, questions should be asked concerning both the symptoms commonly seen during a seizure as well as relating to interictal personality change.

We have now concluded our survey of diagnoses that may demonstrate psychotic symptoms. Figure 11.3 illustrates the rich diversity of etiologic agents that may present with psychotic symptoms. As mentioned at the beginning of the chapter, the word "psychosis"

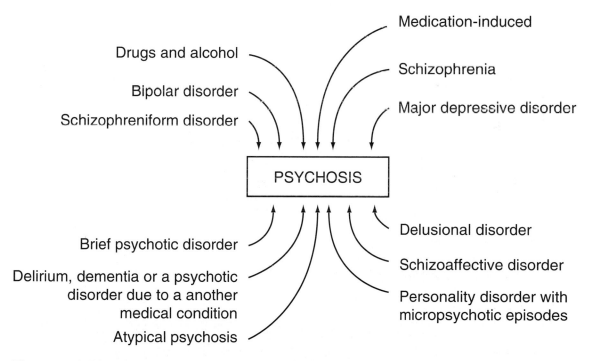

Figure 11.3 Diagnostic possibilities when considering psychosis.

is not a diagnosis. The presence of psychotic symptoms mandates that the clinician try to delineate the possible disorder and the etiologic agent of that disorder.

In order to perform an effective initial assessment, we must possess a sound and flexible knowledge base concerning the differential diagnosis of psychotic process. In this chapter we have attempted to provide just such a base. Hopefully, we have also shown that the performing of differential diagnosis from a person-centered perspective is, indeed, a delicate art in which the clinician always balances the uncovering of diagnostic symptoms with a keen sensitivity to the uniqueness of each patient's experience of those symptoms.

But we have only touched upon how the horrors of psychotic process invade the inner worlds of our patients and disrupt the familial and societal matrix of which these worlds are an integrated part. Much remains to be examined if we are to have the tools necessary to more sensitively explore this world with our patients through the art of interviewing. In this regard, it seems only fitting to end this chapter with the wise quotation that we have seen before from the pen of Sir William Osler, "It is much more important to know what sort of patient has a disease than to know what sort of disease a patient has." With the completion of this chapter, we now know the disease. In the next chapter we will come to know the person beneath it.

REFERENCES

1. Hammacher AM. *Phantoms of the imagination*. New York, NY: Harry N. Abrams; 1981. p. 136–8.
2. Symons A. Essay on Gérard de Nerval. In: *The symbolist movement in literature*. New York, NY: E. P. Dutton; 1985. p. 14–17.
3. American Psychiatric Association. *Diagnostic and statistical manual of mental disorders*. 5th ed, DSM-5. Washington, DC: American Psychiatric Association Publishing; 2013. p. 99–100.
4. Fish F. *Clinical psychopathology*. Bristol, UK: Wright; 1967. p. 19–26.
5. Roberts JK. *Differential diagnosis in neuropsychiatry*. New York, NY: John Wiley; 1984. p. 263.
6. Asaad G, Shapiro B. Hallucinations: theoretical and clinical overview. *Am J Psychiatry* 1986;**143**:1088–97.
7. West LJ. A clinical and theoretical overview of hallucinatory phenomena. In: Siegel RK, West LJ, editors. *Hallucinations: behavior, experience, and theory*. New York, NY: John Wiley; 1975. p. 308.
8. Lehman HE, Canero R. Schizophrenia: clinical features. In: Kaplan HI, Sadock BJ, editors. *Comprehensive textbook of psychiatry IV*. 4th ed. Baltimore, MD: Williams & Wilkins; 1985. p. 683.
9. West LJ. 1975. p. 308.
10. Roberts JK. 1984. p. 262.
11. Sellers EM, Kalant H. Alcohol intoxication and withdrawal. *NEJM* 1976;**294**:757–60.
12. DeBellis R, Smith SB, Choi S, Malloy M. Management of delirium tremens. *J Intensive Care Med* 2005;**20**(3):164–73.
13. Hackett TP. Alcoholism: acute and chronic. In: Hackett TP, Cassem NH, editors. *Massachusetts General Hospital handbook of general hospital psychiatry*. St. Louis, MO: C. V. Mosby; 1978. p. 19.
14. Hackett TP. 1978. p. 20.
15. Goldfrank LR, Lewin NA, Osborn H. Dusted (PCP). *Hosp Physician* 1982;62–7.
16. Fischer GL, Harrison T. *Substance abuse: information for school counselors, social workers, therapists and counselors*. New York, NY: Pearson Education; 2012.
17. Goldfrank LR. 1982. p. 65.
18. Shumard T, Bruijnzeel D. A 56-year-old man with paranoid delusions, auditory hallucinations, and thought blocking. *Psychiatr Ann* 2011;**41**(6):307–9.
19. Akiyama K. Longitudinal clinical course following pharmacological treatment of methamphetamine psychosis which persists after long-term abstinence. *Ann N Y Acad Sci* 2006;**1074**:125–34.
20. McKetin R, Hickey K, Devlin K, Lawrence K. The risk of psychotic symptoms associated with recreational methamphetamine use. *Drug Alcohol Rev* 2010;**29**(4):358–63.

21. Shumard T, Bruijnzeel D. 2011. p. 308.
22. Goodman LS, Gilman A. *The pharmacological basis of therapeutics*. New York, NY: Macmillan; 1975. p. 514–32.
23. Wiffen PJ, Derry S, Moore RA. Impact of morphine, fentanyl, oxycodone, or codeine on patient consciousness, appetite and thirst when used to treat cancer pain. *Cochrane Database Syst Rev* 2014;(5):CD011056.
24. Rajput H. Effects of *Atropa belladonna* as an anti-cholinergic. *Nat Prod Chem Res* 2013;**1**(1):1–2.
25. Kirkpatrick B, Fenton WS, Carpenter WT, Marder SR. The NIMH-Matrics consensus statement on negative symptoms. *Schizophr Bull* 2006;**32**(2):214–19.
26. Rado JT. Management of negative symptoms in schizophrenia. *Psychiatr Ann* 2011;**41**(5):265–70.
27. Guze SB. Schizoaffective disorders. In: Kaplan HI, Sadock BJ, editors. *Comprehensive textbook of psychiatry IV*. 4th ed. Baltimore, MD: Williams & Wilkins; 1985. p. 657.
28. Lehman HE, Canero R. 1985. p. 690.
29. Haier RJ. The diagnosis of schizophrenia: a review of recent development. *Schizophr Bull* 1980;**6**(3):417–27.
30. Guze SG. 1985. p. 757.
31. *DSM-5*. 2013. p. 105–6.
32. Tsuang, Ming T. Schizoaffective disorder. *Arch Gen Psychiatry* 1979;**36**:633–4.
33. Lichtenstein P, Yip BH, Björk C, et al. Common genetic determinants of schizophrenia and bipolar disorder in Swedish families: a population-based study. *Lancet* 2009;**373**(9659):234–9.
34. Kane JM, Perlis RH, Malhotra AK. Clinical insights into pharmacogenetics and schizophrenia, part 2. *J Clin Psychiatry* 2008;**69**(6):1006–13.
35. Malhi GS, Green M, Fagiolini A, et al. Schizoaffective disorder: diagnostic issues and future recommendations. *Bipolar Disord* 2008;**10**(1 Pt 2):215–30.
36. Insel TR. Rethinking schizophrenia. *Nature* 2010;**468**(7321):187–93.
37. Correll CU, Penzner JB, Frederickson AM, et al. Differentiation in the preonset phases of schizophrenia and mood disorders: evidence in support of a bipolar mania prodrome. *Schizophr Bull* 2007;**33**:703–14.
38. Bruijnzeel D, Tandon R. The concept of schizophrenia: from the 1850s to the DSM-V. *Psychiatr Ann* 2011;**41**(5):289–95.
39. Peralta V, Cuesta MJ. Exploring the borders of the schizoaffective spectrum: a categorical and dimensional approach. *J Affect Disord* 2008;**108**(1):71–86.
40. Keshavan MS, Morris DW, Sweeney JA, et al. A dimensional approach to the psychosis spectrum between bipolar disorder and schizophrenia: the schizo-bipolar scale. *Schizophr Res* 2011;**133**(1):250–4.
41. Guze SB. 1985. p. 756–9.
42. *DSM-5*. 2013. p. 90–1.
43. Walker JI, Brodie HK. Paranoid disorders. In: Kaplan HI, Sadock BJ, editors. *Comprehensive textbook of psychiatry*. 4th ed. Baltimore, MD: Williams & Wilkins; 1985. p. 747–55.
44. Walker JI, Brodie HK. 1985. p. 752.
45. Robinson D. My favorite tips for exploring difficult topics such as delusions and substance abuse. *Psychiatr Clin North Am* 2007;**30**(2):239–52.
46. Resnick P. My favorite tips for detecting malingering and violence risk. *Psychiatr Clin North Am* 2007;**30**(2):227–32.
47. Resnick P. 2007. p. 231.
48. Bannister, Sir R. *Brain's clinical neurology*. New York, NY: Oxford University Press; 1978. p. 197.
49. Walker JI, Brodie HK. 1985. p. 751.
50. Raskind M. Paranoid syndromes in the elderly. In: Eisdorfer C, Fann WE, editors. *Treatment of psychopathology in the aging*. New York, NY: Springer Publishing Company; 1982. p. 184–91.
51. Bridge TP, Wyatt RJ. Paraphrenia: Paranoid states of late life: European research. *J Am Geriatr Soc* 1980;**28**(5):193–200.
52. Pearman A, Batra A. Late-onset schizophrenia: a review for clinicians. *Clin Gerontol* 2012;**35**:126–47.
53. Ravindran AV, Yatham LN, Munro A. Parphrenia redefined. *Can J Psychiatry* 1999;**44**(2):133–7.
54. Hassett A. Schizophrenia and delusional disorders with onset in later life. *Rev Bras Psiquiatr* 2002;**24**(Supl 1): 81–6.
55. Castle DJ, Wessely S, Howard R, Murray RM. Schizophrenia with onset at the extremes of adult life. *Int J Geriatr Psychiatry* 1997;**12**:712–17.
56. Hassett. 2002. p. 82.
57. Castle. 1997. p. 715.
58. Lopez-Ibor J. Delusional perception and delusional mood: a phenomenological and existential analysis. In: Koning AJJ, Jenner FA, editors. *Phenomenology and psychiatry*. New York, NY: Grune and Stratton; 1982.
59. Bowers MB. *Retreat from sanity: the structure of emerging psychosis*. Baltimore, MD: Penguin Books; 1974.
60. McDonald N. Living with Schizophrenia. *Can Med Assoc J* 1960;**82**:218–21.
61. Robinson DJ. *Three spheres: a psychiatric interviewing primer*. Port Huron, MI: Rapid Psychler Press; 2000.
62. Robinson DJ. 2007. p. 239–40.
63. Robinson DJ. 2007. p. 241.
64. Dissanaikae L, Agius M. Hearing voices in the normal population. *Cut Edge Psychiatry Pract* 2011;**1**(3.3):50–4.

65. Lawrence C, Jones J, Cooper M. Hearing voices in a non-psychiatric population. *Behav Cogn Psychother* 2010;**38**(3):363–73.
66. Cangas AJ, Langer AI, Moriana JA. Hallucinations and related perceptual disturbance in a non-clinical Spanish population. *Int J Soc Psychiatry* 2011;**57**(2):120–31.
67. Kelleher I, Harley M, Murtagh A, Cannon M. Are screening instruments valid for psychotic-like experiences? A validation study of screening questions for psychotic-like experiences using in-depth clinical interview. *Schizophr Bull* 2011;**37**(2):362–9.
68. Stip E, Letourneau G. Psychotic symptoms as a continuum between normality and pathology. *Can J Psychiatry* 2009;**54**(3):140–51.
69. Morgan C, Fisher H, Hutchinson G, et al. Ethnicity, social disadvantage and psychotic-like experiences in a healthy population based sample. *Acta Psychiatr Scand* 2009;**119**(3):226–35.
70. Sommer IE, Daalman K, Rietkerk T, et al. individuals with auditory verbal hallucinations; who are they? Psychiatric assessments of a selected sample of 103 subjects. *Schizophr Bull* 2010;**36**(3):633–41.
71. Choong C, Hunter MD, Woodruff PW. Auditory hallucinations in those populations that do not suffer from schizophrenia. *Curr Psychiatry Rep* 2007;**9**(3):206–12.
72. Johns LC. Hallucinations in the general population. *Curr Psychiatry Rep* 2005;**7**(3):162–7.
73. van Os J. Is there a continuum of psychotic experiences in the general population? *Epidemiol Psichiatr Soc* 2003;**12**(4):242–52.
74. Johns LC, van Os J. The continuity of psychotic experiences in the general population. *Clin Psychol Rev* 2001;**21**(8):1125–41.
75. Ohayon MM. Prevalence of hallucinations and their pathological associations in the general population. *Psychiatry Res* 2000;**97**(2–3):153–64.
76. Dissanaikae L, Agius M. 2011. p. 50.
77. Waters F. Auditory hallucinations in psychiatric illness. *Psychiatr Times* 2010;**27**(3):54–8.
78. Dewi Rees W. The hallucinations of widowhood. *Br Med J* 1971;**4**(5778):37–41.
79. Roever CP, Vyas BB, Barnett MC, et al. Visual hallucinations in long-term care. *Ann Long Term Care* 2012;**20**(2):25–30.
80. Dissanaikae L, Agius M 2011. p. 50.
81. Lo H, Dzokoto V. Talking to the master: intersection of religion, culture, and counseling in Taiwan and Ghana. *J Ment Health Couns* 2005;**27**(2):117–28.
82. Scott EHM. A study of the contents of delusions and hallucinations in 100 African female psychotics. *S Afr Med J* 1967;**4**:853–8.
83. *DSM-5*. 2013. p. 596–8.
84. Roberts JK. *Differential diagnosis in neuropsychiatry*. New York, NY: John Wiley; 1984. p. 158.
85. Murray GB. Confusion, delirium, and dementia. In: Hackett TP, Cassem NH, editors. *Massachusetts General Hospital handbook of general psychiatry*. St. Louis, MO: C. V. Mosby; 1978. p. 98.
86. Roberts JK. 1984. p. 164.
87. Murray GB. 1978. p. 96.
88. Inouye SK, van Dyck CH, Alessi CA, et al. Clarifying confusion: the confusion assessment method. a new method for detecting delirium. *Ann Intern Med* 1990;**113**:941–8.
89. Inouye SK. *The Confusion Assessment Method (CAM) training manual and coding guide*. 2003. Hospital Elder Life Program. Available at <http://www.hospitalelderlifeprogram.org/uploads/disclaimers/Long_CAM_Training_Manual_10-9-14.pdf> [accessed September 2015].
90. Murray GB. 1978. p. 93–116.
91. Roberts JK. 1984. p. 161–4.
92. Querques J, Fernandez-Roberts C, Quinn D, et al. Evaluation and management of delirium. In: Amos J, Robinson RG, editors. *Psychosomatic medicine: an introduction to consultation-liaison psychiatry*. New York, NY: Cambridge University Press; 2010. p. 64–72.
93. Barsky A. Acute psychoses. In: Bassuk EF, Beck AW, editors. *Emergency psychiatry: concepts, methods, and practices*. New York, NY: Plenum Press; 1984. p. 195–218.
94. Barsky A. 1984. p. 195–218.
95. Bear D, Freeman R, Schiff BA, Greenberg M. Interictal behavioral changes in patients with temporal lobe epilepsy. In: Hales RE, Frances AJ, editors. *APA annual review*, vol. 14. Washington, DC: APA; 1985. p. 190–210.

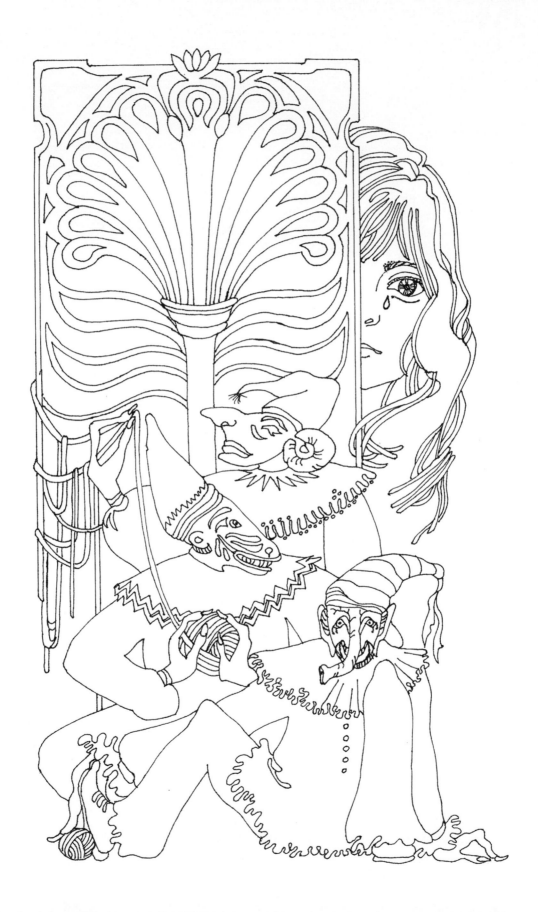

CHAPTER 12

Interviewing Techniques for Understanding the Person Beneath the Psychosis

---

In this unnerved – in this pitiable condition – I feel that the period will sooner or later arrive when I must abandon life and reason together, in some struggle with the grim phantasm, Fear.

Edgar Allan Poe
The Fall of the House of Usher

Poe aptly describes the fear and anxiety that so frequently walk hand-in-hand with the process known as psychosis. Amidst this tapestry of fear and anxiety, a plethora of psychological traps are interwoven, including hallucinatory phenomena, oddities of perception, and difficulties in language formation and cognition. In this chapter we will attempt to move, wing by wing, through the matrices of our patients to better understand the destruction that psychotic process causes the people beneath these diagnoses.

As we saw in Chapter 10 where we discovered that depression can cause widespread disruption across a patient's matrix, psychotic process spreads throughout each and every wing of our patients' matrices like a virus, wreaking havoc on each wing, from the biological to the familial and the spiritual. The more we understand the nuances of this destruction and its movement, the more likely we will be able to develop interviewing techniques and strategies that can help our patients to share their pain with us; this is the goal of this chapter. We will also discover that psychotic process can impact on the interview process itself.

Our abilities to navigate these hurdles and to sensitively spot the subtle emergence of psychotic process is one of the most pivotal and sophisticated skills that any mental health professional can bring to the table. It is a skill that can help us to begin the healing process, whether one is a college counselor sitting with a student experiencing a first break of schizophrenia, a social worker functioning as a crisis worker in an emergency room encountering a patient with a drug-induced psychosis, or a psychiatrist working with a patient admitted to an inpatient unit with command hallucinations to kill himself.

THE PAIN BENEATH PSYCHOTIC PROCESS

Fields of Interaction

I. The Biological Wing of the Matrix

Sleep Disturbances in Psychosis

One of the major physiologic moorings of our daily lives is the routine appearance of the phenomenon known as sleep. If one's sleep patterns are disturbed, one quickly begins to feel "not quite oneself." It appears as no surprise then that a sleep disturbance often appears early in the psychotic process.

As psychotic process begins to gain momentum, the patient often experiences severe problems falling asleep. In some instances the patient will eventually undergo a day/night reversal, in which sleep occurs during the daylight hours and the night becomes a time of agitation. The patient may also experience other sleep disturbances, such as early morning awakening, especially if the psychosis is part of a major depression.

This difficulty with falling asleep stands as a sensitive sign of impending psychosis, frequently appearing during periods of delusional mood or delusional perception. The patient sometimes denies this sleep disturbance. Consequently, it is useful to ask family members about the patient's sleep, because they have frequently been awake themselves, coping with the growing restlessness of their family member.

Psychotic Disruption of the "Sensation of the Physical Boundaries of the Body" and the Concept of a "Porous Ego"

Leaving the area of sleep disruption, one is confronted with another set of somatic concerns created by psychotic process, and these concerns are far removed from normal experiences like sleep: Psychotic patients frequently have problems with determining the limits of their bodies, and in a parallel sense, the limits of their sense of self, their "realness," or sense of "mineness," so to speak.

It has been suggested that patients experiencing psychotic process often regress to an infantile state in which the body is viewed as part self and part object.[1] At such points, the person may experience such intense feelings of depersonalization or derealization that they actually move past these phenomena into odd psychotic experiences in which the patient loses the sense of self or autonomy of self. One such type of experience is known as a "made volitional act," vividly described by one patient as follows:

> I look at my arms and they aren't mine. They move without my direction. Somebody else moves them: All my limbs and my thoughts are attached to strings and these strings are pulled by others. I know not who I am. I have no control. I don't live in me. The outside and I are all the same.[2]

When intense, such feelings may be associated with a terrifying sense of impending annihilation. Perhaps, this blurring of inner and outer reality is the almost otherworldly fear that Roderick Usher felt was his destiny in Poe's story. It is important to realize the intensity of these fears, because they provide insight into the sometimes violent and drastic measures of psychotic patients.

The above quotation leads us into a more sophisticated exploration of psychotic disruptions in the boundaries of the ego. In essence, one can view psychotic patients as possessing a "porous ego." The world seems to invade their skins in a distinctly unpleasant fashion. They experience a variety of sensations, which seem to enter from the outside world while becoming one with them. It is this unidirectional invasion of their integrity that is partially responsible for their fear and anxiety.[3] It is this feeling of invasion, and the dissolution of the integrity of the body, that characterizes many of what have come to be known as Schneiderian symptoms.

Schneiderian First-Rank Symptoms of Psychosis

Kurt Schneider, one of the 20th century's leading European psychiatric innovators, was a pupil of the great phenomenologist Karl Jaspers. Schneider descriptively captured the weird sensations of these invasion experiences. He mistakenly thought that the presence of any of these symptoms, if not caused by another medical condition, *almost* guaranteed the presence of schizophrenia. He consequently called these symptoms "first-rank symptoms" of schizophrenia (often referred to as FRS in the clinical literature). The notion of these symptoms as near confirmation of the presence of schizophrenia proved to be incorrect, for these symptoms can be seen fairly frequently with other diagnoses in which there is psychotic process. But Schneider's symptoms are an excellent inventory of common psychotic phenomena, whatever their etiology, and questions concerning them should be part of any interviewer's repertoire. There is considerable evidence that they are, indeed, more common in schizophrenia than in other causes of psychosis such as mood disorders or in psychotic disorders caused by a medical condition.

Schneider described 11 symptoms, of which seven are characterized by feelings of invasion by the outside world. These seven symptoms are: (1) somatic passivity experiences, (2) made feelings, (3) made impulses, (4) made volitional acts, (5) thought withdrawal, (6) thought insertion, and (7) thought broadcasting. The remaining four Schneiderian symptoms are delusional perception (a symptom we discussed in great detail in the previous chapter) and several types of auditory hallucinations – audible thoughts, voices arguing, and voices commenting upon one's actions.

The literature on Schneiderian FRS can be confusing, for Schneider, to some degree, did not clearly define them in his own writings, resulting in various interpretations being given by subsequent writers.[4,5] To me, the symptoms are best understood by remembering that Schneider was greatly influenced by the philosophy and psychology of phenomenology. Phenomenologists are primarily interested in understanding the fashion in which human beings *experience* being in the world, including the individual's unique concerns as to how their experiences are related to their sense of self and to others. In a general sense, phenomenologists are less interested in secondarily categorizing experiences as specific "things" such as delusions or hallucinations than in trying to understand, as best they can, how a unique human being has experienced a unique phenomenon within his or her mind. Let me clarify this somewhat-confusing abstraction with a specific Schneiderian symptom – thought withdrawal.

A patient can *experience* thought withdrawal in different ways. A patient may literally *feel* a thought being withdrawn from his or her brain/skull as a perception (a haptic hallucination) or a patient could cognitively believe that his or her thoughts are being withdrawn, without necessarily feeling it as a sensation (a delusion, without any precipitating hallucination). Both of these are experienced by patients as real inner phenomena or truths. I believe that for Schneider, it was this inner experience of thought withdrawal that was most important, not whether the patient's experience could be subsequently classified as a hallucination versus a delusion.

Likewise, a patient could interpret this inner phenomenon in various fashions. The patient could, in a nebulous way, simply *feel* as if a nonspecific, non-identified outside agent had done the withdrawing (a feeling state *not* a delusion); or the patient might vaguely believe that an outside entity had withdrawn the thought (an over-valued idea); alternatively, he or she could *definitely believe* that an outside agent had withdrawn the thought (a true delusion); further yet, he or she could arrive at a specific belief as to who (a neighbor) or what (a demon) had withdrawn the thought (an elaboration and refinement of the patient's delusion).

In my opinion, Schneider, as a phenomenologist, was most likely interested in all of these aspects, viewing them as integral parts of the patient's inner experience. It was not that the person had either a hallucination and/or a delusion that would matter most to a classic phenomenologist. It was the fact that a person had experienced the phenomenon of thought withdrawal and had been concerned about it (in whatever unique fashion it was experienced and in whatever unique fashion the patient had experienced the concern) that raised Schneider's suspicion that the patient was experiencing a psychotic world.

It is also important to understand that Schneider did not believe that the mere presence of one of these symptoms indicated the existence of psychotic process or even psychopathology. The symptom had to be embedded within a psychotic matrix, as we described in our previous chapter. He warned, "a psychotic phenomenon is not like a defective stone in an otherwise perfect mosaic."[6] The need to examine the specific symptom within the overall context of the patient's experience Schneider described as the requirement for the presence of "phenomenological leverage." This leverage (psychotic matrix) had to be present in order to determine that a symptom was truly psychotic in nature.[7] With these clarifications in mind, let's take a closer look at Schneider's first-rank symptoms.

Exploring Somatic Passivity and "Made Feelings": The World of the Porous Ego

Schneider did a marvelous job of capturing the essence of these psychotic sensations, which, traditionally, clinicians have a hard time uncovering because they are so foreign to normal experience. A clinician can empathize with paranoia to some extent, because we have all experienced fear of other people to some degree or another. But "somatic passivity" and "made feelings" are something altogether different. They are psychologically foreign phenomena to most clinicians, hence are easily missed. Moreover, despite the damaging power of these symptoms (and the consequent value of targeting them for relief via supportive reassurance, cognitive–behavioral therapy, or medications, etc.), many patients – because the symptoms sound so "crazy" to others in the patient's everyday culture – will not share them unless directly asked about them by the interviewer.

With somatic passivity experiences, the patient is the reluctant recipient of bodily sensations against his will by a force outside of his control such as suddenly feeling that his intestines are wriggling about inside his abdomen or that his organs are shifting about. It is easy to see how such peculiar sensations could plant the seeds of delusional material such as a paranoid fear that someone is purposely twisting the patient's insides or that parasites or snakes have infested his intestines. The following type of question can help to bring such sensations to light:

"Do you ever feel that something is moving or squirming inside of your body?"

Similarly, in made feelings, made impulses, and made volitional acts, the patient once again feels that something is "being done *to* them." Personal control is taken from the patient (sometimes referred to in the literature as delusions of control). This distinct and remarkably unnerving feeling that "I am being made to feel something, made to want to do something, or actually being made to do a specific act against my will" (such as assaulting or killing someone), is the unifying perception of all three of Schneider's "made" symptoms. It is a poignant example of a "porous ego," made vulnerable to invasion at any moment by psychotic process. Mellor, in a classic article on Schneiderian FRS, quotes a patient who describes the oddness of a "made feeling":

> *I cry, tears roll down my cheeks and I look unhappy, but inside I have a cold anger because they are using me in this way, and it is not me who is unhappy, but they are projecting unhappiness into my brain.*[8]

Another of Mellor's patients insightfully describes the sensation of "made volitional acts" of which we already saw one example above. In this instance, the patient is describing that his fingers pick up objects but, "I don't control them … I sit there watching them move, and they are quite independent, what they do has nothing to do with me. I am just a puppet … I am just a puppet who is manipulated by cosmic strings."[9]

Notice how it would be natural for any person experiencing these "made sensations" or somatic passivity experiences to wonder who or what is causing them. This drive to figure out, "what is happening to me?" is totally normal. Unfortunately, as the patient seeks out an answer, they will inevitably come upon an unrealistic answer for the original sensation is psychotic in nature. Their resulting explanation for the made feeling or somatic passivity experience – a demon is making me feel hate or parasites have invaded my intestines – is a delusion. *Thus we see that delusions are often the result of a person's natural hunt for answers to an unnatural, psychotic experience.* This sequential understanding complements what we saw in the last chapter when we described the "life cycle of a delusion" and the concept that the presence of delusions is evidence of an old psychosis.

Armed with an understanding of this life cycle of a delusion, an interviewer may be better able to spot the emergence of subtle psychotic process. This could result in lower anti-psychotic dosages, and perhaps a much less virulent episode of psychosis, for the patient. For instance, a talented interviewer may uncover an insidiously emerging first break of schizophrenia or the earliest signs of a break-through in a patient's psychotic process (previously well-controlled by medications) despite the fact that the patient is denying the presence of delusions. The clinician can accomplish this task by utilizing questions that are designed to uncover the type of made symptoms or somatic passivity *experiences* that often pre-date delusional *thoughts*.

The following questions can be of value in uncovering these unsettling sensations, all of which can lead to the development of delusional material:

"Have you ever felt that something or someone is making you feel an emotion, as if something is making you feel angry, sad, or bitter?" (uncovers made feelings)

"Does it sometimes feel like something or someone is giving you urges that you would never want to do normally, like the urge to yell out at a stranger, use a profanity, or even hurt someone physically?" (uncovers made impulses)

"Right before you assaulted your boss, and I know you feel very badly about that now, what were you feeling, right before you hit him? (an open-ended *indirect* method of potentially uncovering made volitional acts)

"Have you ever felt that something or someone made you actually assault your boss?" (a closed-ended *direct* method of uncovering made volitional acts)

Thought Withdrawal and Thought Insertion

Two other Schneiderian symptoms – thought withdrawal and thought insertion – are reflections of a porous ego. Both sensations are extraordinarily unsettling.

Once again, the operative words are "to me," in that the patient feels that these phenomena are being done "to me" by some outside force. In normal day-to-day functioning, all of us have the discrete sensation that we exist and that we do things to the world about us and even to ourselves. It is a distinct sensation of intentionality. This sensation of intentionality is so innate that people are generally unaware of it. It simply is. But with all of the Schneiderian symptoms discussed thus far, the patient feels that there is some external, disembodied force that is capable of causing them to feel and do things, creating a penultimate fear of loss of control.

So it is with thought withdrawal and thought insertion. In the former, the patients feel, become suspicious, or believe that their thoughts are literally being pulled out of their minds by an alien force. If not present immediately, paranoid delusions are usually quick to follow, as the patient tries to understand or explain the etiology of his or her sensations. Inwardly the patient may feel that his or her mind has had a thought removed, sometimes even in mid-sentence. In an interview, this inward experience may show itself outwardly. The patient may demonstrate thought blocking, in which a sentence is disrupted before completion and the patient cannot recover his or her train of thought. Thought withdrawal can be addressed as follows:

"Have you ever felt that some person or perhaps something like a demon or perhaps the web can pull or remove your thoughts from you, you know, against your will?"

In contrast, with thought insertion, the patient feels or believes that thoughts from a different entity are being forced or pushed into his or her mind. The phenomenon is a truly weird experience, often accompanied by over-valued ideas or delusions frequently tied into demon possession or other types of paranoid delusions, such as a computer or smart phone pushing thoughts into the patient's mind. I have found the following questions to be of use in exploring these sensations:

"You mentioned that your neighbor, Ben, is trying to control you. Does he try to do things like control your thoughts or even literally push his own thoughts into your mind?"
"Does it ever feel to you that you can literally feel Satan pushing these feelings into your mind, against your will?"
"Have you ever felt that thoughts are being pushed into your mind through your smart phone that aren't your own?"

Thought Broadcasting (Unintentional and Intentional)

Unfortunately, the patient's porous ego may also allow for the passive escape of thoughts, feelings, and desires. The result may be fears that aggressive fantasies will be heard by others in the room or, even worse, that in a magical sense, these violent ideas may automatically become reality. A common feeling is that the patient's thoughts are leaking, as elegantly described below:

> *My difficulty is an outgo of my silent thought. It goes as it comes. I may think whatever I please, but whatever I do think goes as it comes. I suppose the constant irritation and annoyance they have kept up around me has affected the tension of nerve, so that unlike others who have the same phenomenal power, it goes as rapidly as my mind thinks. I have but to think a thought and it reaches other minds in sound without an effort on my part, and is sounded for a distance, I suppose, of 2 or 3 miles.*[10]

This type of passive thought broadcasting is sometimes called "thought diffusion." I find the term "thought leakage" more descriptive of the fear attached to the phenomenon by the people experiencing it. One can imagine the intense concern accompanying such a phenomenon, for suddenly there is no privacy whatsoever. What one thinks, others can hear. Generally, thought leaking is experienced in very negative terms. Patients may even feel that their thoughts are being beamed out on radio or television, or simultaneously magically posted on Facebook or other social media.

Note that thought broadcasting is a decidedly different sensation to thought withdrawal. The locus of the experience is not that something is being *actively* done to oneself (an agent is pulling my thoughts out), but that one's thoughts are leaking outwards through a porous ego.

In some rarer instances of thought broadcasting, it feels to patients that they are capable of intentionally sending thoughts from their minds. In such instances, the thought broadcasting may be viewed in a pleasurable light – as a special ability or skill. The following questions can be used to uncover both types of thought broadcasting (unintentional leakage or an intentional sending of thoughts):

"Jim, are you ever worried that other people can read or hear your thoughts without your awareness, or perhaps your inner thoughts are somehow posted on the web without your knowing it?"

"Sometimes people have told me that they have been lucky enough to develop some unusual or special powers, like ESP. For instance, some people have told me that they have the ability to send their thoughts outward into the minds of others, sometimes great distances. Have you ever experienced anything like that, even just a little bit?"

One can quickly sense the inherent strangeness of a world encountered with a porous ego. One can more easily intuit why these patients frequently seem preoccupied or lost in thought. It requires tremendous attention to try to sort out the meanings of so odd and intrusive a world. The clinician must also bear in mind that these patients are frequently attempting to determine which of their sensations are real and which are false. To the degree that they possess a "distance" from their psychosis, they will realize that much is unreal. As the psychosis deepens, this distance is lost, and the inexplicable becomes a reality that needs no explanations.

Spotting Medication-Induced Akathisia

Thus far, the focus has been on the somatic sensations and physiologic ramifications of psychotic process. However, with the advent of antipsychotic medications, which have remarkably enhanced our ability to decrease psychotic process, a new set of problems has unfortunately appeared. Antipsychotics can negatively impact on the extrapyramidal structures of the brain known as the basal ganglia (areas such as the globus pallidus and putamen) that lie deep within the brain beneath the cortex; they are important brain centers, regulating movement and many other activities.

Patients may develop significant movement-related side effects, especially with traditional antipsychotics such as Haldol and Prolixin, when the physiology of these brain structures is adversely effected. These side effects are less common with newer atypical antipsychotics such as Risperdol, Clozaril, and Seroquel, but certainly can still be seen with these medications, sometimes quite severely. We already discussed one of these extrapyramidal side effects in which the patient's affect becomes blunted or flat (no expression) secondary to an antipsychotic-induced Parkinson's syndrome. We saw that this blunting could be easily mistaken by an interviewer for the blunted affect so characteristic of schizophrenia.

A second side effect, akathisia, can also confuse the initial interviewer, because it can be mistaken for evidence of psychotic agitation. Akathisia is most commonly caused by both typical and atypical antipsychotics, but it can also be triggered by other medications including selective serotonin reuptake inhibitor (SSRI) antidepressants, as well as two antiemetics. Akathisia represents a symptom in which patients feel that a part or all of their body needs to move. It is a deep-seated feeling of restlessness. Generally it will show itself as the physical sign of moving about in an agitated fashion, sometimes with a smallish, prance-like step.

It is important to remember that akathisia is a subjective symptom, not a physical sign. In this sense the patient may not always appear agitated or be pacing. Instead, the person may only experience the unpleasant sensation of feeling intensely restless. By way of illustration, if in addition to akathisia the patient has also developed the stiff-like Parkinson's syndrome described above, the patient may move very little, despite an intense drive to move. Needless to say, this type of paradoxical situation creates an extremely discordant sensation for the patient.

It is easy to mistake akathisia for psychotic agitation; consequently the interviewer must be alert for it. When severe, akathisia represents a new and bizarre sensation that a patient already having problems with psychotic process certainly could do without. Some authors have reported incidents in which they felt that akathisia either worsened a psychotic state or, at times, predisposed the patient to inflict self-damage, including suicide.

In the following direct transcription, a young professional describes his experiences with akathisia. At the time of the transcript he was no longer psychotic. When the medication had been utilized, he had been suffering from a frightening delusional system. He had also been told about akathisia and its transitory nature, but his psychotic process appears to have disrupted this information. I have never heard akathisia or its interplay with psychotic process so eloquently described:

> **Pt.:** I was very aware of a different kind of feeling from what I usually have. It felt as if it was most immediately recognizable in the morning, in that I felt that I just couldn't go through with my normal morning routine, like taking a shower and shaving and everything I do to get ready for work. It felt more like I couldn't do it because I couldn't stand to wait that long, to go through those things which were such routine motion.
>
> **Clin.:** Like, what are some of things that were routine?
>
> **Pt.:** Well, like standing under the shower. It just seemed impossible to stand under the shower for any much longer and once I got done with the shower it seemed impossible to stand there and dry myself.
>
> **Clin.:** Okay. What do you mean when you say it wasn't possible. What was it that you felt would happen if you did stay there?
>
> **Pt.:** That I would break out of my skin or something like that. But, uh, that I would be so upset and unsettled that I would just be totally destroyed I think. It's just very unsettling.
>
> **Clin.:** Now, did the experience change over time? In other words, were there parts of the day where you would feel worse than other parts?
>
> **Pt.:** It was pretty much general all day. When I got to work, I have a sit-down job. I do remember that it was hard to stay put. It was really hard to sit. I do a lot of reading in my job and it was very hard to concentrate on the things I have to read, and as a consequence it made me feel ineffectual in my work. I just felt totally wiped out at work. I felt like I really couldn't keep working if I were to keep having this feeling.

Clin.: You mentioned the ineffectual feeling. Did you start to feel upset about being ineffectual?

Pt.: Oh, sure. Yeah, I felt that I was going to be a failure, really, if I were to keep feeling this way. I thought it would become evident right away to all the people around me that I was really screwing this up and that I really couldn't do my job anymore. And, in fact, I even got a little panicky about that.

Clin.: Describe that to me.

Pt.: Yeah, I just felt like being between a rock and a hard place because the feeling was that I had to sit there and keep doing my work because I was at work. On the other hand, my body felt like I just couldn't keep doing that anymore, and, uh, it was like you were in a crisis every second is what it was really like. Between wanting to stay there and do your job and being unable to do so.

Clin.: Did you have any fears that somehow or other that this state would not go away? You know, that this was going to continue?

Pt.: Definitely. I had the fear that the drug had set off something in my system whereby, even if I stopped the drug, that I was going to continue to have this feeling. What was definitely very much a part of the feeling was the fact that how could I go through the rest of my life feeling this way? That was very much a part of it.

Clin.: Now, what types of things did this sort of lead you to think then, that you couldn't do your work and that this state might not change?

Pt.: Uhmm, I felt depressed about it, and, uh, it led me to feel scared and afraid that something was going to happen.

Clin.: Do you think that you got more frightened or nervous than you had been before? In other words, did the unpleasant sensation increase your own anxiety just because you were having it?

Pt.: Oh, yes. Definitely. I was very anxious being around other people, that they might perceive that I was in this agitated state.

Clin.: Did you have any feelings that you should try to hurt yourself or that you might hurt yourself? … because of the …

Pt.: Yes, it did seem, it did occur to me that it would be easier not to live than to live this way. That probably seems really heavy, but that did occur to me. I did, I had a resurgence of suicidal thoughts during those feelings.

Clin.: What kinds of things were you thinking at the time?

Pt.: Uh, usually blowing my head off. Really, I was thinking about that and just ending it all because it just, I think every drug I ever took, I always had the fear that it would do something, … that it would never go away again.

One aspect that can help the interviewer attempt to sort out akathisia from psychotic agitation is the fact that akathisia represents a true bodily sensation. Patients will generally describe a need to move, an actual restlessness within the limbs. This is not generally the case when the agitation is caused by psychotic process. If the patient lacks other psychotic symptoms that could be triggering intense anxiety, then it is also more likely that akathisia is the main problem. But at times the only way to distinguish akathisia from psychotic agitation is to attempt to treat one or the other process. Fortunately with the patient described above, the akathisia was greatly relieved by lowering the dose of the antipsychotic.

Interviewing patients who are experiencing extrapyramidal side effects is often a daily experience for mental health professionals across disciplines, especially if one works in a community mental health center, an inpatient unit, or an emergency room. Let us now turn our attention to a puzzling syndrome that a clinician is a great deal less likely to see on a frequent basis, but is nevertheless important to understand. Indeed, it is its relative rarity that makes it important that we review interviewing techniques that can help us to reach these patients when we do encounter it.

Establishing an Alliance With a Patient Experiencing Catatonia

In the 1800s, catatonia was a relatively frequently seen syndrome, especially if one was walking the back wards of "insane asylums." It is much less frequently encountered by the clinicians of today. Nevertheless, it is encountered. When it is, contemporary clinicians must be prepared to help patients suffering from it. Skilled interviewing may be the first step towards breaking the psychological chains that bind these patients so tightly to a world beyond human interaction.

Psychotic process can disrupt the normal control of activity levels to an extreme degree, resulting in aberrant patient behavior ranging from agitated catatonia, in which the patient cannot stop moving, to stuporous catatonia, in which the patient shows little movement at all. It is to this peculiar state of stuporous catatonia that we shall turn our attention.

At one time, catatonia was generally believed to be primarily associated with schizophrenia. More recently, it has been viewed as a symptom complex that is not only seen in schizophrenia but also in mood disorders, hysterical dissociation, and in a variety of medical illnesses including autoimmune encephalitides triggered by infectious agents and cancers.[11]

Stuporous catatonia is often associated with mutism, lack of movement, negativism (as shown by a tendency to not comply with any requests), and ambitendency. This latter trait reveals itself as a hesitancy to complete behaviors, demonstrated by actions such as extending one's hand to shake and then removing it. All of these behaviors have been referred to as the "negative symptoms of catatonia" (not to be confused with the negative symptoms of schizophrenia, described in the previous chapter).

Stuporous catatonia is also associated with the so-called positive symptoms of catatonia (once again not to be confused with the positive symptoms of schizophrenia), such as the holding of bizarre postures, the senseless repetition of the clinician's words, and waxy flexibility. This latter phenomenon manifests itself as a bizarre willingness to hold one's body in any position to which it is moved.

The initial interviewer is faced with the question of how to approach a catatonic patient. It is not clear exactly what such patients are experiencing, and most likely the experience varies from one patient to another. Apparently some patients seem well aware of what is going on around them whereas others may be lost in peculiar feelings of timelessness and autism.

When speaking with a patient experiencing catatonia, gentleness is imperative. It can seem second nature to talk more loudly if someone is not responding to your questions. Remain gentle in tone, calm in pace of your speech. Always keep in mind that the patient may be processing your words quite effectively, either consciously or unconsciously. One simply does not know. Consequently, speak normally and be sure to say whatever you want to communicate, for the patient may not acknowledge what you are saying on the spot, but he or she may be silently processing it in the moment or later that day. A simple comment such as, "It's okay not to talk now, but any time you feel like talking, please do so. And feel free to ask any of the staff if I'm around. I'll try to talk with you as soon as I am available. It would be a nice thing to do."

A logical question arises as to whether one should attempt a nonverbal technique such as touching the patient. Generally speaking, I believe that in an initial interview the answer is no, primarily because one simply does not know what these patients are experiencing. If delusional or actively hallucinating, the patient may perceive the clinician as attacking. Moreover, some of these patients can move almost immediately from stillness into hyperactive states.

I am reminded of one such patient who I inadvisedly touched. She was lying on the floor in an unresponsive state. We were concerned about the possibility of an overdose. When she did not respond to loud questions, I shook her shoulders. To my shock she immediately grabbed me and attempted to bite me. Apparently, drugs were not the issue.

However, in certain unusual instances the clinician may decide that it would be useful to touch a catatonic patient. If such a decision is reached, then some simple principles should be followed. In the first place, someone else should be in the room, and safety officers should be aware that the patient may be unpredictable. The patient should be told in a calm and reassuring voice exactly who the clinician is and what the clinician is about to do. Patients should also be told why they are being touched and that if at any point they want to be left alone they should simply say so. The clinician should be prepared to quickly take evasive action.

I am reminded of a woman in her mid-30s, suffering from schizophrenia. During the interview she sat with her head wrenched straight back while wincing with apparent pain. For about 10 minutes she refused to answer any questions. Her neck continued to hyperextend, as her face further contorted in pain. A second clinician stepped in at this point and said the following, "Ms. Jackson, I am one of the physicians here. I can see that you are in some kind of pain. I am concerned that you may be having a type of drug side effect (dystonic response to her antipsychotic), and I would like to see if I can help relieve your pain. In a moment you will feel me touching the back of your head. I will be trying to see if I can get your neck to move more freely. If you want me to stop, just tell me." The clinician proceeded to do just as he said, while continuously informing the patient as to his next move. In about a minute, the patient's neck straightened, allowing the interview to continue, although she went on to speak in a disorganized fashion. Her neck spasm was hysterical, not medication related.

II. The Psychological Wing of the Matrix

Auditory Hallucinations: Their Nature, Phenomenology, and Exploration

Auditory hallucinations are false perceptions of sounds, both human and non-human. They represent one of the trademarks of psychotic process. To the layperson, the presence of "voices" is practically synonymous with madness. To the clinician, auditory hallucinations are one of the true hard signs of psychosis, although, as we have already seen, they can be experienced by people without psychopathology.

As described by Waters in an excellent overview of auditory hallucinations, the most common type of hallucination in psychiatric disorders is a voice.[12] These voices may be of people known to the patient, unknown to the patient, reality based (as with a family member, political leader, or celebrity), or imagined (as with a god, a demon, or an angel). The voices are commonly single words, but often contain complete sentences or questions and, at times, are quite complex, including multiple voices conversing (often commenting on the patient's behavior) as well as voices with which the patient engages in an ongoing conversation.

Hallucinations may also be nonverbal, composed of grunting sounds, machine noises, unrecognizable sounds, and music.[13] One of my patients, a college student suffering from a psychotic bipolar disorder, told me that about 30 minutes before he would descend into his most harrowing psychotic periods (characterized by vicious demonic voices), he would often hear, very distinctly, the pleasant music of an ice-cream truck. He related he could hear the truck approaching and leaving, and the music was indistinguishable from the real thing.

He would later discover that he could creatively use this phenomenon as an early warning sign of an acute psychotic worsening. As soon as he heard the ice-cream truck, he took a prn (i.e., as needed) dose of his antipsychotic medication often effectively short-circuiting the demonic voices. Quite remarkable and quite resourceful! It highlights that each person must determine how to interact with his or her unique hallucinatory processes. In this case the patient used one type of pleasurable hallucination – the music of an ice-cream truck – to help him prevent the occurrence of a disturbing type of hallucination – demonic voices.

Auditory hallucinations are commonly seen in psychiatric disorders. It has been reported that 75% of patients with schizophrenia and between 20 to 50% of patients with bipolar disorder experience auditory hallucinations. Many clinicians think of auditory hallucinations in association with these two disorders, but it is important to realize that they can appear with many other disorders. Approximately 10% of patients with major depressive disorder experience auditory hallucinations and prevalence rates of up to 40% have been reported for patients with post-traumatic stress disorder, generally experienced during intense flashbacks.[14]

Determining whether a patient is having hallucinations, whether abnormal or normal, is not as easy as one might think, because, for the most part, the clinician must depend upon the patient's self-report. As we have seen, errors in validity appear more frequently when one must depend upon patient opinion as opposed to the elucidation of behavioral incidents. Because of this, it may be best to start with a basic question regarding the nature of auditory hallucinations, such as "Are they heard inside your head or outside of your head?" The answer may come as a bit of a surprise.

The Directional Location of Auditory Hallucinations

For quite some time, clinicians tended to clump reports of auditory hallucinations into two categories: pseudohallucinations and true hallucinations. This distinction may well have found its most fertile roots in the writings of Karl Jaspers, whose work we encountered before in Chapter 10. Jaspers seemed to believe that there was no continuum between hearing one's thoughts and hearing true hallucinations. Patients either had hallucinations or they did not. With true hallucinations he felt that two elements were always present. First, the hallucination was substantial in the sense that it seemed real and had many of the sensory qualities of a real perception. Second, the hallucination seemed to occupy space. With an auditory hallucination, this suggests that the voice came from a given area outside the head.

But Jaspers was incorrect, as Fish and others have pointed out, and modern clinical experience has borne out.[15–17] There does appear to be a continuum, and I have talked with many patients with schizophrenia who describe their voices as "being in my head." In some instances, as the psychotic process progresses, these voices move out into space and truly seem more real at that point. In other cases, the voices seem to be originating either from inside or outside the patient's head, often appearing to be quite real in either circumstance. But the bottom line remains that auditory hallucinations can be experienced in both ways. And the DSM-5 accepts both voices from inside and outside the head as representing hallucinatory phenomena.

The concept of the apparent localizability of a hallucination might be better viewed with regard to whether a voice is heard within the mind (which has no location) or outside the mind (where a location can be assigned). With some patients, the voice is heard only within the mind. In contrast, with many hallucinations the voice can be physically located, and this location may even be reported as being inside the patient's head as with "A radio transmitter is broadcasting from inside my head, where my neighbor implanted it." The internal terrain of the body can actually represent a geographic space and a source of hallucinatory phenomena in this regard. With other patients, the voice is heard as coming through the ear, on the surface of the body, or anywhere in external space.[18]

Copolov and colleagues reviewed the literature devoted to the location of auditory hallucinations and performed a study on these phenomena. They found that 34.5% of their patients reported hearing the voices inside their heads, 27.9% outside their heads, and 37.6% both inside and outside; these proportions were similar to the previous studies they reviewed.[19] There appeared to be little clinical significance – in terms of severity of symptoms and the patient distress – when comparing where the patients perceived their voices originating.

There was evidence that patients who heard their voices internally tended to exhibit better reality testing and distance from their psychotic process than patients who heard their voices externally. Counter-intuitively, however, patients who heard command hallucinations only *externally*, reported being able *to resist the commands more effectively* than patients who heard them only internally or both internally and externally. We will discuss the significance and techniques for exploring command hallucinations shortly.

On a diagnostic note, it is important to be on the lookout for the relatively rare disorder of dissociative identity disorder (DID; previously known as multiple personality disorder). In this disorder, patients may internally hear the voices of their alters. Keep in mind that if a patient reports hearing voices internally, it is unlikely that he or she has dissociative identity disorder. It is *much* more likely that the patient has schizophrenia or some other psychotic disorder. Note that in DID the voices will generally not be imbedded in a psychotic matrix as described in Chapter 11. Thus in DID one does not tend to see elements such as delusional mood, delusional perception, and other phenomena suggestive of a budding psychotic process, a useful point for discriminating between the voices of DID and the voices seen in psychotic disorders such as schizophrenia.

The Reality of Auditory Hallucinations to the Patient

Auditory hallucinations are viewed as veridical perceptual phenomena, a term that simply means that patients frequently are convinced of the veracity or realness of the hallucinations. On the other hand, each patient is a unique individual and their distance (insight) from these hallucinatory phenomena can vary. In an interview it is useful to explore what a patient means if he or she comments that his or her voices sound real. Such patients, upon more detailed interviewing, may tell the clinician that the voices are quite real but do not sound exactly like normal voices. It is not uncommon for psychotic patients to be able to identify their hallucinations as abnormal. Sometimes they may even have names for them.

If a clinician is attempting to decide whether or not a patient is faking hallucinations, these points become important. A patient who is malingering may tend to describe the voices as sounding exactly like normal voices, which remains possible in psychosis but is not typical. The malingerer may also describe the voices as happening all of a sudden, unaware that hard psychotic symptoms usually have subtle prodromal phases such as delusional mood and delusional perception. Moreover, the voices found in processes such as schizophrenia are frequently hostile in nature and often hurl nasty and/or obscene insults at the patient.

The following type of question can be useful in recognizing malingered hallucinations:

"Have you ever found that, on a very good day when you have really been feeling fine, out of nowhere, the voices start in on you, just like that, out of nowhere?" (a positive response is suggestive of malingering)

Distinction Between Auditory Hallucinations and Auditory Illusions

The difference between auditory hallucinations and auditory illusions is the same as the difference between visual hallucinations and visual illusions; this latter we discussed in Chapter 11. An auditory hallucination occurs *without* any auditory stimulus, whereas an auditory illusion is a distortion of an actual sound. Thus, an example of an *auditory illusion* would be a paranoid patient hearing the words, "I hate you. I'm going to slit your throat" when his friend actually said, "I'd never be late for you. I'm going to be exactly where I told you I'd be before." Obviously, an auditory illusion can be as frightening or as dangerous as an actual auditory hallucination.

Another distinction should be made. There is an odd phenomenon known as a functional auditory hallucination. In this process, an external sound triggers, sometimes fairly consistently, an actual auditory hallucination. Both the triggering sound and the auditory hallucination are heard quite clearly without any distortion.[20] For instance, the sound of a phone ringing triggers a hallucination of a neighbor's voice denigrating the patient from the next apartment. Both the sound of the phone ringing and the sound of the neighbor's voice are distinct and heard clearly without distorting one another. Thus, in a functional hallucination, the extraneous environmental sound merely functions as a trigger for the auditory hallucination.

The Uniqueness of Auditory Hallucinations

From the perspective of person-centered interviewing, it is critical to understand that hallucinations, although they may share various characteristics among patients as we have been describing, are, ultimately, phenomenologically unique to each person experiencing them. In a wonderful paper, Stephane and colleagues[21] have described the phenomenological structure of auditory verbal hallucinations.

They found that voices vary along 20 phenomena and continua. For instance, voices differ in their acoustic qualities from clear (like external speech) to deep (like internal speech or thinking in words). Other acoustic qualities included the personification (male, female, robot) and loudness. Another variable is of the time course of the hallucinatory process (constant versus episodic). The linguistics of the voices can clearly vary as in the syntax (first person, second person, or third person) and the complexity of the communication (hearing words versus sentences versus conversations). Yet another prominent feature was what Stephane called the "affective relatedness," a rather fancy name for whether the voices were comforting or pleasurable versus frightening or bothersome. Considering that Stephane and colleagues found over 15 other characteristics, one can see that voices can present with remarkable variation from person to person. Table 12.1 summarizes Stephanes's phenomenological categories.

Schneiderian Symptoms Related to Auditory Hallucinations

Kurt Schneider provides further insight into the qualities that may impact on how a particular patient experiences his or her voices. As you will recall, three of Schneider's 11 first-rank symptoms concern voices. One of these symptoms consists of the patient experiencing audible thoughts. In this phenomenon, the patient hears his or her thoughts just after having the thought, almost like an internal echo. Alternatively, the patient may hear an undecipherable voice, the content of the speech only becoming clear a few seconds after hearing it. The other two Schneiderian symptoms consist of arguing voices and multiple voices commenting on the patient's activities, patterns of hallucinatory dialogue that are not uncommon in schizophrenia.

The Relationship Between the Patient and the Patient's Voices

It is not only the clinician that has many questions to ask regarding voices. Each patient experiencing voices is seeking answers to a plethora of pressing questions relating to his or her personal relationship to the voices themselves. To the patient, each voice has its own demands and supposed expectations, much like a family member or friend. Patients are frequently searching for answers to the following types of questions: (1) Is this voice real or unreal? (2) Who or what is creating it? (3) Does it mean me harm or good?

Table 12.1 Phenomenological Forms of Auditory Verbal Hallucinations.

FORMS	DIMENSIONS	CHARACTERISTICS
Acoustic qualities	Clarity	Clear (like external speech) vs. deep (like internal speech/thinking in words)
	Personification	Man's voice, woman's voice, or other agent (alien, robot, etc.)
	Loudness	Softer vs. louder vs. similar to normal conversational volume
Location	Inner space	In the head, or other parts of the body
	Outer space	
Number of voices	One, more than one	
Direction	Voices talk among themselves	
	Voices talk to the patient	
Linguistic	Syntax	First (I) vs. second (you, name) vs. third person (he/she, name)
	Complexity	Hearing words vs. hearing sentences vs. hearing conversations
Content	Range	Repetitive vs. systematized
	Focus	Self vs. non-self
Order	First order (hear voices)	
	Second order (talk back to the voices)	
	Third order (converse with the voices)	
Replay	Experiential (heard in real life)	
	Arising from patient's speech	
	Arising from patient's thoughts	
Source attribution	Self	
	Other	Someone familiar, God/spiritual being, or deceased person
Time course	Time dimension	Constant vs. episodic
	Modulation	Worsening vs. improving
Mode of occurrence	Spontaneous	
	Triggered	By intentional will or by other triggers
Happens when	Speaking or listening to speech	
	Listening to non-speech sounds	
	Doing activities requiring attention	
Control strategies	Listening to speech or speaking	
	Listening to non-speech sounds	
	Doing activities requiring attention	
Affective relatedness	Comforting	
	Bothersome/intrusive	

From Waters F. Auditory hallucinations in psychiatric illness. *Psychiatr Times* 2010;**27**(3):54–58. Based on Stephane M, Thuras P, Nasrallah H, Georgopoulos AP. The internal structure of the phenomenology of auditory verbal hallucinations. *Schizophr Res* 2003;**61**:185–193.

(4) Will it go away when I want it to go away or am I stuck with it? (5) Do other people hear it? (6) Can it read my thoughts? (7) Does it want me to do something? (8) Must I do what it wants?

Waters elegantly describes how the answers to such questions coalesce to create a powerful relationship for the patient, a relationship that can match or exceed the importance of relationships with actual family members, friends, or society at large:

> *The content of voices is usually highly personalized. The voices frequently express what the person is feeling or thinking and speak about his or her fears or worries. Psychiatric patients view the content of voices to be meaningful and to have personal relevance. The voices are interpreted to be the manifestation of real people or entities, and this experience contributes to the intense emotional response to the voices. The personalized content and subjective reality of voices play a role in the development of strong beliefs about the intent and power of the voices, and a complicated and intense relationship frequently ensues between patients and their voices.*[22]

Patients search for answers to their questions about the nature of their voices upon their very first "contact" with them. The following excerpt lucidly presents the eerie world created by such a first meeting:

> *Seated on a steamer chair on the boardwalk of Coney Island, I heard the voice for the first time. It was as positive and persistent as any voice I had ever heard. It said slowly, "Jayson, you are worthless. You've never been useful, and you've never been any good." I shook my head unbelievingly, trying to drive out the sound of the words, and as if I had heard nothing, continued to talk with my neighbor. Suddenly, clearer, deeper, and even louder than before, the deep voice came at me again, right in my ear this time, and getting me tight and shivery inside. "Larry Jayson, I told you before you weren't any good. Why are you sitting here making believe you're as good as anyone else when you're not? Whom are you fooling? You're no good," the voice said slowly in the same deep tones. "You've never been any good or use on earth. There is the ocean. You might as well drown yourself. Just walk in and keep walking." As soon as the voice was through, I knew, by its cold command, I had to obey it.*[23]

Uncovering and Sensitively Exploring Auditory Hallucinations

I find that sensitively and thoroughly exploring with a patient his or her hallucinatory phenomena frequently enhances engagement significantly. Patients can sense when a clinician truly wants to find out the nuances of their experiences and is not viewing the patient as a mere "case" with symptomatic DSM-5 criteria, but as a unique individual with highly personalized symptoms and beliefs about those symptoms. In addition, it can be immensely useful to uncover the phenomenology of the patient's hallucinations, for subtle changes in this phenomenology may provide the first signs that a particular antipsychotic or behavioral technique for minimizing the impact of voices is working (decreases in the frequency or intensity of the voices, movements of the voices inwards, increased distance from the voices, etc.).

In the last analysis, there exists no better method of learning about this topic than the experience of asking questions about auditory hallucinations to numerous people, ranging from psychotic to normal. Only in this manner will the clinician develop a sound sense of the range of normal and abnormal responses.

The question now becomes one of, "How do we approach uncovering the vast array of phenomena we have discussed above in a sensitive and effective manner?"

Sensitively Raising the Topic of Auditory Hallucinations

At the moment that an interviewer decides to raise the topic of auditory hallucinations in a interview, one of two very different situations may exist: (1) to that point in the interview, the patient has given no indication of being psychotic (the interviewer is not particularly suspicious of psychosis, but is screening to see if psychotic process may be present or has been experienced in the past), or (2) the patient has already given evidence of psychotic process in the interview.

Let us explore the first situation. We have already seen that psychotic process, even in disorders such as schizophrenia, can fluctuate greatly. The fact that a patient has not appeared psychotic to that point in the interview does not necessarily prove that the patient is not psychotic. Moreover, we have also seen that patients with personality disorders such as borderline, schizotypal, paranoid, narcissistic, and histrionic personality disorders may have experienced micropsychotic states in the past while appearing completely normal during the initial interview itself. Thus, all patients should be screened for psychotic process in an initial interview; the trick is to raise the topic of hallucinations in a sensitive fashion without disengaging them.

As we discussed, and I demonstrated in Video Module 4.1 in our chapter on facilics, the following type of question is one of my favorite ways of raising the topic of voices:

"When you are feeling very depressed, do your thoughts ever get so intense that they sound almost like a voice to you?"

The clinician can substitute words such as "anxious" or "stressed" or "upset" for the word "depressed" in the above question, choosing whatever emotion seems most appropriate for a specific patient.

The wording of this question allows the topic to be broached in a non-affrontive fashion, because the interviewer is tying the phenomenon directly into the patient's pain. It is further softened by the clinician's use of the words *"like a voice,"* a phrasing that offers a reassuring "backdoor" to the reluctant patient who might fear being viewed as "crazy." He or she might respond with something like, "Not really a voice, but sort of like one." If this is the case, further inquiry by the interviewer may reveal that the patient is actually experiencing hallucinations.

Various other options exist for unobtrusively raising the topic of hallucinations in a patient who has not demonstrated psychotic process to that point in the interview. The following question is used in the *Schedules for Clinical Assessment in Neuropsychiatry*[24]:

"Do you ever seem to hear noises or voices when there is nobody about, and no ordinary explanation seems possible?"

Now let us turn our attention to the second situation – the patient has already demonstrated psychotic material in the interview. For instance, a patient may already have talked about a delusional system. In such situations, it is useful to try to seamlessly tie the inquiry about auditory hallucinations to the patient's delusional story. Thus, a patient who has been describing paranoid delusions about a neighbor named Fred can be asked the following question, "Do you ever hear Fred's voice when he is not actually present in the room with you?" or "Do you ever feel that Fred is trying to talk with you or direct your thoughts from his house or when you are at work?"

Sensitively Exploring the Phenomenology of Auditory Hallucinations Once Raised

Once the topic of auditory hallucinations has been sensitively raised, the clinician faces the important task of exploring the patient's voices phenomenologically. This means that an effort is made to better understand the uniqueness of the specific patient's hallucinations as described above, ranging from concrete characteristics (such as loudness, frequency, and content) to more abstract characteristics (such as the patient's relationship with the voice or voices). The following questions, *in whatever order seems natural to use with a specific patient*, can be used to explore the phenomenology of the patient's voices once raised in the initial interview and in subsequent sessions. Generally, it is not possible to ask all of these questions in an initial interview because of time constraints, but you can pick and choose from this list:

a. "Tell me what the voices sound like to you."
b. "Do they sound just like real voices or can you tell the difference?"
c. "How do you tell the difference?"
d. "Some patients tell me they hear their voices only inside their heads, and other patients tell me they hear them only outside their heads, and some patients tell me they hear them both inside and outside of their heads. How do you hear your voices?"
e. "Are they loud or soft?"
f. "How often do you hear them?"
g. "Are they male or female or something else?"
h. "Do you recognize who is talking to you?"
i. "Do you have a name for the voice?"
j. "What does the voice say to you?"
k. "Do your voices sometimes taunt you or say mean things about you?"
l. "Do they ever say nice things to you?"
m. "Does the voice ever tell you to hurt yourself?" (looking for command hallucinations to self-mutilate such as enucleation of an eye or castration)
n. "Does the voice ever tell you to kill yourself?"
o. "Does the voice ever tell you hurt someone else or kill someone else?"
p. "Do you think they are real or do you think they are created by your imagination?"
q. "Do you wish they would stay or go away?"

r. "Do you do anything to try to stop them or make them go away?"

s. "When you first heard the voices, what did you think they were?"

t. "What feelings do you have as you hear the voices?"

u. "Do you ever hear several voices talking to each other about you?"

Although it is not possible, nor perhaps advisable, to cover all of these questions in an initial assessment, *when a patient relates hearing voices, one should always ask about command hallucinations.* Furthermore, if one becomes the treating clinician for the patient, the above list becomes an excellent doorway, over the course of ensuing sessions, for achieving a better understanding of the patient's hallucinatory phenomena.

Illustrative Transcript of a Clinician Exploring Auditory Hallucinations

To bring the above techniques and interviewing strategies to life, let us examine a brief, direct transcript from one of my interviews. The patient, whom we shall call Kenney, self-referred to a psychiatric assessment center during summer school. He was dressed in a casual short-sleeved shirt with shorts that seemed to be a bit tighter than necessary. Kenney presented with a pleasant affect, and an engaging naiveté, telling the charge nurse, "I just stopped by because I think I might benefit from some counseling, I'm really feeling uptight." Apparently, Kenney had benefited from counseling provided by the outpatient department associated with this assessment center a year earlier.

For the first 15 minutes of the interview, Kenney appeared like many other anxious and over-worked college students, complaining of feeling overwhelmed at school and overwhelmed by the prospect of dating, which he was terrified of doing but really wanted to be doing.

Deeper into the interview, I decided to use a technique for indirectly uncovering psychotic process, described earlier (tapping odd language or idiosyncratic phrasing – see Chapter 11, page 474). I asked Kenney to explain in more detail what he had meant when he had said earlier in the interview that, "the pressure I feel in my head to achieve is so intense it's like there is a guy inside me pushing me all the time." I didn't expect to find anything psychotic, but I was just making sure, for the intensity of Kenney's anxiety represented a "soft sign" of potential psychotic process. I gently asked Kenney to explain what he meant by the statement. To my surprise, my question tapped a veritable powder keg of psychotic process. Kenney shared a highly disturbing delusional system in which he believed he was possessed by a demon.

We will pickup the interview at a point where Kenney had been describing in some detail the demon that had invaded him and at which juncture I decided to raise the topic of auditory hallucinations. I used some of the questions listed above to better understand the phenomenology of Kenney's hallucinations. Note the way in which these questions can help a patient to share the unique personal quality of their hallucinations. In this instance, from a psychodynamic perspective, Kenney's exceptionally overactive superego distinctly flavors his hallucinatory process:

> **Pt.:** The only way to describe it is … it's another guy. And that's a very good way to describe it – it is another guy.
>
> **Clin.:** Once again to me, it sounds like a very frightening type of experience – to feel like there is this thing inside you. (said gently)

> **Pt.:** Yeah, it is, like (pauses) … like, I mean I feel sorry for other people that it's happening to.
>
> **Clin.:** Do you ever hear his voice?
>
> **Pt.:** I don't actually hear it. Well, I don't actually hear it in my ears, but somehow I hear it.
>
> **Clin.:** When you are having that experience, does it sound exactly like your normal thoughts, or are you quite aware that something different is happening and you are hearing his voice?
>
> **Pt.:** It's a feeling, like … it sounds like my thoughts, but they're a little bit different, the way I hear them.
>
> **Clin.:** And how do you hear them?
>
> **Pt.:** They just seem to come to me. (reflects for a moment) … They just seem to come to me.
>
> **Clin.:** Does the voice ever tell you to hurt yourself?
>
> **Pt.:** Yeah, that's what it's telling me.
>
> **Clin.:** What exactly will it say?
>
> **Pt.:** Well, he'll say (pauses) … he'll find another way to do it … Like he'll say, like don't study, do bad on the test. And that's his way of saying, "Hurt myself." And once I do bad on the test, it will be easy for him to talk to me. It will be hard to not listen to him.
>
> **Clin.:** It changes if you feel you have failed at some level?
>
> **Pt.:** I can hear him louder.
>
> **Clin.:** Does he ever tell you to cut yourself or to take pills or anything like that?
>
> **Pt.:** He tells me a little bit, and it makes me feel that way also. He'll hint sort of. No, he'll tell me, he'll tell me.
>
> **Clin.:** What will he say?
>
> **Pt.:** He'll say mostly, (whispers) "Do it." He'll say, "Do it." Scary …
>
> **Clin.:** Yeah, it is, I'm sure it is. (Kenney nervously smiles)

When first asked about command hallucinations ("Does the voice ever tell you to hurt yourself"), it is fascinating to see that Kenney's first response is that the voices command him to hurt himself by hurting his grades, a clever punitive superego if ever there was one! Only upon subsequent, specific questioning about physically dangerous commands ("Does he ever tell you to cut yourself or to take pills or anything like that?") am I able to uncover commands that are much more dangerous in nature.

Exploring Command Hallucinations

Command hallucinations are defined as any voice that tells a patient to perform a specific act. Such commands may range from telling the patient to go for a walk to imploring the patient to harm himself or others. Their presence, in some instances (e.g., when suggesting violence), may strongly suggest the need for prompt hospitalization, sometimes immediately. Often knowledge of dangerous command hallucinations is not volunteered by the patient, as witnessed by Kenney above. Consequently, the clinician must actively inquire about their existence.

In the 1980s various papers purported that there appeared to be little or no statistical correlation between command hallucinations and dangerous activities such as suicide.[25-28] However, if one looks at these papers, it becomes evident that none of the research carefully categorized the hallucinatory phenomena along the critical predictive phenomenological variables that we shall examine below. Indeed, the research was generally based on hospital charts, which are notorious for poor reporting of the nuances of patient phenomenology. No one knows whether these voices were at one end or the other end of the continuum of dangerousness. Consequently, the statistical analyses were, in my opinion, essentially meaningless.

In contrast, a well-designed quantitative study by Shawyer and colleagues demonstrated that some patients do, indeed, act upon command hallucinations, exactly as clinicians have reported over decades of experience.[29] Furthermore, they isolated several statistical factors that were correlated with an increased likelihood of a patient acting upon his or her command hallucinations, including: increased age of the patient, the view by the patient that the command is positive and will have beneficial results (e.g., killing a neighbor will end poverty), and that the command hallucination is tied in tightly with a well-developed delusional system. In their study, antipsychotic medication proved to be protective.

In addition, using a phenomenological research framework, Junginger directly interviewed patients in great detail who had recently experienced command hallucinations, to investigate the likelihood that a patient might act upon the command.[30] Of the 20 patients who experienced dangerous command hallucinations, eight acted on them, providing rather striking support for the potential dangerousness of command hallucinations.

It is hoped that future research, well grounded both in phenomenology and empirical studies, will provide better guidelines for predicting the dangerousness of command hallucinations. However, even if better statistics become available, it is crucial to remember that an act of violence is not merely a statistical event. It is a phenomenological one as well, determined by the unique processes at work during a specific moment in time in a unique individual's psyche. Any given patient may kill himself or herself or another person, whether the statistics suggest that he or she is at risk to do so or not. Apparently, patients are not always aware of the statistical rules that they are meant to follow.

As we await better research studies to guide our predictions of dangerousness related to command hallucinations, it remains the task of each individual interviewer to explore the personal nature of the patient's experience of his or her command hallucinations. Such explorations, admittedly subjective in nature, may still represent our best chance to reasonably foresee a dangerous act and potentially prevent it.

Phenomenologically speaking, command hallucinations are not black or white experiences, in the sense that the patient either has them or does not. In actuality, command hallucinations can differ in numerous ways. Some of the defining characteristics include the content of the commands, the auditory quality of the commands (loudness, duration, and frequency), the degree to which the patient feels able to resist the commands, and the emotional impact on the patient (does the patient know the voice and what is the patient's perceived attitude of the voice towards himself or herself). In my opinion, all of these variables could have an impact on how dangerous the command hallucinations might be.

With these variables in mind, command hallucinations can vary from being relatively innocuous phenomena with little frequency and impact on the patient to dangerous phenomena in which the voices incessantly hammer at the patient in an effort to provoke violence. Some people who suffer from chronic schizophrenia have adapted to their voices and pay them little heed. I am reminded of a 65-year-old vet I was initially interviewing to follow in a VA clinic, who, when asked about command hallucinations, responded, with a twinkle in his eye, "Doc, don't get bent out of shape. The Devil has been telling me to kill myself since I was 16 years old. I didn't listen to him then, and I'm sure as hell not gonna listen to him now." His command hallucinations, even though related to violence, were of minimal concern. At the other end of the continuum, command hallucinations can be acutely harassing, loud, insistent, and dangerous. The question now is: How do we explore the characteristics of these potentially dangerous phenomena?

Exploring the Content of Command Hallucinations

Command hallucinations can clearly vary in dangerousness depending upon their content. Any voice that tells the patient to do something is a command hallucination. On the benign side, the voice might command the patient to "Shut the door," or "Change your profile picture on Facebook." On a more humorous note regarding ourselves, it is not uncommon for a voice to tell a patient during an interview, "Don't listen to this guy," or "Don't answer his questions, he's an idiot!" At the other end of the continuum, command hallucinations can push for highly dangerous activities towards the self ("Cut your eye out!" or "Just shoot yourself, just pull the damn trigger, you asshole!") or towards other people ("Push him in front of the subway!" or "Slit his throat!"). Swearing and viciousness commonly accompany command hallucinations, in some instances increasing the likelihood that the patient may act upon them because of the ferocity of their tone.

Clearly, the more dangerous the content, the more concern for safety the clinician will have. However, even if the commands are quite benign, once a voice has begun to give commands the clinician should routinely follow up with the patient in future sessions, to see if the voice advances from benign to dangerous content. Once command hallucinations have begun, such an advance towards violent content may be forthcoming.

With command hallucinations, the simplest of questions is often the best for their elicitation, such as, "Do your voices ever tell you to do things?" If the patient answers yes, then one can simply follow up with, "What do they tell you to do?" No matter what the patient says, at some point it is important to ask specifically about dangerousness, as with, "Do the voices ever tell you to hurt yourself or kill yourself?" This can then be followed by, "Do the voices ever tell you to hurt others or that you should kill someone?"

Exploring the Auditory Quality of Command Hallucinations

To some degree, the auditory quality of hallucinations can influence the amount of pressure they place upon the patient to act on them. I have been surprised at how loud patients report some hallucinations to be. Loudness, long repetitive duration of the commands, and high frequency of occurrence, especially if the patient reports being incessantly barraged by the voices, may all contribute to a greater likelihood of a patient acting upon the commands.

Once again, simple questioning around these issues are often the best such as, "How loud do the voices get?", "How often do you hear the commands?", "Does the voice repeat the commands to kill yourself over and over?", "Does the voice insist that you do so?"

Keep in mind that even though louder more frequent voices may be more compelling with most patients, for some patients even a whispered command may be enough to trigger violence, especially if it is being whispered by a highly valued or respected source.

Exploring the Degree to Which a Patient Feels Able to Resist a Command Hallucination

Patients may have surprisingly good insight into their ability to resist the entreaties of a command hallucination. It behooves clinicians to collaboratively tap their potential wisdom. Patient reassurances that they will not act are important, but limited in reliability. Conversely, patients' perspectives that they are not going to be able to control their urges to act should be taken very seriously. Indeed, sometimes the fear a patient has that he or she is about to do something that, at heart, he or she does not want to do is almost palpable to a clinician. Such patients are often relieved to be hospitalized; indeed, hospitalization is often required in these situations, whether voluntary or involuntary.

I find the following questions to be of value, and the interviewer can use any one or a combination of them. (Let us assume here, for the sake of clarity, that the patient has been describing voices coming from Satan.)

1. "To what extent do you think you can stop yourself from doing what Satan is asking you to do?"
2. "How concerned are you that you are going to do what Satan is asking you to do?"
3. "Should I, you, or your family be worried that you are going to do what Satan wants you to do?"

Another useful follow-up to these questions is, "Have you done anything to stop yourself from doing what Satan is asking you to do?" To such a question, a patient might respond, "Yeah, I took all of the knives in my house and put them in a shoebox and taped it all up with duct tape. Then I put it away up in the attic in a spot that is really hard to get to." Such a response provides some hints of safety, for it clearly shows that the patient is trying to protect himself and/or others. Looking at the dangerous side, however, the answer reveals how real the voice appears to the patient and the extent of the patient's own concern that he or she may act upon the command hallucinations. In either case, it is worthwhile information for the interviewer to know.

Exploring the Emotional Impact of Command Hallucinations on a Patient

Patients can respond with surprising diversity to their command hallucinations. If you will recall the 65-year-old vet I described earlier, he had grown accustomed to the Devil's jabber and essentially ignored it. His unconcerned response to a voice ascribed to a figure as culturally potent as the Devil is atypical in my experience, yet nicely highlights the uniqueness of each patient's response.

One avenue to explore is the importance and/or authority that the patient ascribes to the owner of the voice. When the voice is attributed to a powerful personal figure, whether alive or deceased (father, mother, spouse, intimate friend), well-known cultural icon (political figure, president, pope, or revered Hollywood icon), or an imagined supernatural figure (God, Satan, demon or angel), the patient may feel more pressure to comply with the orders of the voice.

This can be particularly dangerous, as implied by the research of Shawyer and colleagues, if the authoritative figure is tied into a concrete delusional system in which some greater good will occur if the patient complies with the entreaties of the voice. For instance, the patient may hear God saying that, "world peace will occur, if only you would slay your newborn child." Or a similar but contrasting example might be that during a postpartum psychotic episode, a mother believes that her newborn has been possessed by Satan and hears Satan yelling incessantly, "If you don't slit your own throat, I will torture your baby forever here and in eternity."

In addition to the patient's view of his or her relationship to the voice and the appropriateness to do what the voice wants to be done, the patient's perceived relationship to the owner of the voice as reflected by the actual tone of voice of the hallucination, may play a role in the dangerousness of the command hallucinations. In this respect, particularly vicious voices with denigrations, exhortations, and a malevolent tone of voice can, in my opinion, break down a person's natural desires to resist a voice. Indeed, a patient harangued incessantly by a voice may kill themselves to escape the voice or because the person is worried that he or she is about to give in to the voice's exhortations to hurt or kill another person. Throw some alcohol, street drugs, or sleeplessness into the picture and we may have an imminently dangerous situation.

Psychotic Disruptions in Cognition, Logic, and Communication

Besides abnormalities of perception, the psychotic patient's thought process itself is often disrupted by the psychotic process. Thoughts may become speeded up and racing in nature, as is also seen in mania. It becomes difficult to concentrate as evidenced by the following patient description:

> I just can't concentrate on anything. There's too much going on in my head and I can't sort it out. My thoughts wander around in circles without getting anywhere. I try to read even a paragraph in a book but it takes me ages because each bit I read starts me thinking in 10 different directions at once.[31]

This excerpt also hints at another disquieting characteristic sometimes seen. Psychotic thinking has an internally "contagious" quality to it, in the sense that it triggers a multitude of associations, sometimes close in nature and at other times distant and disjointed. This trend of creative but dystonic associations, which are not under the patient's control, is nicely captured in the following excerpt:

My trouble is that I've got too many thoughts. You might think about something – let's say that ashtray – and just think, oh yes, that's for putting my cigarette in, but I would think of it and then I would think of a dozen different things connected with it at the same time.[32]

This internal abnormality in thought process will frequently show itself externally with a loosening of associations (derailment) in the patient's speech. The characteristics of derailment will be examined in detail in Chapter 16 on the mental status.

At other times, thought processes may become, perhaps because of the previously mentioned abnormalities, somewhat disrupted. Patients may stop in midsentence and be unable to return to their original topic. This process, mentioned earlier, is known as thought blocking. It represents a strongly suggestive sign of psychosis. It is useful to quietly ask patients what has happened at these moments. Sometimes the patient's thought has been disrupted by an auditory hallucination. At other times the disruption is related to the patient experiencing thought withdrawal.

It is important to know if a patient is actively hearing voices during the interview, because the patient may feel that the clinician is producing the messages. Generally, it is not good for rapport to be perceived as commenting, "You're a drunken slob," or threatening, "I'm going to chop off your fingers." This actively hallucinatory state represents the type of situation in which violence can erupt towards the interviewer.

It has already become apparent that the patient's thought processes are frequently affected during a psychosis. Another common problem is the presence of truly illogical thought. One of the more frequent breakdowns in formal logic is the appearance of what Rosenbaum has called predicative thinking. This means that the person views things as similar or identical because they are connected by the same predicate (verb). The following example shows this process at work:

Major premise: Jesus Christ was persecuted.
Minor premise: I am persecuted.
Conclusion: Therefore, I am Jesus Christ.[33]

Other distinct problems with logic, as well as the emergence of magical thought as seen in young children, frequently accompany psychotic process. But it is not necessarily a phenomenon that is either present or not present. Many patients will demonstrate varying degrees of normal logic.

How to Safely Interact With an Illogical, Agitated Psychotic Patient

The recognition that a psychotic patient may be losing their ability to think logically is of immediate practical use when approaching a patient who is both psychotic and agitated. It is probably a mistake to assume, before talking with the patient, that he or she either can or cannot be talked down. Instead the interviewer should gently attempt to engage the patient in conversation. While doing this, the clinician can decide to what degree the patient's logic is intact. If it is reasonably intact, the interviewer may try to talk with the patient and perhaps alleviate some of the patient's anger. If, with this technique, the patient's anger begins to escalate or if it becomes subsequently apparent that the patient's logic is severely impaired, it is probably best to quickly back off from the patient and proceed with appropriate safety procedures.

To further attempt to reason with such a patient does not make much sense, because the patient is not processing the clinician's words in a normal fashion. Further interaction may push the patient towards violence. The key lies in carefully assessing the impact of one's interaction and proceeding appropriately.

A similar situation arises if the clinician discovers that the patient has incorporated the clinician into a delusional system. This brings to mind a patient whom I observed in an interview as a supervisor. She had a ragged appearance and sat in her chair spitting her words into a hostile world. As soon as I sat down she yelled out, "You're the one who called me a prostitute the other day. You're the one who has been spying on me!" I had never seen her before, and even if I had, I would not have spoken to her as she was suggesting.

No matter what I said in my defense she immediately grew angrier, and so I quickly shut up. Such a retreat is not only the better part of valor, but also represents a sound clinical maneuver, because this patient was not hearing a word that I was saying. It becomes easier to understand her hostile position if one realizes that she truly believed that I had belittled her publicly. Clinicians cannot quickly detach themselves from such a delusional web.

Unobtrusively Screening for Paranoid Process, Delusions, and Other Psychotic Process

The initial interviewer has much more access to the process of blending with non-agitated patients than with agitated patients. The question then becomes one of: How does one broach the subject of paranoia without offending a patient who has not shown signs of psychotic process to that point in the interview? The art is to enter the topic of paranoia by keying off the content of the patient's conversation, utilizing natural, implied, or referred gates as follows:

> **Pt.:** I don't know what to do with myself. I just, I just feel the whole thing is a mess. Probably, I don't know, probably the baby is not even aware of our arguments. When we were first married, everything was so much better. But when the mill shut down a third time and he lost his job for good, well it all became history.
>
> **Clin.:** It sounds like an ugly situation at home. Has the tension ever gotten so bad that he has struck you?
>
> **Pt.:** Thank God no. I'd leave him, honestly I would.
>
> **Clin.:** Do you think that in any way he is trying to hurt you, perhaps even trying to get your friends against you?
>
> **Pt.:** Oh he's tried to hurt me in the sense of making me feel guilt, but he knows better than to mess with me or my friends.

In this subtle fashion, the clinician has smoothly made a foray into the region of paranoid process. The patient's comments do not suggest the presence of paranoid ideation. There is probably no need to explore further for paranoia. With questioning such as that shown above, most paranoid patients would probably have nibbled at the "bait." The clinician has scouted for paranoid ideation without the patient having any idea that such an exploration of psychotic material has occurred.

This leads to the issue of broaching psychotic topics other than paranoia in a non-threatening fashion. For most interviewers this type of questioning is most difficult when interviewing a patient in whom the clinician doubts the presence of psychotic process. Some authors have suggested that interviewers should never ask questions about voices and other psychotic phenomena unless they strongly suspect their presence. To do so, they argue, will disengage the patient.

But, as we have already noted when we were discussing the life cycle of a psychotic process in the previous chapter, damaging psychopathology may be missed with such an approach. Psychotic process can fluctuate in disorders such as schizophrenia and bipolar disorder. Or it can be infrequently experienced as micropsychotic episodes seen with some personality disorders. Such patients may look remarkably intact during any given interview. For instance, if the interviewer chooses to not screen for psychotic process in the initial interview, he or she risks missing a painful yet treatable disorder such as schizotypal personality disorder.

There are other reasons that I have my doubts about such blanket avoidance of this area of questioning. In the first place, I have seldom, if ever, seen such questioning result in any lasting problems with engagement in a nonpsychotic patient. I have seen a handful of patients balk at it, but with skillful engagement techniques, the blending is quickly restored. Moreover, most patients do not seem offended at all. Thus I generally ask all my patients about psychotic process at some point in the initial interview

But there is another reason to ask about psychotic phenomena, even when psychosis is not apparent – a very practical one. When patients do initially balk at such questioning, their emotional over-reactions provide a window into their defenses and psychodynamics, as seen in the following reconstructed dialogue. Let's return for a moment to an interviewer raising the topic of auditory hallucinations. The interviewer happened to be me, and I was using one of my favorite questions for doing so:

> Pt.: Let's get it straight, things have been tough all over for everybody involved and I've been damn upset.
>
> Clin.: When you are really feeling upset, have your thoughts ever gotten so intense and bothersome that they sound almost like a voice?
>
> Pt.: Oh great, here come the crazy questions (said angrily). Well I got news for you. I'm not crazy and I've been asked all those questions before. (The patient reaches over and squeezes her boyfriend's hand, smiling at him while subsequently tossing a little sneer towards me.)

This hostile display was far from the typical response that I generally receive to this question. Indeed, it suggested to me that, from a psychodynamic perspective, this patient was experiencing a narcissistic insult from my question. It led me to wonder why she might need to do so, opening a window into an interior pain that might lie just below the surface of her anger.

Her atypical response alerted me to be particularly gentle with future questions as well as suggesting the wisdom of looking for possible personality dysfunction in my subsequent social history later in that same interview. Such idiosyncratic responses may suggest the expansion of diagnostic categories not considered earlier. In this case, further interviewing revealed that she was coping with a full-blown borderline personality.

Once entering the facilic content region regarding psychotic process, it is not necessary to beat it into the ground. Quickly, the clinician will achieve some idea as to whether the region is worth expanding further. If hints of psychotic process emerge, then a full expansion may be warranted. If no hints emerge, the topic may be left after only a few probe questions. Part of the art lies in learning how to smoothly enter these psychotic regions.

Some questions that may be used effectively as gates into psychotic material are shown below:

a. "Have you had experiences that seemed odd or frightening to you?"
b. "Earlier we talked about your nightmares. Have you ever had similar types of frightening images bothering you during the day?"
c. "You had been talking about some of your talents. Have you ever felt that you had some unusual abilities such as ESP?"
d. "You mentioned earlier that one of your favorite activities is watching TV (or YouTube). Have you ever been frightened by the TV (or YouTube)?" Depending on what the patient says, one might pursue this with a question such as: "Did it ever seem like the people on TV (or YouTube) were watching you or that they literally were aware of private aspects of your life?"
e. "When you are on Twitter, do you ever feel that tweets from strangers or famous people are actually about you or directed to you personally?"
f. "You had mentioned earlier that your sister had apparently been hearing voices. Have you ever had similar experiences?"

Another excellent method of entering psychotic material is through the discussion of religious issues as shown below:

> **Pt.:** I have always been a fairly religious person. My father was a devout Lutheran. Religion runs in our family.
>
> **Clin.:** On a moment-by-moment basis, how much is God a part of your life?
>
> **Pt.:** (long pause) He is my life and my breath, so be it.
>
> **Clin.:** It sounds like He is a very important part of your life. Sometimes people who are close to God feel that He has a special mission or role for them to play. Do you feel that you may be lucky enough that God has such a role for you?
>
> **Pt.:** Yes, I do. I am to bring peace to all nations. And I shall bring a calmness to all that I touch.

Clearly it would be worth exploring the psychotic region more thoroughly with this patient. But the important issue from our viewpoint is the naturalness of the gate provided by religious discussion. Even as the topic was first entered, the intensity of the patient's feelings probably suggested to the clinician that something was up.

Understanding the Demoralization and Self-Denigration Spurred by Psychotic Process

Thus far we have focused on the complex impact of psychotic process on specific aspects of psychological functioning, such as perception and thought process. This impact is indeed both terrifying and terrible. But what of the "self"? What is the impact of chronic psychotic process and of the deficit (negative) symptoms of diseases like schizophrenia upon a person's self-image and self-respect?

In many ways, I feel that this impact is the most damaging of all. As we saw earlier, the negative symptoms of schizophrenia, such as low interest, low drive, and low energy are powerful and insidious, often lingering indefinitely, long after the voices and delusions have faded. Almost all people coping with schizophrenia initially view these symptoms not as part of the disease but as symbols of their own inadequacy as people. As the deficit symptoms make it difficult, and at times impossible, to work, people frequently get caught up in a vicious process of self-belittlement. Sometimes frustrated and weary family members feed this cycle by misinterpreting these negative symptoms as laziness and psychological weakness, and they wonder, "The voices are gone so why doesn't he just get a job and get on with his life?"

As patients watch their siblings and friends go on to develop successful marriages, careers, and identities, they find themselves left behind in a race that seems unwinnable. It is very easy, and all too human, to decide it is not worth the risk of failure to enter such a race. The patient soon finds himself or herself intensely afraid of further humiliation. Many patients find themselves lost in a labyrinth of self-doubt, and they often adopt a role as "the black sheep" of the family. This intense demoralization, which is often at its worst between psychotic episodes (when the negative symptoms adamantly persist), is often the prelude to suicide, as we shall discuss in Chapter 17.

Schizophrenia rapes the soul. From the very first interview, it is important for the clinician to remember that one of the main tasks in intervention is to help the patient heal this pain and to believe in himself or herself again. People with schizophrenia should not be pitied. Indeed, some of the most courageous and "tough" individuals whom I have had the pleasure to meet are coping with this traumatizing disease with dignity and resourcefulness. This recovery process begins in the very first interview.

For the clinician it begins with the realization that we are all "people" first. The patient's "diagnosis," albeit very important, plays a secondary role in our understanding. This feeling grows, with experience, as we clinicians truly realize that the person in front of us is not a medical term but a person just like ourselves. We, too, or our friends or family members, could develop bipolar disorder or schizophrenia. Like death, mental illness respects no social, educational, or economic boundaries.

For the patient, it begins with a realization that he or she is not a disease entity but a person coping with a disease. In this sense, I think that it is best for both the clinician and the patient to abandon terms such as "schizophrenic." Such terms insidiously lead to stigmatization and identification with the disease. I have never met a schizophrenic. But I have met many different people coping with schizophrenia. This distinction may be subtle, but it is telling.

I am convinced that this sense of respect and empowerment from a clinician shows through in the very first encounter with the patient. Clinicians who convey this perspective often have much more success both in the initial interview and in all subsequent work. Clinicians who do *not* convey this feeling are often sitting alone in their offices during follow-up appointments.

This perspective is elegantly described by Patricia Deegan in an article that I highly recommend, "Recovery: The Lived Experience of Rehabilitation":

> *It is important to understand that persons with a disability do not "get rehabilitated" in the sense that cars "get" tuned up or televisions "get repaired." Disabled persons are not passive recipients of rehabilitation services. Rather, they experience themselves as recovering a new sense of self and of purpose within and beyond the limits of the disability. This distinction between rehabilitation and recovery is important. Rehabilitation refers to the services and technologies that are made available to disabled persons so that they might learn to adapt to their world. Recovery refers to the lived or real life experience of persons as they accept and overcome the challenge of the disability.*[34]

The understanding, from this section, of the damage incurred on the psychological wing of a patient's matrix is at the very heart of the healing process that first begins in the initial interview. It also conveys the delicate interplays that occur between individuals dealing with chronic psychotic disorders and the people around them. Let's take a closer look at these interactions in a broader sense.

III. The Dyadic Wing of the Matrix

Uncovering Social Withdrawal and Recognizing Social Inappropriateness

It is not infrequent for people with psychotic process to become socially withdrawn. In particular, when the psychosis is secondary to schizophrenia, episodes of social withdrawal are extremely frequent.[35] This social withdrawal could be related to the tendency for the patient to enter a more autistic world. In an effort to sort out the tremendous number of peculiar sensations and thoughts, the person suffering from a psychotic process may find it necessary to withdraw. Social contact becomes painfully disruptive. In other patients in whom aggressive drives may be building to a pitch, people may be avoided because of a fear of loss of control.

However, there is another aspect to this entire issue that brings us directly to the dyadic system itself. Frequently, people coping with schizophrenia will display behaviors that are socially inappropriate. As we saw in Chapter 8 on nonverbal behavior, psychotic patients often show some disturbance in the normal nonverbal rules of conversation. This may range from sitting or standing inappropriately close to the clinician (creating an uncomfortable sense of immediacy in other people) to displaying odd or restricted affects (creating a sense of puzzlement or disconnectedness in other people). Because of the tremendous need of these patients to attend to the troubled thoughts in their own minds their ability to empathize is frequently strikingly diminished.

The Impact of Psychotic Process on the Interviewer's Emotions and Behaviors

Clinicians should also be aware of their own feelings of confusion that may develop as they interview patients experiencing psychotic process. This confusion in the clinician may be caused by psychotic processes in the patient, such as a subtle loosening of associations or bits of illogical thought. If the clinician can recognize his or her own subjective feeling of confusion, then a more thorough pursuit of psychotic process and content may be wise. The confusion in the clinician mirrors the confusion or disorganization of the patient.

A word of caution seems in order here. Clinicians lucky enough to be gifted with a particularly intuitive sense of empathy can fall into a trap. The patient may be displaying subtle signs of disorganized thought, but the clinician ignores these signs because he or she understands "what the patient is thinking." Indeed the clinician might understand; however, the patient is still psychotic. When hunting for evidence of formal thought disorder (problems in the formation of thought such as a loosening of associations), the question is not whether we understand the patient but whether a non-professional, perhaps sitting beside the patient on a bus, would understand the patient. At the other extreme, sometimes a well-trained clinician will recognize a formal thought disorder before it would even be evident to a layperson.

All of the above disturbances in dyadic communication may lead to an uncomfortable sensation in a clinician. The sensation has been described as not being able "to feel" with the patient, in short, an inability to experience an empathic bond with the patient. This peculiar sensation has been called the "precox feeling."[36] It is felt to be particularly suggestive of schizophrenia. Used appropriately, as an intuitive guide suggesting the need to carefully explore for the criteria of schizophrenia, the precox feeling is a useful tool. It should never be used as a criterion of schizophrenia or as a justification for labeling someone as having schizophrenia.

People with psychotic process can also create feelings of frustration in the initial interviewer. This may result when the patient's lack of insight results in the patient rejecting avenues of help such as case management, psychotherapy, medication, or hospitalization. It can be particularly frustrating to work with a paranoid patient who clearly needs help but feels strongly that "nothing is wrong with me."

In these instances, it is important to accept the naturalness of one's frustration while avoiding a demonstration of this frustration to the patient. These countertransference problems tend to surface as extensive and sometimes heated attempts to convince the patient of his or her illness. Such attempts are probably far more counterproductive than they are productive. It is often best to calmly discuss one's views and then acknowledge openly that the patient and oneself seem to have a difference of opinion as with:

"Well, we obviously disagree on whether or not you have bipolar disorder, and that's okay, we can agree to disagree (said calmly and with a genuine sincerity). I will always share with you what I really believe, and I know that you will do the same with me. And I appreciate your doing so today. We simply have differing opinions on this, and you are certainly entitled to your own opinion. And, of course, I could be wrong. Only time will help both of us to sort out exactly what is going on."

The patient should know that if he or she feels a desire to talk again or experiences a change of opinion, that the clinician is always available for another meeting.

Frustration may also evolve when the interviewer feels that a patient is somehow in control of the psychotic process, "flipping it on" when it is advantageous to do so. At some level this manipulation may actually occur on both the conscious and unconscious plane.

I remember a man about 30 years old who initially spoke in a disorganized and delusion-littered fashion. As he felt more comfortable with me his thinking became more organized. When I subsequently probed even in a subtle fashion into his personal life, he would quickly become disorganized and mumble about "the cheesedogs that were going to drop a nuclear warhead on Pittsburgh." Oddly enough I do not think he was particularly conscious of this process.

One can better conceptualize such behavior if one assumes that at some level, to the degree that the patient has both insight and motivation, the patient may be able to partially rein in psychotic process. I believe that this tendency to hide potentially embarrassing psychotic material would be a natural one. This self-modulation must require a considerable amount of effort and concentration. Perhaps at times, and depending on the interpersonal situation, the patient might find it simply easier to just let things go as they may. At such points, the psychotic process may emerge in a more pressing fashion as seen above. To the degree that we understand this process, our frustration levels may decrease.

Frustration may also arise with patients suffering from schizophrenia who are persistently negative during the interview. As Michels suggests, the interviewer may gently point out that automatically saying "No" to everything is as much a relinquishment of control as saying "Yes" to all the clinician's requests.[37] Jointly agreeing upon a topic to discuss may also open up avenues for better engagement.

The Impact of the Interviewer's Behaviors on Psychotic Process

Thus far the emphasis has been on the patient's effect on the clinician. With patients dealing with psychotic process, it is also important to realize that clinicians may need to monitor their own impact on the patient. In Chapter 1 (see pages 23–27) we discussed in detail some of the changes in style that may help to facilitate blending with paranoid patients, such as decreasing the use of empathic statements with a high valence regarding implied certainty or intuited attribution. It is also important to realize that, because of disturbances in logic and reality testing, normally well-received statements by a clinician may be hostilely received. Michels points out, for instance, that with one of his patients the word "leg" had taken on a highly sexualized meaning.[38] Consequently, when the clinician would use the word, it was received as a sexual topic, probably carrying a variety of unwanted overtones.

Sometimes when people struggling with psychotic process are cooperative but frightened, it goes a long way to simply reassure them that they are in a safe environment. Especially if such patients are disorganized as well as frightened, it is useful to tell them what is happening, to ask them to raise any questions they may have, and to structure the interview for them. If the patient is forced to handle an unstructured interview, filled with open-ended questions, gentle commands, and pregnant pauses, the interview itself may become traumatizing. Gentle structuring will sometimes actually result in a more organized production of speech as the psychotic defenses recede.

Along similar lines, in some instances an empathic interviewer may so decrease the anxiety level of a subtly psychotic patient that the observable psychotic process temporarily disappears or recedes significantly. Ironically, the clinician's style will have distorted the clinical picture, amply reminding us that as the interview proceeds we become a part of the dyadic system, whether we intend to or not. In a similar fashion, an involvement with the psychotic process itself awaits the friends and family members of the patient. Unfortunately, unlike clinicians, they are not generally trained to handle such bizarre interactions.

IV. The Familial, Cultural, and Societal Wing of the Matrix

Understanding the Exquisite Pain of Family Members

Psychosis, despite its propensity for autistic withdrawal, is a family matter. No person in the immediate vicinity of the patient will be able to remain uninvolved for long. Few processes can so ravage a family and its underlying structure. This is particularly true when the process is chronic in nature such as with schizophrenia or bipolar disorder.

It is hard to put into words the exquisite pain of watching a child or spouse being tortured by psychotic process. The pain is heightened further once a family member understands that the heart-rending process may continue for years or even be life-long in nature. Both the dreams of the patient and of his family are sometimes forever destroyed, a remarkably traumatizing experience for parents, siblings, and the patient.

This devastation will rapidly intensify as the family members try to cope with the damaging matrix effects caused by the psychotic process in their loved one: potential financial ruin for themselves, the need for their child to sometimes live at home even as an adult, and stigmatization from both culture and friends. In addition, almost all parents must cope with two powerfully demoralizing processes: a numbing feeling of helplessness and a sometimes-overwhelming caretaker fatigue. For these reasons, family members will be not only an invaluable source of information for helping our patients but also a targeted group for therapeutic intervention and healing by our teams.

Many of the readers of this book are all-too-well aware of these pains, for they have a loved one stricken by a severe mental illness. Those readers who do not, may very well be destined to experience such pain with a loved one in the future, whether it be a spouse, a partner, a child, a friend, or a fellow mental health professional. But unlike ourselves, most family members are ill equipped with the knowledge that could help them understand and cope with the bizarre behaviors of their loved ones.

One can imagine what it is like for family members to become the object of the penetrating hatred that may erupt when one is perceived as part of a patient's delusional system. In some instances, family members are physically assaulted, and in rare instances they are killed by the very people they have loved most. Obviously, both family and friends must cope with powerfully conflicting feelings, including embarrassment, guilt, fear, compassion, helplessness, bitterness, love, and the desire to abandon the patient.

I remember working with one family whose plight illustrates some of the many processes at work in the family system. The family was of Creole background. The patient was an attractive woman in her mid-30s who sat with a defiant jut to her jaw. Upon her head she wore a faded scarf that lent a sad elegance to her. She had become progressively depressed, and her mind was swarming with religious delusions. She had had to stop work and had been living with her mother and a brother, both of whom were taking care of her children. These family members had not wanted her to seek professional help because they felt that she would get over it with God's help.

But she had recently spent several days with another brother who had angrily insisted that help be sought. Already the psychosis was beginning to dig its claws into the structural foundations of the family. It is common for family tensions to crystallize around issues such as, "What to do with Jim (or Sandy)."

While waiting in the emergency room, the patient, whom we shall call Ms. Jenkins, stood up and began to perform a ritualistic chant. It was sad indeed to watch the mother and brother hide their embarrassment as they struggled to get her back into her seat. Later, this same mother and brother would undercut our efforts to hospitalize Ms. Jenkins. Her mother wearily looked at us saying, "I don't think there is much really wrong with her. I don't think she needs to be in a hospital. She'll pull out of it on her own. But thank you for your help." Her thanks were sincerely given.

The next day the Jenkins family was back. Ms. Jenkins had been acting bizarrely throughout the night. In the waiting room the mother sat with her arm around her daughter, her eyes red from the painful recognition that her daughter was no longer the same person she had raised. Schizoaffective disorder had shifted the matrix. Perhaps forever.

In this regard, it appears useful to remember that, at some level, family members will be mourning the loss of "the person they knew." As with any mourning process, various stages such as denial, anger, bargaining, depression, and acceptance will intermingle and be experienced at different times. The Jenkins family highlights a common problem facing the initial interviewer – the presence of a powerful system of denial among family members. By understanding the mourning of family members, it may help decrease the angry countertransference feelings that can naturally arise in a clinician when encountering a frustrating rejection of their help prompted by a parent or spouse in denial.

From the above discussion, it can be seen that in few cases does the initial interview with a psychotic patient end with the patient. At some early point, the family warrants an assessment, as well as a chance for later counseling and the potential for the healing that we can offer. Keep in mind that some family members may become seriously depressed and perhaps even suicidal, a powerful example of a damaging matrix effect. Psychosis is, indeed, a family affair.

The tensions of the family may, at some level, precipitate or aggravate the psychotic process itself, sometimes unintentionally. Research such as the Environmental/Personal Indicators in the Course of Schizophrenia (EPICS) Project has shown that families in which members are overly involved with the patient, whether in a hostile way or, perhaps, even in an overly concerned caring fashion, may hinder recovery, even when the patient complies with medication use.[39] Family counseling seems to significantly decrease relapse rates. This emphasizes the importance of assessing the family and beginning an alliance with them. Frequently, the initial interviewer is the first person to meet the family and consequently represents a key person in the attempts to build the much-needed alliance described above.

Not only is the family affected, but also other important social networks may begin to collapse around the patient. Jobs may be lost and friendships may become strained and decline. It is difficult to remain friends with a person who has developed a severe psychotic process. Frequently, both friends and family members will be dealing with feelings of guilt. A simple phrase said early during an interview may be comforting such as, "I just finished talking with your friend, who seems very disturbed. I bet you've gone through a lot recently. It was nice of you to come with him today." As with the patient, engagement issues remain critical during the opening phases of collaborative interviews.

Practical Techniques for Engaging Family Members in the Initial Interview

Along these lines, it is important to remember that many parents (as well as siblings and children) of patients with schizophrenia and bipolar disorder come to us with a checkered history with mental health professionals. They have often met many fine professionals, but, not infrequently, they have also unfortunately "been put through the wringer," not only by the disease afflicting their children but also by some of the professionals supposedly helping with this disease.

It is critical in the initial meeting to win over these parents, as well as other family members/friends. The goal is to help them with their immense pain and also to set the stage for a joint effort to help their loved one as he or she recovers.

Opening the Conversation in an Initial Encounter With a Family Member

Murray Swank and colleagues, in their outstanding article "Practical Strategies for Building an Alliance with the Families of Patients who have Severe Mental Illness" (complete article available in Appendix IV), point out that it is helpful to meet the family "where they are at" by both inviting the family's participation and exploring their opinions on what is happening, as illustrated below[40]:

"Thanks for taking the time to meet with me today about [name's] treatment. To begin, it would be helpful to get your thoughts about the problems that [name] is seeking treatment for. If it is OK with you, I would like to ask you a couple questions to get your input and learn about your understanding of things. Can you tell me a little bit about what you think about [name's] problems?"

Follow-up inquiries can include more focused questions such as:

1. "What do you think has caused [name] to have these problems?"
2. "Has anybody ever given you a diagnosis for his/her problems?" If they have been told of a diagnosis, it is useful to follow-up with two questions:
   "What is your understanding of what that diagnosis means?"
   "Do you agree with the diagnosis?"

3. "Are there things that make things better for [name]?"
4. "Are there things that make things worse?"

Questions such as these can help the interviewer learn about family members' views about their relative's psychiatric problems. In addition, such questions can provide useful information to guide the patient's treatment. For example, family members often have valuable observations about prodromal symptoms that signal a risk for relapse in the patient.[41]

During the course of this first meeting, many parents will have some of the following unexpressed fears. Some will have all of these fears, and some will have none. However, as the interview proceeds, the clinician should take the time to try to sensitively address and dismantle these concerns. Some of these concerns are listed, directly followed by samples of clinician statements that can help to allay them:

1. *This clinician doesn't really care what I have to say.*
    Clinician intervention: "One of the things I want to emphasize early on is how important your input and background information is in our helping John. There is no one in the world who knows him better than you. We are dependent on your input. I also really want to know what you think has worked and what you think doesn't work."
2. *This clinician thinks that we are the problem.*
    Clinician intervention: "You know, there are some people out there who think parents somehow cause schizophrenia. Let me assure you of one thing. I don't buy that for one minute. Schizophrenia is a brain disease like epilepsy. Some of the most loving parents whom I have ever met have children who develop schizophrenia. Just in talking with you today, I am struck by how much you love John. I think he is very lucky to have you. Some parents would have abandoned him by now."
3. *This guy is not going to understand how much pain we've been through.*
    Clinician intervention: "You must have gone through a lot over the years. I'm sure it just must seem like it goes on and on. I have no miracles to offer, but I promise you that we will do our very best to help you and your son. How have you coped with all this? Have you had very much support?"
4. *This "Bozo" is going to change these meds.*
    Clinician intervention: "One of the most foolish things a physician [nurse clinician] can do is to change meds before talking with parents and the patient about what is working. Your input is vital. I have no intention of making a recommendation regarding your son's meds until after we talk in detail. By the way, if your son agrees, I would like to always try to talk with you and get your thoughts about any potential major med changes. What is your opinion about this particular set of medications?"
5. *This guy is closed to our ideas and thinks he knows it all.*
    Clinician intervention: "If you have any new ideas about helping John, please let me or the case manager know. If you find interesting articles or hear about new treatments, please let me know, and I'll find out about them, if I'm not familiar with them for some reason. I like to stay on top of new treatments."

It always pays to find out at an early stage what the family has experienced with other mental health professionals. The best way to find out is to simply ask. Your inquiry also metacommunicates that it matters to you what they think of your care. A question such as the following can help, "I'm wondering what your experience with previous psychiatrists (substitute whatever your own professional discipline might be) has been like?" It is also useful to ask, "What are some of the things I can do that would help you? For instance, how frequently would you like to meet with me?"

The first meeting is also a good time to provide family members with avenues of support outside of professional help. One of the best places to start is by providing family members with the telephone number of the local chapter of the National Alliance for the Mentally Ill (NAMI) if they are not already aware of it. NAMI (www.nami.org) is an ongoing support group originated by family members who have a relative with a serious mental illness. Its membership may also include people coping with mental illnesses and mental health professionals, thus creating a well-rounded representation of people affected by mental illnesses. It is a superb organization and has chapters all over the United States. Similar organizations exist in countries throughout the world.

A second platform of support can be found in the many excellent books designed to help family members who have a loved one coping with a mental illness. Two of my favorites are Mueser's *The Complete Family Guide to Schizophrenia*[42] and Torrey's *Surviving Schizophrenia: A Manual for Families.*[43]

Tips for Initial Interviews With Family Members on Inpatient Units

Once again we shall turn our attention to the wisdom of Murray-Swank and colleagues, who emphasize the importance of "taking a read" on the emotional state of family members upon admitting a child or other loved one. Especially if the family member has never been on an inpatient unit, the environment can appear frightening and overwhelming; these feelings are often magnified if the unit is a locked one. The following sensitive acknowledgement of the jarring nature of the situation can be greatly appreciated:

"I realize that you have really been through a lot during this time – you may be feeling anxious, worried, overwhelmed, angry, or maybe a combination of many different feelings – this is certainly understandable, normal, and to be expected as you are dealing with everything going on with [consumer's name]."[44]

This shock of encountering the environment of a locked inpatient unit for the first time is amplified if the parent or loved one has participated in an involuntary hospitalization. Experiencing their child's rage and sense of betrayal creates a pain that is beyond words. Parents, or other family members, are often besieged by guilt and second thoughts about having done the right thing. As Murray-Swank asserts, a reassuring comment, such as that below, at the right moment can be comforting:

"Naturally it can be disturbing to see [name] in the hospital. I just want to emphasize that you really did the right thing bringing [name] into the hospital, even though he didn't want to come in. I think you might have saved his life. It took real courage and love to do

what you did. And we are going to do everything we can to help him get better. He is very lucky he has you, and that you were there to do what needed to be done to help him."[45]

Obviously, we could spend many more pages addressing interviewing techniques and strategies for interviewing family members in a variety of clinical settings, including community mental health center clinics, inpatient units, private practices, and emergency rooms, but we are limited by space and time. As the reader works with family members in these situations, I have found the following three interviewing principles, created by Mueser and Glynn, to be of help in guiding my interventions: (1) try to let the family know they are not alone, (2) provide support and allow relatives to vent, and (3) attempt to instill hope.[46]

Talking With Patients About Involving Their Family Members in Assessment and Treatment

To initiate contact with families of adult patients, it is necessary to ask a patient to identify members of his or her family and to obtain the patient's permission to speak with them. This process is not always an easy task, for psychotic process has often strained family relations markedly through no fault of anyone involved. Once again, the insights of Murray-Swank and colleagues provide an outstanding platform for navigating this delicate tightrope. Consequently, the remaining paragraphs of this section are directly adapted from their work.[47]

Patients will have a wide range of family experiences and preferences with regard to family involvement in their mental health care. As an initial starting point, it is important to find out who, if anybody, the patient considers to be their "family support system," and what role these individuals may play in helping them manage their psychiatric disorder (if any). For example:

"I would like to ask you some questions to better understand your family relationships and support system. Do you have people you would consider to be your family or like family to you? Who would those people be for you?"

For many patients, significant "family" and potential allies in treatment may include members of their support network who are not relatives (e.g., friend, pastor, Alcoholics Anonymous/Narcotics Anonymous sponsor). After identifying the key members of the support network, it is helpful to learn about patients' level of contact with these individuals – for example: (1) Does the patient live with a family member? (2) If not, how close do family members live? and (3) How often does the patient talk, text, e-mail, communicate via Facebook, or get together with family members. Next, it is important to understand the role that these individuals play in supporting the patient, including any involvement in their mental health treatment. For example:

"So, you have said that you are closest to your two brothers, who you get together with every couple of weeks. I'm wondering if your brothers have been supportive as you have been dealing with your mental illness?"

Patients may have a variety of experiences with family in relation to their illness. Interviewers should use techniques such as summaries and reflections to gain an understanding of the patient's experience and help him or her feel supported. Finally, if not yet known, the interviewer can assess the degree to which family members have been involved in the patient's mental health treatment in the past and the patient's preferences with regard to involving family in the present. For example, the following questions might be of use regarding a patient's siblings:

1. "Have your brothers or sisters been involved in your mental health care by coming in to meet with your doctor or team in the past?
2. "Have they ever attended any kind of educational programs or groups?"
3. "Would you like to have some or all of your brothers and sisters involved in your mental health treatment?
4. "What might be the possible benefits?"
5. "What, if any, are your concerns about having them involved?"

Overall, the goals of this discussion are to help the patient: (1) identify family members who could be allies in their treatment; (2) consider the potential advantages of family involvement in treatment; and (3) identify concerns they might have about family participation.

In some instances, the patient may be ambivalent about involving their family. This is understandable, given the complexity of family relationships and the possibility of the presence of abusive family members, as well as the personal nature of mental health treatment. When the patient experiences mixed feelings about involving family in their mental health care, the primary task of the interviewer is to help the patient make informed choices, considering the potential advantages and disadvantages of family involvement in care.

Personally, I feel that if genuinely caring family members would like to be involved, it can be of immense comfort and support to have appropriately open channels of communication. It is terribly frustrating, and sometimes quite frightening, for a family member to be told that they cannot hear anything about treatment "because of confidentiality."

If such is the case, the pain of exclusion can be softened with sensitive interventions such as the following, which skillfully employs Leston Haven's counterprojection technique (see pages e169–e173):

"As you probably know, medical information is private and protected. Therefore, I can't share any specific information about [name's] treatment at this time without her permission. I know it's hard for family members in these kind of situations; it is difficult for us, too, because we really value the opportunity to include patients' families as part of the treatment whenever we can. What I can do is talk with [name] the next chance that I get to try to get her permission to talk with you more about her treatment."

On a final note, it should be remembered that in a situation where there are concerns that the patient may be at risk for suicide or violence, confidentiality is trumped by the need to procure the information necessary to perform a sound risk assessment. Information from family members may be life saving in this regard; at such times, confidentiality must be broken. If at all possible, in such situations, consult with a supervisor or colleague to decide whether the crisis requires an over-riding of confidentiality, and document the reasons for such an over-ride carefully.

Cultural and Societal Impacts on Psychotic Process

Encountering Culture-Bound Syndromes and Behaviors

Psychotic process can show itself in different fashions depending upon the matrix effects of any given culture. These distinctive presentations are often called "culture-bound syndromes," a term that I hope will someday be replaced, for, in my opinion, all diagnoses are culture bound. The DSM-5 diagnoses are, by definition, defined by Western culture and, hence, culture bound by it. Indeed, contemporary cultural psychiatry recognizes that all classification systems are inherently culture bound.[48] Perhaps it is simply more accurate to state that these syndromes are not found in Western culture unless they are being experienced by an immigrant or visitor.

What is important to take from these syndromes is the realization that cultures shape psychotic process. Consequently, a talented interviewer must always be aware of the culture of origin of the patient and keep an eye out for cultural variations and symptoms that may be out of the ordinary for the clinician. Without such an awareness, an interviewer may miss a psychotic process, or, equally problematic, misread a patient's behavior as psychotic when it is a normal experience within the patient's culture of origin, an issue we have addressed in earlier chapters.

Missing Culturally Specific Psychotic Process

Let us look at our first problem facing an initial interviewer – missing a psychotic process that is limited to a specific culture. Picture a young Chinese graduate student attending a major university in the United States, who has brought his reluctant father into a community mental health center commenting, "I don't know what's wrong with my Dad. He's been visiting me for the past 2 weeks and he's really wound up about something, but he won't tell me what's going on. At night he locks himself up in the guest bedroom and gets really mad if I knock or try to talk to him. I'm really worried about him."

The student's 55-year-old father presents in a friendly, yet clearly hesitant fashion. He reluctantly describes being upset and anxious, relates marked problems with sleep, and demonstrates an unusually intense affect. He admits to some episodes of yelling at his son, highly atypical for him and terribly embarrassing to admit.

The clinician wisely realizes that the patient is demonstrating some soft signs of psychosis, indicated by the intensity of his anxiety and the presence of his atypical, angry outbursts. Consequently, the interviewer delicately asks about a variety of psychotic symptoms including auditory hallucinations, paranoid feelings, and delusions, concerns about alien control, as well as sensitively probing for psychotic hyper-religiosity. Nothing.

The clinician believes that a psychotic process is unlikely and feels that some variant of a severe generalized anxiety disorder or social phobia may be present. Alternatively, perhaps there is a powerful situational stress present that the patient is hesitant to share, such as financial concerns or marital distress. All of these are reasonable speculations. Unfortunately, all of them are wrong.

What the interviewer doesn't know to ask is the following question, which a clinician in China might know would be worth an inquiry in a potentially psychotic male: "Sometimes when we least expect it, we can have fears that are really quite frightening, but might seem sort of strange to us or embarrassing because they are very private fears. They are so private, it makes them hard to talk about. For instance, sometimes people will get really worried about their bodies. Back in China I know that some men will get worried about their penis being damaged or somehow being pulled up into their bodies. I know that, sometimes in China, some men are even frightened that this could cause them to die. I'm wondering if you have heard of that or might even be worried about it?"

Bingo. The student's father looks up and shyly nods his head yes. He is experiencing a syndrome known as *koro*. *Koro* is generally seen in China and South East Asia. Depending upon locale, it is variously called *shuk yang*, *shook yong*, *suo yang* (Chinese), *jinjinia bemar* (Assam), or *rok-joo* (Thailand).[49] In women, the syndrome revolves around a fear of retraction of the vulva or nipples. Our point is that, because of the sexually intimate nature of this delusional fear, it would probably never have been spontaneously mentioned by the patient above unless he was directly asked about it. Our graduate student's father easily could have left this clinic without anyone knowing what he was experiencing and, consequently, no hope for effective attention and treatment.

Before leaving the problem of missing psychotic syndromes, let us look at an actual clinical example of a culturally specific syndrome that could be puzzling to an interviewer familiar only with Western psychotic presentations. It is described by Mezzich and colleagues:

> *A 28-year-old mainland Chinese man living in the United States for several years was hospitalized in a psychiatric ward with delusions and hallucinations of 2 to 3 week's duration. These began after he took up the practice of* qi-gong, *a form of meditation, as treatment for his severe intermittent backaches and chronic exhaustion. According to the patient, feelings of* qi *("vital energy") were circulating in the "wrong direction" in his body, and he heard the voices of supernatural beings commenting on how he should practice* qi-gong. *He denied depressed mood, appetite or weight changes, substance abuse, or a history of psychosis. The results of extensive medical evaluation, including electroencephalography and magnetic resonance imaging, were normal. Haloperidol substantially reduced his delusions and hallucinations, but follow-up information is unavailable because he did not keep his appointment after discharge.*

> *Transient psychotic symptoms in connection with* qi-gong *practices are not uncommon, but duration for more than a few days is unusual. The patient's picture meets criteria in the Chinese classification system for* qi-gong-*induced psychosis …"*[50]

There are numerous other culturally specific disorders, some of which are psychotic: *locura* (Latinos); occasionally psychotic: *amok* (Malaysia), *iich'aa* (Navajo), *boufee delirante* (West Africa and Haiti), *Taijin kyofusho* (South Asia); and non-psychotic: *billis, colera, muina* (Latino), *Kufungisisa* (Shona of Zimbabwe), *hwa-byung* (Korean). The interested reader can find nice descriptions of the symptoms seen in these disorders in the appendices of the DSM-IV-TR[51] and the DSM-5.[52]

Our goal here is not to review all the culturally specific syndromes, a task far beyond the reaches of our book, but to alert the clinician of the need to be aware of such disorders and the role they may play in an initial interview.

Mistaking Culturally Normal Phenomena for Psychotic Process Redux

Let us now look at our second problem facing an initial interviewer – mistaking a normal process that is specific to a local culture for a psychotic process. We have addressed this issue several times before, yet I feel it is important to review it, for it is quite likely that a contemporary clinician will need to thoroughly understand this phenomenon and its clinical ramifications. World travel, immigration and emigration, and the development of the web have intermixed cultures to a far greater degree than the world has ever before experienced.

By way of example, let us picture a recently graduated psychiatrist, psychiatric nurse, or social worker who is either Black, White, or Hispanic in cultural heritage. Following graduation from an esteemed program in the Southwest of the United States, he or she moves to Minnesota for an excellent job opportunity that has become available at a local community mental health center in Minneapolis. It is highly likely that such a young professional will quickly find himself or herself in a room interviewing a Hmong immigrant.

Asian Americans and Pacific Islanders (AAPIs) are one of the fastest growing and the most diverse ethnic groups in the United States. The Asian American population has increased from 7 million in 1990 to 12 million in 2004. The Hmong are a significant subgroup of this influx. They have a relatively recent history in the U.S. with many of them being war refugees following the Vietnam War. One of their main destinations has been the Twin Cities of Minnesota, this area having the fastest growth rate of South East Asian immigrants.

As Lee and colleagues have noted, many of the Hmong are victims of multiple psychological insults from years spent in refugee camps, traumas related to war, poverty, unemployment, and forced relocation.[53] The psychological impact of all these experiences is further exacerbated by the loss of social networks, traditional roles, and social status. As one can imagine, mental health problems are high, with 50% of Cambodian refugees experiencing depression even after living in the United States for 20 years.

And here our clinician, whether he or she is Black, White, or Hispanic, will stumble upon a potential problem: the misidentification of a Hmong patient with a major depression as being actively psychotic when he or she is not. Frankly, it's an easy mistake to make if one is not aware of certain cross-cultural factors. It is a classic kulturbrille effect as we delineated in Chapter 6 (see pages 210–212).

Although most Hmong have a word for feeling emotionally "very distressed" – *nyuaj siab* [nu-shea] – it is not the same syndrome as the Western term for depression. In fact, they don't really have a word for depression *per se*. The situation is further complicated by the fact that the Hmong believe that *nyuaj siab* and what Western clinicians would call depression, as well as many other illnesses, are often caused by the presence of spirits and ghosts.[54]

As Al-Issa has pointed out, many non-Western cultures do not make as clear a distinction between what is real and what is imagined as Western cultures maintain.[55] Consequently, a patient from a non-Western culture, such as the Hmong, may be predisposed to talk more openly with a clinician about such things as spirits and ghosts, relating matter-of-factly that they see such entities and indeed hear their voices. An interviewer not familiar with these cultural traditions could easily view the Hmong patient's talk of voices as evidence of psychotic process, a striking kulturbrille effect.

Of course, some Hmong patients who are talking about spirit voices may actually be psychotic. A savvy interviewer will be able to spot such patients, because, if psychotic in nature, the voices will be embedded in a matrix of the prodromal signs of psychotic process. Such a patient would most likely, upon careful interviewing, describe symptoms such as delusional mood and delusional perception while demonstrating a plethora of the soft signs of psychosis.

The Community Mental Health Center as a Subculture

In Chapter 10 on depression and its impact on the patient's matrix, we talked about the importance of understanding the patient's specific subculture. This is equally true with patients dealing with chronic psychotic process. Here, though, we encounter a new and somewhat expected, but often ignored, twist.

Patients with chronic psychotic processes such as schizophrenia, schizoaffective disorder, and bipolar disorder frequently become members of a new subculture. As these patients lose their friends, spend long stays in hospitals, and wear out their welcome with relatives, they end up spending progressively more time with each other. If actively engaged in treatment, these patients may spend large amounts of time at the community mental health center itself, or perhaps at local clubhouses and patient-run support centers or at government-supported residential centers.

In addition, our society, through stigmatization, fear, and ignorance, gradually pushes people with chronic mental illnesses into a social caste of sorts. Patients frequently become outcasts from the mainstream of society. It is important for the initial interviewer to understand the dynamics of this, because it can manifest as a veiled hostility from the patient. And sometimes this animosity is not so veiled.

Whatever the causes, community mental health centers are important subcultures that can strongly influence the views of our patients with regard to their treatment. It is useful for clinicians to learn about these biases. For example, the local patients may develop prejudicial views on certain medications. If all of a patient's friends hate the drug Risperdol (respiridone), it does not make a lot of sense to send the patient home on Risperdol, when a different antipsychotic may be just as effective and is not a medication that is blackballed by that subculture.

In this regard, when talking with patients about the potential use of a particular medication, I find it useful to inquire, "Do you know anybody around here that is taking Risperdol [replace with whatever med is being considered]?" If the patient says yes,

I simply ask, "What do they think about it?" and often follow up with, "What do patients in general seem to think about [whatever the medication might be] around here?"

Such a question can provide considerable insight into the gestalt of the community mental health center subculture of the patient. I once asked a patient about Paxil and was quite fascinated by the response, "Oh Paxil, Paxil causes a real nasty side effect. We have a name for it, we call it 'Paxil-head' it really gets you wound up." Paxil was clearly not the choice for this patient.

Language and Culture: Potential Roadblocks When Uncovering Psychotic Process

As our final topic regarding culture and its impact on how people experience psychotic process and subsequently communicate that experience with others, we shall look at an often overlooked barrier to uncovering psychotic process: language. Other than the abnormalities in nonverbal behaviors that sometimes indicate the presence of psychotic process, the clinician is dependent upon the self-report of the patient and/or the reports of concerned loved ones for uncovering psychotic process. For this reason, psychotic process can be an elusive phenomenon to spot. Patients may be hesitant to share psychotic processes for numerous reasons, ranging from fear of stigmatization to misinterpretation of what is being asked by the clinician.

We have already seen that the words we choose can play a pivotal role as to whether a patient feels safe enough to share psychotic process, but our words are always embedded in the complexities of our personal languages. Language can limit what can be easily shared with a clinician and what is difficult to share with a clinician who does not speak the patient's native language. For instance, we have already seen that with certain Hmong patients it is hard for them to share depression for the simple reason that they do not have a word for depression.

Let us now look at a brilliant example of this phenomenon from an actual clinical vignette shared by Junji Takeshita from the University of Hawaii:

> *A 79-year-old Filipino male was admitted to an inpatient psychiatric unit through the court system. He had a delusional belief that his wife was trying to kill him, so he decided to murder her first. When interviewed in English by a non-Filipino psychiatrist, no delusions or other odd beliefs were noted. He was cooperative and was a model patient on the ward. However, the psychiatrist felt that poor fluency in English limited the interview.*

> *As a result, the psychiatrist asked several members of the Filipino nursing staff to serve as interpreters. They noted that the patient was fluent in Ilocano, but had significantly less understanding of Tagalog, both of which are Filipino dialects. Fixed and extensive delusions about multiple family members trying to kill him were elaborated in Ilocano, while only fragments of paranoid thoughts were revealed in Tagalog. Interestingly enough, no delusions were detected when he was interviewed in English.*[56]

Money is tight in all mental health centers. Consequently, interpreters, as well as mental health professionals who can also interpret, are precious commodities. The above illustration from Takeshita shows us one place to prioritize their use – the uncovering of psychotic process.

Generally, when interviewing a patient whose language you do not speak fluently, if you are suspicious of psychotic process, strongly consider having the patient re-interviewed. Try to find an interpreter who speaks the exact language of the patient, or as close as possible to this. In the above vignette we saw that even the differences between two local dialects (Ilocano and Tagalog in the Filipino culture) determined whether psychotic process was shared or not shared. The nuances created by language when discussing the delusional content of psychotic process, as well as the presence of hallucinatory phenomena, tend to be lost when patients are not conversing in their native tongue. As we can see with the strikingly paranoid delusions of the above patient, the breakdown in communication caused by language barriers can leave potentially dangerous, or even lethal, psychotic process untapped.

Takeshita further points out a curious, but important, occurrence occasionally seen in initial interviews. During psychotic episodes, otherwise-bilingual patients may be less able, or even unable, to communicate effectively in whatever their second language may be, in the above case English. With greater and greater disorganization in thinking, some patients regress and may rely entirely upon their primary language.[57]

Another potential problem with language is how it relates to and reflects stigmatization. For example, in some cultures, serious mental illnesses such as schizophrenia or psychotic bipolar disorder are viewed as signs of family or personal failure; thus, these illnesses are sometimes alluded to by the use of euphemisms. If the initial interviewer is not familiar with these euphemisms, major psychiatric disorders can be missed when exploring a patient's past psychiatric history or when taking a family history. Also be aware that family members may hide serious disorders in relatives when providing a family history.

By way of illustration, in Japan *neurasthenia* continues to be used as a euphemism for serious disorders such as schizophrenia. Another Japanese term, *shinshinsho*, directly relates to psychosomatic concerns, but frequently this "psychosomatic" label serves as a euphemism for a more serious mental illness in the relative. In this instance, a psychosomatic illness is significantly less stigmatizing than admitting that one's loved one has schizophrenia.[58]

When interviewing White Americans in the United States, I have sometimes found that the term "nervous breakdown" is proffered when I am taking a family history. Upon careful questioning, this term often belies the necessity of a psychiatric hospitalization in the relative. At a minimum, I have found that the term "nervous breakdown" is generally used to describe an episode of agitated major depression and, at a maximum, a psychotic or manic episode.

V. The Wing of the Matrix Encompassing Worldview and Spirituality

Psychotic Destruction of the Patient's Religious Worldview

Through the window of psychosis, the problem is not so much that the world is meaningless, but rather the world is too meaningful. As the patient copes with a suffocating mixture of bizarre and unscreened sensory experiences, the world is gradually transformed into a desert filled with burning bushes. The patient finds little rest from the intensity of the delusional world, and this intensity creates the driven quality so characteristic of psychotic process.

One of the saddest aspects of psychotic process remains the irony that it can make a patient so religiously preoccupied, that religion is no longer a practical support system. Instead of providing a calm guidance, religious issues become disturbing. This type of overzealous religious ideation is frequently seen with schizophrenia and mania.

Psychotic religious preoccupation may represent an unconscious effort to replace previous areas that had provided a sense of meaning to the patient. For instance, the patient's family ties may have become critically weakened, thus depriving the patient of a powerful framework for meaning. In some unfortunate instances, patients may actually come to view themselves as burdens upon their families. In such situations, one can easily see why a grandiose religious delusion may serve as a source of much needed solace. It could represent a very real resurrection of sorts, a resurrection of the patient's self-esteem.

This process brings to light a curious aspect of the psychotic patient's search for a framework for meaning. With some patients, the psychotic delusions literally become the focal points of their lives. When these delusions disappear, so can the meaning behind life.

The Personalized Meaning of Psychotic Symptoms to Patients

Regarding the potential loss of meaning precipitated by the break-up of a delusional belief, I am reminded of a young man with whom I worked who was suffering from schizophrenia. We shall call him Jake. Jake had been admitted to my unit during a particularly severe initial psychotic break heralding the onset of schizophrenia. I found him to be very likeable and very sad.

Lean and wispy-haired, Jake spoke with an almost child-like innocence. To me, his outlook and demeanor were, indeed, almost more akin to a child than an adult. On the other hand his social responsibilities were all-too adult. He was married to a tough, yet loving, 17-year-old girl who was pregnant with Jake's child. Neither expectant parent was employed, both were without marketable skills, and both were about to be thrown out of their housing. In addition, both were estranged from their families of origin. Put bluntly, the social and interpersonal wings of their matrices were a tragic shambles. Jake knew it. And Jake felt it was all his fault.

Jake was beset by a bevy of horrifying hallucinations and delusions of persecution. Demons of retribution and judgment were flying about the chambers of his mind. Their voices echoed loudly in the hallways of his consciousness. It was a tough inner landscape. And it was terrifying.

On the other hand, there was one delusion that Jake accepted with open arms. He believed that he could intentionally broadcast his thoughts. As he phrased it during my initial interview with him, "I'm the best there is, Dr. Shea. Nobody can send their thoughts faster or further than me." As he came out of his psychosis, in addition to all of his disturbing delusions disappearing, his delusion of thought broadcasting also began to fade. One evening as we were talking by his bedside, he seemed out of sorts. I asked him what was the matter. Jake turned to me, his eyes almost frightened – as if they sensed something bad was about to happen; he said, "I can't do it, can I, Dr. Shea?"

Puzzled, I asked him what he meant. He replied, "Send my thoughts out. I can't do that, can I?" I responded, "Well, that particular belief is probably part of your schizophrenia too. I'm sorry it wasn't true for you." Jake paused for moment, and then he began to weep profusely. Apparently his delusion was serving as a last-ditch prop for a severely battered ego. Several years later, I heard that Jake had died from a self-inflicted gunshot.

As clinicians we will undoubtedly be working with patients in various stages of belief and disbelief concerning their delusions. Jake reminds us that it is important to try to understand the significance of these beliefs to the patient at the time of their presentation. He reminds us that there is always a person beneath the psychosis, beneath each and every delusion.

Even if the patient's psychosis is being caused primarily by biologic dysfunction, the fact remains that the content of the delusions are directly related to the patient's psychological constitution, including the patient's upbringing, memories, values, culture, and spirituality. In that sense, one may find important clues to underlying fears, strengths, and issues in these seemingly illogical fantasies.

Finally, it cannot be emphasized enough that the presence of a chronic, severe mental illness often leads to a quiet desperation that is to be expected when one's dreams are being shattered. Accompanied by the intense guilt and shame of "having become a failure" – a misconception often enhanced by a stigmatizing culture – patients often lose a belief that there is a purpose and meaning for their existence. The shattering of such a critical spiritual support is undoubtedly one of the precipitants of the suicidal ideation we frequently see in patients afflicted by severe psychotic illnesses, as witnessed by Jake.

It is time to end our survey of methods for exploring psychosis. You might recall that we began our two chapters dedicated to uncovering psychotic process by visiting the writings of Gérard De Nerval. De Nerval was the symbolist poet who, unfortunately, was found hanging from an iron gate in a darkened alleyway of Paris. On that dismal night, who knows what the voices were saying to him or in what personal hell he found himself. What we do have are his words. As we reread them now, perhaps aided by our enhanced understanding of psychotic process from the last two chapters, we will hear them with a new respect for both their brilliance and the pain that brilliance echoes:

I seemed to myself a hero living under the very eyes of the gods; everything in nature assumed new aspects, and secret voices came to me from the plants, the trees, animals, the meanest insects, to warn and to encourage me. The words of my companions had mysterious messages, the sense of which I alone understood.

REFERENCES

1. Hedges LE. *Listening perspectives in psychotherapy*. New York, NY: Jason Aronson; 1983. p. 239–43.
2. Mendel WM. A phenomenological theory of schizophrenia. In: Burton A, Lopez-Ibor JJ, Mendel WM, editors. *Schizophrenia as a lifestyle*. New York, NY: Springer Publishers; 1974. p. 106–55.
3. Lopez-Ibor J. Delusional perception and delusional mood: a phenomenological and existential analysis. In: Koning AJJ, Jenner FA, editors. *Phenomenology and psychiatry*. New York, NY: Grune and Stratton; 1982. p. 135–52.

4. Saddichha S, Kumar R, Sur S, Sinha BN. First rank symptoms: concepts and diagnostic utility. *Afr J Psychiatry (Johannesbg)* 2010;**13**:263–6.

5. eMedMD. *Descriptive Clinical Features of Schizophrenia.* http://www.emedmd.com/content/descriptive-clinical-features-schizophrenia [accessed May 2016].

6. Schneider K. *Clinical psychopathology.* [Hamilton MW, Trans.] New York, NY: Grune & Stratton; 1959.

7. Hembram M, Simlai J, Chaudhury S, Biswas P. First rank symptoms and neurological soft signs in schizophrenia. *Psychiatry J* 2014;**2014**:931014.

8. Mellor CS. First rank symptoms of schizophrenia. *Br J Psychiatry* 1970;**156**:15–23.

9. Mellor CS. 1970. p. 15–23.

10. Landis C, Mettler FA. *Varieties of psychopathological experience.* New York, NY: Holt, Rinehart and Winston; 1964.

11. Roberts JK. *Differential diagnosis in neuropsychiatry.* New York, NY: John Wiley; 1984. p. 263.

12. Waters F. Auditory hallucinations in psychiatric illness. *Psychiatr Times* 2010;**27**(3):54–8.

13. Waters F. 2010. p. 55.

14. Waters F. 2010. p. 55.

15. Fish F. *Clinical psychopathology.* Bristol, UK: Wright; 1967. p. 19–26.

16. Asaad G, Shapiro B. Hallucinations: theoretical and clinical overview. *Am J Psychiatry* 1986;**143**:1088–97.

17. West LJ. A clinical and theoretical overview of hallucinatory phenomena. In: Siegel RK, West LJ, editors. *Hallucinations: behavior, experience, and theory.* New York, NY: John Wiley; 1975.

18. Waters F. 2010. p. 55.

19. Copolov D, Trauer T, Mackinnon A. On the non-significance of internal versus external auditory hallucinations. *Schizophr Res* 2004;**69**(1):1–6.

20. Waters F. 2010. p. 55.

21. Stephane M, Thuras P, Nasrallah H, Georgopoulos AP. The internal structure of the phenomenology of auditory verbal hallucinations. *Schizophr Res* 2003;**61**:185–93.

22. Waters F. 2010. p. 55.

23. Landis C, Mettler FA. 1964.

24. Wing JK, Babor T, Brugha T, et al. SCAN: schedule for clinical assessment in neuropsychiatry. *Arch Gen Psychiatry* 1990;**47**(6):589–93.

25. Roy A. Depression, attempted suicide, and suicide in patients with chronic schizophrenia. *Psychiatr Clin North Am* 1986;**9**(1):193–206.

26. Wilkinson G, Bacon NA. A clinical and epidemiological survey of parasuicide and suicide in Edinburgh schizophrenics. *Psychol Med* 1984;**14**:899–912.

27. Breier A, Astrachan BM. Characterization of schizophrenic patients who commit suicide. *Am J Psychiatry* 1984;**141**:206–9.

28. Hellerstein D, Frosch W, Koenigsberg HW. The clinical significance of command hallucinations. *Am J Psychiatry* 1987;**144**(2):219–21.

29. Shawyer F. Command hallucinations and violence: implications for detection and treatment. *Psychiat Psychol Law* 2003;**10**(1):97–107.

30. Junginger J. Predicting compliance with command hallucinations. *Am J Psychiatry* 1990;**147**(2):245–7.

31. McGhie A, Chapman J. Disorders of attention and perception in early schizophrenia. *Br J Med Psychol* 1961;**34**:103–17.

32. McGhie A, Chapman J. 1961. p. 103–17.

33. Rosenbaum P. *The meaning of madness.* New York, NY: Science House; 1970. p. 73–99.

34. Deegan PE. Recovery: The lived experience of rehabilitation. *Psychosoc Rehabil J* 1988;**11**:11–19.

35. Lehman HE, Cancro R. Schizophrenia: Clinical features. In: Kaplan H, Sadock B, editors. *Comprehensive textbook of psychiatry IV.* Baltimore, MD: Williams & Wilkins; 1985. p. 680–713.

36. Lehman HE, Cancro R. 1985. p. 704.

37. MacKinnon R, Michels RP. *The psychiatric interview in clinical practice.* Philadelphia, PA: W. B. Saunders; 1971. p. 236.

38. MacKinnon R, Michels R, Buckley PJ. *The psychiatric interview in clinical practice.* 2nd ed. Washington, DC: American Psychiatric Association Publishing; 2006. p. 431.

39. Hogarty GE, Anderson CM, Reiss DJ, et al. Family education, social skills training, and maintenance chemotherapy in the aftercare treatment of schizophrenia. *Arch Gen Psychiatry* 1986;**43**:633–42.

40. Murray-Swank A, Dixon LB, Stewart B. Practical strategies for building an alliance with the families of patients who have severe mental illness. *Psychiatr Clin North Am* 2007;**30**(2):167–80.

41. Murray-Swank A, Dixon LB, Stewart B. 2007. p. 173.

42. Mueser KT, Gingerich S. *The complete family guide to schizophrenia.* New York, NY: The Guilford Press; 2006.

43. Torrey EF. *Surviving schizophrenia: a manual for families.* 5th ed. New York, NY: Harper Perennial; 2006.

44. Murray-Swank A, Dixon LB, Stewart B. 2007. p. 168.

45. Murray-Swank A, Dixon LB, Stewart B. 2007. p. 169.

46. Mueser KT, Glynn SM. *Behavioral family therapy for psychiatric disorders.* Oakland, CA: New Harbinger Publications; 1999.

47. Murray-Swank A, Dixon LB, Stewart B. 2007. p. 176-7.
48. Mezzich JE, Lewis-Fernandez R. Cultural considerations in psychopathology. In: Tasman Allan, Kay Jerald, Lieberman Jeffrey A., editors. *Psychiatry*, vol. 1. Philadelphia, PA: W. B. Saunders; 1997. p. 563–71.
49. American Psychiatric Association. *Diagnostic and statistical manual of mental disorders*. Text Revised. *DSM-IV-TR*. Washington, DC: American Psychiatric Publishing, Inc.; 2000. p. 900.
50. Mezzich JE, Lewis-Fernandez R. 1997. p. 564.
51. *DSM-IV-TR*. 2000. p. 897-903.
52. American Psychiatric Association. *Diagnostic and statistical manual of mental disorders*. 5th ed. *DSM-5*. Washington, DC: American Psychiatric Publishing, Inc.; 2013. p. 833–7.
53. Lee HY, Lytle K, Yang PN, Lum T. Mental health literacy in Hmong and Cambodian elderly refugees: a barrier to understanding, recognizing, and responding to depression. *Int J Aging Hum Dev* 2010;**71**(4):323–44.
54. Lee HY, Lytle K, Yang PN, Lum T. 2010. p. 330-4.
55. Al-Issa I. The illusion of reality or the reality of illusion: hallucinations and culture. *Br J Psychiatry* 1995;**166**:368–73.
56. Takeshita J. Psychosis. In: Tseng Wen-Shing, Streltzer Jon, editors. *Culture and psychopathology*. New York, NY: Brunner/Mazel; 1997.
57. Takeshita J. 1997. p. 135.
58. Takeshita J. 1997. p. 134.

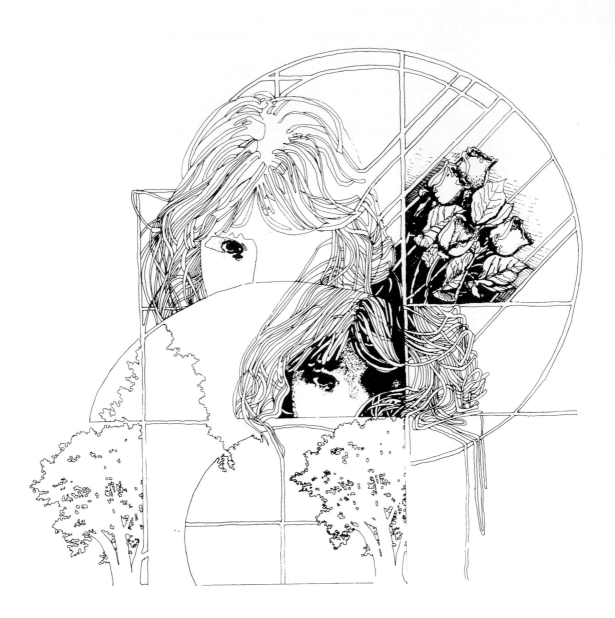

CHAPTER 13

Personality Disorders: Before the Interview Begins – Core Concepts

The passionate hand is fleshy, resisting, hard, sometimes dry, always strong. The fingers are thick and rather short. … The passionate character is believing, powerful, active, inspired. It proceeds by a feeling for things and produced by a natural abundance. Capacity for work. Keen, enthusiastic, absorbed worker.

Anonymous
The Encyclopedia of Occult Sciences

INTRODUCTION

As the above quotation illustrates, for ages humans have enthusiastically attempted to classify each other. Such behavior seems to represent a trademark of the species, for better or worse. In previous centuries, cheirologists attempted to determine the currents of personality in the physical characteristics of the hand. Today, cheirology has been appropriately relegated to the niche of the historically curious – an intellectual antique of sorts.

However, personality theory remains as intriguing today as it did for the cheirologists of the 18th century. On the one hand, tremendous advances have been made in understanding both the normal and abnormal aspects of personality development. On the other hand, much remains to be learned. To be successful in the art of personality assessment, it is important to understand the limitations of current conceptualizations. It is also of value to be familiar with some of the controversies surrounding personality disorders and the systems developed for categorizing them.

Taking into consideration both the presence of these controversies and the fact that there are 10 specific personality disorders in the DSM-5, we will utilize a slightly different approach in the following chapters than was used when we explored mood disorders and psychotic process. Rather than attempt the exhaustive task of representing each diagnosis by a separate clinical presentation, smaller clinical illustrations will be liberally used to delineate diagnostic principles that may be generalizable to any personality disorder.

The emphasis will remain on practical techniques and strategies, brought to life with clinical illustrations, sample questions, and excerpts from initial interviews. My aim here is to acknowledge the controversies and nuances of these diagnoses while simultaneously developing a user-friendly approach for arriving at a differential diagnosis regarding personality dysfunction. My goal is to provide psychiatric residents and graduate students in social work, nursing, clinical psychology, and counseling with the practical tools to effectively and sensitively arrive at a personality disorder diagnosis in the real world of everyday practice as experienced in community mental health centers, hospitals, and private practices.

To achieve this goal, two chapters are devoted to the art of uncovering personality dysfunction and the complexities of differential diagnosis. A third, and final, chapter will explore the fascinating phenomenology and psychodynamics that ultimately drive the behaviors of the people who carry these enigmatic diagnoses.

In this chapter, *Personality Disorders: Before the Interview Begins – Core Concepts*, we will be introduced to the theoretical aspects regarding personality disorders that most directly impact upon our ability to effectively uncover them during an initial interview, including basic definitions, the pros and cons of making personality diagnoses, and the etiology of personality dysfunction. In Chapter 14, *Personality Disorders: How to Sensitively Arrive at a Differential Diagnosis*, practical interviewing techniques and strategies for sensitively performing a differential diagnosis will be addressed in a comprehensive fashion. The set of chapters on personality disorders concludes with Chapter 15, *Understanding and Effectively Engaging People With Difficult Personality Disorders: The Psychodynamic Lens*. It will be in this chapter that our diagnostic illustrations will step out of the pages of this book to become fully realized people, whom we will meet, interact with, and care for in our counseling centers, inpatient units, and emergency rooms.

THE MYSTERY OF PERSONALITY DISORDERS REVEALED: CORE PRINCIPLES AND DEFINITIONS

In Search of a Definition

The Gestalt of Personality Dysfunction

To achieve a better feel for how personality dysfunction presents and is experienced by both the patient and the clinician, let us begin by looking at an exchange in an initial interview between a therapist and a person coping with significant personality dysfunction. As is commonly seen with personality dysfunction, the problematic perceptions, attitudes, and behaviors shadow the patient across time zones, locations, and interpersonal relationships. They impact upon almost every person with whom they develop a relationship, sometimes even with a total stranger encountered on a subway or in a bar, or even in a chat room on the internet. On the day of this interview, they would quickly make themselves known to the unsuspecting initial interviewer – me. We will refer to the patient as Mr. Fellows and begin by examining his history, which will then be complemented by a re-creation of a brief bit of dialogue from the interview itself.

Mr. Fellows was referred for outpatient psychotherapy. He had originally been seen in the emergency room with a subsequent referral for possible group therapy. After attending two group sessions, he left because "the therapist spent too much time listening to all those screwball people. And he was also an inexperienced therapist, that's for sure. I just didn't like him."

Mr. Fellows presented in a dirty plaid shirt encased by an unkempt army jacket. He was short in stature with a balding head from which his black hair sprouted. His hair had clearly met a comb, but the liaison had been a brief one. He quickly conveyed a feeling that he did not really want to be in the room. His handshake was overly firm and then suddenly weak as if purposely avoiding prolonged contact. He had entered the room sporting a jaunty cap, which was a little worse for wear, and had now found itself in his lap, a plaything for his fidgeting hands.

With regard to his history he had come from a tough neighborhood, and he had seldom felt at home there. "I didn't belong there, I'm a sensitive guy, and I felt things those other kids could never feel. But I beat it." He related having a very high IQ, and he indeed appeared quite knowledgeable and well read. However, he had always encountered intermittent problems in school. He had frequently been involved in arguments with teachers and tended to be a loner. He had had no problems with the law and seemed strongly opposed to violence and criminal activity. He considered taking drugs to be bad, yet he hesitantly admitted to drinking problems in the past.

He had never liked his father, who considered him to be a complete failure and had beaten him in the past. Over the years he had lost contact with most of his family, and he was generally not welcome in their homes.

He viewed himself as talented, especially with regard to writing. Indeed, he had been working on a novel for years. He also boasted of his ability to protect others, as well as himself, from violence. To this point he always carried a small canister of pepper spray with him.

Despite his abhorrence of physical conflict, he reported a life-long history of "finding the nearest argument." Apparently he often tended to dominate conversations, because "in all honesty I'm smarter than most of the people I meet." In short, he had developed the rather nifty habit of alienating people almost upon first contact. I would prove to be no different. The following dialogue occurred during the early phases of the body of the interview:

Pt.:   That last therapist was a real loser. And I really don't see much sense in group therapy anyway. In fact, if I really look at this realistically, I don't really need any help at this time.

Clin.:   With that idea in mind what were some of your reasons for coming in for an evaluation today? Apparently you had been referred for outpatient psychotherapy.

Pt.:   In the first place I don't really like psychotherapists. I don't think you guys really know what you're doing anyway. I mean I had seen a therapist off and on for 6 or 7 years. He was okay, but he charged more than he was worth. What you need to do for me today is to write a note saying that for medical reasons I need to live in a new halfway house. The one I'm at is situated in too dangerous a neighborhood. And that's all I need or want from you.

Mr. Fellows was clearly not meant for public relations work. At least he quickly got to his point. In the next session, when he was reminded that further evaluation was needed before I could legitimately address his request, he became actively hostile and commented, "You don't give a damn do you, Doctor! For all you care, I could be mugged tomorrow, and it would be no sweat off your back. I hope someday you're being murdered and when you call the police, they say further inquiry will be necessary before we respond to your call!" His words were said with such vehemence and disdain that I felt a twinge of fear.

With regard to diagnosis, further interviewing revealed that Mr. Fellows met the criteria for a narcissistic personality disorder. He also displayed antisocial, borderline, and paranoid traits. Indeed, a rule-out secondary diagnosis was "other specified personality disorder" (i.e., mixed personality features: antisocial, borderline, and paranoid traits). Concerning other psychiatric diagnoses, he was still having intermittent problems with excessive alcohol use, although he had not been drinking for several months.

Subsequent therapy revealed that throughout his life Mr. Fellows had suffered from an intense feeling of vulnerability. The question, "Am I really worth loving?" was a rather constant companion, a shadow from which he could not step away, no matter how hard he tried to inflate his self-esteem. He developed a series of defenses to protect himself from this pain, including a sense of entitlement, a tendency to put others down, fantasies and preoccupations with grandiosity, and a coolness in interpersonal contacts. This coolness could serve to protect him from the danger of imminent rejection, a rejection that had first surfaced in the form of abuse from his father.

We are now beginning to perceive the subtle workings of disordered personality structure. In these conditions, the individual develops a series of defenses that can temporarily and in certain circumstances protect them from significant pain. Unfortunately, these same defenses become rigid and limited in number. The patient is left with a defensive structure that is inflexible and frequently ineffective in decreasing pain in the long term; in fact, often it creates new pains (in the form of lost friends, shattered marriages, and blown job opportunities).

Mr. Fellow's cool indifference and his tendency to put others down may indeed protect him from the potential pain of losing a loving figure, but, ironically, it will also prevent him from ever developing such a relationship in the first place. Mr. Fellows does not know how to function otherwise, and therein lies the tragedy of the situation. The intensity of the loneliness and self-loathing can be enormous. Mr. Fellows is not choosing to have a personality disorder. It has bloomed inside him, a product of his environment, pains, and psychological limitations.

This point is important for the clinician, because it serves to reframe the irritating and sometimes, if one is frank, obnoxious behaviors that some people with personality disorders display in response to their pain and anxiety. Such a realization can help to decrease angry countertransference feelings, while serving to increase a sense of compassion. For instance, the same Mr. Fellows who was initially so patently rude and demanding, would later cry from his sense of loss during the termination phase of his time-limited psychotherapy with me, a mere 12 sessions after our initial handshake.

The story of Mr. Fellows also highlights another, easily missed point. The key to understanding adult psychopathology lies in an understanding of childhood and adolescent development. An adult psychiatrist cannot work in an intellectual vacuum, as if adult patients spontaneously appeared at 18 years of age. Many critical therapeutic interactions parallel parent–child behaviors and feelings. Indeed, these patients can quickly arouse parental responses in the clinician even during the initial interview. If unaware of these psychodynamic concerns, initial interviewers can inadvertently disrupt blending.

DSM-5 Definitions of a Personality Disorder

With these ideas in mind let us look at the definition of a personality disorder (or character disorder, as it has sometimes been described in the past) as viewed in the DSM-5:

> *A personality disorder is an enduring pattern of inner experience and behavior that deviates markedly from the expectations of the individual's culture, is pervasive and inflexible, has an onset in adolescence or early adulthood, is stable over time, and leads to distress or impairment.*[1]

The actual diagnostic criteria[2] are as follows:

DSM-5 DIAGNOSTIC CRITERIA FOR GENERAL PERSONALITY DISORDER

A. An enduring pattern of inner experience and behavior that deviates markedly from the expectations of the individual's culture. This pattern is manifested in two (or more) of the following areas:
  1. Cognition (i.e., ways of perceiving and interpreting self, other people, and events).
  2. Affectivity (i.e., the range, intensity, lability, and appropriateness of emotional response).
  3. Interpersonal functioning.
  4. Impulse control.
B. The enduring pattern is inflexible and pervasive across a broad range of personal and social situations.
C. The enduring pattern leads to clinically significant distress or impairment in social, occupational, or other important areas of functioning.
D. The pattern is stable and of long duration, and its onset can be traced back at least to adolescence or early adulthood.
E. The enduring pattern is not better explained as manifestation or consequence of another mental disorder.
F. The enduring pattern is not attributable to the physiological effects of a substance (e.g., a drug of abuse, a medication) or another medical condition (e.g., head trauma).

Reprinted with permission from the *Diagnostic and Statistical Manual of Mental Disorders, Fifth Edition*, (Copyright ©2013). American Psychiatric Association. All Rights Reserved.

Personality Disorders as Reflections of the Social History

The DSM-5 insists that the pathological feelings and behaviors to be used as diagnostic criteria must be consistent and persistent over time. *From the perspective of an interviewer, this fact emphasizes that a personality disorder is a historical diagnosis. The critical criteria for making the diagnosis lie in the patient's history, not in the patient's behavior in the interview itself.* The patient's immediate behavior in the interview often provides important clues to underlying psychopathology, as it did with Mr. Fellows, but the criteria for establishing the diagnosis lie in historical evidence, for the onset must be traced back to adolescence or young adulthood. In a sense, a personality disorder leaves historical artifacts. These artifacts are often buried in the patient's social history.

The nature of these artifacts varies significantly, but one of two elements will be present: (1) either the patient's rigid defenses result in behaviors/feelings/consequences that are disturbing to other people, and/or (2) the patient's rigid defenses result in behaviors/feelings/consequences that are unsettling to the patient. By way of illustration, a person with an antisocial personality may steal the life savings of an employer who trusted the patient implicitly. The patient may have no regrets about such actions, but clearly the patient's behavior will have had a disastrous effect on the employer. Such behaviors are called ego-syntonic, because they do not disturb the patient.

At the other extreme, a person with an avoidant personality may shun almost all social contact while living in a self-imposed interpersonal exile. This behavior may not really harm anyone else *per se* but results in significant personal distress. These types of behaviors are referred to as ego-dystonic, because they directly create subjective pain in the patient and are viewed by the patient as a problem. Some patients show a combination of ego-dystonic and ego-syntonic symptoms. Moreover, some ego-syntonic behaviors may morph into ego-dystonic behaviors as the patient begins to realize the damaging consequences of their behaviors to themselves over the course of time.

In patients who display primarily ego-syntonic behaviors, an important issue arises. These patients frequently are not strongly invested in receiving help, because their behaviors are not disturbing to them. Family members, lawyers, or employers may have pressured such patients into therapy; consequently, these patients may be unusually difficult to engage, both in the initial interview and in subsequent therapy. Thus, if an interviewer happens to be functioning as a consultant or triage agent, the presence of primarily ego-syntonic behaviors may suggest that the interviewer should ultimately recommend that an experienced staff member be responsible for ongoing therapy as opposed to a trainee.

But whether ego-syntonic or ego-dystonic, the behavioral manifestations of a personality disorder tend to result in specific types of dysfunctional interpersonal patterns within parental, sibling, dating, marital, employment, and friendship relationships. Consequently, as mentioned earlier, the historical evidence of a disordered personality is usually reflected in the patient's social history. To an experienced interviewer, the social history is like a snowfield, in which the characteristics of the patient's personality dysfunction can be read in the tracks criss-crossing its surface.

Thus the social history is not merely a sterile recording of "what job was held when," but represents a sensitive mirror in which the reflections of a personality disorder may first appear to the alert clinician. Stated even more boldly, a totally normal social history, if accurately related by the patient, is not consistent with a personality disorder. Somewhere along the line, the pathologic personality traits will disrupt interpersonal relationships.

From the DSM-5 definitions we can see that when performing a differential diagnosis in the initial interview, the clinician must actively search for consistent patterns of behavior, demonstrated from adolescence or early adulthood onward, without major disruption of these patterns. In this regard, Mr. Fellows serves as a suitable illustration. His defensive patterns appeared early in his life. His social history was littered with weak relationships, a poor job history, an unending string of arguments, and a maladaptive grandiosity. These behaviors were consistent over time and were undeniably crystallized by late adolescence.

The Nature of Personality Diagnoses: Abuses and Uses

A Cautionary Note

The first thing to note about personality diagnoses across all diagnostic systems (from the DSM systems of the United States to the ICD systems used internationally) is the simple fact that they are fictions. There are no such things as "borderlines" and "narcissists." In reality, there are people whose cognitions, emotions, and behaviors fit specific clusters or patterns that have been identified, classified, and named by a body of mental health professionals. From our person-centered interviewing perspective, this fact-check has important cautionary implications.

As fictions, personality diagnoses are, by definition, labels, and the potential problems described in the literature on "label theory" holds true with diagnostic labels, especially for personality diagnoses. These clinical traps coalesce around the following four phenomena: (1) the diagnosis serves as a stereotype, (2) the diagnosis functions as a pejorative label, (3) the diagnosis is viewed as an overly simplistic answer to all of the patient's behavioral problems, and (4) the patient is tagged with the label indefinitely.

First, when misused, personality diagnoses can become stereotypes. Clinicians can inadvertently decide that people fitting the diagnosis of an antisocial personality disorder are very similar to each other. Sometimes true, sometimes not true. For instance, many people coping with an antisocial structure (because it is filled with ego-syntonic symptoms) often do not benefit as quickly or as well to individual psychotherapy as do patients without this diagnosis. But some people with these diagnoses do. Consequently, if an initial interviewer decides that people with an antisocial personality disorder should routinely not be referred to individual therapy, the interviewer may be doing a marked disservice to the particular patient who might benefit. One size does not fit all.

Second, another common problem with diagnostic labels is that they may carry a pejorative connotation that predisposes clinicians to immediately feel hesitant about working with people carrying these diagnoses. Diagnoses such as borderline personality, narcissistic personality, histrionic personality, and antisocial personality come to mind. I have seen patients, given the diagnosis of borderline personality disorder in an initial interview, subsequently encounter marked difficulties finding therapists who "have room in their practices" at the moment of their call.

In a similar vein, some clinicians can have surprisingly powerful countertransference feelings towards a patient, just because the patient carries one of these diagnoses. It is not uncommon in an emergency room or on an inpatient unit to hear a staff member say something along the lines of, "Oh God, not another borderline." In truth, if we are totally honest with ourselves, most of us probably have, ingrained in our clinical psyches, a bit of this type of bias. These prejudices are powerful baggage, emphasizing the importance of not placing these labels on people unless they clearly meet the diagnostic criteria warranting them.

A third problem arises when clinicians simplistically view all of the patient's problems as caused by their diagnostic label. By way of example, a growing upsurge in grandiosity of a patient with a narcissistic personality disorder will be immediately attributed to the patient's personality disorder. However, in reality, it may be an early harbinger of a first-time manic break, which will consequently go untreated until it is too late.

Finally, personality diagnoses have a nasty habit of becoming permanent. It should be remembered that whether attributable to therapy or merely the passage of time, some people grow out of personality disorders. A person who has transformed his or her borderline processes, once they have achieved this difficult transformation, should have the diagnosis of borderline personality moved to the category of past psychiatric disorders.

The potential for outgrowing a personality disorder diagnosis also emphasizes that when "picking up" a new patient who carries such a diagnosis – if a clinician has been trained to perform differential diagnoses, whether a psychiatrist, psychologist, social worker, counselor, or nurse clinician – it is important that the clinician performs his or her own differential diagnosis. Such a clinician may discover that a given diagnosis is outdated and should be removed as described above. In addition, one should respect other clinician's diagnoses, but that does not mean that one should automatically agree with them. Even the best diagnostician can make mistakes or have a bad day. Diagnoses regarding personality dysfunction carry great weight and should be routinely re-evaluated.

At this point we have reviewed so many problems with these diagnoses that one might wonder, "Should we even use them?" My answer is a simple "yes," because when used appropriately they can be immensely helpful to people.

The Beneficial Uses of Personality Diagnoses

The positive benefits of recognizing both personality diagnoses and/or personality traits can be summarized as follows: (1) such an understanding can provide significant hints for choosing an effective psychotherapy; (2) it can provide practical suggestions for the use of specific psychoactive medications; (3) it can help the clinician to more collaboratively talk with patients about medications and other treatment interventions; (4) it can provide immediate tips for engagement in the initial interview (as well as ongoing therapy); (5) it can alert the clinician to potential psychotherapeutic missteps; (6) it can help a clinician to better understand the psychodynamics of a patient, resulting in less countertransference and an increased sense of comfort working with the patient; (7) it can provide a gateway to clinical literature that can help the clinician to provide better care; and (8) personality disorders, as part of a well-delineated diagnostic system, are essential for ongoing research leading to improved therapeutic interventions.

First, an accurate personality diagnosis can point towards the use of specific psychotherapies. Perhaps the best example of this advantage is the variety of current psychotherapies that appear to provide more effective relief for patients with a borderline personality disorder including dialectical behavioral therapy (DBT), mentalization-based therapy (MBT), systems training for emotional predictability and problem-solving systems (STEPPS), transference-focused psychotherapy (TFP), and schema-focused therapy.[3] Recognizing that a given patient meets the criteria for a borderline personality disorder and then subsequently referring the patient to appropriate therapy and an appropriate therapist (someone who likes working with such patients and is trained to effectively do so) can be pivotal to the patient's recovery, and, with regard to suicide, potentially life saving.

A less striking, yet more commonly encountered, benefit is that in the age of managed care, clinicians frequently have a limited number of sessions in which to help a patient. If one is limited to only 12 sessions with a patient, it is important to maximize the healing process within those time limits. Being unique individuals, patients may possess innate proclivities as to which psychotherapy works best for them. Once again, one size does not fit all.

I am reminded of an analogous situation with teachers in which some pupils learn best with visual presentation, others with verbal, emotional, or experiential approaches. In a similar regard, if the clinician determines that a patient meets the criteria for a histrionic personality disorder, it may suggest that one particular time limited intervention may be more likely to succeed than another.

A histrionic patient who is overly dramatic, dislikes details, loathes structure, and has a history of very negative past experiences with school, testing, and homework, may find the structure of cognitive–behavioral therapy (CBT) or solution-focused therapy an uneasy fit that might slow progress. Both of these therapies emphasize homework assignments, which could have bad connotations for such a patient; at best, this could slow acceptance of the therapy, and, at worst, it could result in discontinuation of the therapy. However, such a patient may both enjoy and gain more benefit from a psychodynamic time-limited model or a narrative-based model in which he or she gets a chance "to tell their story." In stark contrast, a patient who, in an initial session, displays many of the hallmarks of an obsessive–compulsive personality disorder, replete with a love of details, direction, and task assignment (who also has history of loving school), is practically begging the therapist to recommend a structured therapy such as CBT.

Second, and in a similar vein, an accurate personality diagnosis can suggest important psychopharmacologic interventions. Perhaps the most striking example is the significant benefit that people with schizotypal personality disorders sometimes report with the use of low-dose antipsychotics when coupled with supportive therapy and psychoeducation. I believe that with some of these patients, the addition of the antipsychotic can be life transforming. In patients in which the schizotypal process is a prodrome of schizophrenia, future research may show that the addition of the antipsychotic may soften the severity of the schizophrenia and/or prevent its full-blown emergence.

Specific elements of borderline personality disorder may also benefit from the use of medications. Research is inconclusive in this regard at present, but is promising, as reflected in a meta-analysis by Ingenhoven and colleagues.[4] Perhaps the most consistent finding is the power of mood stabilizers to positively impact on impulse control, anger expression, anxiety, mood, and global functioning. Some antipsychotics, such as olanzapine, may help with aggression and irritability.[5]

But, of course, no medication can work inside a bottle. Interest in taking a medication and following through on its use is crucial to healing. In an analogous situation, no psychotherapy can work if the patient does not buy into its use. This point raises the third benefit of recognizing personality dysfunction and/or traits. Psychiatric disorders such as schizophrenia, bipolar disorder, and depression do not arise in empty shells. They manifest in people who have distinctive personalities. These disorders must show themselves within the confines of that unique personality and that unique personality will have a unique perspective on the disorder and what it means. Each person must cope with the pains of bipolar disorder and post-traumatic stress disorder in his or her own fashion, including how they approach treatment.

In this regard, I have found an understanding of my patient's personality traits, both healthy and problematic, to be of use in talking with them about interventions such as medications and various psychotherapies. People process information uniquely, learn uniquely, and make choices uniquely. If I have a patient with schizophrenia with whom I am suggesting the use of an antipsychotic, I find it useful to present my thoughts in a fashion that resonates with the patient's personality proclivities.

Thus, if a person coping with schizophrenia has an underlying obsessive–compulsive personality disorder or traits, I might suggest that he or she read some available patient education material on the pros and cons of antipsychotics or refer them to a non-biased website on the medications. On the other hand, if my patient with schizophrenia has a histrionic personality disorder, in which they demonstrate a love of personal dramas and an aversion to homework and assignments (e.g., reading therapist-assigned psychoeducation materials) I might choose a different track, such as suggesting that the patient talk with another patient of mine who has taken the medication and feels that it has been beneficial. The use of stories and personal sharing may be much more effective with such a patient than a reading assignment on the web.

Frequently, prescribers such as psychiatrists and nurse clinicians are expected to discuss medications in the closing phase of the initial interview. An astute interviewer who has attempted to understand the patient's personality proclivities earlier in the interview, may have a significantly better chance of helping the patient to consider treatment options with an open mind.

We have emphasized repeatedly in this book that one of the most important, if not *the* most important, goal of the first interview is to ensure that there is a second interview. The success of this goal is intimately related to the sense of comfortableness and psychological safety the patient feels by the end of the initial encounter. This concept leads us directly to the fourth benefit of an understanding of the patient's personality structures and traits.

If a clinician recognizes that the patient has many narcissistic needs, the clinician will be careful not to be overly challenging to the patient, for such premature challenges in an initial interview may be perceived by the patient as a narcissistic insult resulting in a "no show" at the next appointment. Likewise, if the interviewer recognizes that the patient has more than his or her fair share of histrionic traits, then the following statement in the closing phase, "You have a fascinating story, and I'll be very interested to hear more of it in our next session" may seal the deal for a next appointment, for such a patient is usually eager to tell more of his or her drama to an interested ear.

The fifth benefit of rapidly recognizing personality dysfunction is its ability to help the initial interviewer to avoid therapeutic missteps when collaboratively treatment planning. For instance, let us picture a clinician that is about to leave a clinical position in 6 months to go to a different area of the country. One can be certain that this clinician will be kept busy by their clinical director up to his or her last day. If this clinician avoids performing a differential diagnosis regarding personality structure with a patient until many sessions have unfolded, or simply does not do one, he or she may miss that the patient fits the criteria for a borderline personality disorder (or may make the diagnosis only after powerful clinician-dependency issues have developed). Such a diagnostic omission could be a costly one for the patient.

The early recognition of such a diagnosis can have pertinent treatment ramifications. In short, if the diagnosis had been determined in the first or second interview, it would probably have been best to immediately refer the patient to a therapist who is not leaving the area in the near future. Such a therapist could provide an ongoing and stable relationship for the patient. If the initial interviewer misses this diagnosis and provides ongoing therapy for this patient, from our knowledge of people with borderline process, there is a significant chance that the patient will have developed an intensely dependent relationship by the end of the 6 months. Despite their reassurances that, "don't worry, I won't get too dependent on you," this patient may experience the loss of the clinician as an intense abandonment. Suicidal behavior and/or a completed suicide is a possibility. This type of unnecessary complication could have been avoided if the clinician had recognized the borderline diagnosis in the first or second interview, appropriately referring the patient to a therapist who could provide consistent long-term care.

The sixth advantage arises from the complementary nature of DSM diagnoses and psychodynamic diagnoses. Although it can be argued that these two systems oppose each other, I have found them to nicely re-enforce one another. In clinical practice, when I can make a DSM-5 diagnosis, upon deeper interviewing in subsequent sessions, I have generally found that the patient subsequently demonstrated the psychodynamics associated more traditionally with the same psychoanalytic diagnosis.

Thus a patient who met the criteria for a borderline personality disorder by DSM-5 criteria, upon subsequent psychotherapy showed the psychodynamics associated with borderline process (such as splitting, lack of object constancy). Such a psychodynamic understanding, as we shall see in Chapter 15, can help an interviewer feel more comfortable with a patient's erratic behaviors such as self-cutting or rage responses. The psychodynamic framework makes the unexplainable appear understandable and the unexpected seem more predictable. The advantage of the DSM/ICD diagnostic systems lies in their ability to allow clinicians to more quickly determine personality diagnoses, thus allowing an interviewer to more swiftly apply psychodynamic principles to further engagement and to foster psychological safety for the patient.

The seventh advantage of the effective use of differential personality diagnosis is obvious, but warrants emphasis. For psychiatric residents and graduate students (and experienced clinicians as well), the vicissitudes and therapeutic dilemmas that arise when providing therapy for people coping with severe personality dysfunction are many and sometimes daunting in nature. Accurate diagnosis opens the door for effective literature reviews, web resources, and discussions with experienced supervisors and colleagues on how to work with these patients.

Finally, the eighth benefit follows hot on the heels of the seventh. For clinicians to benefit from the literature and from ongoing research, the researchers and clinicians must be speaking the same language as one another. Thus a research protocol that indicates the effectiveness of a particular psychotherapy for borderline patients is worthless to me unless I know that the researcher means the same thing as I do by the term "borderline." A reliable diagnostic system is absolutely necessary for research to progress. The result is an increased array of tools for healing.

A Useful Metaphor

To use personality diagnoses effectively, one must understand their limitations as described above. Only when a clinician understands the limitations of a diagnostic system can he or she utilize its benefits wisely. In this light, I have found the following metaphor to be of use.

Imagine that you are about to go on a "survival weekend" in which you will be dropped off in one of the deserts of the American Southwest with a friend. Further imagine that neither one of you has ever set foot into a desert. In the weeks before the trip, it is likely that you would procure a map of the desert. From this map you would be able to learn about a variety of important local features that could prove to be invaluable, such as locations of water supplies, first aid, highways, and even positions of cell-phone towers that could ensure communication with potential rescuers. But even after reviewing this map for hours, neither you nor your friend would turn to the other and say, "Now that I've looked at this map, I know exactly what it will be like to be in a desert."

You would know nothing about what it is like to actually be in a desert, despite all of the valuable information gleaned from the map. The only way to know what it is like to be in a desert is to be in a desert. You must experience a desert to know what it is like to be in a desert. In short, one would never mistake a map for the terrain the map is describing.

Personality diagnoses are maps. They can provide invaluable information when used with appropriate caution. They can alert an interviewer to use specific engagement techniques to create safety (avoiding putting a person with narcissistic tendencies on the spot), they can predict specific therapeutic interventions (such as DBT for borderline process or an antipsychotic for schizotypal process), they can predict likely future problematic behaviors (over-dependency in a person with borderline process), or even save a life (suggesting effective ways for helping a person with borderline process transform suicidal crises).

In effect, like a map to a hiker in a desert, they can are invaluable tools. But they do not tell you anything about the person beneath the diagnosis. The only way to understand a person with serious personality psychopathology is to sensitively listen and listen and listen. A personality diagnosis can sometimes be made in a single session; compassionate understanding will necessitate many sessions.

As long as a clinician understands to never mistake the map for the terrain beneath the map – the diagnosis for the person beneath the diagnosis – these diagnoses can be used to greatly enhance engagement, care, and treatment.

The Etiology of Personality Disorders

"Where do they come from?" This question easily demands attention at this point in our discussion. Alas, the answer itself does not come so easily. Theoreticians could spend – and have spent – a large amount of time discussing conflicting theories regarding etiology. However, a recapitulation of their work would not be time well spent in a text of this type. Instead a simplified and unifying approach will be described, which can guide us toward a more sophisticated understanding of the person seeking our help.

Fortunately this unifying approach is a concept with which we are already well acquainted, for the human matrix provides a sound framework for understanding how personalities, both normal and abnormal, evolve. Each wing of the matrix (biological, psychological, dyadic, familial/cultural/societal, and worldview) contributes in an ongoing fashion to the shaping of a human personality, with each wing impacting upon the others as well as being impacted by the others. Together, these fluctuating influences will eventually determine the anxieties and need states that will result in the development of the specific unconscious defense mechanisms and conscious coping strategies of the individual.

On the biological wing, Thomas and Chess have emphasized the point that small infants display characteristic temperaments, which can persist into later stages of life.[6] These variables include intensity of reaction, activity level, attention span, threshold of response to stimulation, mood, and distractibility. Both genetics and intrauterine factors could influence the development of such traits. Indeed, several studies have suggested that, by school age, children often have a personality structure similar to that which they will demonstrate as adolescents and even as adults.[7,8] Both normal and abnormal personality trait domains are moderately heritable with estimates usually around 50%.[9,10] One can easily see how biological factors can play a significant part in the determination of personality structure. In the age-old debate of which determines human behaviors – nature versus nurture – it is clear that nature plays a major contributing role as it spins out from the biological wing of the matrix, creating both healing and damaging effects on the other wings.

For example, let us imagine a child. We shall call him Khalid. Imagine that Khalid was born with a biological propensity to be easily distracted. He subsequently may have significant problems with learning and school performance. But the negative impact of his biological deficit in attention does not stop with the obvious problems directly caused by his biological deficits in concentration.

Indirect consequences may create equally (or perhaps even more) devastating long-term effects for Khalid. Because he has no idea why he is having problems learning (a biological deficit), his low grades will probably be interpreted by him as being a failure on his part. The result might be a punishing sense of low self-esteem. In addition, Khalid's concentration deficit may impact not only on his ability to perform in school but also on his ability to obey his parents.

And here we see the immense power of matrix effects to shape, and potentially damage, personality development. Khalid's biological deficit has already impacted on his psychological wing, creating problems with task completion and perhaps, indirectly, with self-esteem. These damaging psychological processes may be further amplified by reciprocating matrix effects between his psychological wing and his familial/cultural/societal wing.

Khalid's seemingly intentional disobedience and poor school performance may disturb his parents' equilibrium and happiness as they are summoned into the school to address Khalid's "lack of effort" and "clear underachievement" (a damaging matrix effect from Khalid's psychological wing onto his familial wing). Frustration and anger may result, even in high-functioning parents, who may tend to show displeasure and subtle rejection of Khalid (a reciprocal damaging matrix effect from the familial wing back onto Khalid's psychological wing). It is a vicious cycle that is likely to tatter Khalid's sense of self-worth yet further. Perhaps a sibling will now become "the apple of Daddy's eye," a fact surely not missed by Khalid.

We can also readily imagine that considerably more problems would arise if our theoretical child, Khalid, had been born into a family already steeped in psychopathology or grew up in a neighborhood ripe with animosity towards Khalid's ethnic or religious background. Abuse – whether societal or familial in origin – can further the need for Khalid to develop a rigid set of psychological defenses in order to survive.

An alcoholic parent may beat Khalid, probably resulting in a child who is further unable to concentrate and learn secondary to fear and agitation. The pathologic cycles begin to feed upon each other, with damaging matrix effects resonating across wings. Marital disharmony may intensify as arguments ensue regarding the management of Khalid's bad behavior.

As time passes, Khalid's chances for developing a reasonably healthy personality structure are dimming. The only question that remains is which defense mechanisms, coping skills, and compensatory personality traits will arise to help Khalid navigate the storms inherent in his matrix. These defenses and coping skills will be key in shaping Khalid's personality structure, and hence, his personality diagnosis.

It should be kept in mind that a child without any biological deficits regarding attention, if born into an abusive family with alcoholic traits, could soon develop personality deficits of his or her own, including damage to the attention centers of his or her brain. For instance, there is compelling evidence that early childhood trauma can cause lasting changes in the physiology of various structures in the limbic system of the brain (a fascinating example of a damaging matrix effect from the family wing to the biological wing of the matrix).[11,12] A chaotic home environment with abusive parents can quickly damage a developing personality. Such a child may become chronically anxious, and, in this instance, environmental influences will actually change the neurophysiology – and perhaps even cytoarchitecture.

In any case, an abused child will begin to develop psychological defenses in order to function at a reasonable level of anxiety. Such a theoretical child could easily become more reclusive and timid; or the child may develop a conception of himself or herself as being inferior and unwanted. The result may be the development of distancing tactics that protect the child from rejection or the development of grandiose thinking that serves to shore up a fragile self-esteem. These tactics function to buffer the child from feelings of worthlessness. Perhaps these were the types of factors that jointly combined to create Mr. Fellows, the theoretical child in the flesh.

No easy explanations exist. It is relatively meaningless to deliberate over which wing of the matrix was most instrumental, because with each individual this mixture will vary. Moreover, with most people, the resultant personality is a reasonably healthy one. The following chapters concern themselves with those instances in which an inflexible set of defenses emerge, such as with Khalid or Mr. Fellows. The result is not so healthy.

Having procured a sound introduction to the concepts shaping the assessment of personality dysfunction – from core definitions to etiology – we are now ready to explore the practical art of uncovering these diagnoses in a clinical setting, the topic of our next chapter.

REFERENCES

1. American Psychiatric Association. *Diagnostic and statistical manual of mental disorders*. 5th ed. (DSM-5). Washington, DC: American Psychiatric Publishing; 2013. p. 645.
2. DSM-5. 2013. p. 646–7.
3. Nelson JN, Schulz SC. Treatment advances in borderline personality disorder. *Psychiatr Ann* 2012;**42**(2):59–64.
4. Ingenhoven T, Lafay P, Rinne T, et al. Effectiveness of pharmacotherapy for severe personality disorders: meta-analysis of randomized controlled trials. *J Clin Psychiatry* 2010;**71**(1):14–25.
5. Linehan MM, McDavid JD, Brown MZ, et al. Olanzapine plus dialectical behavior therapy for women with high irritability who meet criteria for borderline personality disorder: a double-blind placebo-controlled study. *J Clin Psychiatry* 2008;**69**(6):999–1005.
6. Siever LJ, Insel TR, Ulde TW. Biogenetic factors in personalities. In: Frosch JP, editor. *Personality disorders*. Washington, DC: APA Press; 1983. p. 42–65.
7. Shiner RL. The development of personality disorders: perspectives from normal personality development in childhood and adolescence. *Dev Psychopathol* 2009;**21**:715–34.
8. Tackett JL, Balsis S, Oltmanns TF, Krueger RF. A unifying perspective on personality pathology across the life span: developmental considerations for the fifth edition of the Diagnostic and Statistical Model of Mental Disorders. *Dev Psychopathol* 2009;**21**:687–713.
9. Bouchard TJ Jr, Loehlin JC. Genes, evolution, and personality. *Behav Genet* 2001;**31**:243–73.
10. Jang KL, Livesley WJ, Vernon PA, Jackson DN. Heritability of personality disorder traits: a twin study. *Acta Psychiatr Scand* 1996;**94**:438–44.
11. Dannlowski U, Stuhrmann A, Beutelmann V, et al. Limbic scars: long-term consequences of childhood maltreatment revealed by functional and structural magnetic resonance imaging. *Biol Psychiatry* 2012;**71**(4):286–93.
12. van der Kolk BA, Saporta JW. Biological responses to psychic trauma. In: Preston J, Raphael B, editors. *International handbook of traumatic stress syndromes*. New York, NY: Plenum Press; 1993.

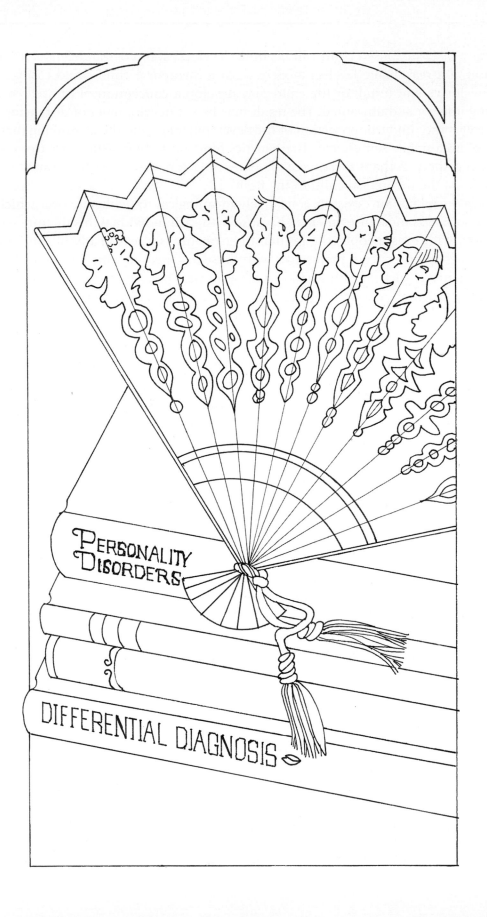

CHAPTER 14

Personality Disorders: How to Sensitively Arrive at a Differential Diagnosis

Sometimes she [Emily Dickinson] would only talk to acquaintances from behind a closed door. She fled from approaching visitors and refused to appear when friends or guests came to see her. She surprised one visitor, who was permitted to see her, by allowing him to choose between a glass of wine or a rose from the garden. Whenever possible, she avoided conversation, preferring to communicate with people in writing.

A. M. Hammacher
Phantoms of the Imagination[1]

INTRODUCTION

I cannot say whether Emily Dickinson was coping with a personality disorder or not, but I can say that she was both wonderfully fascinating and creatively gifted. I can also say from our biographical knowledge of her that she experienced great pain and loneliness in her life.

If she was suffering from something such as an avoidant personality disorder and had lived today, one would like to think that a contemporary clinician could help her to share her pain in a productive fashion. One would like to think that with the outstanding psychotherapeutic and psychopharmacologic tools that we now have available to us, we could relieve at least some of her suffering. To do so, we would need to pull upon the core engagement skills that we mastered in the opening chapters of our book. These core engagement skills would allow us to create a safe enough interpersonal space to tempt her to "move from behind her door" into a therapeutic alliance. In addition, we would need a variety of advanced interviewing skills. These advanced skills would sculpt the gateway through which we could sensitively delineate the vague outlines of her personality, and to uncover a personality disorder, if there was one from which we could have helped her to find relief. This chapter is about those skills.

Emily Dickinson is a shadow of the past. We cannot help her now. Although there may be only a few people today who possess the creative genius of Emily Dickinson, there are innumerable people today who share her pains. These people enter our offices seeking our help. But to help them, within the substantial time constraints of today's clinical culture, and to do so with sensitivity and compassion, requires great interviewing skill.

The ability to delineate a differential diagnosis of personality dysfunction in the initial interview is a daunting task at first glance. But, upon closer inspection, we will find that there are specific interviewing strategies and techniques that can allow us to succeed in this task.

To accomplish our task this chapter is divided into four sections: (1) a survey of the DSM-5 diagnoses, (2) common problems encountered when arriving at a personality diagnosis, (3) an interviewing strategy for using the DSM-5 to arrive at a diagnosis, and (4) a look at the future of the differential diagnosis of personality disorders and the usefulness of dimensionality.

SECTION I: A SURVEY OF THE DSM-5 PERSONALITY DISORDERS

Goals and Limitations of the Survey

In undertaking a differential diagnosis, it is crucial that the clinician becomes thoroughly familiar with the actual diagnostic criteria, because the diagnoses are made by a careful expansion of these criteria. However, the criteria utilized in the DSM-5 are somewhat sterile sounding in nature. One of the first steps in gaining an interviewing proficiency for delineating personality disorders is the development of a general sense of what the core characteristics of each disorder actually look like. The clinician must gain a familiarity of these disorders not as checklists but as they manifest in living individuals.

To jumpstart us on this process, let us examine the fashion in which patients coping with these disorders tend to think, feel, and respond to others. In this survey, based upon the clinical literature as well as my own clinical experiences, I have attempted to provide some flesh to the individual personality disorders, while pointing out some of the distinguishing characteristics between them. To accomplish this task, I have also borrowed from the narrative structure and descriptive style of an alternative diagnostic schema for personality dysfunction called the Shedler–Westen Assessment Procedure (SWAP-II),[2] which adds a nice dimensionality to the DSM-5 approach and of which we will hear more later in the chapter. These brief vignettes are designed to highlight the prototypic characteristics with which people with these disorders present.

As a note of caution, I must emphasize that these vignettes are characterizations, and, as such, represent particularly vivid depictions of people who meet the diagnostic criteria for these disorders. Although some people do, indeed, present with such intensity, many present with less severity. It is important to keep in mind that the following vignettes are not meant to be used as stereotypes. The actual presentations of people with these disorders can vary widely within the margins, and even beyond the margins, of these cross-sectional depictions. Only by listening carefully to many patients, while attempting to actively empathize, can the clinician gain a clearer understanding of the individuality of each person seated across from him or her.

Keeping these cautions in mind, I believe that the vivid nature of our presentations will serve us well in two ways: (1) the descriptions are designed to provide a rapid and realistic introduction to the remarkable diversity and nuance in presentation of people with these disorders, and (2) the vividness of the depictions will hopefully make it easier for readers to recall the needed diagnostic traits *during* interviews, a task that can be daunting unless one has a clear picture in one's mind of how these traits actually manifest in the real world. The reader should supplement these descriptions with parallel reading of the actual DSM-5 criteria.

To aid in the familiarization process, I have placed the 10 specific personality disorders recognized by the DSM-5 into three broad groups. These groups contain disorders that have similar core characteristics with regard to how the patient experiences life. If, during the course of the initial interview, the clinician recognizes these pervasive worldviews, then an immediate cluster of diagnostic regions for more extensive expansion suggests itself. Each clinician can determine his or her own ways of organizing the personality disorders. The following system merely represents a method that I have found practical. The three broad categorizations are as follows: (1) anxiety-prone disorders, (2) poorly empathic disorders, and (3) psychotic-prone disorders (referring to a more frequent tendency to develop micropsychotic episodes, as described in Chapter 11). It should be noted that the DSM-5 officially uses a fairly similar, yet different, set of clusters (i.e., odd–eccentric [Cluster A], dramatic–emotional [Cluster B], and anxious–fearful [Cluster C]).

1. Anxiety-Prone Disorders

This cluster includes the following three disorders: the obsessive–compulsive personality, the dependent personality, and the avoidant personality. All three of these disorders share the common thread of an existence riddled with tension and anxiety. They differ in how this anxiety manifests itself and with which methods it is controlled. This is not to say that people with other personality disorders do not experience anxiety, because they do. Instead, it merely suggests that anxiety is often a keynote feature of these three disorders. These patients are also susceptible to intermittent bouts of depression, which may occur when their needs are not met or their defenses are not adequate.

Obsessive–Compulsive Personality Disorder

A person who has an obsessive–compulsive personality sees life from the inside of a pressure cooker. It is a pressure cooker often constructed from the patient's own set of perfectionistic goals and demands. In short, these patients are hard on themselves. Driven by an internal sense that any failure is an ultimate failure, they help to form the army of workaholics who both love and resent their work. In a sad sense, these people frequently function under a covert belief system that they must prove themselves worthy of being loved. Thus there is no time for fun, and they often appear too serious for their own good while presenting a somewhat cool and distant exterior.

They tend to control their anxiety through the use of an abstract and overly intellectualized style of thinking. Deep inside, there seems to be a fear that they are about to lose control. Consequently, life becomes a series of contests that are won through discipline and endless lists and work schedules. Patients with an obsessive–compulsive personality truly show their colors when they produce a splendidly paradoxical "schedule for play." Even free time is a commodity to be well spent. Moreover, major decisions rapidly become major hurdles, because the patient becomes terrified of the prospect of making a wrong decision. Life is viewed as a long corridor of one-way doors few of which lead to "success." It is a costly lifestyle, filled with stress. It is a way of life in which tears may not be shown but are felt nevertheless.

Dependent Personality Disorder

As with the previous disorder, a person with a dependent personality views the world as a place fraught with potential disaster; however, the resultant anxiety is handled in a different fashion. The compulsive person throttles the anxiety by fiercely attempting to control all possible situations, including the behaviors of others. The passive-aggressive individual mutes the anxiety by saying, "I never expected much from this lousy show anyway." In contrast, the dependent personality runs from the anxiety, straight into the arms of some unsuspecting surrogate parent. Life is spent hunting for this savior. White knights are not the inhabitants of fairy tales; they are the invited dinner guest.

These patients are exquisitely sensitive to rejection, but they are willing to risk humiliation if the reward is eventual safety. Consequently, they are often warm and giving, bordering precariously on the cusp of obsequiousness. They are more than willing to bend to the needs of others; indeed, they thrive on the chance to prove their irreplaceable devotion by doing just about anything they are asked to do. They can be coerced to do things they find to be objectionable, or even illegal, if such activities are necessary to be accepted or loved. They invented the concept of bending to peer pressure.

Having a fear of showing anger, because it could result in rejection, they display their anger passively by making mistakes, procrastinating, or "forgetting" to do requested tasks. Because they view themselves as weak and ineffectual, they do not want to make decisions. Moreover, their intensely low self-esteem traps them into a fear that they could not make it on their own. This type of person is often unable to leave the spouse-abuser, and his or her unfortunate answer to insecurity is the safety of interpersonal dependency.

Avoidant Personality Disorder

Affection and love are two conditions that people with an avoidant personality hope for desperately. Unfortunately these goals remain mere dreams, because these patients suffer from such low self-esteem that they dare not risk making an attempt at friendship. If ever there were people who followed the credo "Any club that would accept me, I wouldn't want to belong to," it is this group of patients. Like people with dependent personalities, they feel inadequate, but their low self-esteem seems laced with a more brutal self-ridicule. These people do not generally trust themselves and essentially become socially phobic. Unlike the person with a dependent personality, they frequently appear aloof and cool, so as to protect themselves from the rejection they feel is a future certainty. They also tend to alienate other people with self-denigrating comments such as, "You probably don't want me along, but can I come to the movies too?" Such testing comments beg for a statement of acceptance from their targets, who may quickly tire of providing reassurance.

Their timid demeanor may provoke ridicule from bullies and those predisposed to cruelty. Moreover, they do not search for the "white knight" so valued by people with dependent personalities, because they would not even dare to address such a figure if found. It is a lonely existence. These are the patients who live in cities for years without making an effort to secure a friendship unless they feel absolutely certain that rejection will not occur. Every night is lost in the anonymity of online exchanges or in the white flickering of television characters, who have no method of inflicting pain and who will reliably show up for the next date.

2. Poorly Empathic Disorders

People with these personality disorders (the schizoid personality, the antisocial personality, the histrionic personality, and the narcissistic personality) share a peculiar inability to empathize in the same sense, or with the same regularity, as most people. Their personal history may be littered with a trail of people who have felt betrayed and manipulated. Alternatively, their lack of empathy may be a reflection of a true lack of interest in human contact, as seen with the schizoid personality. In any case, during the initial interview, one may catch glimmers of a world in which the feelings of other people are of little worth to the patient.

As Westen and Shedler point out, the manner in which this self-centered approach manifests may vary strikingly among the four disorders.[3] Narcissistic patients are often oblivious to the needs of others. However, people with an antisocial bent may well recognize the needs of others, but will use them to manipulate them. In contrast, the person with a histrionic style may simply miss the needs of others because they are swept away by the self-created drama of the moment. Meanwhile, the schizoid personality so lacks an interior world of pronounced emotions and needs that they literally can't recognize such feelings in others.

Schizoid Personality Disorder

The person presenting with a schizoid personality structure represents the classic picture of the quiet loner. If one were to picture an animal analogue, some type of mollusk comes to mind – a creature that is slow moving, has limited ability to reach out, yet is more than capable of living a shell-like existence, content to function as an isolated unit. There is a blandness to the world of these patients, both in their internal and external worlds. They tend to form few relationships and prefer the role of a wallflower. Emotions run neither high nor deep. Tenderness tends to be neither felt nor sought. They exhibit a relatively bland indifference to what others may think of them. Their lack of affective color may suggest the cool stamp of one looking down from the pedestal of superiority. This is seldom the case. In actuality, their "colorless" quality represents a muted palette. These people tend to lack both the need and the social skills to actively engage other people.

On the surface, they may sound somewhat like people with avoidant personalities. But the avoidant personality is a hotbed of anxious emotions stirred by a perpetual duel with predicted humiliation. A person with an avoidant personality actively avoids people, whereas a person with a schizoid personality effortlessly glides through people with a minimum of contact. There is no fear of rejection because there is no desire for acceptance.

Some mention should be made of another diagnosis with which the schizoid disorder is sometimes associated, but which, in my opinion, shares little overt resemblance, except with regard to the spelling of their names. A person with a *schizotypal* personality disorder (which we will examine in detail in a few pages), like a person with a schizoid personality, may also have few friends and appear somewhat aloof and distant. But patients with a schizotypal personality disorder are generally, but not always, rejection sensitive, much more like a person with an avoidant personality. Moreover, their world is seldom bland. On the contrary, it is extremely active, rich with bizarre and idiosyncratic emotions and conceptualizations, a bit like a dream on feet. Furthermore, the diagnosis of the schizotypal personality seems to be related to schizophrenia and people with such personality traits may later develop this psychotic disorder. Indeed, in the DSM-5, the schizotypal personality disorder is viewed as being part of the schizophrenia spectrum as well as being a personality disorder.

In contrast, there appears to be no striking relationship between the person with a *schizoid* personality and the occurrence of schizophrenia. Indeed the person with a schizoid personality disorder is not generally prone to micropsychotic episodes, as seen in schizotypal personality disorders.

Antisocial Personality Disorder

A person with an antisocial personality is a chameleon. At times he or she may appear somewhat withdrawn like a person with a schizoid personality disorder, but more frequently the person appears actively involved with others. With certain people this individual may appear belligerent and nasty. On a different night or with a different person, he or she may be the epitome of charm. The reason for the deftness in style lies primarily in the fact that these patients are participating in a continual game in which other individuals exist as pieces to be manipulated and utilized as deemed fit.

As a result, people with antisocial personalities are frequently at odds with the law and are noted for lying, cheating, drug fencing, job hopping, and paternity suits. They can be particularly nasty on the web, wrapping their cruelty in the anonymity of a false internet identity. Sex is a one-night affair, and the word "responsibility" is not listed in their dictionary. At their worst, these patients may be cruel, sadistic, and violent (a subcategory of this disorder is referred to in the literature as "sociopathy"). It has been suggested that they seldom feel anxiety and certainly infrequently feel the anxiety born from guilt. Indeed, they live a life in which a superego seems to have never set foot in their psyche. In a surprising sense, these people frequently see their problems as arising from flaws in other people, as opposed to their own inadequacies. They have an almost uncanny knack at convincing others to give them yet another chance, leaving people to feel convinced that "this time is really different." It isn't.

Obnoxious as these patients may sound, Vaillant makes the humanizing point that, in reality, they probably do, or at least did at some point, feel pain.[4] Indeed, their amoral behaviors and worldview probably are, at least in part, a reflection of defenses developed to deflect relatively intense pain. For instance, the apparent callousness of their relationships may in some cases represent a defense, protecting the patient from a fear of being engulfed by intense dependency needs. Ironically, people with an antisocial personality may very well be as entrapped as their victims, their distancing defenses taking them so far from human emotion that they may appear as monsters. But in the last analysis, they are all too human.

Histrionic Personality Disorder

There are probably few people who are as exhilarating to be around as a histrionic person "on a good day" and few as miserable to encounter as an unhappy one "on a bad day." On this adult see-saw, these patients attempt to live life as a child, hoping to find a perch on Daddy or Mommy's knee. The world is seen through the eyes of an Impressionist painter, popping an occasional hallucinogen. They do not look at details and seldom remember them. The past is a blur of impressionistic images. Whereas the person dealing with an obsessive–compulsive personality collects the world in neat categories and cages, the histrionic patient gleefully unlocks the doors of any cages within sight.

These patients feel little responsibility and demonstrate an unnerving sense of devil-may-care. With a forced eviction lying only days ahead, the histrionic patient may be focusing attention on landing a date with someone he or she met in a pick-up bar or encountered in a risqué chat room. Somehow or another a new apartment is supposed to simply materialize in the meantime. Their impulsive nature is often also manifested in flirtatiousness and even promiscuity. They are frequently drawn to people who are already attached or sought by someone else.

There is no doubt that life is exciting for them, because they view themselves as if their life were part of a movie. They tend to demand center stage, and if lucky enough to be good-looking or talented, they may well end up center stage. Their life is a long string of over-reactions, tantrums, and lost loves. Many a Hollywood train-wreck is pulled by the locomotive of an underlying histrionic personality. Fascinating people to read about; painful people to befriend.

Beneath the dramatics is a fragile self-esteem that is easily crushed. Behind the glamour, intense feelings of inferiority and neediness hide. They are powerfully dependent upon the applause of others for their own sense of self-worth. Keenly sensitive to rejection, they are constantly searching for reassurance and praise. People are manipulated to achieve these needs, and a person with a histrionic personality can little afford to empathize with the needs of those who may lie in his or her way.

Mild suicidal behaviors without intent to die are not uncommon. But these suicidal behaviors may be followed several days later by a bright smile if "Mr. or Mrs. Right" has entered the picture. This ability to change moods rapidly, depending on environmental circumstances, is a hallmark feature. Like a child throwing a tantrum, one needs only to distract a person with a histrionic personality in order to make things better. Somehow, there is tragedy in all this glamour. Adults were not made to live as children.

Narcissistic Personality Disorder

As mentioned earlier, this category seems to house two rather distinctive types, which, for want of a better title, can be referred to as the stable and unstable variants. In the stable variant, the patient's narcissism appears to be well rooted. These patients actually view themselves as superior and frequently enjoy their own company. In contrast to this picture, with the unstable variant, the narcissism appears more as a defensive front, a type of pseudo-narcissism. With these patients, the grandiosity is more of a charade, hiding an intensely frightened ego.

Let us look at people with a stable narcissistic personality first. To these patients, other people exist as objects, whose reason for existence is to comfort the patient. A person with this type of narcissism finds it difficult to view others as having needs. The world revolves around one god, and the god is "I."

Like a small child, the stable narcissist's views of others may rapidly change from idealizing to denigrating. Mother is great if she buys the toy airplane and is a hated object if she denies the purchase. People with a stable narcissism are often the product of a spoiled upbringing, in which sharing was not common. Consequently, they never develop the ability to think of other's needs. It simply does not cross their minds.

Naturally, few people locked into a narcissistic perspective are born with the abundance of talents and skills they feel they have. Daddy's little girl may merely be another average kid to the rest of the world. To deflect this painful realization, these patients may preoccupy themselves with grandiose fantasies. On the other hand, some people with a stable narcissistic personality structure, especially if talented, may be reasonably happy, although they may be difficult to get along with. Problems arise if, for whatever reason, adulation and subservience do not come their way. In such instances, they may pout, stomp about, become depressed, and/or turn to inappropriate substance use for comfort.

In contrast, a person with an unstable narcissistic personality tends to live in a much more hostile world. The sense of ego is actually poorly developed, and life is a constant threat. There lurks an incipient feeling of annihilation and a piercing feeling that the individual is truly worthless. This is defended against by the production of a grandiose style, not unlike that seen in the person with a histrionic personality. But the stakes are high, and these patients are easily wounded. Their defense may consist of a vicious rage, and they can turn on a friend in moments. Few people are trusted and bitterness becomes a way of life.

They are constantly fleeing humiliation, while gloating over the embarrassment of others. If dinner is not on the table on time, then one may find it angrily thrown on the floor. Tantrums and rages become second nature. They expect to be at the head of the line, and when this does not happen, a scene is to be expected. They are almost impossible to please and are prone to severe depressive episodes when their needs are not met. Their personality structure is quite primitive, and they are prone to micropsychotic episodes. People with unstable narcissism are often not successful in life, because their behavior prevents advancement, while their mood swings make consistent work difficult. In some instances, they may demonstrate reasonably good impulse control in public or on the job, but display their more primitive qualities in their intimate relationships such as with their spouse or their therapist.

Unlike the stable narcissist, the unstable narcissist is frequently sad and angry. Every day is a battlefield. They pretend to be Napoleon, but deep in their hearts they know they are a sham. Worse yet, they unconsciously fear that others will recognize the sham as well.

3. Psychotic-Prone Disorders

This collection of disorders includes the borderline personality, the schizotypal personality, and the paranoid personality. If one looks at the patient's sense of self in these disorders, as indicated by their ego structure and spontaneous coping defenses, one finds these people to be seriously developmentally delayed. Their defensive structure is reminiscent of the defenses used by children, including magical thinking, preoccupation with internal fantasy worlds, and tendencies to act impulsively or out of rage.

When pressured, they may experience micropsychotic episodes, as these defenses sweep them into a false reality. For this reason they are clustered as "psychotic-prone." They could just as easily be referred to as the regressed personality disorders, referring to the developmental immaturity of their ego structure. In this regard, the histrionic personality and the unstable narcissistic personality (both of which, during extreme moments of stress, can also demonstrate micropsychotic episodes) may also function as regressed personalities. Let us begin our survey of these disorders by giving special attention to the intense pain that coats their reality with a distinctive sense of impending chaos.

Borderline Personality Disorder

The person coping with a borderline personality structure experiences life as if there were no sense of inner self. If one could feel inanimate, like a piece of clothing hanging forlornly in a closet, then one can begin to appreciate the hollowness that haunts these people. Like the clothing, they feel empty unless filled by the presence of others. Like the clothing, they depend on others to give meaning to life. Consequently, they often intensely dislike being alone, because it can lead to sensations of impending annihilation and destruction. As a friend leaves the apartment, they may literally feel empty, as if a part of themselves were now absent.

Their need for others is so great that they cannot understand how anyone who really cares about them could leave them alone. Thus their dependency quickly becomes a hostile one as they resent the pain that others inflict upon them. When they feel slighted, they can rapidly escalate into rages, throwing glasses, breaking furniture, and screaming profanities. In this sense, they are unpredictable. Because they are so exquisitely sensitive to being hurt, friends and lovers may quickly tire of apologizing, eventually growing angry themselves. A high level of interpersonal stress is the standard price required to befriend these patients.

Without the presence of others, these patients frequently view life as colorless and boring. Consequently, coupled with their intense feelings of weakness and self-loathing, they may ceaselessly seek stimulation using drugs, sex, and eating to satisfy their feelings of emptiness. Their impulsive behaviors unfortunately may bring them into contact with superficial people, who promptly proceed to abuse them, thus fulfilling their worst fears. Fear of abandonment becomes a nagging companion, stoked by the fact that their unpredictable behavior and manipulative attitude frequently result in actual rejection.

Their thinking often has a black/white quality to it, in which they have problems seeing the grey both in situations and in the actions of others. This can result in a tendency to "catastrophize," seeing problems and relationships as disastrous or untenable. Their catastrophizing tendency is frequently accompanied by an inability to soothe or comfort themselves without the help of another person.

Suicidal thought arises almost with a predictability. It may be coupled with a tendency to use self-cutting and other forms of non-lethal self-harm such as burning themselves with cigarette butts and matches, striking themselves, or head banging. When cutting themselves, they frequently feel no pain. The self-cutting seems to serve as a surprisingly reliable method for relieving their feelings of intense pain or anger. Such episodes often follow an argument or perceived slight. These periods of analgesia, while cutting themselves, probably represent fleeting periods of psychotic depersonalization. Other common micropsychotic processes include derealization and paranoia.

In the last analysis, these patients face a harsh world, over which they feel they have little control. The picture is further darkened by the sense that they themselves are also out of control. They represent the stuff of which soap operas are made. They are "the glass people," delicate to touch, easily broken, and dangerous when shattered.

Schizotypal Personality Disorder

Like the person with a borderline personality, the individual with a schizotypal personality seems to lack a core. This person also is stalked by a rather unsettling sensation that he or she is somehow empty. This blandness becomes an invitation to an in-pouring of vivid fantasy and psychotic-like process. The world becomes peopled with clairvoyant messages, ghost-like presences, magical hunches, and secretive glances. Like a child withdrawn into a world peopled with pretend playmates, the person with a schizotypal personality silently retreats from life. Unlike a person with a schizoid personality described earlier, a person struggling with a schizotypal personality disorder is frequently sensitive to rejection. This person wants contact but does not know how to make it. There is a desperate quality here, in which the eccentric professor finds more solace in his books than with others of his species. They may find that the only safe place to fulfill their needs for intimacy lies in the addictive world of massively multiplayer online gaming (MMO). Here in the world of MMOs they find it easier to befriend an avatar than the human who created it. One of my adolescent patients would spend endless days running with stray dogs in the woods near his house. Apparently, they were kinder companions than the children at his school. Moreover, he was "the king" of his dogs, whereas he was merely "the dog boy" at his school. Thus these fantasy wanderings may provide a firmer sense of self-esteem to these patients.

Because of the withdrawal into their private worlds, these patients may develop idiosyncratic ways of thinking and using words, tending to become metaphoric and vague.

There may have been a tiny bit of schizotypal flair to the oddness of Emily Dickinson. Unfortunately, these traits may result in further problems with socialization, as reflected by Ms. Dickinson suggesting to her guest that he choose between a glass of wine or a rose from the garden. With the right guest, this eccentric gesture is endearing; with the wrong guest, it is puzzling if not downright bizarre. When stressed, the person with a schizotypal personality may decompensate into micropsychotic episodes including delusions and hallucinations. And as part of the schizophrenia spectrum, people with this personality disorder can be more likely to develop schizophrenia itself, or they may have relatives afflicted by it. In a sense, this individual lives life from "the inside of the bottle," peering at others as if watching a different species, worried that someone may poke a finger or two into his or her private world.

Paranoid Personality Disorder

The world of the person with a paranoid personality is blanketed by a thick covering of restless worrying. Probably more than any other disorder discussed so far, these patients see the world as a hostile environment. These patients have never evolved the ability to trust other people. As a consequence, they are suspicious and guarded by nature. They scour their interactions with others for the subtlest hints of deception, often ignoring the bigger picture as they fixate on a slip of the tongue or an errant look. They tend to be over-controlling and prone to intense jealousy.

Their paranoid ideation, except during micropsychotic episodes, is not delusional in quality, but nevertheless, they seem driven by it. It is as if they feed on their own concerns. One is left with the feeling that without their fears, they would feel awkward and without purpose.

Their defensive guardedness has generally arisen to protect them from a deep-rooted sense of inferiority. Moreover, they fear that their weaknesses will leave them vulnerable to attack. In response, they become haughty, finding it extremely difficult to admit mistakes. All new faces represent potential enemies, not potential friends. Everything needs to be checked out. By way of illustration, during an initial interview one of my patients suddenly produced a notebook in which he began vigorously scribbling down our dialogue. He related that, "I'm just keeping a record so that people on the outside know what's going on in here."

It is a lonely existence. It is also one in which delusional thinking can erupt, because the paranoid patient's isolation prevents him or her from receiving corrective opinions from others. It is further complicated by their tendency to see their own unacceptable impulses in other people instead of in themselves (a psychodynamic defense known as projection). They are consequently prone to misattribute their own hostility to others. Their brief delusional micropsychotic breaks are often accompanied by tremendous feelings of rage and indignation. These patients are also predisposed to more severe psychiatric disorders, such as a paranoid delusional disorder. In the final analysis, they are exquisitely unhappy. In a true sense, they lead tortured lives, because everywhere that they look they see men with inquisitor's hoods. Ironically, it is the hands of their own projections that weave such ominous raiments.

SECTION II: COMMON PROBLEMS ENCOUNTERED WHEN DIAGNOSING PERSONALITY DISORDERS

Premature Diagnosis: "Label Slapping"

Mistaking Behaviors Shown in the Interview as Personality Traits

In this section we will focus upon those problems related not so much to weaknesses in the diagnostic systems but to clinicians' frequent misconceptions with regard to how to use these systems. The first common problem to be avoided is the tendency to make personality diagnoses too rapidly, without actually determining whether the patient truly fulfills the criteria or not. This problem manifests itself frequently, when clinicians diagnose in an impressionistic fashion, saying to themselves things like, "That patient is clearly a borderline – she was so manipulative during that interview."

The behavior of the patient in the interview and the clinician's intuitive feeling for the patient's pathology are extremely useful tools. But they are tools whose usefulness resides in guiding the clinician towards diagnostic regions that merit further detailed exploration, perhaps, even in future interviews if time does not allow appropriate immediate exploration. As we have emphasized multiple times already, and with good reason, personality disorders are historical diagnoses. The patient's behavior in the interview provides suggestive, not conclusive, evidence of their presence.

Even when one is aware of this important distinction, it can be surprisingly easy to mistake the behaviors of the patient in the interview itself as concrete evidence that the patient has a personality disorder. For example, a patient may present in a dramatic fashion, wearing a seductive blouse and brightly colored pants. The patient may talk with a mild pressure to her speech, demonstrating a knack for telling a colorful tale. The same patient may act coyly and may be caught by the clinician telling several trivial lies. An inexperienced clinician may immediately label this patient as having a histrionic personality, but this diagnosis is being made on the recent and immediate behavior of the patient in the interview.

A careful interviewer might have discovered that this extroverted and overly dramatic behavior is quite atypical for this patient historically, being neither consistent nor persistent in nature. In addition, the patient may have a long history of depressive episodes, as well as a positive family history for bipolar disorder. Indeed, this patient is experiencing the early symptoms of the initial manic episode of a bipolar disorder. With regard to treatment, she may benefit significantly from a trial of lithium or another mood stabilizer. Unfortunately, the impressionistic diagnostician may not "get the point" until the patient turns the corner into a blatant manic crisis.

An overly dramatic patient presentation could also be seen with other classic psychiatric diagnoses, including atypical bipolar disorder, cyclothymic disorder, and amphetamine abuse or some other drug-related disorder. An even more ominous problem would exist if this atypical behavior was secondary to an organic agent such as a brain tumor. A premature diagnosis of histrionic personality disorder could be disastrous in such a situation – leading to the delayed treatment of the tumor.

Problems With Countertransference

The impressionistic diagnostician can also run into problems around the issues of countertransference and labeling theory. As we mentioned in Chapter 13, when we were cautioning against careless labeling with personality disorder diagnoses, these diagnoses often carry negative connotations and may be thought of by some in pejorative terms. If a clinician takes a rapid dislike to an abusive patient, then in the clinician's mind the patient may become "just another damned sociopath." One would like to think that one is "above all that," but few, if any, clinicians actually are. In this sense, it is important for clinicians to explore what these diagnoses mean to them on a personal and emotional level.

It is important to remember that these diagnoses should not be made casually, because they can greatly affect the future course of therapy for the patient. I have certainly seen patients refused by a clinic because "he's a borderline and we don't have room for any more borderlines now or in the near future either." These issues also serve to remind us not to fall into the trap of using these diagnoses as stereotypes.

Indeed, when one speaks of an approach to performing a differential diagnosis concerning personality dysfunction, one is in some sense speaking of the clinician's approach to life as well. More precisely, a clinician who is prone to passing moral judgments will probably have great difficulty in both interviewing and subsequently working with people who have developed the character structures that we label as pathologic. A gentle compassion is needed in order to convey the unconditional positive regard of Carl Rogers, as discussed in Chapter 2.

This point is important because many of the traits that the clinician must explore in order to detect the presence of character pathology are traits that may arouse considerable guilt in the patient. If the clinician conveys a judgmental attitude, this guilt will generally be intensified, frequently to the point that the patient will feel uncomfortable – as if undergoing a public humiliation rather than a therapeutic exchange. A clinician's parental glance may punish as effectively as a scarlet letter.

Besides unsettling the patient, such behaviors by the clinician serve to sabotage the interview itself, because the more that the patient's self-system is activated, the more likely it is that information will be distorted or withheld. Indeed, the skill of a clinician to uncover personality pathology greatly parallels his or her ability to ask questions regarding sensitive material in an unassuming, non-judgmental, and natural fashion.

Inappropriate Hesitation to Make a Personality Diagnosis

The above cautionary points are important in guiding the clinician toward a wise use of these diagnostic labels. But if taken to their extreme interpretation, they become damaging in themselves. By this I mean that clinicians can become almost phobic about the idea of making a personality diagnosis in a single hour. One might hear a clinician state, "I never make a personality diagnosis in an hour; it takes much longer to know a person and make sure they present in the same way over several sessions." Ironically, this misinterpretation of the concept of a personality disorder hinges on the same error in thinking seen with the impressionistic interviewer – specifically, that the diagnosis is being made primarily upon how the patient presents. But, as we have seen, a hypomanic patient could present for months in a style totally consistent with a histrionic personality.

The pertinent point remains that personality disorders are not made primarily upon the basis of the patient's presentation. Once again, we are reminded that they are historical diagnoses. *The issue is not whether the patient presents for seven sessions with histrionic behaviors, but whether the patient has displayed histrionic behavior consistently for years dating back to adolescence.*

In this light, the limiting factors in making a personality diagnosis in the initial interview are twofold: (1) Does the clinician have enough time to explore the past history of the patient appropriately to ensure historical consistency and persistency? (2) Is the patient providing reasonably valid information? If the above two criteria are met, then one can safely make a personality diagnosis in an initial assessment.

The truth of the matter is that some diagnoses are more easily made in an initial assessment and some are difficult to make in this "50-minute hour" timeframe. As one would expect, those diagnoses that are easier to make tend to have behaviorally oriented criteria that do not depend much upon the subjective opinions of the clinician.

For instance, people coping with antisocial, borderline, and schizotypal personality disorders present with fairly concrete, behaviorally specific criteria. As a case in point, either the patient has or has not been suspended from school. Either the patient has consistently demonstrated self-mutilating behaviors or no such behaviors have occurred. Those personality diagnoses characterized primarily by behaviorally specific criteria can frequently be made in a single hour as long as the patient is telling the truth and the symptoms are not "state dependent."

This latter requirement is critically important. By "state dependent," I am referring to the exclusion criteria in the DSM-5, which forbid the use of the criteria as valid if the criteria symptoms or behaviors are directly caused by another mental disorder (such as the hypomania or mania described above that could mimic histrionic behaviors) or by a medical condition (such as a brain tumor, epilepsy, or acute substance-induced intoxication). *Thus, no symptom can be viewed as meeting a personality disorder criterion in the DSM-5 if the symptom can be viewed as being state dependent.*

In contrast to those diagnoses whose criteria are highly behavioral and concrete, those disorders whose diagnostic criteria are highly subjective may be quite difficult to make in an hour, for the clinician must cover a wide variety of historical circumstances in order to determine whether or not the patient demonstrates these features or behaviors consistently. This category of disorders (diagnoses that are difficult to make in the 7 to 12 minutes available for personality disorder delineation in the typical 50-minute initial assessment) include entities such as the histrionic personality and the narcissistic personality, both of which have predominantly subjective diagnostic criteria.

In real-life practice, a talented clinician who actively pursues clues to personality dysfunction and who persistently hunts for diagnostic criteria will usually have a good idea as to whether a personality disorder is present or not in an hour. With the more behavioral diagnoses, this may result in an actual diagnosis or perhaps a provisional diagnosis; or at least, a set of possible rule-out diagnoses. In the more elusive diagnoses, the clinician should at least have a feeling for possible rule-out diagnoses and, at times, even an actual or provisional diagnosis in an initial assessment. *Interviews with family members and other sources are particularly valuable in clarifying personality diagnoses when the picture is unclear.*

An interviewer who is overly cautious risks a variety of consequences. In the first place, the attitude itself tends to make these interviewers sloppy in approaching these diagnoses because, "if you can't make the diagnosis, then why try?" In a sense, they generate self-fulfilling prophecies. Because they do not practice the skills needed to make these diagnoses efficiently, they, indeed, cannot make them efficiently in one or two interviews. But even more important is the fact that to fail to spot these diagnoses until it is too late is a disservice to the patient.

This is particularly true in the case of a consultant or an intake interviewer who is being asked to suggest treatment approaches or may actually determine the triage of the patient to other services. If the interviewer determines that the patient either fulfills or nearly fulfills the criteria for a borderline personality, the head of an outpatient psychotherapy clinic would be ill advised to refer this patient to one of the inexperienced clinicians or, worse yet, to a clinician demonstrating serious psychopathology. The consequences of the patient being assigned to an unsuitable clinician without the necessary skills and insight could be very problematic. In short, it is of value to recognize these diagnoses as early as possible.

These diagnoses are useful in other ways too. For example, a psychotherapist may think twice about making significant changes to parameters such as the frequency of sessions with patients with a borderline disorder or a severely dependent personality disorder. Also, as noted in Chapter 13, it might be detrimental to accept for therapy such a patient if the clinician intends to move from the area in the next 6 months. It may be best to refer such a patient to a therapist who will be remaining at the clinic.

We have ended our discussion of the numerous factors that can affect the clinician's ability to perform a differential diagnosis regarding personality disorders. It is hoped that, coupled with our prototypic survey of the disorders, we have secured an appreciation of the enormous pain that sometimes envelops these patients and the people who care about them. Let us now examine the actual art of delineating a differential diagnosis with these patients, a process that represents a complicated challenge even for experienced clinicians.

SECTION III: USING THE DSM-5 TO ARRIVE AT A PERSONALITY DIAGNOSIS

In the following section we will explore a practical and sensitive interviewing strategy that I have found to be very useful over the years for arriving at a reasonable differential diagnosis during an initial interview. Using these sequential steps, by the end of the initial interview one will often have delineated one or more specific personality diagnoses (especially if the diagnoses tend to have particularly objective diagnostic criteria). At the very least, these steps will have gone a long way towards uncovering probable diagnoses – greatly facilitating their final determination in the next interview – while providing pivotal information for effective engagement, safe triage, and collaborative treatment planning.

Step #1: Limiting the Field of Diagnostic Choices

There are two steps involved in delineating a personality diagnosis in the initial interview using the DSM-5: (1) The first step consists of limiting the field of diagnostic possibilities. No clinician could gracefully and sensitively explore the criteria of all 10 personality disorders in 50 minutes. The resulting interview would be hurried, stilted, and inviting of a "no show" at the next appointment. Instead, the clinician must figure out one or two (maybe three) diagnoses that are most probable. (2) The second step consists of subsequently exploring these diagnoses in a thorough and sensitive fashion to see if the patient's history adequately meets the diagnostic criteria for those diagnoses. It is to the first step that we now turn our attention.

Passively Scouting for Clues to Personality Dysfunction

Throughout the interview, the clinician has the opportunity to reflect upon both the patient's words and actions. In this way, without actively searching for clues to personality dysfunction, the astute clinician frequently picks up on a variety of hints as to which disorders may be worth pursuing in more detail.

In this regard, the clinician can focus on the patient's *observable* behaviors and style of interaction (signal signs) or on the patient's *reported* complaints (signal symptoms). Both areas are rich with implication, providing pertinent clinical hints that point toward the personality diagnoses or traits that are most likely present. Keep in mind that the presence of signal signs or signal symptoms does not indicate that a personality disorder (or even a specific personality criterion) is present. They merely indicate that it is worth looking for a particular disorder or trait historically in the available timeframe.

Signal Signs

Since personality disorders represent long-standing patterns of behavior, it is not unusual for patients to reveal some of their pathologic behaviors during the interview itself. This does not *always* occur, but it frequently does. I am consistently amazed by the regularity with which these signal signs occur in the first 5 to 8 minutes of the interview, during the scouting period. This early appearance of characteristic defensive behaviors may result from the patient's anxiety stimulated by meeting a clinician. This self-system anxiety probably triggers many of the most ingrained defenses of the patient.

In Chapter 3 (see pages 68–97) we discussed the mnemonic PACE as representing the mental activities of the clinician during the scouting period. If the reader will recall, the "A" stands for an assessment of the patient's mental state and behaviors. An important part of this assessment process is the clinician's careful openness to the presence of signal signs (observable behaviors). Signal signs may also appear during any subsequent phase of the interview as well.

The signal signs represent behaviors suggestive of specific personality disorders that may warrant further investigation. As noted earlier, they do not indicate that the patient necessarily has these disorders, because these behaviors may be present in personality disorders other than the ones listed or in people without character pathology at all, sometimes caused by state-dependent factors such as the presence of bipolar disorder or schizophrenia. But what the signal signs do suggest is the increased likelihood that a particular disorder may be present and may be worth exploring later in the interview, perhaps while eliciting the social history.

Each clinician could probably develop a long list of signal signs gleaned from experience. In this chapter, I am sharing some of those that have been most useful for me. Many others exist, and I am not attempting an exhaustive study here. The following observations are derived from clinical experience and do not represent research-validated data. Nevertheless, I think that they provide a useful jumping-off point for clinicians who are attempting to master the art of delineating a differential diagnosis regarding personality.

One of the more peculiar signal signs is the presence of comments made by the patient during the interview about the interview itself or the interviewer. Most patients do not make such process comments, because they are inhibited by the newness of the situation and do not want to do something that is wrong. I remember a young man who was being interviewed by a student in front of a group of fellow students. The patient had a dramatic intensity and related several times that he was an extremely sensitive individual. It has been said that if one has a good trait, one never needs to tell others about it. Such was the case with this "sensitive" patient, for in the middle of the interview he turned to the obviously struggling interviewer saying, "You sure seem to be having a lot more trouble with this interview than me." If the clinician was not feeling awkward enough already, then this statement certainly pulled out a few more beads of sweat.

This practice of commenting on the process of the interview, frequently in a somewhat caustic fashion, is often a dead giveaway that the clinician is speaking with a person exhibiting one of the following four disorders: an antisocial personality, a narcissistic personality, a histrionic personality, or a borderline personality (it may also manifest in people with passive-aggressive traits).

A somewhat-related behavior that can signal the presence of personality dysfunction arises when the patient makes some type of unwarranted complaint during the interview itself. These complaints may be coupled with demands of a subtle nature and sometimes of a not-so-subtle nature. For example, a patient may walk in the door for the first appointment announcing that he or she does not intend to sit in the waiting room so long the next time. Or the patient may begin, "You really should get better parking arrangements for your patients, although I'm sure you've already looked into this matter before" (topped off with a pleasant smile). Such behaviors are often the "window dressings" of a person with one of the following disorders: a narcissistic personality, a borderline personality, a paranoid personality, or an antisocial personality.

At the other extreme, one may encounter patients who seems a little too pleased with the clinician. These are the patients who make sexual innuendoes or references throughout the interview. This may consist of overly frank discussions of sexual adventures or overt offers for a date or the request of a telephone number. In other instances, the patient may turn on the charm with phrases such as, "Well, I've always seemed to be fairly attractive to the opposite sex, as I'm sure you've found to be true for yourself." These types of comments represent signal signs consistent with the following: an antisocial personality, a histrionic personality, and a narcissistic personality. If the innuendoes become more lewd or intrusive, one should become even more alert to the possible presence of an antisocial personality structure. I have found that males with an antisocial personality disorder will not infrequently use this type of sexual innuendo for putting female interviewers on-guard as a means of attempting to control the interview.

This type of behavior is similar to the patient who presents with a dramatic bravado. The patient may be boldly dressed in bright colors or a sinewy scarf. If male, the patient may be encased in clothing so tight that one cannot help but notice he is a gold card member at the local gym and has the muscles to prove it. If female, provocative clothing and sexual innuendo may rule the day. The patient is frequently quite enthralled with the very act of talking about the history of the present illness while animatedly gesturing. Such patients may rapidly become tearful and even more rapidly shut off the tears when the clinician embarks on a new line of questioning. These types of behaviors should serve as an indication that one may be in the presence of a person with a histrionic personality or a borderline personality.

Another type of signal sign consists of the patient who appears child-like and helpless. These patients may speak with a quiet meekness, accompanied by an earnest attempt to please the interviewer with statements such as, "Is this what you wanted to hear?" As one would suspect, such behaviors are often the trademarks of a dependent personality structure. Such helplessness is sometimes also seen episodically in people with histrionic personalities and with borderline personalities.

As a final example of a signal sign, we turn to those patients who become openly manipulative during the interview itself. They may attempt to make the clinician grant them a request or make a condemnation of another clinician. For instance, the patient may say, "My current therapist is very bossy. Don't you think that is strange for a therapist?" The patient then waits anxiously for the clinician to make a disparaging comment that will undoubtedly be fired as a verbal salvo at the therapist in question. Other types of manipulations may consist of various methods of controlling the interview or bargaining with the clinician, such as, "Look it's getting late, if we must talk let's do it quickly and I need a cigarette first." Once again, we've hit the province of disorders such as the borderline personality, the histrionic personality, and the narcissistic personality. Such "sighing compliance" may also mark a person presenting with passive-aggressive traits. (See Figure 14.1 for a summary of signal signs)

To wrap up this discussion of signal signs, an actual clinical example may serve to consolidate some of the ideas. The following activities occurred primarily in the minutes directly preceding the interview and in the first few minutes of the interview itself. The interview was taped for supervision purposes. The patient, who we discussed earlier in

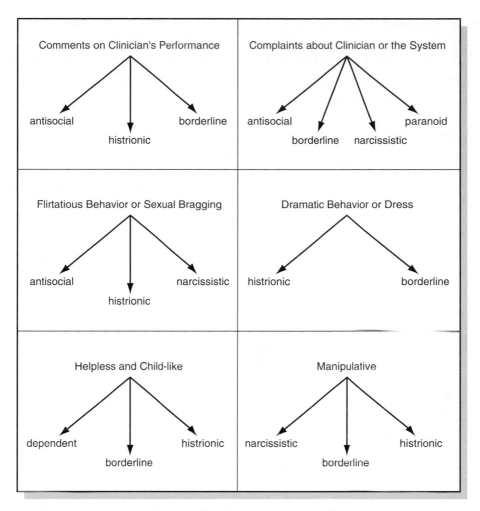

Figure 14.1 Signal signs suggesting fan-like diagnostic possibilities.

the chapter on nonverbal behavior, had come to the Diagnostic and Evaluation Center because "I'm having problems coping." For the sake of convenience, the patient will be called Ms. Dole. Ms. Dole was dressed somewhat shabbily in worn-out corduroy trousers and a faded blouse. Her dull brown hair seemed to "come with the outfit," in the sense that it too had seen better days, as it hung in long folds. Her lengthy hair accented her lanky body.

Both she and the clinician began placing their respective microphones. Ms. Dole fumbled repeatedly with her microphone, until her awkward actions attracted the eye of the interviewer. However, immediately before the clinician looked at Ms. Dole, a most curious process unfolded. Ms. Dole had actually managed to get the microphone on, but she promptly pulled it off. As the clinician asked if she could manage, Ms. Dole looked up with pleading eyes and shook her head from side to side, never saying a word. She looked like a 3-year-old asking her mother for help. And help was quickly on the way, because the clinician proceeded to attach the microphone for her. Earlier we had mentioned this interactive process as a nice example of a parent–child nonverbal reciprocal.

When the interviewer began the actual interview, Ms. Dole quietly handed her some notes, mumbling that these would help the interviewer to understand. "I wrote them a few days ago," she meekly related. At which point the interviewer watched as Ms. Dole fumbled with the papers, taking about a minute to find the passage she wanted read.

Ms. Dole was managing to rapidly gain control of the interview by utilizing a mixture of helpless ineffectuality and manipulative staging. Her helplessness may have been a signal sign suggestive of the presence of a borderline personality or a dependent personality. Her manipulative gestures would also be consistent with a histrionic personality, a borderline personality, or a dependent personality. Subsequent detailed interviewing resulted in a diagnosis of a mixed personality disorder with histrionic and dependent traits. Thus the first 3 minutes of interaction provided powerful clues as to which diagnostic regions needed further exploration. Sometimes an interviewer's eyes are more useful than his or her questions.

Signal Symptoms

As the interview proceeds, the patient frequently relates symptoms or pieces of history that may function to guide the clinician toward consideration of specific personality disorders. Once again, as with signal signs, the clinician is not actively eliciting these symptoms. Instead, the patient is spontaneously providing them; the clinician needs only to recognize their importance.

Some signal symptoms are classic for certain disorders. This does not suggest that these symptoms are seen only in these disorders, but rather that they are frequently characteristic of these disorders. For instance, the presence of a history of self-mutilation or of frequent suicidal behaviors should alert the clinician to the possibility of a borderline personality disorder. People with borderline personalities are well known for self-damaging non-lethal behaviors such as wrist cutting, burning themselves with cigarettes, head banging, and frequent overdoses.

Another classic signal symptom is the reporting by the patient of an extreme need for perfectionism. This is frequently accompanied by a nagging sensation that the patient has never done enough. It is the mark of a superego run amok, and should strongly suggest the presence of an obsessive–compulsive personality or at least some compulsive traits.

A third relatively classic signal symptom is the reporting of a history of run-ins with the law. Repeated arrests, burglary, or frequent fights all strongly suggest the need to expand the antisocial personality region. Other areas to explore include fencing drugs, prostitution, and arrests for disorderly conduct or drunken driving. When asked about arrests, patients often conveniently fail to mention the last two types of incidents. It is often best to specifically inquire about disorderly conduct and drunken driving, as well as speeding.

Other signal symptoms suggest not just one disorder, but a variety of disorders. In a sense, these signal symptoms suggest a fan-like differential diagnosis. The presence of frequent feelings of anger, sometimes accompanied by actual physical violence, alerts the clinician to the likely presence of either an antisocial personality or a borderline personality. Other less likely components of the fan include the paranoid personality, the narcissistic personality, and the histrionic personality.

A different signal symptom consists of an extreme feeling of low self-esteem. Such intense feelings of worthlessness and inadequacy are frequently seen in people with a dependent personality, avoidant personality, schizotypal personality, or borderline personality. Figure 14.2 illustrates some of the various signal symptoms and the possible diagnoses they suggest.

It should be kept in mind that the characteristics that I used earlier to group the various personality disorders (anxiety-prone, poorly empathic, and psychotic-prone) may also serve as signal symptoms. Thus the reporting by the patient of powerful and persistent feelings of anxiety should alert the clinician to the possible presence of the obsessive–compulsive personality, the dependent personality, and the avoidant personality. In a similar fashion, the antisocial personality, the histrionic personality, the schizoid

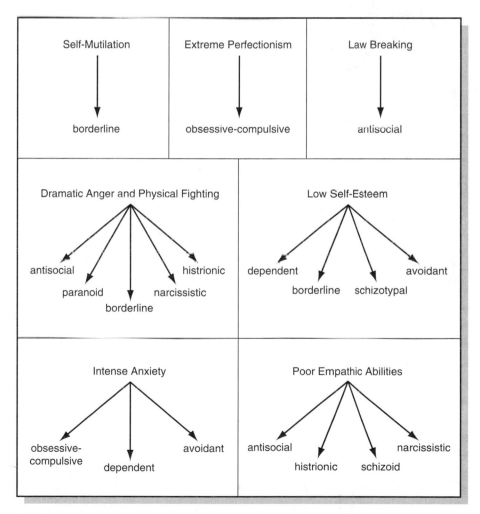

Figure 14.2 Signal symptoms suggesting diagnostic possibilities.

personality, and the narcissistic personality are all suggested by a tendency for the patient to demonstrate a poor ability to empathize effectively. Finally, the presence of frequent micropsychotic breaks should alert the clinician to the potential presence of personality disorders such as the borderline personality, the schizotypal personality, and the paranoid personality.

It takes some time for clinicians to begin to routinely recognize the significance of signal signs and signal symptoms; however, with experience, the ability to utilize these invaluable clues becomes almost second nature. It should be readily apparent that many patients will, in the course of 30 minutes, practically point the way to the most likely paths that will provide concrete evidence of personality psychopathology. Note that this part of the differential diagnostic process requires no additional time, for these signal signs and symptoms are passively spotted while the interviewer is merely asking questions regarding the patient's stresses, history of presenting problems, and uncovering other psychiatric symptoms.

However, a clinician does not have to rely solely on passively noting signal signs and symptoms; the interviewer can also actively try to draw out evidence of personality dysfunction that can further limit the field of diagnostic possibilities.

Actively Limiting the Diagnostic Field With Probe Questions

There is one other method of accomplishing the first step in personality assessment of limiting the field. This technique consists of asking probe questions concerning a specific disorder. If the patient's answers to the probe questions are not consistent with the presence of the disorder, the clinician may decide that no further expansion of that specific disorder is indicated. On the other hand, answers consistent with the diagnosis suggest that further questioning may uncover the specific disorder. The craft of delicately and thoroughly substantiating a personality diagnosis requires both skill and a sense of timing. The talented interviewer doggedly pursues the evidence needed to make the diagnosis but does so in a manner that fosters both a more powerful blending and an increased understanding of the patient not as a label but as an individual.

First let us examine a list of probe questions for personality disorders, several of which were developed by Jeremy Roberts.[5]

1. Obsessive–compulsive personality:
   a. "Do you tend to drive yourself pretty hard, frequently feeling like you need to do just a little more?" (yes)
   b. "Do you think that most people would view you as witty and light-hearted?" (no)
   c. "Do you tend towards being perfectionistic?" (yes)"
   d. "Do you tend to keep lists or sometimes feel a need to keep checking things, like is the door locked?" (yes)
2. Passive-aggressive personality (described in DSM-IV-TR Appendix)
   a. "Do you frequently feel like your friends or employers tend to take you a little too much for granted?" (yes)
   b. "Sometimes have bosses tended to nag you, you know, ask you to do something a couple of times?" (yes)

   c. "If your boss asks you to do something that is stupid or that you disagree with, do you sometimes try to make a point by doing it slowly or without your full effort?" (yes)

   d. "When others are overly optimistic, do you tend to be the one who shows them the problems with their plans?" (yes)

3. Dependent personality

   a. "Is it sort of hard for you to argue with your spouse (use whatever term is appropriate, e.g., partner, significant other, boyfriend, etc.), because you're worried that he or she will really get mad at you and start to dislike you?" (yes)

   b. "When you wake up in the morning, do you tend to plan your day around the activities of your spouse (use whatever term is appropriate, e.g., partner, significant other, boyfriend, etc.)?" (yes)

   c. "Do you enjoy making most decisions in your house or would you prefer that others make most important decisions?" (prefers others to make the decisions)

   d. "When you were younger, did you often dream of finding someone who would take care of you and guide you?" (yes)

4. Avoidant personality

   a. "Throughout most of your life, have you found yourself being worried that people won't like you?" (yes)

   b. "Do you often find yourself sort of feeling inadequate and not up to new challenges or tasks?" (yes)

   c. "Do you tend to be very careful about selecting friends, perhaps only having one or two close friends in your whole life?" (yes)

   d. "Have you often felt hurt by others, so that you are pretty wary of opening yourself to other people?" (yes)

5. Schizoid personality

   a. "Do you tend to really enjoy being around people, or do you much prefer being alone?" (much prefers being alone)

   b. "Do you care a lot about what people think about you as a person?" (tends not to care)

   c. "Are you a real emotional person?" (no, feels strongly that he or she is not emotional)

   d. "During the course of your life have you had only about one or two friends?" (yes)

6. Antisocial personality

   a. "If you felt like the situation really warranted it, do you think that you would find it pretty easy to lie?" (yes)

   b. "Have you ever been arrested or been pulled over by the police for unruly behavior, the use of drugs, or drinking while driving?" (yes)

   c. "Over the years have you found yourself able to take care of yourself in physical fights?" (yes)

   d. "Do you sometimes find yourself resenting people who give you orders?" (yes)

7. Histrionic personality

   a. "Do people of the opposite sex frequently find you attractive?" (answered with an unabashed "yes")

     b. "Do you frequently find yourself being the center of attention, even if you don't want to?" (yes)

     c. "Do you view yourself as being a powerfully emotional person?" (yes)

     d. "Do you think that you'd make a reasonably good actor or actress?" (yes)

8. Narcissistic personality

     a. "Do you find that when you really get down to it, most people aren't quite up to your standards?" (yes)

     b. "If people give you a hard time, do you tend to put them in their place quickly?" (yes)

     c. "If someone criticizes you, do you find yourself getting angry pretty quickly?" (yes)

     d. "Do you think that compared with other people you are a very special person?" (answered with a self-assured "yes")

9. Borderline personality

     a. "Do you frequently feel let down by people?" (yes)

     b. "If a friend or a family member hurts you, do you sometimes feel like hurting yourself, perhaps by cutting at yourself or burning yourself?" (yes)

     c. "Do you find that other people cause you to feel angry a couple of times per week?" (yes)

     d. "Do you think that your friends would view you as sort of moody?" (yes)

10. Schizotypal personality

     a. "Do you think that you have sort of special, even sort of unusual thoughts that others may not have?" (yes)

     b. "Do you sometimes feel like other people are watching you or have some sort of special interest in you?" (yes)

     c. "Have you ever felt like you had some special powers like ESP or some sort of magical influence over others?" (yes)

     d. "Do you feel that people often want to reject you or that they find you odd?" (yes)

11. Paranoid personality

     a. "Do you find that people often have a tendency to be disloyal or dishonest?" (yes)

     b. "Is it fairly easy for you to get jealous, especially if someone is flirting with your spouse (use whatever term is appropriate, e.g., partner, significant other, boyfriend, etc.)?" (yes)

     c. "Do you tend to keep things to yourself just to make sure the wrong people don't get the right information?" (yes)

     d. "Do you feel that other people take advantage of you?" (yes)

Responses in the indicated direction to one or two of these questions generally suggest that it would be worth the clinician's time to pursue the personality disorder in more detail. Some of these questions may overlap, and positive answers may be consistent with several different diagnoses. For example, if the patient responds positively to the probe question for the paranoid personality concerning jealousy, several other disorders may also be worth considering. Jealousy is commonly seen in people with narcissistic personalities, histrionic personalities, and borderline personalities. But an effort has been made in compiling these questions to list those questions that tend to be more specific for each of the diagnoses for which the question serves as a probe. If the patient responds positively to several or all of the probe questions for a given diagnosis, then it is significantly more likely that this diagnosis will eventually prove to be valid.

These probe questions are *never* used in a checklist fashion but are quietly woven into the fabric of the natural flow of the interview using graceful facilic transitions, such as natural gates or referred gates, as described in Chapter 4. The clinician will probably only have time to utilize a few of the specific probes for each diagnosis. Fortunately, these probe questions can often serve to quickly eliminate certain diagnoses.

If one asks the following probe for schizoid qualities, "Do you really enjoy being around people or do you much prefer being alone?" and the patient responds, "Oh I love being around people, I'm a party animal," one can safely assume that a person with a schizoid personality is not in the room – unless it happens to be the interviewer! All levity aside, the point of the matter is that certain answers are inconsistent with certain diagnoses and no further probing will be required.

Keep in mind one caveat concerning the potentially misleading quality of state-dependent "traits." On occasion, a state-dependent process will not just mimic a personality disorder as we have discussed (a manic state creating the impression that the patient is histrionic), it will hide it. For instance, a patient with a schizoid personality may claim to be a "party animal" if the patient is currently manic.

In point of fact, the clinician will probably not have a need to ask most of these questions, because the passively observed signal signs and symptoms given by the patient will have already eliminated many diagnoses while pointing the way toward those with more potential. Those diagnostic areas with more potential can then be actively scouted by using several of the probe questions; and, if the diagnosis appears likely, the clinician will proceed with a more thorough exploration in order to substantiate it.

One may wonder whether there are regions of the interview where it is best to utilize probe questions and to explore for personality dysfunction. The answer to this question is that the interviewer can utilize these techniques essentially anywhere in the body of the interview. However, as one would expect, there is one area – the social history – in which personality pathology virtually leaps out at the interviewer, if it has not already done so in the history of the present illness.

As mentioned before, the social history represents the region of the interview in which patients inadvertently discuss the impact of their personalities on the people and jobs in their past. Many signal symptoms will be given here, and probe questions can be utilized effectively to determine which personality disorders warrant a more thorough exploration. Since the social history is often not taken in detail until later in the body of the interview, the blending has usually had time to develop strongly, thus allowing the clinician to more effectively explore the sensitive types of material frequently associated with personality disorders.

Illustration of a Clinician Limiting the Field of Diagnostic Possibilities

Let us picture a 30-year-old man seeking psychotherapy, whose initial assessment is underway.

In the following example we will watch his clinician as she delineates which areas of personality dysfunction warrant more careful exploration. The dialogue occurs during the social history. Some of the clinical thinking that might be guiding such an interview is presented in brackets.

Clin.: After you left college what happened?

Pt.: Let's see, uh, I think the first job I took was with the electric company, but that job didn't really pan out to be what I was promised.

Clin.: In what sort of ways?

Pt.: Oh, the job was really boring and the pay wasn't so hot either. So I left after about 3 months and eventually got a job in sales. I liked that much better. I stayed there for, let me see, maybe a year, and then I had a whole string of jobs.

Clin.: In the 5 years following that time how many jobs do you think you had, a couple, 20, 30? (symptom amplification)

Pt.: Oh, pretty many, maybe close to 20 jobs. (The large number of jobs in a relatively short period of time certainly suggests that something is up here. An erratic job history is a signal symptom frequently suggesting the presence of an underlying antisocial personality, as well as a personality with a tendency for erratic relationships and impulsivity. Consequently, the clinician asks several probe questions concerning antisocial hallmarks.)

Clin.: Did anything ever happen on some of these jobs, like having a problem with the law or an arrest, *that made you have to leave*, because sometimes that's why people leave jobs quickly? (shame attenuation)

Pt.: Oh no, not with me. I don't like the police. They terrify me. I've never been arrested or even pulled over for running a light.

Clin.: Doesn't sound like you have a very extensive criminal record. (clinician smiles and patient laughs)

Pt.: No, it sure doesn't. I don't break the laws. In that regard, I'm a pretty straight arrow.

Clin.: What about things like using drugs or selling drugs?

Pt.: Nope, I wouldn't touch them, never even tried them. I just don't think it's right to use illegal drugs, that may sound sort of corny but it's true. (This patient shows little evidence of antisocial proclivities; in fact, he seems to have a fairly strong superego sense of what is right or wrong. Thus there must be something else going on. The clinician will now switch the focus more toward social interaction and friendships.)

Clin.: What kinds of things do you like to do for fun?

Pt.: Now that's a good question, because I don't have a lot of fun. I'm really pretty much of a loner. Sometimes I think that I just wasn't made to get along well with people, so I keep to myself pretty much. (Here various options are opening up. A person with a schizoid personality classically describes himself or herself as being a "loner," but such a person frequently holds jobs down well. Moreover, the openness and talkativeness of this patient earlier in the interview are uncharacteristic of the schizoid personality disorder. However, some of the disorders that are rejection sensitive lead to the avoidance of people as a means of protection. The clinician decides to figure out, by the use of a probe question, if the patient shuns people because he does not really want the company of people [as with a schizoid personality] or because he fears the company of people [as with an avoidant personality].)

Clin.: If you had some better skills at being around people, do you think you would like to do that?

Pt.: Oh yes, I have always wanted to be popular and sometimes I really do enjoy people. I love to laugh, but somehow I always end up getting hurt. (The schizoid personality disorder has essentially been eliminated with the use of the probe question, because such patients seldom, if ever, strive for social interaction in the fashion that this patient is describing. The feelings of inferiority and inadequacy expressed by this patient also make it unlikely that we are dealing with an entity like a narcissistic personality disorder.)

Clin.: Do you frequently feel let down or hurt by people?

Pt.: Very frequently. And, to be quite frank, it angers me, and that's why I've basically decided to keep my distance, but that's no fun either. And I resent that. Why should I be the one that suffers, what do they want from me anyway? (Plenty of important information is coming to light here. The patient truly sounds rejection sensitive. Entities come to mind such as the schizotypal personality, the dependent personality, the avoidant personality, the histrionic personality, and the borderline personality. That is quite a string of possibilities, but they can be decreased relatively rapidly. First, in an earlier part of the interview not shown here, when the region of psychotic material was being reviewed, the patient denied any psychotic material, even of a subtle nature. Consequently, the schizotypal personality is not worth pursuing. A careful sensitivity to the material already uncovered reveals another interesting point. People with dependent personalities and with avoidant personalities tend to stay in jobs for a long time, because they fear new situations and they tend to dislike the process of job interviewing or meeting new co-workers. To sort out this situation better, the clinician refers back to the job history, to see if the erratic history may be related to interpersonal problems with bosses or with co-workers. If frequent angry interactions are uncovered, then one could essentially rule out more timid entities such as the dependent personality and the avoidant personality.)

Clin.: Earlier you mentioned that you changed jobs frequently. Did you find that some of the people you were around were difficult people to work with? (utilization of shame attenuation)

Pt.: As a matter of fact, I did. Some of them were very difficult.

Clin.: What types of arguments would you get into?

Pt.: The usual kind, you know, a boss who can't let you do your own work and who asks you to do things one way one time and another the next. I hate that. I never know what they want. Now don't get me wrong, I sometimes had something to do with it too, but not usually, at least I don't think so.

Clin.: Did some of the bosses get angry and ask you to leave?

Pt.: Yeah, I've been fired a couple of times if that's what you mean. And I think it's been 50–50.

Clin.: How do you mean?

Pt.: Fifty percent of the time my fault and 50% of the time their fault. (The demonstration of open anger, the firings, and the tendency to see a lot of other people at fault all essentially eliminate the dependent personality and the avoidant personality as suggested before. This pattern is also certainly not the job history of a person with a compulsive personality.)

Clin.: When you get angry, what do you do?

Pt.: Sometimes I really get furious. I go home and I let off steam.

Clin.: How do you mean?

Pt.: I don't know, break things, throw things … people just treat me like shit sometimes and it's not fair. It's not fair. That's why I get depressed all the time (angry tone of voice).

At this point, the differential is becoming a good deal more manageable. We are left with the histrionic personality and the borderline personality. The patient's history is thus far consistent with both, but the histrionic personality seems less likely for several reasons. In the first place, few people with histrionic personalities view themselves as socially inept, and, despite repeated painful experiences, they seldom become more reclusive. The better bet is probably the borderline personality.

The anger-control problems are certainly consistent with borderline process. We are also starting to see, with his last statement, the possibility of the marked moodiness so often seen in people with borderline process. At this point, the clinician has successfully limited the field. Time is probably best spent exploring the borderline criteria thoroughly and further checking for histrionic criteria. There is, of course, the possibility that the patient has a mixed personality disorder with borderline and histrionic traits. One could also add that this patient seems to have some fairly striking passive-aggressive traits.

This example illustrates how quickly the clinician can begin to develop a differential regarding personality dysfunction by utilizing passive techniques, such as recognizing signal behaviors and signal symptoms, in conjunction with the more active technique of asking probe questions. In this interview, the interviewer accomplished the task in 2½ minutes. What remains now is for the clinician to skillfully expand the most likely diagnosis in a graceful and non-invasive manner – step #2 of performing a differential diagnosis regarding personality disorders.

Step #2: Actively Expanding the Diagnostic Criteria for a Specific Diagnosis

You will recall that earlier we mentioned that the limiting factors in making a personality diagnosis in the timeframe of an initial interview are twofold: (1) Does the clinician have enough time to explore the past history of the patient appropriately to ensure historical consistency and persistency? (2) Is the patient providing reasonably valid information? The importance of these two factors is no better demonstrated than during the clinician's attempt to expand the specific diagnostic criteria within a single diagnosis – step #2 of our strategy for arriving at a differential diagnosis regarding personality dysfunction after having limited the field in step #1.

As one can imagine, an immediate problem is the need to ensure, within the tight time constraints of an initial interview, that the pathologic personality behavior is manifested by the patient from adolescence onwards (i.e., it meets the historical nature of the criteria). A second problem is attempting to ensure that the reporting of the behavior is valid.

Validity can be especially problematic with diagnostic criteria that are more subjective than objective in nature. One of the problems is that the patient and the interviewer may mean different things by a particular phrase. If a patient responds with a "yes" to the question, "Are you overly perfectionistic?" what does the patient's positive response really mean? Does the patient really know what the interviewer would consider as being overly perfectionistic? Two people can legitimately differ on this point. It is here that invalid information can be an issue. Fortunately, as we shall see below, there are specific interviewing techniques that can help with both of these types of challenging concerns.

In addition, to perform the second step in diagnosis – expanding the diagnostic criteria – the clinician must become intimately familiar with the specific criteria for each personality diagnosis in the DSM-5. Such familiarity comes both from conscientious study and, more powerfully, from experience. The process is greatly enhanced as the clinician develops a more sophisticated feel for the manner in which people with these diagnoses present and what it is like to be this particular patient with this particular style of "being in the world" in a phenomenological sense. Once again, the skillful blending of empathy, intuition, and analytic reasoning remains critical to the art of crafting a successful interview.

In order to delineate the principles behind performing a sensitive and thorough expansion of a personality disorder, we will focus on a single example to serve as an illustration. We will use the enigmatic diagnosis of borderline personality disorder as our example. It stands as one of the diagnoses that, in certain instances, may more readily be made in a single interview, because many of its criteria are behavioral in nature. Those criteria that are of a more subjective nature tend to be unique enough that they are fairly easy to spot.

There is another reason to focus on this particular diagnosis. Exciting therapeutic advances have been made in helping people with borderline structure, such as dialectical behavioral therapy (DBT),[6] as well as several other approaches as mentioned in Chapter 13. DBT, which utilizes both individual and group therapy, was developed by Marsha Linehan and has a robust evidence base demonstrating its efficacy. However, you can't use it or any of the other approaches unless you spot the diagnosis first. Fortunately, this diagnosis can frequently be made early on, even in the first session, if one knows what to look for.

With these ideas in mind, let us imagine a clinician expanding the diagnostic region of a borderline personality. The patient was a casually dressed woman with dark brown hair that was somewhat unkempt. She spoke with a curious blandness, as if commenting on a character viewed from afar, as opposed to her own life. She tended to have poor eye contact, which seemed purposeful, as if she would look at you if she felt moved to do so. Earlier aspects of the interview had demonstrated that the patient had experienced, besides her current episode, only a single bout of major depression in her life. She also denied a history of manic episodes. The immediate reason for her presentation involved her transfer from another hospital. Apparently, she had been doing reasonably well, but when she went out on a brief pass, she bought a bottle of aspirin, and promptly ingested all 24 tablets. Upon returning to the unit, she conveniently waited a while before she proceeded to casually inform the nursing staff that she had just overdosed. We will join the conversation roughly midway through the body of the interview being undertaken upon transfer to a new unit at a different hospital.

Illustration of a Clinician Expanding the Diagnostic Criteria of a Specific Diagnosis

Clin.: Mrs. Jacobs, tell me a little more about what led up to your overdose at the hospital you were just at.

Pt.: In the first place, I told him I was going to do it, Dr. Johnson I mean. I really did, but I guess nobody wanted to believe me. Now Dr. Johnson claims I said that I was all done hurting myself – maybe I did, but I sure don't remember telling him that. In fact, I told him I was feeling impulsive, like I might overdose, maybe he was just thinking differently, I don't know. But my husband thinks he blew it, and he's real mad that Dr. Johnson let me go out on that pass. And it was so easy, I just cut off my patient wristband, went to the drugstore right around the corner, and they sold me a bottle of aspirin (patient smiles).

Clin.: You seem to have some mixed feelings about Dr. Johnson.

Pt.: Do I? … Well I suppose I do. I really like him but I think he's dumping me by sending me here. He says he'll take me back, as an outpatient, I don't know. (pauses) I liked my psychologist before Dr. Johnson and I never would have believed I could work with anyone but him, but I got along well eventually with Dr. Johnson too. I guess he'll take me back, but he's mad at me even though I told him I was gonna do it.

Clin.: With both Dr. Johnson and your previous therapist you seem to have formed strong relationships. Has that been typical of yourself, say back in junior high and high school?

Pt.: Oh yeah (said in a somewhat disinterested fashion). I always seem to have this thing for an older man who will sort of guide me, help me with my development. That's happened a lot with me, maybe I have a thing for father figures, I don't know. But I had several teachers who I was very close to and there was a minister of our church group who helped a lot too. I'd rather spend my time with these kinds of men.

Clin.: Did you ever find that some of these people would later let you down and you learned to dislike them?

Pt.: Oh yeah, people use me for a doormat. Reverend Jenkins was a good example. I viewed him as very special, like almost a saint or something, but I wasn't special to him. He saw hundreds of other people in his congregation, I mean there I was sharing my deepest feelings and he'd soon be listening to another person's problems, just like I was one of them.

Clin.: Back around that time, during your school years, what were your friendships like?

Pt.: They weren't so hot. My mother always told me I was the most gifted kid, but look how I turned out. I wasn't that popular, and people are all basically bastards, trust me.

Clin.: Did you form any friendships in your life that have lasted for over 4 or 5 years?

Pt.: Not really … let me … no … not real friends.

Clin.: What usually happens to your friendships?

Pt.: We end up having an argument or something like that, and I tell them off or they tell me off. For some reason people always seem to take advantage of me and it makes me angry.

Clin.: When you get angry, do you tend to keep your anger bottled up inside or do you tend to let it out, maybe by yelling at the person or throwing something?

Pt.: I keep a lot of it in, but when I let go I can get pretty mean, I mean I have thrown things. I threw a plate at my husband when I was on a pass from the hospital about 2 weeks ago.

Clin.: I know you've been feeling pretty depressed recently, how about just when you're feeling your normal self, how many times do you think you've broken things when someone angered you?

Pt.: Oh I've done that, probably more times than I could count easily. I remember throwing down my husband's camera – that set him off.

Clin.: Sounds like it would. What's the biggest thing you've ever broken?

Pt.: My husband's nose (patient smiles and both the patient and clinician chuckle).

Clin.: Pretty big nose huh?

Pt.: Yeah and it got bigger.

Clin.: Well, what about when you're feeling very angry, say back in your school days again, did you ever pound your fists into a wall?

Pt.: Oh yeah, I put my fist through the wall once; my mother almost screamed, but then she needed shaking up a bit.

Clin.: Some patients tell me that when they get really angry, they might even pound their heads against the wall, just to get the anger out. Have you ever felt that way?

Pt.: I think I've done that, yeah I think I've done that.

Clin.: What do you remember?

Pt.: A long time ago I used to do that, not a lot though, sort of sounds silly, hurt too. You know, I've done this too. (Mrs. Jacobs rolls up her sleeve and reveals some small scars on her wrist, her affect also hardens a bit, with a very mildly angry undertone.)

Clin.: Looks like you've cut at yourself at times. Is that what these marks are?

Pt.: Yeah, that's what they are all right.

Clin.: Did it hurt when you cut at yourself?

Pt.: Not really, I just sort of like to watch it bleed.

Clin.: What makes you stop?

Pt.: I've never figured that one out, somehow it just feels better, I feel like it's all over.

Clin.: Like what's all over?

Pt.: The anger, the pain, I don't know, all I know is I'm probably going to do it again, 'cause I like it. And you're not going to stop me.

Clin.: Are you worried that I'm going to try to stop you?

Pt.: No I'm not, 'cause I know you can't.

Clin.: I think you're right about the fact that I can't ultimately stop you, only you would be able to do that and right now you don't want to. So let's not focus on that right now, we'll come back to it a little later on. With all these tough times you've had, and you've had some tough ones, do you feel that your moods change pretty rapidly?

Pt.: Yeah that's something I don't like. And if you could help me with that, I'd appreciate it.

Clin.: Do your moods ever change rapidly in a single day, you know, you might wake up in one mood and somebody says something and boom you're in a bad mood and 3 hours later you're okay again.

Pt.: Oh yeah, I'm moody, just like that.

Clin.: Do you think your parents or friends in high school viewed you as moody?

> Pt.: Sure, I've always been a moody person and people just have to learn to live with my moods. I don't try to be irritable, but sometimes I can't help it. If you can't deal with a person who gets depressed and gets pissed then you better not hang out with me. (smiles sheepishly)
>
> Clin.: What about when you're alone, what is your mood like for you when you are all by yourself, say back in your apartment?
>
> Pt.: Sometimes I like it and sometimes I don't.
>
> Clin.: When you don't like it, what does it feel like?
>
> Pt.: I just don't like it, I get depressed.
>
> Clin.: Say a friend of yours just left for the evening. As the door shuts and you suddenly find yourself alone, does your mood ever change as that door shuts?
>
> Pt.: Yes it does, sometimes I feel really bad, like a piece of me has been torn away, and sometimes I get angry, sometimes that's when I cut myself. I really am a moody person, and I don't know what to do about it. I guess that's why Dr. Johnson hates me now. (Mrs. Jacobs becomes quietly sadder.)
>
> Clin.: When you feel depressed like that, do you ever start to feel almost empty inside, like a piece of you is missing?
>
> Pt.: Sort of, I don't know if I would phrase it that way.
>
> Clin.: What does it feel like to you, that's what I'm most interested in understanding.
>
> Pt.: Dead. I feel dead.
>
> Clin.: With the deadness, do you frequently feel bored?
>
> Pt.: No, not really. But it's as if a part of me were not in the room, it's very hard to explain, but it is very unpleasant. My husband just simply can't understand it. He can be such a mean person, but then I guess I've let him down. I let all the people down at the hospital.
>
> Clin.: How do you mean?
>
> Pt.: I think my friends back at the hospital were disappointed that I tried to hurt myself. Maybe they're worried I might lose control. Will I be on a locked ward?
>
> Clin.: Yes, the ward will be locked. I guess that can be sort of scary, are you worried about it?
>
> Pt.: Yeah, but I guess they better lock me up.

Although this illustration is somewhat lengthy, it probably only required around 10 minutes of interviewing time. In this relatively short period of time, the clinician has uncovered a variety of characteristics seen in the borderline personality, including mood instability, chronic feelings of emptiness, tendencies for idealization alternating with devaluation (as seen with her minister), inappropriate outbursts of anger, tendencies for self-damaging acts, and a general dislike of being alone. In fact, the clinician has probably already gathered close to enough data to fulfill the criteria for a borderline personality disorder by DSM-5 standards, all in a matter of 10 minutes. In addition, the blending seemed reasonably high, as indicated by shared periods of levity and a report by the patient, when the interview had ended, that she liked this clinician.

What is of particular note is the fashion in which the clinician gently and persistently pursued the criteria needed for the diagnosis. Specifically, the clinician utilized specific interviewing strategies and techniques for addressing issues related to effectively verifying historic consistency and persistency and for checking on the validity of the patient's reported diagnostic criteria. Interviewers need to ascertain that the behavior in question is severe enough that it is pathologic. Let us now examine in more detail the interviewing principles, strategies, and techniques that the interviewer utilized in the above interview to address these validity concerns.

Verifying the Validity of Patient-Reported Diagnostic Traits

Enhancing Validity by Maintaining Engagement

One secret to enhancing validity lies within the skillful and sensitive structuring employed by the clinician when expanding the diagnostic region of a specific personality disorder. As emphasized in Chapter 4, an effective expansion must be done with a naturally engaging flow, never as a checklist. To create a natural expansion of a personality diagnosis it is important for the interviewer to be flexible, demonstrating an ability to sidetrack when the patient has a need to sidetrack, as opposed to doggedly pursing diagnostic criteria. For instance, this clinician spent some well-used time when he joked with the patient about her husband's nose. This brief interlude helped the patient to feel more at ease, while also conveying to her the clinician's own sense of humor. This clinician was truly listening to the patient, not just attempting to complete a diagnostic checklist.

Even when Mrs. Jacobs begins to turn on the so-called borderline charm with the interviewer, the interviewer does not over-react. For example, when on the subject of wrist cutting she challenges the interviewer with, "I don't know, all I know is I'm probably going to do it again, 'cause I like it. And you're not going to stop me," the interviewer does not reflexively counter-attack immediately telling the patient not to undertake such activity. Such a display of clinician fear would be "just what the doctor ordered" for a person with a borderline personality. If fear had been displayed, the patient would then begin to push the clinician in a war on nerves. Instead, this clinician calmly acknowledged the dilemma, agreed with Mrs. Jacobs' impression, and gracefully proceeded with the pertinent exploration of diagnostic information. At a later point in the interview, the issue of self-cutting would be more thoroughly explored.

Keeping in mind the characteristics of non-lethal self-cutting described earlier in this chapter, at this later point in the interview, the following questions could be of value in validating the presence of non-lethal self-cutting: "What did you feel when you were cutting?", "What did you feel when you stopped cutting?", and "Were you trying to kill yourself?"

Besides demonstrating a method of unobtrusively expanding a specific diagnostic region, this excerpt serves to remind us of the intensely unsettling world of people with the personality structure we refer to as "borderline." Mrs. Jacobs' world is one of ceaselessly circular contradictions. Her husband is at one moment the good guy who will protect her from the carelessness of Dr. Johnson; at another moment, he has been transformed, by her tendency to see only black or white, into "such a mean person." Her minister is transmuted from a saint into a demon merely because he does not devote all of his attention to her.

She is truly frightened of the world because she must battle back an insistent feeling of "deadness," which threatens to swallow her and those around her for all she knows. Consequently, she resorts to the age-old axiom that the best defense is a good offense. She attacks. Even during this first encounter with a new clinician, she quickly challenges him to a duel of sorts over the issue of who will rule her wrists. Wisely he declined the verbal glove that so unexpectedly slapped his face.

Even at a subtle level, she antagonizes because of her unpredictability. By way of illustration, at the end of the excerpt she suggests a fear of being placed on a locked ward. The clinician attempts to calm this fear with an empathic inquiry. No sooner does the clinician extend his concern than Mrs. Jacobs coolly responds, "Yeah, but I guess they better lock me up." This type of inconsistent interaction is what clinicians frequently report as being "jerked around" by borderline patients. Just as the clinician tries to be nice, the patient conveys a cool nonchalance. It is always important to remember that such behaviors are less manipulative than they are defensive – inadequate, yet sometimes useful – methods for deflecting pain.

The compassionate interviewer tries to see beneath this type of anger, realizing that the patient is coping with an ominous sense of impending doom and cannot find anything to grab hold of to prevent a lethal plummet. In this sense, Mrs. Jacobs represents a child trapped in an adult's body, and no one wants to play her game. The art is for the clinician to understand both the child and the adult, helping the patient to recognize that they do not need to be enemies. By doing so, powerful engagement can be maintained with minimal countertransference on the interviewer's part. The result will be an enhanced validity of what the patient is willing to share about the intimacies of their personality.

Techniques for Verifying Historical Persistency

To establish that a criterion has been met in a valid fashion, a clinician must show that it has been relatively consistent and persistent in nature. To assure this historical quality, I find that when delineating any one personality disorder, I will introduce many of my questions with phrases such as, "From high school onwards, have you found that …?" and, "Looking over your life from adolescence onwards, and up until the present, is it typical for you to feel …?" I would estimate that I use such phrasing around five times, and often more, within each diagnostic expansion of a personality disorder, to better ensure that I am hearing about enduring personality traits that are historically consistent for the patient.

We actually saw this interviewing technique used in the above illustration when the interviewer carefully searched for historical validity by utilizing focusing statements such as, "Back around that time, during your school years, what were your friendships like?" or, "Well, what about when you're feeling very angry, say back in your school days again, did you ever pound your fists into a wall?" or "Do you think that your parents or friends in high school viewed you as moody?"

Techniques for Ruling Out State Dependency

As we mentioned earlier, if a behavior is clearly caused by a non-personality related psychiatric disorder such as a mania, schizophrenia, or a substance use disorder it is viewed as being "state dependent," meaning that it is caused by a state or circumstance not related to the patient's personality. Any behavior that is state dependent is logically eliminated as fulfilling a diagnostic criterion for a personality disorder in the DSM-5. To avoid mistaking a behavioral problem as being a pathologic personality trait criterion when it is actually state dependent, a clinician can use clarifying phrases, as the dialogue below illustrates:

> Clin.: I know you've been feeling pretty depressed recently, *how about just when you're feeling your normal self*, how many times do you think you've broken things when someone angered you?
>
> Pt.: Oh I've done that, probably more times than I could count easily. I remember throwing down my husband's camera – that set him off.
>
> Clin.: Sounds like it would. What's the biggest thing you've ever broken?

In this fashion, the clinician is trying to uncover episodes of impulsive anger that are not related to the patient's depressive episodes, which had been well delineated as being present earlier in the interview. Sure enough, Mrs. Jacobs proceeds to describe a long-standing pattern of angry and hostile feelings *sans* depressive symptoms. If the interviewer does not frequently make it explicit to the patient which periods of time are being discussed, then patients almost invariably begin to merge time periods. Once this inadvertent blurring occurs, the clinician is likely to gather a history that is considerably distorted.

Verifying Pathological Severity

As the designers of the DSM-5 have emphasized, human behaviors often have a dimensional quality to them. A given trait may range from being beneficial to damaging, depending upon its frequency, severity, and rigidness.

Take, for example, the trait of obsessive attention to detail. When rigid and uncontrolled, it can be a remarkably problematic trait, resulting in an inability to function at a job because one is constantly slowed by an attention to detail that hinders performance. Imagine an emergency department nurse crippled with a rigid need to "get all the facts" trying to rapidly triage patients after a natural disaster. Not good. On the other hand, if one were designing an ideal emergency room nurse, one would want the nurse to exhibit significantly better-than average attention to detail, but in a flexible fashion. One does not want an emergency room nurse who has a rather flip attitude towards details – who, after assessing a patient for suicidal risk, would walk out of the room comfortably thinking, "I don't know, maybe yes, maybe no. It's basically a coin toss." No. One wants a nurse who is obsessive enough to stay in that room until he or she has the best read possible on the patient's suicide risk within reasonable time limits.

The DSM-5 (although it is *not* a dimensional personality diagnostic system) *indirectly* requires a dimensional assessment regarding all of its diagnostic criteria. In the DSM-5, no behavior or personality trait can be viewed as meeting any of the individual diagnostic criteria of any personality diagnosis unless the interviewer feels that it is severe enough and rigid enough that it causes significant pain to the patient and/or others. Unless a trait meets this requirement, it is not viewed as pathologic.

The DSM-5 cautions clinicians against the mislabeling of a trait in a patient as being pathological when it is merely at the upper limits of normal severity, or perhaps even slightly beyond normal, but does not interfere with that person's ability to function within his or her job or social role. Not all actors are pathologically histrionic, but all actors must be at ease with being center stage more than is normal, in order to function. Not all surgeons are narcissists, but all surgeons must have a greater-than-normal sense of "being right" or they could not function in an operating room with confidence, where life and death decisions are routine.

It all comes down to validity. The DSM/ICD systems demand that the clinician use an appropriate degree of accuracy in delineating the difference between normal personality traits and abnormal ones (which are to be viewed as meeting the requirements for specific diagnostic criteria). Although such a determination might sound complicated, and potentially time consuming, at first glance, it is, surprisingly, neither. Let's see why.

Tapping for Epiphenomena

We will focus upon the criteria for obsessive–compulsive personality disorder, for the interviewing strategy and techniques for quickly ascertaining whether or not a trait is pathologic or within normal limits is nicely illustrated with these diagnostic criteria.

The first step is to ask a patient whether or not a particular diagnostic trait is present or not. For instance, regarding the criterion of "over-perfectionism," one might simply ask, "Do you feel that you are particularly perfectionistic, perhaps to the point of it being a problem?" If the patient answers with a chuckle, "I wish. I hate details. Bosses always accuse me of being sloppy at my work," then one can move on to the next criterion, for over-perfectionism is clearly not present. But what if the patient answers "yes"?

It would be a mistake to immediately assume that the patient meets the diagnostic criterion for being over-perfectionistic, for the patient's self-appraisal may be accurate or inaccurate. Probably many readers, being trainees or graduates of difficult training programs, would answer "yes" to this question, for we need more than a bit of perfectionism to adequately achieve within our fields of study. But does that mean we all actually demonstrate the pathologic severity to meet the DSM-5 criterion for over-perfectionism? The answer is no. To meet this criterion, we must display the trait with enough severity and rigidity that it causes us or other people problems.

There is a trick of the trade to rapidly establishing a trait's degree of severity (i.e., does the patient's trait reach a pathological level of severity?). If a person's perfectionism is truly of a pathologic nature, then it should result in a cluster of associated experiences caused by the patient's over-perfectionism that are reflections of the pathologic nature of the trait. If these so-called "epiphenomena" are present, then one can more reliably conclude that the given trait or behavior is of pathologic proportions. If the epiphenomena are not present, it is probably best to view the trait as falling within normal limits. This interview strategy is called "tapping for epiphenomena." In reality, the strategy employs a special type of behavioral incident, as defined by Gerald Pascal (see Chapter 5), called a "*generic* epiphenomena question."

To utilize the strategy of tapping for epiphenomena, the interviewer asks a generic epiphenomena question whenever a patient answers "yes" to a probe question regarding a specific diagnostic criterion (such as over-perfectionism). These questions are designed to see whether the patient is experiencing the type of associated phenomena that often accompany over-perfectionism. Generic epiphenomena questions are usually of a simple nature such as "What makes you say that?" or "Can you give me an example of your over-perfectionism?"

Most patients who truly have a pathological quality to their behavior (in this case over-perfectionism) will generally be able to quite readily rattle off an example or two of associated phenomena. The trick is to be nonspecific and simply see if the patient can relate, from their own experiences, convincing examples that the trait is causing the patient, and/or other people, some problems.

People who are pathologically over-perfectionistic may tell a clinician that, "I've got to get things right. I hate to be criticized. I need to be perfect, just perfect," or "I'm always the last guy done with anything, because I'm always going over my answers or second guessing that I've done the job well. I drove my wife nuts painting our library. By the time I was done painting the door to the library, when I turned around, she had finished three of the walls, including the book shelves!" Such graphic examples are telling.

When tapping for epiphenomena, be sure to watch the patient's nonverbal behaviors as well. If the trait is truly of pathologic proportions, the patient will frequently respond quickly to the question and show a naturalness of facial expression that reflects that the presence of the trait resonates with the patient, for it is well known to the patient. Thus a trained clinician can use both the content and the process of the patient's response to more accurately determine the severity of a trait.

Following the patient's response to the *generic* epiphenomena question, if it remains unclear to the interviewer whether or not the severity of the trait meets the threshold for being viewed as pathologic (thus meeting the diagnostic criterion), the interviewer can ask a *"specific* epiphenomena question." With a specific epiphenomena question, the interviewer asks about specific experiences that are common epiphenomena for the pathologic trait in question. For instance, regarding over-perfectionism, the clinician might ask, "Do you have trouble finishing tasks on time?" or "Has anyone complained to you that you are way too slow in finishing assignments or tasks?"

With the strategic use of both generic and specific epiphenomena questions, interviewers can often determine the presence of a specific personality trait, as well as whether it is severe enough to be viewed as pathologic (hence meeting the diagnostic criterion), in a surprisingly short amount of time. Let's see the strategy of tapping for epiphenomena at work in a direct transcript from one of my own interviews with an actual patient.

Tommy was a college student who self-referred, complaining, "I'm pretty wound up with my anxiety, especially around my school work." He was dressed with a neat casualness in shorts and an attractive sport shirt. He had short-clipped hair, his teeth were sparkling, and his manners meticulous. We will pick up the interview about 30 minutes in, as I was exploring his social history. I had already limited the diagnostic field to obsessive–compulsive personality disorder and avoidant personality disorder using signal signs and symptoms. I had decided to begin my diagnostic expansion of obsessive–compulsive disorder:

Clin.:   Now you talked a little bit earlier about your studies and that you work hard; that's very apparent to me – it shows from your very excellent grade point average. Do

	you find that it is, that you are fairly perfectionistic? (referred gate used to enter the diagnostic region of obsessive–compulsive personality smoothly)
Pt.:	Yeah, yeah, I am.
Clin.:	How do you know that? (tapping with a generic epiphenomena question)
Pt.:	Like, say someone gives me something to do, one of the reasons I won't do it is because I feel I won't do it right.
Clin.:	Uh-hmmmm (nodding head as with 'Go on')
Pt.:	And then if I do it and I'm criticized. I'm not good at … I guess that it's part of my not being good at accepting criticism.
Clin.:	Now, once again, is this a new trait for you or is this something that you noticed even when you were a kid or an adolescent, that you were perfectionistic? (checking for historical persistency)
Pt.:	My whole life. (said quickly in response to the question and with sincerity)
Clin.:	Now, some people also carry that over in the sense that if someone else tries to do something for them they don't like that feeling, because they feel that the other person won't do it well enough or good enough. Do you have those kinds of feelings? (smoothly transitioning, with a normalization, to the diagnostic criterion related to reluctance to delegate work)
Pt.:	Yeah. Yeah. … Like if I could do something myself … If I don't have to ask someone to do something, I won't let them do it. If I could do it myself, I won't ask someone else to do it.
Clin.:	And why is that? (tapping with a generic epiphenomena question)
Pt.:	Because they might not do it as. (cuts himself off) … I don't like talking like this … because they might not do it as good as me. I don't like talking like this (clearly looks ill-at-ease).
Clin.:	And why? (asked gently)
Pt.:	Because I know it is rude.
Clin.:	Oh, once again, because you feel that you're sort of complimenting yourself?
Pt.:	Yeah. (almost blushing)
Clin.:	You know, during the course of a day do you frequently have thoughts like "I should be doing this," or "I should be doing that," and often think about what you ought to be doing? (transitioning to the obsessive–compulsive diagnostic criterion of being excessively concerned with work and productivity)
Pt.:	That happens – like say I'm, say there'll be a time I'm doing nothing, I'll be saying to myself, "I should be doing such and such."
Clin.:	Can you give me an example? (tapping with a generic epiphenomena question)
Pt.:	I'll be on a break at work, and I'll be saying "right now I should be studying." (Note that many people who do not really meet the severity for this criterion might also answer as Tommy just did. I decided to ask a *specific* epiphenomena question that would give me more concrete evidence that his inability to relax and preoccupation with work was truly of pathologic dimensions.)
Clin.:	Do you laugh a lot? (specific epiphenomena question related to taking work too seriously)
Pt.:	Never. (pauses) … Well I'll laugh, but it's not, it's just, it's just like, just like a little laugh. Like a laugh you'll see when someone says a joke on the TV. You laugh. That's the only kind of laugh I have.

Clin.: That sounds sort of sad? (said gently)

Pt.: Yeah …Yeah … It is.

Clin.: Once again, is that a life-long trait for you, or is that something that has just happened in the past month or so, the inability to laugh real freely? (checking for historical persistency and consistency)

Pt.: (mulls it over) … It's been a few years. (Note that, although many of us might say that we think about what we should be doing when on a study break, not many people would say that they take work so seriously that they never laugh. Tommy's response to my specific epiphenomena question points to a pathologic severity – his over-seriousness clearly causes him pain.)

This entire excerpt required slightly less than 3 minutes of interviewing time. In that 3 minutes, three of the diagnostic criteria for meeting the diagnosis of an obsessive–compulsive personality disorder have been met in my opinion (over-perfectionism, problems with delegating tasks, and an overly serious dedication to work). Hopefully, they have been met in a sensitive and conversational manner. In addition, I believe they are valid both regarding severity and persistency over time. No label slapping here. This diagnosis only requires one more criterion to be met to fulfill it. I actually spent another 5 minutes exploring these diagnostic criteria with Tommy and he met all but one.

Now that we have seen the potential to effectively delineate a specific personality disorder – in this case obsessive personality disorder – within the 7 to 12 minutes available for personality exploration in a typical initial interview, it might be nice to view such a delineation in real time in one of our video modules. Let's take a look at the delineation of a specific personality disorder that you will frequently come across in your future, or current, clinical practice. It is a diagnosis that many clinicians find difficult to pin down in an initial interview. But, we will find it is often surprisingly easy to delineate this disorder in the first meeting by effectively utilizing the validity techniques we previously acquired in Chapter 5 in conjunction with the principles and strategies that we have just acquired in the pages of this chapter:

VIDEO MODULE 14.1

Title: Sensitively Uncovering Criteria for Antisocial Personality Disorder

Contents: Contains both expanded didactics and an annotated interview excerpt demonstrating the expansion of the criteria for an antisocial personality disorder.

SECTION IV: FUTURE DIAGNOSTIC SYSTEMS OF PERSONALITY DYSFUNCTION AND THE USEFULNESS OF DIMENSIONALITY TODAY

Dimensionality: A Note of Caution

Originally, the DSM-5 was going to introduce – as its required standard approach to differential diagnosis – a system that was a hybrid of a categorical and dimensional diagnostic system but emphasized a highly dimensional approach to diagnosis. They subsequently decided to present this innovative system as an alternative system to their standard system. If you will recall from our chapters on mood disorders, dimensional diagnostic systems tend to paint a clearer picture of the unique qualities of the patient than can be achieved by categorical diagnostic systems. Arguably, this need to be more accurate and nuanced is of the utmost importance in understanding personality structure, for we are all highly individualized. The downside to highly dimensional systems is the simple fact that the more detailed one becomes about specific personality traits and the larger the number of traits explored, the longer the interview takes.

We have now seen that the categorical personality approach used in the DSM-5 (which is identical to the one used in the DSM-IV system) is surprisingly good at allowing a clinician to arrive at a reasonable (although far from perfect) differential diagnosis of personality dysfunction *in the 7 to 12 minutes that are available for such explorations in a standard 50-minute initial intake in today's clinical environment.*

The dimensionally oriented system originally developed for the DSM-5 (now appearing in the Appendix of the DSM-5 as the "Alternative DSM-5 Model for Personality Disorders") undoubtedly paints a more vivid picture of the patient than the system we have just examined (requiring that the clinician explore in detail 25 specific personality trait facets, including characteristics such as emotional lability, submissiveness, intimacy avoidance, deceitfulness, and impulsivity).

Unfortunately, in my opinion, it has a significant weakness for use in the real world of everyday clinical interviewing, related to the length of time it takes to employ. For use in a typical clinic or hospital setting, to be effective, an interviewer needs a diagnostic system that can be used to arrive at a reasonable personality diagnosis in the "50-minute hour" of a standard initial assessment (as is exemplified by the DSM-5 system we have just examined). The prototypic dimensionally oriented system for making a personality disorder diagnosis that appears in the Appendix of the DSM-5 would, in my opinion, take a sophisticated interviewer at least 1 hour to do well. This makes it impractical for use in the 7 to 12 minute framework available in an initial intake for personality exploration in an everyday clinical practice. Indeed, a wealth of reasonable criticisms regarding the time requirement and other aspects of the proposed system have appeared in the clinical literature.[7-19]

Despite these limitations, there is much to learn from the innovative and pioneering dimensional aspects of the Alternative DSM-5 Model for Personality Disorders. The approach may help us to make improvements to future DSM systems. More importantly, some useful tips can be derived from this system for immediate application. Furthermore, in situations where there is enough time to use the Alternative DSM-5 Model – perhaps if a clinician is functioning as the long-term therapist for the patient – the DSM-5 allows this alternative system to be used *instead* of the standard system described in the main body of the DSM-5. When time is available, some readers may find that they prefer this alternative system.

The Power of Dimensionality in the Initial Interview

Although clearly, in my opinion, not applicable for use in the 7 to 12 minutes available in an initial assessment for the differential diagnosis of personality disorders, the

Alternative DSM-5 Model provides an excellent overview of important personality traits that can cause major problems for the patient as well as clear-cut target symptoms that can be agreed upon during collaborative treatment planning. Indeed, the 25 personality traits (referred to as "trait facets") delineated in the system can be used over the course of ongoing therapy as useful entry points for uncovering an in-depth and compassionate understanding of the patient's phenomenological world and everyday encounters. In addition, *as time permits* in the initial assessment, a small sample of these traits can be explored and the results may prove to be of significant value in engagement, initial treatment planning, and even triage. Let's look at such a practical utilization.

In an initial intake, as time constraints allow, an interviewer may decide to raise a specific personality trait or traits that seem to be of pressing significance to the patient. Once the interviewer has gracefully raised a specific trait, he or she can use behavioral incidents to elucidate its severity and position on a continuum of importance for collaborative therapeutic intervention. Moreover, one can use generic and specific epiphenomena questions to make sure that a trait is truly present, pathologic, and valid. Such careful collaborative explorations of personality traits can be surprisingly powerful, both with regard to deepening understanding for the clinician as well as providing insight to the patient concerning possible areas for psychotherapeutic focus. Sometimes our dimensional explorations yield surprises for both the patient and the clinician.

In fact, if an interviewer discovers that a specific personality trait does not seem to be problematic, the reverse is sometimes true. The interviewer may have uncovered an area of unexpected strength and wellness. This unexpectedly discovered pocket of strength can be effectively built upon in the initial or subsequent interviews.

By way of illustration, in the following prototypic dialogue, the clinician is exploring the personality trait of "impulsivity." Let us suppose that this is the clinician's second session with the patient. In the first session, the clinician made the diagnosis of borderline personality disorder. He also shared the diagnosis with the patient, who seemed to appreciate the light the diagnosis shed on her heretofore impossible-to-understand behaviors. The therapy was off to a good start. We will pick up this second session after about 20 minutes have elapsed:

Clin.: Nancy, I'd like to continue our efforts to pin down which problems you think it would be wise to focus upon in our work together. You mentioned earlier that you have regretted a lot of your life decisions, was that because you made them sort of impulsively, you know, sort of acting on the spur of the moment? (enters exploration of the personality trait of impulsivity)

Pt.: (patient laughs) Hardly! I don't think I've made an impulsive decision in my life. It drives Peggy (her spouse) absolutely nuts. I regret my decisions because I'm always second-guessing them.

Clin.: How do you mean?

Pt.: I can't make up my mind. I think everything through, and then I think it through again and again. I weigh every pro and con you can imagine (pauses) ... probably some you couldn't imagine.

Clin.: Sounds like a bit of a problem.

Pt.:   Yeah, sort of (pause) … but not a real bad one, (chuckles) not compared to the screaming, mood swings, temper tantrums, and cutting we've been talking about.

Clin.:   (smiles) Well, that's for sure. You know what?

Pt.:   What?

Clin.:   It's not only *not* much of a problem, I think it's a hidden strength.

Pt.:   How do you mean?

Clin.:   I've interviewed an awful lot of people coping with a borderline personality disorder over the years. Most of them have tremendous problems with impulsivity as far as life decisions and even important daily decisions. And you don't. Somehow you have figured out a system for reining that type of problem in. And it's a system, a trait of yours, that works, and works well. I rarely see it with people coping with borderline process.

Pt.:   Really? (perks up) Hmmm. I never thought of it that way.

Clin.:   Not only that. I think we might be able to tap this strength of yours, your ability to weigh the pro and cons, as a method that might help you tamp down some of your angry outbursts, if we can just figure out a way to help you weigh the pros and cons of your angry outbursts before you have them, because they have consequences, usually not good ones. But I think this is a good insight we've had today. What do you think?

Pt.:   I'm not sure what to think. But I'm pretty game to try anything. I sure never viewed that as a strength, but I guess it is.

Clin.:   Well, let's put that on the back-burner for right now and see what else we might want to work on together. You are clearly not an impulsive thinker. Has that tended to limit your risk taking? (clinician has deftly begun to explore another personality trait – risk taking)

Pt.:   Oh yeah. I don't take risks. I'm a scaredy cat.

Such dimensional explorations remind us that not all people who fit the diagnostic criteria for a specific personality disorder (in this case borderline personality disorder) will show all of the same traits.

In this instance, Nancy happens to be a person meeting the criteria for a borderline personality disorder who has developed a compulsive tendency. In some situations, this compulsivity might be somewhat pathologic. But, for Nancy, it is usually a beneficial check on the impulsive and risk-taking attributes usually seen with borderline process. Moreover, not only has the interviewer uncovered a unique quality to Nancy's personality structure that might be tagged for use in therapy itself, he has given Nancy, who has chronic feelings of worthlessness, something of which to be proud. Healing has begun.

Entrance Questions for Exploring Personality Traits

Having acknowledged that time restraints severely limit our ability to explore numerous personality traits in the first encounter, we can now turn our attention to effective questions for exploring them as time permits, both in the initial assessment and in subsequent counseling sessions. We will utilize as our focus the prototypic dimensionally oriented traits described in the Alternative DSM-5 Model for Personality Disorders, for they represent an outstanding starting point phenomenologically.

Naturally, a clinician can use whatever questions he or she feels are suitable for raising the subject of these personality traits. But the following list provides various options that may be of use. Note the utility of reminding the patient of the historical nature of the inquiry (exposing long-term persistence of the quality as would be expected in a true personality trait not caused by a state-dependent factor such as alcohol or bipolar disorder).

By the way, if you discover particularly useful entrance questions, be sure to share them with myself and my readers for potential inclusion in our Interviewing Tip of the Month feature on our website at the Training Institute for Suicide Assessment and Clinical Interviewing (www.suicideassessment.com). You will find the dimensional entrance questions listed in Table 14.1 to be similar in style and principle to the probe questions that were described earlier for uncovering promising categorical diagnostic regions.

Table 14.1 Entrance Questions for Exploring DSM-5 Personality Trait Domains and Facets

I. Trait Domain of Negative Affectivity

A. Emotional lability
1. From adolescence onwards to the present have you found that you usually find yourself to be particularly moody compared to others, with your moods changing several times throughout a day?
2. Have you found that people often tell you that you over-react to things or actually say things to you like, "Just calm down, everything is fine?"

B. Anxiousness
1. From adolescence onwards to the present have you found that you are almost routinely worrying or fretting about something or other?
2. Outside of actually having a panic attack, do you find that from adolescence onwards, you find yourself throughout most days having feelings that you are going to "lose it" or "fall apart"?
3. Have you had people tell you that you are a worrywart?

C. Separation insecurity
1. From the time you were in middle school to now, would you say that you are generally quite worried that people will not like you or will make fun of you?
2. Are you the type of person that feels a consistent need to be around other people to the point that you seldom if ever like being alone?

D. Perseveration
1. From the time you were in middle school to now, do you think that you spend too much time trying to get things just right, you know, a real detail person?
2. Do people tend to tell you that you are just too perfectionistic?
3. Do you rigidly stay with a task even though you keep failing at it and your time would be better spent doing something else?

E. Submissiveness
1. From your mid-teens onwards, would you describe yourself as being the type of person that always puts the needs of other people ahead of your own?
2. Are you the type of person who tends to make sacrifices for others, when sometimes you should be looking out a bit more for yourself?

Continued

Table 14.1 Entrance Questions for Exploring DSM-5 Personality Trait Domains and Facets—cont'd

F. Hostility
1. From your mid-teens onwards, would you say that you get really angry multiple times a week, even over small things like the way people drive or things your friends have done to you?
2. Have a fair number of people told you that you are a bit of a bitch or a bastard?
3. Has anyone from a friend to a boss told you that you have an attitude problem?
4. From adolescence onwards, how many physical fights have you been in?
5. How many times, if any, have you been arrested for assault or disorderly conduct?

G. Depressivity
1. From adolescence onwards to the present have you found that you almost routinely feel depressed or down?
2. Do you think it is your nature to be a depressed person?
3. From middle school onwards, would you say that, to you, life is basically a drag?
4. Do your friends or family view you as a negative kind of person or make jokes about your half-empty way of seeing things?

H. Suspiciousness
1. From middle school up to the present, do you generally feel that people can't be trusted and you look at everyone with a fairly wary eye?
2. Has anyone ever accused you of being jealous?
3. Have you found it to be useful over the years to frequently keep notes on other's behaviors or to tape telephone calls?
4. Do you tend to feel that other people are out to get you?

II. Trait Domain of Detachment

Note that in the DSM-5, because two of these facets are rated earlier, as part of Negative Affectivity, Depressivity and Suspiciousness, are not listed again under the Detachment heading, but should be evaluated in rating the overall Detachment domain.

A. Restricted affectivity
1. From middle school up to the present, would you say that you are unusually calm and unemotional when compared to other people?
2. From adolescence onwards to the present, have you found that you are a pretty cool character, you know, you don't show much emotion?
3. Has anyone told you that you are a cold person or unfeeling?

B. Withdrawal
1. From your mid-teens onwards, have you persistently preferred being alone to being around others?
2. Have you found it hard to make friends in the sense that you really don't try?
3. Do you or other people view you as a loner or a wallflower?

C. Anhedonia
1. Since you were younger, from around 15 or 16, have you found that on a daily basis you just don't find yourself able to enjoy things, even things you think might interest you?
2. Do you find that as a baseline for years you just don't tend to look forward to doing things even if you would think they would appeal to you?
3. Do you tend to view yourself as fun loving?

D. Intimacy avoidance
1. From adolescence onwards to the present, have you found that it is hard for you to develop intimacy with people whether as friends or even lovers?
2. If I asked people who knew you, would they say you were hard or easy to get to know?
3. Generally speaking, if you are feeling hurt or in pain, do you like to talk to other people about it to get some comfort or perspective or do you tend to keep your troubles to yourself?

Table 14.1 Entrance Questions for Exploring DSM-5 Personality Trait Domains and Facets—cont'd

III. Trait Domain of Antagonism

   A. Manipulativeness

      1. Over the years, do you think that people might see you, even if you disagree with their opinion, as being a bit manipulative?

      2. You know, from your adolescence onwards, have you found that it is pretty easy for you to get people to do what you want?

      3. People vary on how good they are at flirting, where would you place yourself in that regard?

   B. Deceitfulness

      1. From your mid-teens onwards, do you think you have developed a bit of a tendency, perhaps out of habit, of being just a wee bit deceitful?

      2. Over the years, have you posted things on the web that weren't really totally true about yourself?

      3. Have you ever cheated on your taxes, or misrepresented yourself or your qualifications, perhaps when dating or on a job application?

      4. Have you ever been accused or charged with fraud or of "ripping somebody off"?

      5. Have you ever had an affair?

   C. Grandiosity

      1. Generally speaking, have you found that most people you meet, not that you are bragging or anything, are simply not as smart as you or talented as you?

      2. Has anyone ever told you that you were pompous or "a big-shot"?

   D. Attention seeking

      1. When you look back on yourself from adolescence to now, would you view yourself as someone who can get the attention of others, who can bring a little needed drama to life?

      2. Over the years, have you had the reputation for being the life of the party and unusually fun to have at a gathering?

      3. Do you like to post things on the web that really get people upset or angry?

   E. Callousness

      1. Over the years, from your adolescence to now, would you view yourself as being fairly callous, maybe even a bit cruel at times?

      2. Tell me about some times when you felt a lot of guilt about something you did?

IV. Trait Domain of Disinhibition

   A. Irresponsibility

      1. Over the years, how often do you think you needed to shade the truth a bit so that you could get something that you deserved, if ever?

      2. Has anyone ever accused you of not keeping your promises?

   B. Impulsivity

      1. When you look back at yourself from adolescence to the present, are you the kind of person who likes to plan everything out in life or are you a fairly carefree agent, who just lets life happen?

      2. Is it typical throughout your life to regret decisions that you feel were impulsive in nature, you know, were made on the spur of the moment?

      3. Has anyone in your family, friends, teachers or employers told you that you are too impulsive or don't take life seriously enough?

Continued

Table 14.1 Entrance Questions for Exploring DSM-5 Personality Trait Domains and Facets—cont'd

   C. Distractibility
      1. From middle school onwards, or even before, have you found that you are easily distractible, making it very hard to read or perhaps it even hurt your grades?
      2. Has anyone ever joked that you are like a "nutty professor" because you are always forgetting things or forgetting what you were trying to do because you got distracted?

   D. Risk taking
      1. Is it typical of you, over the years, to be a risk taker?
      2. Have you gotten more than a couple of speeding tickets or been charged with drinking while driving or had your license suspended or taken?
      3. Do friends tend to view you as a pretty wild person?

   E. (Lack of) rigid perfectionism
      1. When you look back at your typical way of approaching tasks throughout most of your life, do you tend to be particularly neat or particularly sloppy at school or work?
      2. When you are given a task do you get it done much faster than most people because you've learned how to cut corners and not get hung up on details?

V. Trait Domain of Psychoticism

   A. Unusual beliefs and experiences
      1. Over the years have you frequently felt that things magically seemed to happen to you or felt like you might have some special powers that others don't have?
      2. Has it been typical of you, from adolescence onwards, that others have viewed your thoughts as being quite strange?
      3. Have a lot of people thought that your ideas were a "little bit nuts" and really believed that you had irrational thoughts and told you that you needed help?

   B. Eccentricity
      1. Over the years, even as an adult, have people tended to view you as "kinda weird"?
      2. Have people teased you or accused you of being eccentric or the town "crazy"?

   C. Cognitive and perceptual dysregulation
      1. Has it been fairly frequent for you over the years to wonder whether or not you might be hearing voices or seeing things that other people do not see?
      2. Do people ever tell you that they can't follow your thoughts or that what you are saying, doesn't make sense to them and they literally mean that your words are so odd that they seem strange to them?

Differential Diagnosis of Personality Disorders: A Glimpse Into the Future

Building Upon the DSM-5 Categorical System

The DSM-5 used an identical system and set of criteria for the differential diagnosis of personality dysfunction as was utilized in the DSM-IV-TR. This decision probably pivoted upon the fact that, as we have seen in this chapter, this categorical system provides a surprisingly robust method of delineating a personality differential of reasonable validity in the remarkably short amount of time available in the "50-minute hour" typical for initial intakes.

Much of the initial hour must be spent on a plethora of critical explorations, ranging from a scouting phase focused upon engagement, the delineation of the presenting problem, and the differential diagnosis of the non-personality psychiatric diagnoses from the DSM-5, to the uncovering of a family history, treatment history, medical history, mental status, suicide and violence assessment, and an exploration of the various wings of the patient's matrix from cultural and spiritual to psychological concerns. Thus there is, at best, about 7 to 12 minutes available for an exploration of the social history and its reflections – the personality disorders.

I believe that the best innovations for the future may well lie in directly building upon the categorical system currently in use by simply adding the exploration of dimensional traits as optional specifiers to be investigated as time permits. This addition of personality traits as specifiers, such as those in the list above from the Alternative DSM-5 Model for Personality Disorders, resonates with the use of specifiers in the other non-personality related psychiatric diagnoses such as depressive disorder, bipolar disorder, schizophrenia, substance use disorders, and post-traumatic stress disorder.

Undoubtedly, clinicians will only have time to explore a small number, if any, of these optional traits in the initial interview, but in later sessions (and during ongoing therapy) a more sculpted and accurate picture of the patient can be uncovered through the use of these specifiers. In essence, a secondary diagnosis of a more sophisticated and tailored personality description will emerge. We have already seen how this process can also be used to better collaboratively target specific problematic personality traits for intervention in ongoing psychotherapy.

Yet another way of improving the validity of future systems may be to move away from criteria *per se*. As we have seen, the DSM-5 utilizes a categorical system for differential diagnosis. It also happens to be a categorical system that uses lists of "diagnostic criteria" for determining the appropriateness of the diagnosis for a specific patient. In contrast, categorical systems that use a "prototype-based" approach do not have individualized diagnostic criteria. These narrative prototypes read very much like the introductory descriptions I used earlier in the chapter when first introducing the reader to the specific personality disorders. Prototypic diagnostic systems provide a brief narrative description of how people with a specified personality disorder behave, appear, feel, and think. The diagnosis is made if the interviewer *feels* that the patient seems to match the description for the most part.

One way of building onto of the foundations made by the DSM-IV and DSM-5 would be to create a prototype-based system that is centered upon the DSM-5 criteria but adds depth and dimensionality through the use of narrative prototypes conveying the way in which patients with these disorders experience the world and present with symptoms. In my opinion, a particularly promising prototype-based system has been proposed by Jonathan Shedler and Drew Westen. Known as the Shedler–Westen Assessment Procedure - II (SWAP-II), it builds upon the personality categories used in the DSM-IV-TR.[20–25] Below is a nice illustration of a prototype-based diagnosis from the SWAP-II describing what they call the Borderline-Dysregulated Personality[26]:

Summary Statement: Individuals with Borderline-Dysregulated Personality have impaired ability to regulate their emotions, have unstable perceptions of self and others that lead to intense and chaotic relationships, and are prone to act on impulses, including self-destructive impulses.

Individuals who match this prototype have emotions that can change rapidly and spiral out of control, leading to extremes of sadness, anxiety, and rage. They tend to "catastroph-ize," seeing problems as disastrous or unsolvable, and are often unable to soothe or comfort themselves without the help of another person. They tend to become irrational when strong emotions are stirred up, showing a significant decline from their usual level of functioning. Individuals who match this prototype lack a stable sense of self: Their attitudes, values, goals, and feelings about themselves may seem unstable or ever-changing, and they are prone to painful feelings of emptiness. They similarly have difficulty maintaining stable, balanced views of others: When upset, they have trouble perceiving positive and negative qualities in the same person at the same time, seeing others in extreme, black-or-white terms. Consequently, their relationships tend to be unstable, chaotic, and rapidly changing. They fear rejection and abandonment, fear being alone, and tend to become attached quickly and intensely. They are prone to feeling misunderstood, mistreated, or victimized. They often elicit intense emotions in other people and may draw them into roles or "scripts" that feel alien and unfamiliar (e.g., being uncharacteristically cruel, or making "heroic" efforts to rescue them). They may likewise stir up conflict or animosity between other people. Individuals who match this prototype tend to act impulsively. Their work life or living arrangements may be chaotic and unstable. They may act on self-destructive impulses, including self-mutilating behavior, suicidal threats or gestures, and genuine suicidality, especially when an attachment relationship is disrupted or threatened.

Unlike most criterion-based categorical systems, which have strong reliability but some weaknesses regarding validity, the great strength of these prototype-based categorical systems is their validity. In my opinion, the narrative descriptions used in prototype-based systems such as the SWAP-II exhibit a high degree of *descriptive essence*, allowing for nuance, realism, and variation in presentation within a specific personality type. I think one would be hard pressed to find a better description of a person exhibiting a borderline personality disorder than the one above.

CONCLUSION

I think stories are important, stories are vital, storytellers are in some sense very vital.
Neil Gaiman, graphic novelist[27]

Our patients with severe personality disorders are, indeed, storytellers. As Neil Gaiman writes, their stories are vital. In this instance, they are vital to their healing. Unlike Neil Gaiman, who is creating fictional stories, our patients are relating, to the best of their abilities, stories that are all too real. They are stories filled with histories of physical and sexual abuse, divorces, deaths, illnesses, and the advent of terrifying symptoms ranging from disabling depressions to hallucinations and episodes of self-cutting.

Such patients live lives of remarkable complexity and pain. Their behaviors – none of which they asked for – create maelstroms of interpersonal chaos and rejection. These behaviors, such as angry outbursts, wrist slashing, help rejection, rages, and suicidal plunges sometimes impact not only their family, friends, and employers; they impact clinicians.

Unlike Neil Gaiman, we are not storytellers; we are professional story collectors. Our ability to collect comprehensive and valid stories is at the heart of our ability to heal. Unfortunately, the types of behaviors demonstrated by patients with severe personality dysfunction – such as borderline and narcissistic process – can sometimes get in the way of their ability to tell their stories or for their stories to be heard. The intensity of their rage, the thirst of their dependency, or the depth of their suicidal angst, are, if we are honest with ourselves, potentially intimidating. In some instances, the cacophony of emotions stirred by these patients can lead a clinician, even of the best of intentions, to turn off the story before it is fully heard, either consciously or unconsciously.

In our next chapter we will search for an understanding of the people beneath these diagnostic labels that can mute the ferocity of their clinical needs. The understanding that we will gain will help us to be less personally affronted by the behaviors of these patients, feel less pressured by their demands, be less frightened by their cuttings, and become more comfortable with the intensity of their pain. The lens that will provide us with this compassionate patience will prove to be of great value in the initial interview. It is a lens that has guided clinicians for many decades. It is a lens that is always changing, always evolving, always improving. It is a lens that is both intriguing and powerfully healing. It is the lens of psychodynamics.

REFERENCES

1. Hammacher AM. *Phantoms of the imagination.* New York, NY: Harry N. Abrams; 1981. p. 17.
2. Westen D, Shedler J, Bradley B, DeFife JA. An empirically derived taxonomy for personality diagnosis: bridging science and practice in conceptualizing personality. *Am J Psychiatry* 2012;**169**(3):273–84.
3. Westen D, Shedler J. 2012. p. 277–8.
4. Vaillant G. Sociopathy as a human process. In: Guggenheim F, Nadelson C, editors. *Major psychiatric disorders.* New York, NY: Elsevier Biomedical; 1982. p. 179–88.
5. Roberts JKA. *Differential diagnosis in neuropsychiatry.* New York, NY: John Wiley; 1984. p. 26.
6. Linehan M. *Cognitive–behavioral treatment of borderline personality disorder.* New York, NY: Guilford Press; 1993.
7. Wakefield JC. The perils of dimensionalization: challenges in distinguishing negative traits from personality disorders. *Psychiatr Clin North Am* 2008;**31**:379–93.
8. Bornstein RF. Reconceptualizing personality pathology in DSM 5: limitations in evidence for eliminating dependent personality disorder and other DSM-IV syndromes. *J Pers Disord* 2011;**25**:235–47
9. Clarkin JF, Huprich SK. Do DSM-5 personality disorder proposals meet criteria for clinical utility? *J Pers Disord* 2011;**25**:192 205.
10. Costa PT Jr, McCrae RR. Bridging the gap with the five-factor model. *Personal Disord* 2010;**1**:127–30.
11. First MB. Commentary on Krueger and Eaton's "Personality traits and the classification of mental disorders: toward a more complete integration in DSM-5 and an empirical model of psychopathology": real-world considerations in implementing an empirically based dimensional model of personality in DSM-5. *Personal Disord* 2010;**1**:123–6.
12. First MB. Clinical utility: a prerequisite for the adoption of a dimensional approach in DSM. *J Abnorm Psychol* 2005;**114**:560–4.
13. Gunderson JG. Commentary on "Personality traits and the classification of mental disorders: toward a more complete integration in DSM-5 and an empirical model of psychopathology". *Personal Disord* 2010;**1**:119–22.
14. Livesley WJ. The current state of personality disorder classification: introduction to the special feature on the classification. *J Pers Disord* 2011;**25**:269–78.
15. Pilkonis PA, Hallquist MN, Morse JQ, Stepp SD. Striking the (im)proper balance between scientific advances and clinical utility: commentary on the DSM-5 proposal for personality disorders. *Personal Disord* 2011;**2**:68–82.
16. Ronningstam E. Narcissistic personality disorder in DSM-V: in support of retaining a significant diagnosis. *J Pers Disord* 2011;**25**:248–9.
17. Shedler J, Beck A, Fonagy P, et al. Personality disorders in DSM-5. *Am J Psychiatry* 2010;**167**:1026–8.
18. Widiger TA. A shaky future for personality disorders. *Personal Disord* 2011a;**2**:54–67.
19. Widiger TA. The DSM-5 dimensional model of personality disorder: rationale and empirical support. *J Pers Disord* 2011b;**25**:222–34.
20. Westen D, Shedler J, Bradley B, DeFife JA. 2012. p. 273–84.

21. Shedler J, Westen D. The Shedler–Westen Assessment Procedure (SWAP): making personality diagnosis clinically meaningful. *J Pers Assess* 2007;**89**:41–55.
22. Westen D, Muderrisoglu S. Clinical assessment of pathological personality traits. *Am J Psychiatry* 2006;**163**:1285–7.
23. Shedler J, Westen D. Dimensions of personality pathology: an alternative to the five-factor model. *Am J Psychiatry* 2004;**161**:1743–54.
24. Shedler J, Westen D. Refining personality disorder diagnosis: integrating science and practice. *Am J Psychiatry* 2004;**161**:1350–65.
25. Westen D, Shedler J. Revising and assessing axis II, part II: toward an empirically based and clinically useful classification of personality disorders. *Am J Psychiatry* 1999;**156**:273–85.
26. Westen D, Shedler J, Bradley B, DeFife JA. 2012. p. 281–2.
27. Campbell H. *The art of Neil Gaiman*. New York, NY: Harper Design, An Imprint of Harper Collins Publishers; 2014. p. 8.

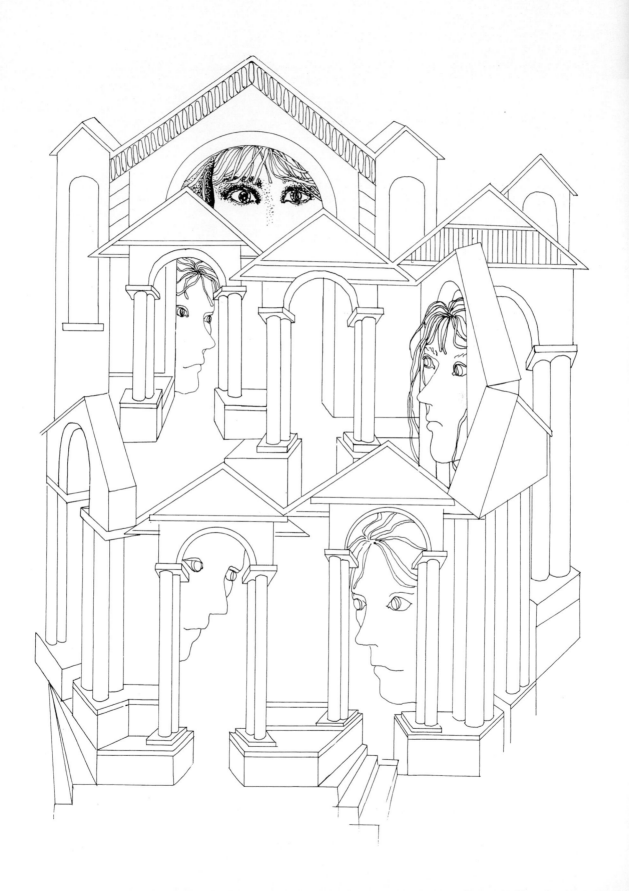

CHAPTER 15

Understanding and Effectively Engaging People With Difficult Personality Disorders: The Psychodynamic Lens

… man can no more survive psychologically in a psychological milieu that does not respond empathetically to him than he can survive physically in an atmosphere that contains no oxygen.

Heinz Kohut
Founder of self psychology[1]

INTRODUCTION TO OBJECT RELATIONS AND SELF PSYCHOLOGY

If we follow the logic in our opening epigram from Kohut, patients who present to us with borderline and narcissistic structure are suffocating on a psychological level. Their behaviors so assault others, that the people they meet, try to befriend, or attempt to engage in intimate relationships cannot, and do not, provide them with an environment rich with empathy. One could argue that with such patients, during the initial interview, the major goal of the interviewer is to create an environment in which they can breathe. The ability for us to create such an environment is dependent upon our ability to empathize with these patients. But empathy is so much easier to feel and convey when patients are nice to us!

To me, it was the insights of the object relation theorists and the self psychologists, such as Otto Kernberg and Heinz Kohut, respectively, who shed light into the dark anger of patients who were wrestling with borderline, narcissistic, and passive-aggressive demons. If we follow the guidance of their lanterns, we find ourselves naturally empathizing with patients who, shall we say, on occasion, are not particularly nice to us. It is a rather startling sleight of hand – a magic of sorts. Of course, the appearance of this empathy decreases our burnout and increases our patients' chances for healing. This chapter is a manual on how to perform this magic. And this magic is an integral part of the person-centered approach to interviewing that has been the foundation of this book.

Part of the magic evolves from the reassuring explanatory framework that these psychodynamic models provide the initial interviewer and/or ongoing therapist. Clinicians, as is the case with people in general, are often caught off-guard when patients exhibit unexpected behaviors whose origins are not easily explained, especially if the behaviors are antagonistic (unexpected rage at the interviewer) or self-damaging (unexpected acts of self-mutilation or cutting).

The seemingly unexplainable quality of the behaviors can easily create an uneasiness in the therapist, who must function while on edge – anticipating that something odd or problematic may arise at any moment. This edginess can cause the therapist to develop an aversion to encounters with the patient, or, in an initial interview, an almost immediate negative countertransference that can disrupt the healing nature of the interview itself.

By way of illustration, in an initial interview that is proceeding well, an interviewer can be caught off-guard and left genuinely puzzled when a patient responds to an interpretive question angrily with, "What the fuck did you mean by that?" An understanding of object relations and self psychology can provide a surprisingly sound framework for not only understanding the origins of such behaviors but creating a framework from which a clinician may even be able to predict and possibly prevent such behaviors proactively. Such a clinician functions with a much-enhanced sense of competency and calmness. This chapter is designed to provide the conceptual framework for such calmness.

Object relations is not really a single unified theory. Rather, it is a collection of psychodynamic perspectives that differ in important ways – sometimes even in contradictory ways.[2] But together they moved the field of psychoanalysis away from a predominant focus upon intrapsychic structures (id, ego, superego) and drive reductions to an additional interest in how the human mind creates internal representations of the people who provide relief for those very same drives.[3]

In a similar fashion, self psychology is composed of varying theories, but it, too, added a specific new dimension to psychoanalytic thought. It emphasized that the interactions with significant caregivers early in life, as well as in subsequent years, had major ramifications upon intrapsychic structures and processes critical to the development of a secure sense of self as reflected by a sense of the continuity of the self, a viable independence of self functioning, a reasonable sense of self-worth, and an ability to empathize with other selves. In essence, both of these perspectives shifted the emphasis of psychoanalysis from a primary focus upon the psychological wing of the human matrix to an emphasis that included the interaction of the psychological wing with the intimate, family, and cultural wings of the matrix.

It has proven to be an exciting expansion that has freed therapists to more readily utilize the principles of what we have called matrix treatment planning. These theories have opened the door to a better understanding of how early family relationships, cultures, and spiritualities can provide critical links in the development of an intrapsychic world in which a person feels safe, wanted, and needed. Indeed, self psychology has even helped us to better appreciate the healing power of a non-human relationship, as with a cherished a pet, to substantially provide components of all three of these critical factors for a person whose personality proclivities, sometimes shaped by early abuse, have robbed them of the ability to bond effectively with people.[4]

Object relations and self psychology have also provided the catalyst for the development of more recent psychodynamic models that emphasize the relational interplay between patient and therapist, including intersubjectivity, interpersonal psychoanalysis, and social constructivism.[5] Most importantly from the perspective of this book, object relations and self psychology provide new interviewing techniques of immediate use to us.

When first encountered by psychiatric residents and graduate students, the fields of object relations and self psychology are often viewed as being a bit difficult to understand. Indeed, the language used can, at first glance, appear odd or even cold (e.g., referring to internal images of people as "objects" or concepts such as mirroring or idealizing transferences). Indeed, that sense of perplexity was a feature of my own experience when encountering these concepts in my early years of training.

Fortunately I came upon the book *Listening Perspectives in Psychotherapy* by Lawrence Hedges, which I cannot recommend enough.[6] In his book, from which I borrow liberally in this section, Hedges integrates object relations and self psychology while simultaneously simplifying and clarifying their application to everyday practice. He does so in a lucid and easy reading style. With the help of Hedges' clarifications and perspectives, I have found these psychodynamic concepts to be useful from the very first handshake to the final good-bye of the initial interview.

Moreover, despite the apparent coldness of terms such as "object relations," these fields provide a person-centered lens for better understanding both our patients' humanity and our own. They allow us to more clearly see the person beneath the diagnostic label of "borderline personality disorder" as well as the person who carries the societal label of "shrink." In an initial interview, both participants can come to the encounter with limiting prejudices regarding both the other person in the room and themselves. The sophisticated understanding afforded by object relations and self psychology can transform these biases, providing a fertile ground in which the healing process can germinate.

Goals of This Chapter and Core Definitions

Hopefully the following chapter is an antidote to the typical confusion encountered when first reading about object relations and self psychology. My goal is to provide a concise, clarifying, easily understood introduction to these psychodynamic topics that is both fun to read and of immediate practical application to the initial interview.

More specifically, in this chapter we will examine, in a simplified fashion, how object relations and self psychology can explain how a human being develops a secure and ultimately high-functioning sense of self. As these developmental stages are explored, we will uncover interviewing techniques that we can use during an initial interview to better achieve a sensitive differential diagnosis as rapidly as possible. Perhaps even more importantly, an understanding of object relations and self psychology will emerge that can help readers to effectively engage patients who present with severe personality dysfunction while simultaneously increasing the enjoyment of working with them.

This more compassionate framework, built upon an empathic groundwork, allows a clinician to understand the why and how of a patient's seemingly inexplicable behaviors. Specifically, an understanding of these two psychodynamic models facilitates the following three clinical interviewing skill sets: (1) it provides new signal *signs* for limiting the diagnostic field, (2) it provides new signal *symptoms* for limiting the diagnostic field, and (3) it provides new tools for enhancing engagement. Deeper into this chapter, as we uncover various psychodynamic concepts related to object relations and the psychology of the self (such as merger objects, splitting, and mirror-transferences), we will sequentially examine practical interviewing techniques from each of these three skill sets. But first we must begin our study by operationally defining object relations and the psychology of the self.

Defining Object Relations and Self Psychology

Object relations and self psychology delineate how human beings, from infancy onwards, develop a concrete inner concept of the fact that they are a separate self (with concrete boundaries and unique needs, feelings, perceptions, and cognitions) and that there are other separate selves in the world (with their own concrete boundaries and unique needs, feelings, perceptions, and cognitions). It also deals with how the human mind maintains these *intrapsychic* constructs in such a way that an individual can interact effectively with his or her counterparts in the real world outside one's mind – the real people that the internal object relations represent.

Put succinctly, we are social animals. To function effectively, we must know who we are, who others are, and how we can effectively understand them and communicate with them. It is our internal object relations and our internal sense of self that allows us to do so.

Theoretically, all of this intrapsychic structure and processing is primarily unconscious. We are not aware of our object relations, nor do we consciously partake in shaping them. Moreover, in a classic reading of object relations/self psychology, the formation of our object relations happens during infancy and early childhood (although later events, such as severe abuse later in childhood, can certainly impact on both object relations and our sense of self and self-worth). The unconscious process that allows one to take an image of another person and bring it into one's own unconscious, where it becomes an object relation, is generally called introjection or internalization. Consequently, in the literature you will sometimes see a specific unconscious object relation called "an introject."

At one level, our sense of self is so secure and natural that the above processes are hardly given a second thought by most of us, for they have been secured during infancy and toddlerhood (often secured at such an early age that we do not have many, if any, memories of the timeframe). Moreover, these unconscious introjects have been used daily since. They appear as "a given" aspect of our daily functioning.

At another level, this developmental process is, in reality, extraordinarily complex and delicate. A newborn probably has essentially no conceptual framework that it exists as a distinct entity from the rest of the world. A newborn will need to discover its own physical boundaries. As time goes on, this very basic sense of self will have to become vastly more sophisticated, to the point that the individual recognizes his or her own needs, feels capable and safe being alone, feels that he or she can safely approach other human beings (who for the infant and toddler are monstrously large and all powerful), generally feels that these other beings do not intend harm, can learn to recognize humans who do intend harm (such as an abusive parent or caretaker), develops a sense of self-worth, enjoys a sense of competency, and develops the ability to empathize and get along with others. This is the core evolution of a human's object relations and his or her self psychology in the opening 4 or 5 years of life.

Once secured, throughout later childhood and adolescence the human being must add on an ultra-sophisticated more adult sense of self and identity beyond basic object relations and a core sense of self. But the healthy sequential development of these more sophisticated identities is strikingly dependent upon the person's core, early object relations. If the sequence is successful, the patient's adult self is reflected in a secure sense of self-worth, self-direction, discovery and acceptance of sexual orientation and gender identification, career track, ability to empathize at a high level (including the ability to sacrifice for others), and the ability to develop intimate relationships based upon trust. Looked at in this light, it is evident that much can go wrong in the development of the core self and the subsequent adult self. In this chapter we will focus upon problems encountered in the early development of human autonomy, the arena of true object relations and self psychology.

To me, the secret to understanding the practical application of object relations and self psychology in everyday interviewing (as well as in psychotherapy) lies in the following realization:

Object relations and self psychology are the study of how an individual comes to feel psychologically safe in the room with another human being.

This ability to feel safe impacts on all relationships, from parental to sibling to spouse to employer to the first encounter with a clinician in an initial intake. If a patient does not feel safe in our presence by the end of the interview, there will probably not be a second interview. It is that simple.

And this sense of safety is necessary not only with patients who have personality disorders and unstable object relations (the subjects of this chapter), it is important to all of us and to any patients seeking our services. Thus, those that have good object relations and healthy personalities must also feel psychologically safe by the end of the initial interview. Consequently, although we will be focusing upon interviewing tips for use with people with damaged personalities in this section, many of these techniques can be of use with a variety of higher functioning patients.

We will see that the self concept seems to evolve over four stages: (1) discovering the boundaries of the body, (2) finding safety by merging with others, (3) finding independence by feeling grandiosely powerful or identifying with powerful idealized figures, and (4) learning to be empathic and self-sacrificing. Although all four stages are fascinating, we will focus upon stages 2 and 3 for they provide a plethora of interviewing techniques with regard to uncovering personality dysfunction and better understanding those people experiencing it.

These four stages are characterized by four specific object relations: (1) part self/part object, (2) merger object, (3) self object, and (4) the stable self. Developmental arrest or regression to each of these four stages may reflect itself with a specific form of psychopathology respectively: (1) psychosis (arrested at part self/part object), (2) borderline personality disorder (arrested at merger object), (3) narcissistic personality disorder (arrested at self object), and (4) neurotic process/normalcy (achieves stable self). All of this will make much more sense as we continue forwards, and I believe that Figure 15.1

will provide a useful roadmap as we proceed to see how a human being develops from lacking a firm self concept at birth to experiencing a firm sense of self as an adult.

Moving from left to right in Figure 15.1, the various sequential stages of development from birth to adulthood are shown. The rows of Figure 15.1 show this movement. Thus one moves from the earliest stage (part self/part object) through the merger object and self object stages, ultimately reaching the stage of a stable sense of self. The columns of Figure 15.1 delineate characteristics typical of each stage. Using the first column as an example (part self/part object), we find the following: psychopathology resulting from a disruption of development at that stage (psychosis), a particularly well-known explicator of that stage (Harold Searles) and a psychodynamic process or construct associated with that stage of development (porous ego of psychosis).

What Propels the Development of the Self?

From a biological standpoint, for a human to function effectively in a social milieu, it is necessary to feel an internal sensation of point (0,0). An infant cannot consciously conceptualize "Mom is over there," unless the infant can conceptualize "I am here." This primitive sensation of self as being point (0,0) from which all other things are referenced is most likely biologically hardwired into the brain. Over time, there is probably a sequential evolution of neural networking that allows a human to develop an ever more sophisticated layering upon this primitive sense of self.

Thus, one of the major drivers for the development of the self is the biological hard-wiring that unfolds at age-appropriate times, allowing an individual to interact socially with parent figures and others in a progressively more complex fashion. This core "biologically induced" sensation of self is obviously dependent upon normally functioning neuroanatomy and neurophysiology. Biological disruptions in these areas, as seen in proactive development (autism) and in retroactive reversals of development (delirium/ dementia), can result in marked disruptions in the sense of self, the importance of others, and the immediate sense of safety.

From a psychological perspective, it has been hypothesized that one of the major drives that ensures an individual will develop a secure sense of self is the fact that without it an individual will, at best, feel an intense sense of being ill-at-ease, and, at worst, an almost catastrophic feeling of impending destruction. In this theory, a human will be driven to do whatever it takes to relieve this sensation of catastrophic annihilation. By way of example, the developing human will be driven towards other humans because when cuddled by them, they feel more whole or safe. Thus the psychological state of intense anxiety drives the infant towards nurturing figures where interactions will occur that further develop the sense of self or wholeness.

Of course, for this interpersonal reaching outwards to work, the other people must be able to provide appropriate support for the infant and toddler. Abusive or neglectful parenting figures can result in severe psychological damage to the nascent sense of self. Continuing with our computer metaphor, one can conceptualize the actions of other people as being the software that determines whether or not the development of the self can proceed normally (as long as the hardware – brain structure and function – is intact).

This portrayal of the biological and psychological factors that provide the driving forces for the development of the self is a gross simplification that a reading of the original innovators of object corrections and self psychology can correct. Nevertheless, it can serve as a useful platform from which to launch our study of interviewing techniques born from these two models.

THE FOUR DEVELOPMENTAL STAGES OF THE SELF AND THEIR CLINICAL APPLICATIONS

Developmental Stage #1: Discovering the Boundaries of the Body

It is unlikely that a newborn baby has much of a cognitive framework for interpreting the world at all. As Hedges points out, a newborn just simply "is"; sort of a pleasantly plump Zen monk. It is doubtful that a newborn has a conceptual idea of its own self existence. It will literally have to discover where it ends and the rest of the world begins.

Most newborns probably succeed at delineating this extremely basic fact by the manipulations of their hands. They will unconsciously realize that there are things in this world that, when you touch them, you get a single sensory input (cribs, blankets, rattles). In contrast, when infants touch their own bodies they discover that there are other "things" in this world (the various parts of their own bodies) that when you touch them you receive two sensory inputs: (1) sensations from the part of their body that they are touching, and (2) sensations from their own fingertips that are doing the touching. Suddenly the world can be divided into two distinct divisions. If you think about it, it is quite a discovery! It is the rudimentary discovery of the self.

Interestingly there are other phenomena that quickly re-enforce these exploratory distinctions made by this young navigator of new worlds. For instance, there exist things that one cannot make move purely by thinking the thought (cribs, blankets, rattles) and there are things that one can voluntarily make move with just one's thoughts (one's own arms, legs and face, etc.). The confirmation that there is a difference between my "self" and the rest of the world is quickly being secured through experience. This *unconscious* recognition of the boundaries of one's body is probably one of the first experiences that allows an infant to carve out the beginnings of a true self concept.

This primitive way of perceiving the world is so foreign to most adults that it is hard to conceptualize or even empathize with it. Object relation theorists have tried to capture its essence by the term "part-self/part-object," suggesting that the infant experiences the world as being initially rather confusing (as boundaries are being explored), so that the infant is not always sure whether something is part of them or not part of them (see Figure 15.1).

And here is where we stumble upon our first bit of insight into the utility of object relations theory as it applies to the initial interview. By understanding the phenomenology of this primitive part-self/part-object way of being in the world, we may spot evidence that psychotic process may be present at very early stages of the interview.

Some adults can retrogress into part-self/part-object states. This regression is generally caused by biological dysfunction that damages the patient's abilities to experience normal object relations. We have already seen that a delirium or dementia can do this (note the loss of orientation, including frequent disorientation to self) seen in both of these states, as well as the accompanying catastrophic anxiety also frequently seen in these states.

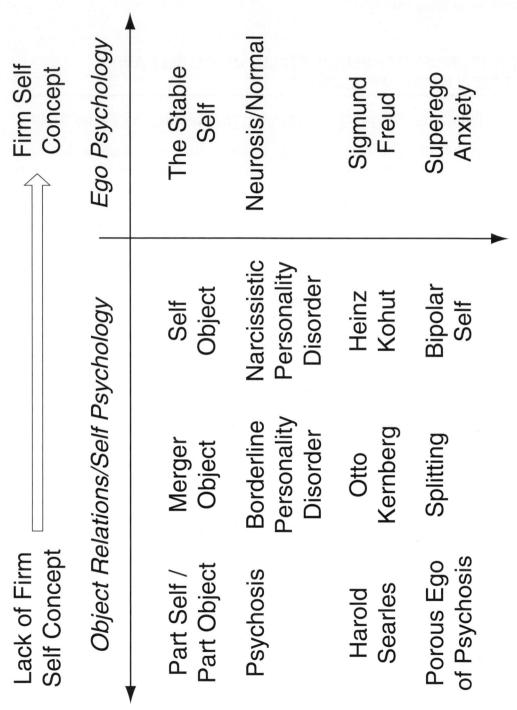

Figure 15.1 The psychodynamic development of the self.

Perhaps even more curious is the damage done to object relations by the biological pathophysiology of processes such as schizophrenia or psychotic bipolar disorder. As the world's boundaries begin to dissolve in such disorders, the world becomes a strange and frightening experience. The "made feelings, made impulses, and made perceptions" described by Kurt Schneider (see pages 510–512) are all probably examples of an adult experiencing the world as part-self/part-object.

In such a frightening condition, a person can experience what can best be called a "porous ego." A psychotic patient may feel that he or she can easily be invaded by objects from the outside world. Alternatively, a person may feel that he or she can extend him- or herself into this outer world (as seen with thought projection) or have bits of them-selves pulled into the world beyond his or her own skin as seen with the extraordinarily unpleasant sensation of thought withdrawal. Obviously, during an initial interview, a patient moving into a psychotic state may show moments of wariness and internal pre-occupation as he or she attempts to make sense of these disturbing sensations of part-self/part-object. Such fleeting moments of patient distraction may be the first warning to an alert interviewer that psychotic process may be present.

Not so obviously, it is important to realize that some patients with schizotypal per-sonality disorders may be experiencing lower grade examples of these phenomena. Con-sequently, intermittent moments of preoccupation or a lack of the nonverbal behaviors typical of engagement may represent signal *signs* alerting the interviewer to pursue the possibility of schizotypal process.

Similarly, patients with schizotypal personality disorders may report signal *symptoms* betraying that they have experienced micropsychotic episodes highlighted by experiences typical of a person regressing to the world of part-self/part-object relations. These patients may describe fleeting sensations of magical thinking (where they or others impact upon each other from a distance) or relate episodes of low-grade paranoia with sensations of people reading their minds or experiencing ideas of reference.

Finally, if an interviewer sees such signal signs or the patient reports such signal symp-toms suggesting potential schizotypal process, it is important to realize that these patients may be exquisitely prone to developing paranoid responses towards the interviewer. A wise clinician, once spotting signal signs or symptoms suggesting a schizotypal process (or perhaps frank psychotic process), should "go slow" and "go carefully." As we dis-cussed in Chapter 1, such patients may respond poorly to high-valence empathic state-ments (see pages 23–27). With such patients, I avoid questions that require the patient to self-reflect, for these can be misinterpreted as being accusatory in nature. I also avoid interpretive questions, for these, too, can trigger wariness in such fragile patients.

Developmental Stage #2: Seeking Safety by Merging With Others

Winnicott, Merger Objects, and Transitional Objects

It is untenable for an infant to function indefinitely by only using part-self/part-object dynamics, for the infant would be in an almost perpetual state of anxiety (often reflected by an infant's screaming when left alone). Obviously, the next step towards a feeling of safety is to not be alone. When cuddled and surrounded by the tactile warmth and nur-turing sounds of a parental figure, an infant feels somehow more whole. As the infant is embraced, his or her sense of self is artificially enhanced. For the ability to keep this construct of an all-encompassing parent "alive," once the parenting figure has left the room intrapsychically, this external thing must be introjected into an object relation.

It is here that one of the theorists from the British school of object relations, Donald W. Winnicott, added some fascinating pieces of the puzzle.[7] These puzzle pieces would prove to hold immediate secrets for interviewing more effectively. Winnicott suggested that this maternal "holding environment" was an essential way-station in the development of the self. Put bluntly, the act of "being held" felt so good, and created such a sense of safety, that unconsciously an infant would discover ways of maintaining it. In this fashion, even when the external person (Mom or Dad) was out of the room, the sensation of comfort would be maintained.

Winnicott coined one of the most famous of all terms in object relations, a term that rapidly entered pop parlance – the transitional object. It would prove to be the Holy Grail for the character Linus from the internationally renowned *Peanuts* comic strip. Linus's ubiquitous blanket or "binky" is *the* transitional object *par excellence*. Wherever Linus ventured, even into the maws of his sister Lucy's rants, he felt safe as long as he had his binky with him. Without it, he melted into a pool of apprehension. Unlike the classic intrapsychic objects of object relations theory, Winnicott's transitional object is a real object outside of the patient's mind. It is not an intrapsychic construct. Moreover, it works. Transitional objects allow one to feel safe when the outside "merger objects" have vanished. (Note that when I bastardize the *intra*psychic term "object" to refer to *external* people or things which are introjected to create true internal objects in a psychoanalytic sense, I will place the terms in quotations, as with his mother was a "merger object" or his big brother was an "idealized self-object").

Sometimes people can get stuck needing to use this very early developmental defense of merger objects in order to feel safe as adults. Such a phenomenon is not uncommon with people who have been abused by a parent. Once that parent has left the room (or perhaps while he or she is abusing the child) the child's unconscious may fixate upon the presence of an internalized caring or imagined "good parent" figure to sustain what sense of safety can be salvaged at the moment. People with borderline personality disorders are particularly prone to using merger objects as a safe holding environment as adults (refer again to Figure 15.1). But it is also often displayed in people with narcissistic and histrionic personality disorders, and occasionally in schizotypal process as well.

Let us now return to the three skill sets that are potentially enhanced by a more sophisticated understanding of object relations and self psychology (new signal signs, new signal symptoms, and new engagement techniques). In this light we will examine how we can utilize the concept of "merger objects" to both facilitate a sensitive differential diagnosis and to bolster engagement from the very first words of the initial interview to the very last.

Signal Signs Arising From Merger Dynamics

Some patients will enter our offices for the first time wearing either a piece of clothing or a piece of jewelry that may, in essence, represent a transitional object. When worn, such an object may represent a signal sign for the clinician to more carefully explore for borderline process as well as narcissistic, histrionic, and schizotypal process. Unknowingly, these adult patients may be depending upon the more child-like use of a transitional object to create a sense of safety when "out and about." We already encountered such a compelling signal sign with my patient Debbie, described in Chapter 7 (see pages 224–225). If you will recall, Debbie had entered my office wearing a handsome leather wristband upon which the name "Paul" had been carefully tooled. Later in the interview I learned that "Paul" stood for the actor Paul Newman.

As I described Chapter 7, Debbie and her partner played a game in which they both pretended that Debbie was Paul Newman. For instance, if a Paul Newman movie came out, Debbie's partner would go to the movie alone, type up a positive movie review, and post-haste send the review to Debbie. As Debbie proactively alerted me in the initial interview, "Don't worry Dr. Shea, we know I'm not Paul Newman. It's not a delusion, but it sure is fun."

In this fantasy world, Debbie powerfully merged with the actor's identity in an admittedly odd but non-psychotic sense. Through the wearing of her "Newman band" she had further wrapped a real life transitional object about her wrist, thus maintaining a sense of safety by merging with the powerful figure of an internationally renowned icon. By the end of the interview, I had uncovered that, as I suspected, Debbie did indeed meet the criteria for a borderline personality disorder. The signal sign of an empty sense of self – the leather transitional object – had proven to be an accurate predictor of borderline process.

It is important to remember that the adult use of transitional objects is not necessarily a sign of psychopathology. Normal adults may revert to merger states during times of stress (it's one of the reasons we like to cuddle with loved ones) or may possess a transitional object that is not relied upon for safety but is merely an adjunctive tool for remembering powerful "merger objects," such as crosses (merging with a godhead), wedding bands (merging with a loved one), jewelry from a deceased loved one (merging with a grandmother or lost child), and, of course, tattoos that include the name or face of a romantic interest (merging with a girlfriend or boyfriend, which, at a later date, alas, depending upon the duration of the romance, may need to be conveniently, yet painfully, removed as a transitional object). When noted during an initial interview, these items invite a careful exploration of their unique significance to the patient. Such an exploration will often reveal whether they represent normal functioning or a pathologic reflection of an overdependence upon merger objects (as seen in borderline process and the other personality disorders described above).

In subsequent sessions, the presence of transitional objects can play a significant role that can be used constructively or destructively in therapy. Specifically, the interviewer must be keenly aware that he or she can become a "merger object." I vividly remember the issue of a transitional object unexpectedly showing itself in a subsequent session with Debbie. As I moved from my third year of training to becoming a chief resident, I needed to move offices. During my last session with Debbie in my old office, I informed her nonchalantly of the upcoming move, thinking nothing of the merger dynamics. Debbie's mood quickly shifted. A troubled look stole across her face within minutes. It was so striking a shift that I felt compelled to address it.

When I asked, "Debbie is there something bothering you?", she looked up pensively – almost anguished – saying, "Is the chair coming?" Genuinely puzzled, I asked, "What do you mean? She answered, "This chair. Are you bringing this chair to the other office?" I answered, "Oh no. I'm not allowed to do that. I have to leave it for the next resident." Without recognizing that a merger dynamic was in play, I cheerfully added, "I bet we will have even nicer chairs in the next office. Why do you ask?" Debbie looked up, "Because (pause) … because I just love sitting in this chair (pause) … I don't know. I can't really explain it. But I just feel safe in this chair."

A more convincing example of an adult using a "merger object" would be hard to imagine. Apparently not only Linus needs transitional objects. Winnicott was onto something.

Signal Symptoms Arising From Merger Dynamics

Through our understanding of the psychodynamics of patients becoming stuck with the need for merger objects – and for the people from which these merger objects arise in the real world – some of the pain seen in the borderline process is more easily recognized. Two signal symptoms are frequently spontaneously reported by these patients during an initial interview: (1) intense feelings of abandonment, and (2) peculiar sensations of emptiness (not being whole). These are not the pains of adults; these are the strikingly terror filled pains of a small child who suddenly finds himself or herself lost in a public park or shopping mall.

Let us look at this pain in more detail. To do so we will utilize a fictional description, for gifted authors often tap the pain of the unconscious with an almost uncanny sensitivity. In his novel *Women in Love*, D. H. Lawrence elegantly captures the pain encountered when one must struggle with an incomplete sense of self and the resulting lack of self-esteem such a struggle engenders:

> *And yet her soul was tortured, exposed. Even walking up the path of the church, confident as she was that in every respect she stood beyond all vulgar judgment, knowing perfectly that her appearance was complete and perfect, according to the first standards, yet she suffered a torture, under her confidence and her pride, feeling herself exposed to wounds and to mockery and to despite. She always felt vulnerable, vulnerable, there was always a secret chink in her armor. She did not know herself what it was. It was a lack of robust self, she had no natural sufficiency, there was a terrible void, a lack, a deficiency of being within her.*

> *And she wanted someone to close up this deficiency, to close it up forever. She craved for Rupert Birkin. When he was there, she felt complete, she was sufficient, whole. For the rest of time she was established on the sand, built over a chasm, and, in spite of all her vanity and securities, any common maid-servant of positive, robust temper could fling her down this bottomless pit of insufficiency, by the slightest movement of jeering or contempt. And all the while the pensive, tortured woman piled up her own defenses of aesthetic knowledge, and culture, and world-visions, and disinterestedness. Yet she could never stop up the terrible gap of insufficiency.*[8]

This particular fictional character may or may not completely fit the designation of a borderline personality, but this description of the hollowness experienced by the person with a borderline personality could not be more convincing.

Let us now look at this same pain in the real world – Debbie's world. In our first session, Debbie described feeling intensely angry at her partner any time her partner would roll over to fall asleep. Suddenly Debbie was left by herself. She immediately experienced a disquieting sense of panic, like a lost child in a department store who suddenly realizes that a parent is not nearby. At these moments she would feel acutely abandoned by her partner and deeply resented her partner's need for sleep. Angry conversations frequently ensued. Debbie confided the following to me with a roiling rage, "I can't believe she would do that to me. … to abandon me like that!"

One can easily see how this defect on the psychological wing often leads directly to severe ramifications on the interpersonal wing of the patient's matrix. Deeply troubled relationships are an almost inevitable consequence of merger object dynamics being predominant in adulthood. The loved ones of these patients are left genuinely perplexed by what appear to be the unexplainable antics of their loved ones. It is a tragic defect for all involved. No one at fault. Everyone damaged.

Enhancing Engagement as Related to Merger Objects

If an initial interviewer recognizes from signal signs and signal symptoms that the patient is predisposed to the need for merger objects and, hence, prone to severe dependency issues with therapists, caution is advised in the initial encounter. In the very first session, such patients can push clinicians to do things for them such as interceding with others or writing various notes or excuses for use at work or school. They may also quickly push for frequent appointments and immediately want to be able to contact the interviewer at home or by e-mail, or may request a cell phone number for 24/7 contact.

Before ever entering the clinician's office for the first time, they may have already googled the clinician, searched for a clinician Facebook page, or may already be posting on their own Facebook page their anticipations about the upcoming meeting. It is surprising how quickly patients with merger object dynamics can become overly dependent upon a therapist, who is immediately viewed as a powerful mother or father figure. Such inappropriate attachments can destroy effective engagement if not recognized by an initial interviewer and gentle, yet appropriate, boundaries and expectations set (including expectations and guidelines on what material is appropriately utilized or viewed by both parties on the web and via e-mail).

With Debbie, her descriptions of dependency, both with intimate others and with former therapists (police needed to be called to remove her from her last therapist's office), led us to a matter-of-fact discussion of her dependency needs (which she recognized) and the use of the following question during the closing phase of her initial assessment, "How will we make sure that you don't become too dependent upon me?" This question led to a productive conversation that laid the foundation for our boundaries for the rest of her psychotherapy.

Kernberg, Splitting, and the Move Towards Mobility

Although the use of merger objects clearly creates a more secure sense of self than the use of part-self/part-object dynamics, it remains highly problematic, as seen with patients coping with borderline personality structure. The problem is a simple one. The toddler cannot feel safe unless Mom or Dad are directly cuddling them or in plain sight. The problem with this is one of mobility – not enough of it. One of the unconscious processes that enables a toddler to gain more mobility while functioning as a bridging mechanism to the next stage in the development of the self is the defense mechanism of splitting.

Splitting, first described by Melanie Klein, and subsequently elaborated by one the greatest of the object relation theorists, Otto Kernberg, is an unconscious mechanism in which internal objects can be split, depending upon the immediate moment, into objects which the person views as either "all good" or "all bad."[9] This process is sometimes referred to as a splitting of affects. As we shall soon see, splitting when seen in adult patients is often problematic (indeed a focus of therapy), but in an infant or toddler, who is developing a sense of self, it is initially very valuable (refer again to Figure 15.1).

In cognitive theory, there is a correlate of sorts to the psychodynamic concept of splitting. In early life, a human cannot see shades of gray: the cortex is not mature enough to make such distinctions, nor has the interpersonal milieu been experienced by the toddler in enough situations that he or she can perceive the existence of various shades of gray. As with splitting, during this early level of cognitive development, things tend to be seen as existing at opposite ends of a continuum (being perceived as either very good or very bad). This style of cognition is sometimes called black/whiting.

Both splitting and black/whiting provide an important tool for the development of the self. In fact, they can be considered as providing a major answer to finding mobility and establishing the initial steps towards more independent functioning. They do so by providing an alerting radar of sorts. As the toddler attempts to step away from the parent "merger object," he or she must be able to quickly identify danger and thus know when to equally quickly run back to the protective arms of the "merger object" when necessary. Armed with its transitional object (creating a sense of security) and with its splitting mechanisms (black/whiting cognitive apparatus), the child can now wander from the parent. During its wanderings, armed with its cognitive radar, the child can immediately make a snap judgment on any new person encountered as being either "safe" or "not safe." If deemed to be "safe," interaction continues. If "not safe," back to Mom or Dad *pronto*.

It is an ingenious, albeit unconsciously employed, developmental tool. In some instances, it might be life saving. For instance, a small toddler living with a physically abusive father has milliseconds, when first entering a room in which his or her father is standing, to determine whether it is "Good Dad" (playful when not drinking) or "Bad Dad" (violent when drinking). Unfortunately for some patients (some of whom go on to develop borderline personality disorders), during their childhood they needed to use this splitting defense in an abnormally frequent fashion, for they risked an encounter with the abusive figure at almost any moment. In addition, they would have needed to maintain this guarded posture for many years. Consequently, in contrast to a person with normal self-development (who rather rapidly moves past the frequent use of splitting into a more sophisticated ability to see the shades of gray), a person requiring the prolonged need for a warning radar to alert them to the presence of an abusive parent or sibling can become stuck with splitting as a common defense mechanism well into adulthood.

Signal Signs Arising From Splitting Defenses

Once we understand that a person with a borderline personality disorder for the most part lacks the ability to see gray, their world becomes at once more comprehensible and intriguing. If the patient with a borderline personality must always clump experiences into extremes, then the simplest of frustrations or rejections may be interpreted quite naturally as a vicious attack.

By way of example, if the clinician must cancel an appointment because of an unexpected illness, then the person with the borderline personality is limited, by his or her inability to see gray, to hearing only one of two messages from the clinician, either "I care about you" or "I don't care about you." In this instance, the words of the clinician are more on the negative side, so they are immediately transformed into the latter cognitive interpretation. In this situation, it is no wonder that the patient with a borderline personality structure slams the phone down yelling, "You really are a son of a bitch aren't you?" Such a response is no different from the small child who berates his mother for not buying the toy airplane with an, "I hate you. I hate you!" The child sees the denial as a true rejection, an act of cruelty.

Meanwhile, at the other end of the phone, the clinician sits dumbfounded, wondering what went wrong. In actuality, the "irrationally" angry response of the patient is not as irrational as it may seem at first glance. It would be irrational for a person with a normal ability to see gray to respond in such a fashion, because the normal response would be to view this cancellation as disappointing but understandable. On the other hand, if a person simply did not have the cognitive ability to see gray, then the angry response is reasonably appropriate, because this patient "heard" the therapist state, rather boldly, that the therapist did not care about the patient. In essence, the primary psychological deficit is more with the patient's cognitive apparatus than with their anger control.

In addition, on the biological wing of the matrix, abused patients may have a physiological predisposition towards affective lability. Sometimes trauma can create changes in the limbic system of the brain that may predispose the patient to such emotional over-reactivity. Considering either or both of these contributing factors, the patient's unsettling rages may be understood from a more compassionate stance. Indeed, limited by an unconscious predisposition for splitting, patients with a borderline structure face a tremendously punishing interpersonal environment on a daily basis.

This tendency for seeing only the black or the white of a situation may present itself in the initial interview, where it represents a signal sign to the interviewer that he or she may be in the presence of a person with borderline psychopathology. Such a developmentally delayed manner of cognitively interpreting the world can also be seen in people with other personality disorders, including the paranoid personality, the schizotypal personality, and the more regressed forms of the narcissistic or histrionic personality. In mild degrees it can be seen in all of us and can lead to a variety of neurotic tensions.

Two classic signal signs resulting from splitting and black/whiting that can first suggest to the clinician the presence of the personality disorders above are: (1) overuse of extreme words during the scouting phase, and (2) idealization–devaluation of others.

With regard to the first signal sign, because a patient with splitting experiences the world as a cascade of "all-good" and "all-bad" experiences, it is entirely natural for the patient to describe his or her world with extreme words. There is no other way to describe the world if one is trying to tell the clinician the truth. These patients are *not* intentionally over-dramatizing the world. It is literally how they are experiencing the world. Their extreme word choices are normal and honest. But the extreme quality of their word choices, a process I like to call "linguistic polarization," can alert the clinician to the potential presence of marked psychopathology such as borderline process.

Patients stuck with splitting as a common defense will often display linguistic polarization during the scouting phase of the interview (the first 5 to 7 minutes), as they are encouraged to tell their stories in an unstructured format. Be on the lookout for an unusually high number of words such as "extremely," "very," "best," "worst," "horrible," "amazing," "unbelievable." You may hear, "I have the worst brother in the world," or "My last therapist was the absolute best" (note that you are already, at best, second-best), or "That was the best movie I ever saw," or "No one has had a worse childhood." We all can use such phrases. It is the frequency of their use that is striking with these patients. Over the years, I have found that recognizing linguistic polarization during the scouting phase has often been my first tip-off that a patient may have a borderline personality disorder or has been abused in childhood.

Let us now examine the second signal sign suggestive of borderline process, stemming from the patient's dependence upon splitting. Patients plagued by splitting may describe loved ones in an idealized fashion followed, sometimes in the same interview, with devaluation that can be to the point of vicious denigration. "Back then my brother was a total asshole." Later in the interview the patient comments, "You know, my brother is one of the kindest people I know now." If the brother happens to say something a bit terse in the coming week, you can bet that in the next session you will hear the patient angrily comment, "What an idiot. He's just a big shot. That's who he thinks he is, a big shot. I hate him."

One can see that patients hampered by splitting or black/whiting are genuinely impaired through no fault of their own. In essence, it is hard for them to maintain a consistent view of their important internal object relations (representing the external people in their lives), for the smallest of gray interactions can swing them towards wildly inaccurate depictions of loved ones as being all good or all bad. This problematic swinging and over-judging of people (in both directions) is sometimes called a deficit in object constancy. It is a painful place from which to view the world. In this regard, having a borderline personality is a little like being a toddler who rolls a ball under a couch and believes that the ball has vanished into non-existence. A good cry will soon follow as the child finds that its favorite play toy has disappeared. People with borderline personality development may have problems believing in the constancy of those who love them.

Sometimes a clinician may even see the patient rapidly change opinions about the interviewer, himself or herself, as the interview unfolds – a classic signal symptom suggesting the possibility of borderline, narcissistic, or histrionic process. I am reminded of a young woman, whom I interviewed directly after another clinician. The patient quickly began, "You know, the person I was just talking with didn't seem to know what she was doing. I didn't like her. I'm not going to have to talk with her again, am I?"

As our interview proceeded, the patient seemed to warm to me relatively quickly, eventually stating that she would not mind working with me. She eventually attempted to demand placement on a specific inpatient unit, which we felt was inappropriate for her. When I told her that she would not be able to go to that particular unit, she angrily pouted. Later her boyfriend came up to me privately, saying, "My girlfriend is very displeased with you, and frankly so am I." More classic borderline behavior could not be found. I jumped from being Prince Charming to Charles Manson in a single bound. This type of rapid idealization–devaluation is a classic signal behavior suggestive of borderline psychopathology or some other personality disorder that is dependent upon the splitting defense.

This patient also displayed a trait commonly seen with borderline pathology in which the unconscious mechanism of splitting has led the patient to consciously pit one person (her boyfriend) against another (me). This was also demonstrated when she relayed to me her complaints about the previous interviewer. Note that the *conscious* attempt to pit one person against another is often called "splitting" by staff. This use of the word "splitting" is okay as long as one remembers that it is really a bastardization of the word, for true splitting in a psychodynamic sense is an *unconscious* defense mechanism.

Signal Symptoms Arising From Splitting Defenses

When listening to the histories and symptom pictures of patients who subsequently, upon further interviewing, prove to have a borderline personality disorder, the presence of splitting may emerge as a signal symptom pointing towards the disorder. As one can imagine, the rollercoaster impressions of people as being either "all good" or "all bad" results in a similar rollercoaster of emotions and symptoms.

Earlier we saw a series of probe questions that were designed to uncover such emotional swings, but it is not uncommon for patients with borderline process to spontaneously betray these swings. Patients plagued by splitting, whether seen with borderline, narcissistic, or histrionic process, may describe a surprisingly fragile sensitivity to "being slighted." Be on the lookout, especially during the scouting phase, for patients to relay an inordinately large number of instances in which they felt intense anger prompted by perceptions of being let down or betrayed by others. Complaints by the patient of being strikingly moody, especially if his or her moodiness is triggered by perceptions of being interpersonally slighted, may be a signal symptom alerting the clinician to search for borderline process later in the interview.

At times, the severe damage done to the patient's psyche by splitting will show itself as genuine surprise on the part of the patient as to how cruel loved ones can be and will be reflected by statements such as, "I just don't get it. People are always cruel to me. You can't trust anybody. In the final analysis, everyone will hurt you deeply." Unfortunately, because of splitting, everyone will be perceived as doing so, even if they love the patient dearly.

Enhancing Engagement as Related to Splitting Defenses

Much as we saw with both schizotypal process and with an over-reliance on merging, if one spots splitting as a predominant defense mechanism early in an interview, it is important to "go slow," to choose one's words carefully. As one can imagine, the attitude of these patients towards the interviewer can change with extreme rapidity. The initial alliance is fragile with these patients.

In the presence of splitting, the interviewer is well advised to avoid interpretive questions or questions that push the patient to view his or her own behavior. In addition, a collaborative approach to determining the goals of the interview, as well as treatment planning, is not only useful, it is critical. If a patient with splitting misinterprets the interviewer's well-intended suggestion for direction to the interview or for subsequent treatment options as an attempt for control, the interviewer can be transformed from an "all-good clinician" to an "all-bad clinician" with the abruptness of a dropped call on a cell phone. Here, perhaps more than with any other type of patient, it is important to remember that the goal of any first interview is to secure a second one. A clinician who recognizes splitting during the scouting phase of an interview, and subsequently responds appropriately, is much more likely to see a second interview than one who does not.

Developmental Stage #3: Securing the Self Through Grandiosity and Idealization

Kohut, the Bipolar Self, and the Search for Independent Functioning

By this stage of development, through the use of merger objects and splitting, a toddler has secured a more stable sense of self than could be dreamed of when limited by the psychodynamics of part-self/part-object (as seen in the infant's first explorations of his or her own boundaries as well as potentially experienced by an adult caught in the storm of psychotic process). Yet a problem remains. The toddler can venture into the world away from the parenting figure, but it is difficult to stay in this world. The unconscious radar provided by splitting can alert the toddler to danger, but the only response possible is immediate retreat into the arms of Mom or Dad. Independence is fleeting. It is limited by a lack of power.

Heinz Kohut, the founding figure in self psychology, proposed a process that explains how a toddler can gain a sense of power, enough power to not necessarily require retreat upon encountering a potential threat. The toddler, through the mechanism Kohut named the "bipolar self,"[10] can gain the ability to stand his or her ground. (Note that this concept is totally unrelated to the diagnosis of bipolar disorder; also note that later in his career, Kohut re-conceptualized the self as being a tripolar process, which the interested reader can learn about in the work of Flanagan.[11] For our current discussion, the concept of the bipolar self may be the most clarifying concept regarding use in an initial interview.) The question now is exactly how does this bipolar self accomplish this critical developmental task?

If faced by a potential threat, a toddler needs to feel powerful enough to feel safe. Two unconscious processes can provide this sense of safety, albeit a rather artificial one in both instances. Nevertheless, these two unconscious mechanisms can provide an adequate launch-pad for increased independence. Put succinctly, one can establish a more powerful sense of self by either of the following mechanisms: (1) inflating one's sense of self by a massive dose of grandiosity (I am incredibly powerful and can handle any threat that comes my way), or (2) idealizing a protective figure who then becomes invincible (that guy over there is incredibly powerful and he is my protector) (Figure 15.2).

Kohut created a term "self-object" (he subsequently removed the hyphen to "selfobject") that explains the role of these two processes. He viewed both of these processes (building self through grandiosity reflected from others and finding a secure sense of self by identifying with idealized others) as being examples of selfobjects.

Interestingly, in Kohut's original conceptualization, a selfobject is not really an object at all, it is a dimension of experience that an individual has with another person that helps to shore up the individual's sense of an ongoing and secure self. There are significant debates in the field of self psychology as to whether Kohut's original distinction of selfobjects as a process, not an object or an object relation, should be strictly enforced or whether it should be expanded to include the idea that a selfobject is also an internal representation (an object relation) of an external object and/or a shared interpersonal experience. These debates, important as they are in their psychotherapeutic implications, go far beyond our current needs. For our purposes we will loosely accept both interpretations.

Thus a selfobject is a person (or even an environmental situation such as a sunny day or a favorite haunt) that when encountered in real time or imagined internally (as an object relation) provides a person with a more secure sense of self characterized by a feeling of wholeness, consistency, and safety. Encounters with these selfobjects often accomplish this task via processes such as grandiosity or idealization as mentioned above.

As we shall soon see, selfobjects play a major role in normal development. They are also part and parcel of a healthy adult's ongoing search for safety. In other more pathological instances, patients can become fixated upon the need for selfobjects, a fixation that often shows itself with narcissistic personality functioning. Before exploring this pathological track and its relevance to the initial interview, let us first shore up our understanding of the role of selfobjects in health. To do so we will look at a thank you note written by the analyst Phyllis Greenacre to Heinz Kohut himself, who had graciously introduced her as a speaker:

> *Something happened to me with your introduction of me that Sunday. I have tried to think of what it was: I thought "I was greatly touched" – "No, I was moved" – and then it occurred to me that perhaps it was not so much one of these, as that I was gently and reassuringly solidified.*[12]

I believe we would be hard pressed to find a more eloquent and insightful description of the experience of encountering a healthy selfobject than that provided by Greenacre's words that she was "gently and reassuringly solidified." Looked at through the lens of common sense, Greenacre – like all of us – seems to have benefited from a dose of positive feedback in a world that often confronts us with more than ample negative feedback.

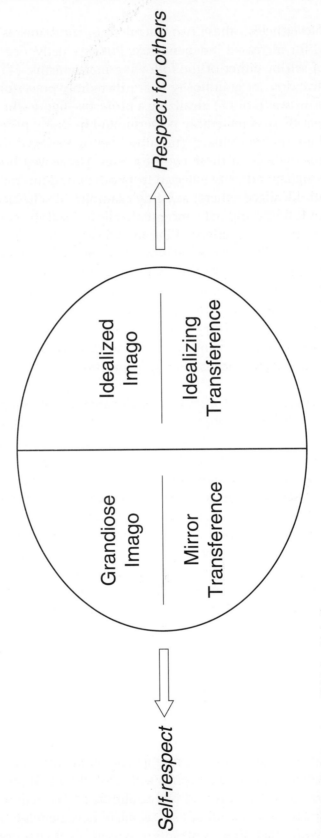

Figure 15.2 Bipolar self (Heinz Kohut).

Financial challenges, opposing viewpoints, and politics as usual all too often remind us of our frailties.

Looked at with the lens of the bipolar self, we can understand Greenacre's experience with a new depth of understanding. We see that Phyllis Greenacre was made more "reassuringly solidified" through the two processes inherent in Kohut's concept of the bipolar self. First, she received an appropriate boost of grandiosity by the kind words of praise from Kohut. Second, I suspect that, in addition, because of Kohut's fame, she probably experienced a solidification of herself through a healthy identification with an idealized figure (Kohut) and his highly respected movement (Self Psychology) of which she was an esteemed member. Kohut had the distinction of simultaneously serving as a selfobject from both ends of the spectrum of the bipolar self!

Let us now see more clearly how healthy movement between the poles of the bipolar self plays a role in early human development, a role that can propel a toddler past an over-reliance on merger objects. It allows a toddler to tolerate potentially threatening people and situations without retreating to the arms of Mom or Dad, thus providing the opportunity for a more independent functioning.

Self psychologists sometimes refer to the first style of selfobject as the "grandiose imago." A child increases his or her sense of safety by unconsciously assuming a grandiose sense of power (see Figure 15.2). Note that the use of an unconscious grandiosity can work surprisingly well, but it has a caveat: A challenging or threatening object must reflect back the grandiosity of the individual. If a toddler meets a bully, he may grandiosely think to himself, "This bully better watch his step. If he tries anything, I'll beat him to a pulp and he'll be one very sorry dude." But, for the toddler's inflated sense of grandiosity to maintain a sense of safety in the toddler, the threatening object (the bully) must back down. If the bully submits, all is well. If the bully punches the toddler in the schnoz, the self shatters as easily as Humpty Dumpty falling off his proverbial wall. The toddler will race back to the protective arms of Mom or Dad, desperately regressing to the comfort of a merger object.

From the perspective of self psychology (and I am greatly simplifying here), this type of relationship (in which a person *reflects* back the grandiosity of another person who happens to be relying upon his or her grandiose imago for a sense of safety) can be conceived as a "mirroring" interaction. When such a process occurs in therapy (e.g., the clinician temporarily mirrors back the grandiosity of the patient to shore up the patient's sense of safety), it is known as a "mirror-transference." As the reader may have already guessed, a pathologic over-dependence upon the use of a grandiose imago by a patient, and the resulting need for ongoing mirroring interactions with people in their everyday lives (or the necessity of temporary mirror-transferences with clinicians), is the hallmark of people meeting the criteria for a narcissistic personality disorder. It is also often seen with histrionic psychodynamics as well.

Note that people with narcissistic personality disorders who happen to be extremely talented may be remarkably happy. They can bask in their own sense of self-importance, for their underlings consistently praise them and idolize them, mirroring back their grandiosity. One can see this process at work with talented narcissistic sports figures, politicians, or Hollywood stars. However, watch what happens when the sports figure ages past his or her prime or the Hollywood star loses his or her looks. The shattered selves that remain are often cradled in the arms of a bottle of alcohol or a line of cocaine, or may self-destruct through a self-inflicted gunshot to the head.

Kohut referred to the second object relation as the "idealizing imago." In self psychology, this object relation represents the other pole of the "bipolar self" (see Figure 15.2). In the mechanism of idealization, a toddler identifies with a powerful idealized figure such as a parent or older sibling, and through this identification, feels better about him- or herself, because the toddler is both identified with the power of this idolized figure and protected by its power.

Adults who are developmentally stuck at this level of self, live a precarious psychological balance. Picture a neurosurgery resident that genuinely believes that the chairperson of her department is, without a doubt, the single greatest neurosurgeon in the world. Now further picture that this neurosurgery resident – who lacks a secure sense of self – unconsciously "says" to herself, "Dr. Jenkins is the greatest neurosurgeon in the world. And he has hand-picked me to be his sole Chief Resident." It's a nifty way to feel very special indeed – all at an unconscious level. With a sense of "specialness" comes an accompanying sense of "safety."

It works. Idealization, with subsequent identification with the idealized person, can create a striking sense of self-importance and subsequent safety. But, once again, as we saw with the use of the grandiose imago, there is a caveat: The idealized "object" better remain ideal. May the gods help our insecure neurosurgery resident if Dr. Jenkins is found to be falsifying research results and/or is being sued by several patients for gross malpractice. This broken idealized "object" leaves a broken neurosurgery Chief Resident as well. The world will collapse for our imagined neurosurgery resident. Like the fuselage of an airplane flying at 30,000 feet that is suddenly violated by breach in its aging structure, the hollow self of the resident will suck in the shame and humiliation of the fallen idealized "object" (Dr. Jenkins) with a stunning rapidity. This need for the idealized "object" to remain idealized – in order for an idealized imago to shore up a person's sense of self-esteem – is an example of an idealizing interaction and when it occurs in therapy is called an "idealizing-transference" (I am, once again, simplifying). It, too, is a hallmark defense of people coping with narcissistic personality function, and is also, perhaps even more so than seen with the overuse of the grandiose imago, a classic defense of people exhibiting a histrionic personality disorder.

Whether in health or in pathology (as encountered with a narcissistic personality), the individual is using grandiosity or idealization to secure a higher degree of safety. Internally, both the grandiose object and the idealized object serve one major function – they complete the sense of self for the person, much like the merger object did. But the difference between a healthy use of selfobjects (high-functioning adult) and an unhealthy use of them (narcissistic personality disorder) depends upon two things: (1) whether the individual *requires* a relatively *consistent and rigid* use of these processes in order to feel safe, and (2) to what degree the person recognizes the needs of the other objects (people) who operate in their lives.

With regard to the first point, in a person with a narcissistic personality disorder, there has been a significant psychological advance in the development of the self. Their sense of self is remarkably more mature than in a person depending upon part-self/part-object dynamics (literally having trouble determining the boundaries of their own self) or a person relying upon merger objects for safety (needing to be in the presence of others in order to feel complete as seen in borderline functioning). Indeed, in contrast to such patients, people with a narcissistic structure have achieved a fairly secure sense that they exist as separate entities, and they have a fairly secure sense that others exist as separate entities. The sense of self has clearly crystallized.

But in contrast to a person who has developed in a healthy fashion, the sense of safety in a person who has a narcissistic personality disorder, *depends* upon a consistent dose of mirroring and idealizing interactions for everyday functioning. Healthy people, such as the speaker Phyllis Greenacre, mentioned above, occasionally benefit from an intermittent dose or two of praise or a chance to idealize, but they are not dependent upon it for normal functioning. Their own grandiosity has been transformed into an appropriate sense of self-respect (see Figure 15.2). Their former idealized objects (Kohut from the perspective of Greenacre) are now appropriately viewed with genuine respect, but are not viewed as being perfect. In short, a person who has developed a healthy sense of self does not need mirroring or idealizing transferences or interactions to maintain that sense of self. They can take them or leave them.

With regard to the second process demarcating healthy personality development from pathological development – the patient's views of other's needs – a striking distinction emerges. In pathologic narcissism, the external selfobjects that are internalized to provide completeness to the self are recognized as separate entities. But the patient cannot perceive them as having their own needs, expectations, and feelings. They have essentially no sense that other selves exist other than to serve their own needs.

In this sense, the term "selfobject" becomes a linguistic reminder that, for narcissists, other people exist solely as "self-objects." They exist for one reason and one reason only: to serve the needs of one's own self. Clinically, and socially, this interpersonal deficiency shows itself in a simple and predictable fashion. People with a narcissistic structure lack an ability to effectively empathize. They really can be bastards.

This lack of empathy is readily apparent in patients dependent upon the grandiose end of the bipolar self. As they tootle about, sharing with others their great achievements, or denigrating the achievements of others, it is clear such individuals lack empathic bonding. But this lack of empathy is also present with patients at the other end of the bipolar self, where idealization secures a sense of safety and importance for the patient.

If one has any doubts as to the lack of empathy in those who idealize others, one merely has to note the rapidity with which a narcissistic or histrionic personality will turn upon an idealized object that has failed to maintain their ideal qualities. Such patients, as the idealizing transference is ruptured, a process that catapults the patient into a painful sense of worthlessness, can verbally attack their former idols with a nasty viciousness. At such moments, the patient may feel a very real sense of being betrayed or let down by their idol, even though their idol continues to be caring towards them. A person with narcissistic structure will have little empathy for the embarrassment or shame being experienced by their former idol. Once off the pedestal, such patients may be the first to trample upon their former idol's shattered remains.

In bringing to a close our look at the theoretical foundations of self psychology as it relates to the initial interview, it is useful to remind ourselves that the bipolar self is not necessarily pathologic. Indeed, as discussed earlier, it is critically useful for the normal development of the self. Normally functioning people use the defenses of the bipolar self throughout much of childhood in order to feel safe enough to test the admittedly turbulent waters of interpersonal relationships. A developing child may flip back and forth between the poles of the bipolar self fluidly many times in a single day.

One can fondly think back upon one of the key functions of fantasy during childhood. During fantasy play, children often assume the identities of grandiosely powerful figures from Spiderman and Wonder Woman to wizards and queens. In addition, children often make idealizations of parent figures, protective big brothers and sisters, playmates, or the latest rock group or winner of American Idol. Indeed, during adolescence, when teenagers enter the threatening world of fellow adolescents raging with hormones, defined by cliques and prone to cruel bullying antics on Twitter and Facebook, many adolescents will regress to the need for grandiose fantasies or idealized protectors.

With this understanding of both the normal and abnormal parameters of the bipolar self, we are now ready to apply this understanding to the initial interview.

Signal Signs Arising From the Psychodynamics of the Bipolar Self

During an initial interview, as well as during subsequent therapy, people dependent upon the bipolar self for safety may show characteristic behaviors or styles of communication. They become "selfies" personified. When using grandiosity, such patients may be surprisingly bold about their own achievements, a clear signal sign to look for the presence of a narcissistic personality later in the social history of the interview. Be on the lookout for patients who use phrases such as, "People are always looking up to me," "To be frank, I am the best there is at what I do," and "I've been gifted all my life" that are conveyed with a nonchalant matter-of-factness. To the narcissist, these words are not pompous – they are merely reflections of the obvious.

A reliance upon the grandiose imago can show itself in rather odd ways as well. A patient may communicate that the therapist is actually lucky to have such a special patient in the room. I vividly remember a patient who happened to also be a psychotherapist himself, who proclaimed with a proud insolence, "Yeah, I'm a narcissist. And there is no therapist in the world who can handle my narcissism." The statement was punctuated with a challenging smile.

In a similar fashion, a patient stuck with grandiose defenses may try to put the therapist down or "in his place" during the initial encounter. Watch out for any patient who refers to you as a "friend," as with a comment such as, "Listen, my friend, here is what's going down." This denigrating use of the word "friend" is almost always a sign of narcissistic grandiosity. The patient clearly does not view you as a friend. You can see this defense wondrously displayed on television when viewing various political pundits and talking heads debating one another.

In the scouting phase, and as the history itself unfolds, people depending upon either a grandiose or idealizing imago will demonstrate their inability to empathize by a surprising lack of affective change when describing other people's plights, points of view, or life circumstances. Tenderness in tone of voice, slowing of speech when reflecting upon another person's difficulties, or a tearful welling up when describing another person's pain are seldom seen in narcissism. Such patients often exude a cool indifference when recounting the troubles of other people. People are only important as pathologic self-objects existing to please the patient. Sometimes narcissism can be so striking that it has a comical flavor to it, as seen in the patient who comments to an old friend (after talking about his own recent achievements for several minutes), "Well, enough about me. Let's talk about you. What do you think about my new iPhone, pretty damn amazing isn't it?"

A person relying upon an idealizing imago for safety will often be predisposed in an initial interview to describe many people in their lives in superlative terms. This may represent a signal sign of histrionic structure as well. In a similar light, people with a histrionic style will often be unusually ardent fans of a variety of popular icons in sports, movies, and music, for they gain a sense of self-wholeness by identifying with such figures.

Finally, many people with narcissistic structure are reluctant patients. They have often entered therapy at the request, or even demand, of other people, such as spouses or employers. Whereas many patients, when spontaneously describing their symptoms during an initial interview, communicate a sense of pain, as well as an admixture of hesitancy and embarrassment, people with narcissistic object relations often communicate a surprising amount of anger towards others, as well as a hesitancy to admit or even consider their own role in their problems. Especially when stuck in a dependency on the use of a grandiose imago for a secure sense of self, people with narcissistic personality disorders often view other people as the root of their problems. Comments such as, "My wife is the real problem here, not my drinking. She's the reason I drink, trust me. She should be here not me," are strong indicators that one is likely to be in the room with a person using a grandiose object relation to secure a sense of safety.

Indeed, people coping with severe inappropriate alcohol and/or drug use often regress to such narcissistic defenses. It should also be mentioned that people with an antisocial personality structure sometimes rely upon a grandiose imago to secure a sense of self, with a particularly intense lack of empathy and a penchant for nastiness and irresponsibility. In its extreme form, as seen in sociopathy, it can manifest as cruelty, sadism, and an uncanny total lack of empathy as seen in serial killers.

Signal Symptoms Arising From the Psychodynamics of the Bipolar Self

With regard to their own symptoms, the fragility of the sense of self – especially with people with a malignant style of narcissism in which the sense of self is extremely tenuous – means that mood swings are commonly reported, especially depressive swings. In this regard, people dependent upon grandiosity for self stability may be particularly sensitive to interpersonal slight. Such slights – even innocuous in nature – can break their interpersonal "mirrors" whose surfaces are desperately needed to reflect back their grandiosity. This is common in both narcissistic and histrionic styles.

As one can imagine, jealousy is often present with the psychodyanmics of Kohut's bipolar self. Both grandiose narcissists (who are jealous of people who seem better than them) and idealizing narcissists (who perceive other people as a threat to become the apple of the eye of the idealized hero or heroine over themselves) are prone to classic bouts of jealousy, with backbiting, scheming, and the political undermining of others. Reports of intense sexual jealousy regarding the patient's significant other (and reports of verbal abuse or violent outbursts of domestic violence) are signal symptoms that one should search for narcissistic structure.

This narcissistic jealousy can show itself in less classic ways as well. MacKinnon points out that people with narcissistic psychodynamics may report envy towards a new baby, a bride at a wedding, and even towards the person being eulogized at a funeral.[13]

Another signal symptom that may slip the attention of the interviewer – for it is not traditionally viewed as an aspect of narcissism – is the presence of hypochondriasis, as well as extreme attention to bodily appearance. In some patients, the constant drawing of attention to their bodily ills or bodily defects serves as an unconscious mechanism for drawing attention to oneself, perhaps as the sickest person in the room, a person needing everyone's attention.

I remember a young woman with a histrionic personality I had been treating in long-term psychotherapy who appeared one day in a distraught manner. When asked what was going on, she replied, "It's my hand, the scar on my hand has just been bothering me a lot recently, and I think I need to see a plastic surgeon." I was puzzled that after months of seeing her in therapy I had been so unobservant as to have never noticed her scar. Consequently, I asked if I could see it. When she presented her hand, with the grandiose poise of a Baroque duchess presenting her hand for a gentleman's kiss, I looked and looked and could not see the scar. She then, with a bit of irritation to her voice, pointed it out to me, commenting, "horrible isn't it?" It was indeed the most horrible looking 1 mm scar I had ever had the pleasure to see. To this day, I'm not certain there was any scar at all.

Enhancing Engagement Via an Understanding of the Bipolar Self

An understanding of the nuanced psychodynamics of the bipolar self may exhibit its highest utility in the arena of engagement. Arguably the greatest challenge in an initial interview with a person exhibiting a narcissistic personality disorder is to secure a second interview. This challenge is particularly evident when working with a person limited by the need for a grandiose object relation in order to feel safe with others (in this instance the interviewer). With such patients, the speed with which a mirror-transference can arise is a bit startling. The subtlest hint that the clinician does not reflect back the patient's grandiosity can jeopardize the likelihood of a return visit.

Complementary Shifts

Over the years, a technique that I like to call a "complementary shift" has proven to be useful in communicating and maintaining a mirror-transference during an initial interview. One of the great fears of a person who requires the use of a grandiose imago is that the clinician perceives himself or herself to be somehow superior or "above" the patient. If the patient leaves the first meeting feeling "one-down" to the interviewer, I think it is quite likely that the interviewer has had the last meeting with this particular patient.

In order to avoid creating the sensation in the patient of being "one-down," the interviewer can employ one or a series of complementary shifts. A complementary shift is a verbal response or a nonverbal gesture that shifts the patient's view of the clinician so that the patient feels superior or one-up on the interviewer. Such maneuvers are called complementary because they complement the patient's need for a mirroring of their grandiosity. In essence, the interviewer temporarily accepts the role of a self-object as a means of complementing or completing the patient's immediate sense of self.

One can employ a variety of complementary shifts. One of the easiest is to literally compliment the patient, thus gently stroking the patient's self-esteem. It is critical that one provides a genuine compliment – one that is truly felt by the interviewer. A false compliment is never appropriate, and such a pretense violates the trust necessary in a healthy therapeutic alliance. Moreover, many patients will see through such a disingenuous compliment immediately. But if one notices an attribute of the patient that one genuinely respects, it can be transformative to share it with the patient.

I recall an initial assessment with a young, lanky 26-year-old man with poorly controlled schizophrenia. We shall call him Dale. He had jet-black hair that hung as a wavy bang over his forehead, nearly covering his eyebrows. It was a forehead behind which there sat an unusually bright brain, as we shall soon see. It was through this thick bang of hair that Dale would angrily swipe his hand as he spoke with me. And Dale was angry with me from the minute he set eyes upon me.

I was picking Dale up as a new patient in a community mental health center. He was on Haldol. There were two things Dale hated most in life, Haldol and psychiatrists. Not necessarily in that order.

Despite my best attempts during the interview to engage Dale, he would return to an ongoing diatribe about the evils of Haldol and all antipsychotic medications. There was nothing wrong with him, he asserted tartly, adding accusations such as, "You have no right to fill me with your poisons." In truth, Dale was a bit frightening. I was contemplating ending the session early in order to avoid further escalation of his anger, for he had a history of some low-grade violence towards staff.

As he continued his diatribe on this particular day, he made a sophisticated point, "Dr. Shea, admit it, you know and I know that your antipsychotics can lead to sub-cortical dementias." As I hastily reviewed in my head the difference between cortical and sub-cortical dementias as related to the use of Haldol, the level of sophistication behind Dale's statement dawned upon me. I then remembered two things: (1) the ferocious pain beneath most anger and its common link with narcissistic insult, and (2) the use of complementary shifts. I paused and the following dialogue, as best I remember it, ensued:

Clin.: You know, Dale, I'm struck by how much you know about Haldol. Where have you learned all this? (said very quietly and with genuine curiosity)

Pt.: I read.

Clin.: That's pretty obvious, because whatever it is you're reading sounds like it must be pretty sophisticated because your knowledge about Haldol is impressive. I'm curious what type of thing you like to read and how you manage to find it. (It actually was impressive. He clearly knew more about the neuroscience of Haldol than most general physicians.)

Pt.: Well, I read articles and stuff. (his tone of voice was softening)

Clin.: Yeah, but they must be sort of hard to find. I'm curious where you find them.

Pt.: Oh, I take a bus out to the medical center.

Clin.: You mean Wilshine Medical Center?

Pt.: Yeah, I go to the medical library there.

Clin.: That's a couple of miles from where you live isn't it?

Pt.: Three. I take the bus to get there. It runs a couple of times a day. (his voice was significantly calmer at this point)

Clin.: What do you read when you get there?

Pt.: My favorite journal is the *American Journal of Psychiatry*.

Clin.: (I had to smile. I barely have time to read it.) That's really impressive. (pause) … I've never had a patient tell me anything like that before, you know, that they were reading professional journal articles as opposed to information written for the general public.

Pt.: Well, I do. (Dale then broke into a smile)

Clin.: That's obvious from your questions and your points. (pause) … Look, we clearly disagree about the Haldol right now, but I genuinely want to listen to any points you may find in your readings. I am open to new ideas. I can't promise that you will change my mind anymore than I can promise that I'll be able to change your mind. But we can always talk, and I promise you I will listen carefully, very carefully, which I hope that you will too. Since this is our very first meeting, let's just back track a bit and try to get to know each other a little better to see what it will be like to work together, because I think we can work together. I really do. Tell me a little bit about how you got involved with the clinic here in the first place.

The interview proceeded much more smoothly from that point onwards.

Another effective type of complementary shift is to ask the patient for help. I have found this to be effective with adolescents when first meeting them. After having spoken with the parents to get an overview of their concerns, when I meet with the patient I will use a complementary shift that goes something like this (depending upon the presenting circumstances), "Jim, I was just speaking with your parents about the problems at school and I need your help. Your parents were not in the room when you had the argument with your principal. Nor was I. Only you and the principal were there. She's not here now. Only you are. And only you and that principal know what actually happened. I need your help here. Tell me, from your perspective, what Mrs. Drake said that you found so upsetting. Clearly she said something that you found really, really upsetting. I want to know what she said and why it pissed you off so much?"

Asking the patient for help is frequently a powerful strategy with people feeling one-down to the clinician. It is a rapid and genuine request that immediately puts the patient one-up (as a dispenser of knowledge unknown to the clinician). Moreover, it is a genuinely person-centered perspective, for the patient's perspective may be the correct one, and the inquiry communicates both respect and a collaborative stance.

Countertransference: Short-Circuiting a Clinical Gremlin

When a patient presents with a heavy reliance on the use of a grandiose imago, especially when it displays itself with a callous cruelty towards others and/or it manifests as an angry sense of entitlement towards the clinician, it is easy to have negative feelings towards the patient. Such feelings are natural. They reflect a healthy sense of ethics and compassion in the interviewer. Nevertheless, it is critical to recognize such seeds of countertransference, and to make sure these feelings don't manifest themselves in negative behaviors towards the patient.

Often, especially when intense, such negative clinician emotions are reasonably easy to spot in ourselves. It is when the negative feelings are subtle or unconscious that they tend to be harder to recognize. In this regard, MacKinnon and colleagues, in their classic exploration of the psychodynamics of the interview, illuminate the significance of boredom in the clinician as a reflection of countertransference. They eloquently delineate the relation of this boredom to the patient's use of a grandiose imago and the subsequent pressure upon the interviewer to mirror back this grandiosity:

> Feeling bored in response to the narcissist's egocentricity is a common reaction for the clinician, who may have the feeling that his function is only that of an appreciative audience. There is often no sense of being engaged in a collaborative enterprise designed to bring some understanding to the troubles that brought the patient to request a consultation in the first place. Considerable effort may be required to remain engaged and not drift off into one's own thoughts, reflecting the same self-preoccupation as the patient.[14]

In the presence of a patient manifesting unpleasant grandiosity, once a clinician has recognized any negative countertransferential feelings, it becomes important to internally process them while continuing to communicate the unconditional positive regard described by Carl Rogers and discussed in the early chapters of this book. It is here that an understanding of the bipolar psychodynamics of the patient can help to mitigate negative feelings towards the patient. According to these concepts, the self-objects of pathological grandiosity and pathological idealization arise as defenses against intense pain. Patients do not choose to be narcissists; they are sculpted by the unique matrices of their lives into becoming narcissists. The intense fears and pain associated with a fragile sense of self are the hammer and chisel that create these living sculptures.

In this sense, the analytical understanding provided by a knowledge of bipolar psychodynamics can help transform a clinician's initial negative responses to the patient into a developing sense of empathy for the patient. Indeed, Kohut emphasized the power of empathy as a healing agent in the treatment of people suffering from narcissism in ongoing therapy. We can see that such empathy can also play a role in transforming countertransference in the initial encounter as well.

Interviewers must also be aware of nonverbal leakage. It is not enough to be aware of one's negative feelings towards the patient if present. It is also important to ensure that nonverbal behaviors do not transmit these feelings without the conscious awareness of the clinician, thus breaking unconditional positive regard. As stated in Chapter 8 on nonverbal communication, much of empathy is communicated nonverbally. Likewise, much of disapproval is communicated without words as well.

Clinicians, even though they have consciously recognized their countertransferential feelings, must make sure that they are not automatically communicating them nonverbally. Such behaviors as decreased smiling, a decrease of warmth in the tone of voice, decreased head nodding, and even rolling one's chair back a bit from the patient, can inadvertently communicate disapproval. Patients can be exquisitely sensitive to such changes in conversational markers.

I am reminded of the actual patient upon which the role play was based that you saw in Video Module 5.1. You might recall that Ben was the late adolescent who had taken little kid's candy bags on Halloween. He and his friends got a real kick out of waiting till the siren went off announcing that trick-or-treating was over, at which point they would steal the full candy bags from the little tots heading home. During the video of my actual interview with Ben, I was so aghast at the action that I almost fell over backwards in my chair. My unintentional, yet inappropriate, response generally results in a great deal of laughter from my audiences when viewing the actual patient video in my workshops. Apparently my unconscious was not on board with Carl Rogers' concept of unconditional positive regard at that exact moment.

Accepting Idealization

As clinicians we attempt to work collaboratively with patients. We are trained to not place ourselves on pedestals. It is good training. However, in initial interviews, there are rare occasions when it is wise to accept being put on a pedestal if it is the patient who has placed us there.

This situation can be the prudent alternative when we are first meeting a patient who is dependent upon an idealized imago (and a subsequent idealizing transference) in order to feel safe. To such fragile patients, their sense of self and safety is dependent upon the clinician being a powerful "white knight" who can help them.

Such patients may say things like, "I hear from a friend that you are the very best therapist in the city," or "I just know that you are going to be able to change everything for me." I believe many of us have an immediate inclination to respond to such overblown statements with comments such as, "Well I don't know if I'm the very best in the city, but I certainly try to do my best with everyone," or "Well, I can't guarantee that your whole life is going to turn around, but I certainly think I might be able to help you."

Such appropriate statements of humility might not be well received by a person who intensely needs an idealized figure in order to effectively function at that moment in time. These statements, completely appropriate with most patients, can shatter the sense of safety and hope in a patient dependent upon an idealizing transference before the therapy has even begun. Indeed, such statements may ensure that there will be no ongoing therapy, for there will be no second appointment. Feeling that they are in the presence of an imperfect knight, they may feel remarkably ill-at-ease, even frightened.

Such patients may be better served by responses that do not destroy the much-needed idealized imago (in this case the interviewer), such as, "Well I'm glad your friend thinks so highly of me," or "We are certainly going to try to look at everything you feel is important and hopefully make some important changes for you."

As the patient's maturation occurs in ongoing sessions, the therapist will subsequently be able to appropriately challenge the patient's idealizations. But it is important to remember that some patients may need us to temporarily stand atop a pedestal. It is alright to accept such a position in the service of the patient's current psychological needs as long as we do not fall into the trap of believing that the patient is correct in placing us there!

Developmental Stage #4: Achieving a Stable Self and the Advent of Empathy

With appropriate parenting, both the toddler's grandiosity and his or her idealization (of parents) will be softened (see Figure 15.2). Grandiose demands such as "I deserve to get all the ice-cream" are muted by parental limit setting that communicates that the child is not the center of the universe but is nevertheless much loved.

In addition, with time children learn that parent figures are not all-powerful. They too make mistakes (blaming the child for a broken window when her brother was the one who kicked the soccer ball through it). As the parent acknowledges the mistake, apologizes to the child, and fairly punishes the little dickens of a brother, the child becomes aware of the limitations of parental figures and shows less of a tendency to idealize them. The idealization of the parents, older siblings, powerful friends, and teachers is gradually transformed into an appropriate respect *sans* idolization. As one can imagine, this process unfolds neither quickly nor smoothly.

As the years go by, there are ups and downs in this process. This is especially true during adolescence, when the sense of a secure self meets a genuine threat from the interpersonal traps set by peers and one's own hormonal turbulence; many regressions towards grandiosity (putting others down) and idealization (rock posters all over the walls) are to be expected. As we all know, adolescence ain't an easy time.

During early childhood, and in later years as well, the child begins to become more adept at intellectually imagining the needs and expectations of others, a process sometimes referred to as "mentalization." This ability to imaginatively picture the thoughts and needs of other people can be an initial step towards the placement of the final piece in the puzzle we call the "stable self" – the ability to empathize. As long as the neural hardware is functioning that provides a rewarding sensation for doing what is empathic and the parenting is good enough to re-enforce caring behaviors towards others, the child begins to associate empathic caring as a good thing that results in good feelings. The last shreds of pathological narcissism fall away and the stable self is born (refer again to Figure 15.1).

Once a person has achieved the evolution of a stable self – capable of empathy and compassion – the patient's words and behaviors in the initial interview will often reflect this achievement. Such a patient will describe symptoms and sensations that signal their genuine ability to care about others. He or she will demonstrate appropriate non-idealized respect for others including the clinician. These signal signs and symptoms suggest that one is in the presence of a patient who has evolved past pathologic object relations and is unlikely to have severe personality dysfunction as seen in narcissistic, histrionic, paranoid, schizotypal, and borderline processes. In this sense, the diagnostic field related to personality dysfunction has been effectively limited in number. If personality dysfunction is present, it will probably be of a developmentally higher order, as seen with obsessive–compulsive process or an avoidant personality disorder.

Concerning engagement, these signal signs and symptoms suggest that one can be more certain of securing a healthy therapeutic alliance. The patient's sense of self is probably reasonably robust, allowing the interviewer to ask interpretive questions, to gently challenge damaging patient assumptions, and to quietly push the patient to self-reflect without a fear of breaking the newly emerging therapeutic alliance.

CONCLUDING COMMENTS: ON THE UTILITY OF MIRRORS

This marks the conclusion of our three chapters devoted to developing effective interviewing strategies and techniques for uncovering personality dysfunction. In these chapters an attempt has been made to examine many of the core principles and intrigues surrounding the issues of personality dysfunction. If effective as intended, the reader comes away with a variety of new perspectives, as well as specific interviewing techniques of immediate practical use.

Hopefully something else has also been achieved – a greater understanding of the suffering and struggles beneath these diagnoses and also within ourselves. It is when working with personality dysfunction that I believe clinicians themselves face some of their greatest challenges in self-understanding and compassion.

If we are honest with ourselves, especially when encountering patients coping with processes such as borderline personality disorder, narcissistic personality disorder, and antisocial personality disorder (disorders in which anger, rage, deceit, and sometimes even cruelty and violence may be manifested towards others and/or the clinician), it can be easy to dislike the patient. Such patients can challenge the limits of our empathy.

But in these chapters we have come to see the psychodynamic factors and historical factors that shape these pathological disorders (from being abused or molested in childhood, or from poverty and tragedies such as the death of parents, to a lack of modeling of empathic behaviors and bullying from peers). As noted in the epigram that opened our chapter, we recognize that many of these patients come to us having been deprived of the psychological oxygen that they needed to breathe. Many have never seen the face of compassion nor the eyes of empathy.

I have found that it is with these patients (who often try me the most) that it has been useful to take a moment to look into my own mirror. Because in that mirror I believe that all of us will see similar factors that we have had to overcome in our own development. Perhaps we too have had to recover from one or several of the challenges that seem to punctuate human life, from our own histories of abuse or poverty or racism, to disease, failure in our marriages, death of loved ones, romantic rejections, or financial stresses. At such moments, I am reminded of one of my favorite quotations by John

Watson: "Be kind; everyone you meet is fighting a hard fight."[15] Few wiser words have been said.

When we work with people struggling with serous personality dysfunction, I believe that we too can often grow as therapists and as people. We see more of ourselves in these patients than at first we may perceive, for who among us, from our own personal struggles, does not have aspects of our personality that might benefit from some modification? Such honest realizations open the door to a more compassionate understanding of these patients and their difficulties.

In the last analysis, the ability to readily recognize the presence of these disorders is probably one of the most difficult tasks facing the initial interviewer. The ability to not only recognize them but to also see the person beneath them is an even greater challenge. Without the latter skill, the former pales considerably in significance.

REFERENCES

1. AZ Quotes at <www.azquotes.com/author/42058-Heinz_Kohut>; [accessed April 2016].
2. Seelig B, Ginsburg SA. Object relations theory. In: Tasman A, Kay J, Lieberman JA, editors. *Psychiatry*. Philadelphia, PA: W. B. Saunders; 1997. p. 420.
3. MacKinnon RA, Michels R, Buckley PJ. *The psychiatric interview*. 2nd ed. Washington, DC: American Psychiatric Publishing, Inc.; 2006. p. 101.
4. Brown S. The human–animal bond and self psychology: toward a new understanding. *Soc Anim* 2004;**12**(1):67–86.
5. Roughton R, Dunn J. Relational perspective, interpersonal psychoanalysis, social constructivism, and intersubjectivity. In: Tasman A, Kay J, Lieberman JA, editors. *Psychiatry*. 2nd ed. Chichester, UK: John Wiley & Sons, Ltd.; 2003. p. 482–5.
6. Hedges LE. *Listening perspectives in psychotherapy*. 20th anniversary ed. New York, NY: Jason Aronson; 1992.
7. Seelig B, Ginsburg SA. 1997. p. 420–7.
8. Lawrence DH. *Women in love*. Franklin Center, PA: The Franklin Library; 1979. p. 12.
9. Seelig B, Ginsburg SA. 1997. p. 426–7.
10. Kohut H. *The restoration of the self*. New York, NY: International Universities Press; 1977.
11. Flanagan LM. The theory of self psychology. In: Berzoff J, Melano Flanagan L, Hertz P, editors. *Inside out & outside in: psychodynamic clinical theory and psychopathology in contemporary multicultural contexts*. 2nd ed. Lanhan, MD: Jason Aronson; 2008. p. 161–88.
12. Flanagan LM. 2008. p. 171.
13. MacKinnon RA, Michels R, Buckley PJ. 2006. p. 179.
14. MacKinnon RA, Michels R, Buckley PJ. 2006. p. 199–200.
15. Shea SC. *Happiness is: unexpected answers to practical questions in curious times*. Deerfield Beach, FL: Health Communications, Inc.; 2004. p. 327.

Part III

Mastering Complex Interviewing Tasks Demanded in Everyday Clinical Practice

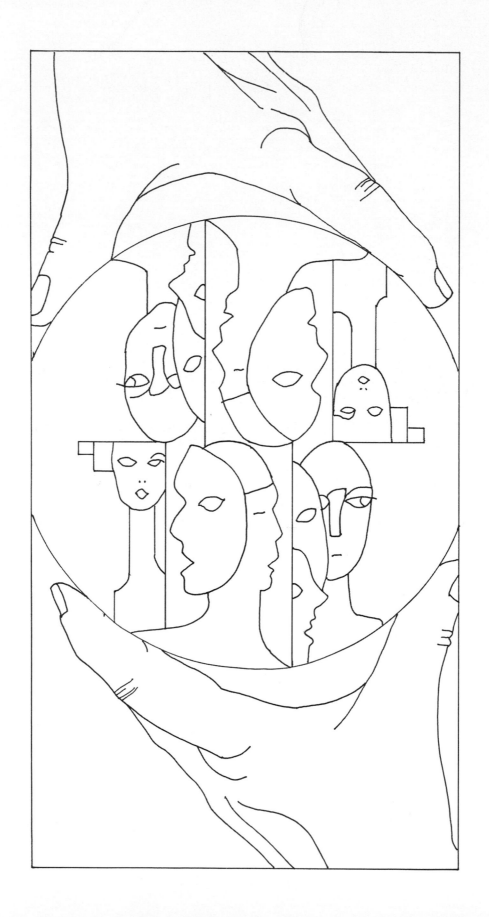

CHAPTER 16

The Mental Status: How to Perform and Document It Effectively

The value of experience is not in seeing much, but in seeing wisely. … The whole art of medicine is in observation.

Sir William Osler, Professor of Medicine[1]
Johns Hopkins University, 1909–1923

INTRODUCTION

To see what one is actually seeing – to see wisely, as Sir William Osler advised – is not necessarily as easy as it might seem at first glance. When performing a mental status we are attempting to accurately observe the patient's appearance, behaviors, and reported symptoms, as we search for both health and pathology. Our picture of the patient would be wondrously accurate, and our resulting interpretations splendidly wise, if we had the recording power of a camera lens and the objectivity of a computer chip. We don't. We are all too human. This simple fact is both to our benefit and to our detriment when performing a mental status. As humans, we are drawn towards empathy and sensitivity. Such predilections are generally very useful in our interviewing – indeed critical to success – as we have emphasized throughout our book. But sometimes our natural proclivities can lead us astray to the detriment of our patients.

By way of illustration, sensitive clinicians are naturally drawn toward the vantage point of looking *with* the patient in an empathic sense. It is our nature. But such an alignment can be a trap if the clinician over-utilizes it to the detriment of seeing what is actually before one's eyes in an objective fashion. Empathic connection can cast a fog over accurate observation. A clinician can begin to see not what is there but what the clinician wishes were there.

In this context, I observed a clinician empathizing with a subtly psychotic patient to the point that the clinician did not recognize that the patient was displaying a loosening of associations and other soft signs of psychosis. In this instance, sole reliance upon empathic listening blocked the clinician from establishing enough distance to observe with an objective compassion. The clinician was drawn into the patient's worldview, with the result that the patient did not receive the appropriate recommendation for antipsychotic medication.

THE IMPACT STATUS

Two slightly different approaches are useful when attempting to observe the patient with a sensitive, yet accurate, eye: (1) the impact status and (2) the mental status. The impact status refers to the immediate behavior and affect of the patient *at any single moment of the interview*. Thus, the impact status represents a quick subjective mental "take" of the patient's presentation, in which the clinician focuses upon the immediate impact on the patient of both the patient's inner world and of the behaviors of the clinician.

In contrast, the mental status is a composite of all the observations made *during the course of the interview*. Metaphorically speaking, if one were to view the patient's reported history as representing an ongoing video of the patient's problems and symptom history, then the mental status is an attempt to create – as best we can – an objective snapshot of the patient's presentation during the interview itself.

In many respects, the impact status was discussed in length in Chapter 8 on nonverbal behavior, but this area is worth a second look. The skilled clinician keenly observes all aspects of the patient's behavior, including mode of dress, hygiene, motor activity, affect and facial expression, mannerisms, and attitude. It is valuable, during the course of the interview, to periodically note the immediate affect of the patient, while asking oneself whether one's own behavior may be affecting the patient negatively, as evidenced by a decrease in the blending process. If such negative interactions are recognized early, one can quickly act to alleviate the stress before significant disengagement has occurred. At other times, one may opt to explore with the patient the reasons behind the change in affect. In this fashion, the clinician may uncover projective defenses or parataxic distortion, as described by Harry Stack Sullivan (see Chapter 6, pages 192–193).

The clinician may also uncover significant unconscious material or attitudes betrayed by the patient's mannerisms. In this regard, it is also useful to consciously make a note of the baseline nonverbal activity of the patient, so that subtle variations can be reflected upon. I am reminded of a young woman who had been in psychotherapy for roughly a year and a half. In one of her sessions she described an upcoming meeting with a supervisor in her graduate program. While she commented, "I guess I better go in and find out what my future is gonna be," she gave a child-like grin, accompanied by a helpless tone of voice. Apparently, at that moment in time, the thought of meeting her supervisor produced an attitude of child-like subservience.

This impact status observation could be immediately put to use. I asked her what she had been feeling while discussing her upcoming supervision. I also shared some of my observations on her appearance at that time. This led to a rich exploration of her tendency to not take herself seriously. As she became more aware of her facial expressions, she was also able to successfully role-play meeting this supervisor while displaying an adult affect and attitude.

Throughout the book, much has already been discussed with regard to nonverbal behavior, the behavioral indicators of blending, and other aspects key to the concept of the impact status. Consequently, it may be of value to shift our emphasis to the numerous considerations involved in uncovering a sound mental status.

THE MENTAL STATUS

General Characteristics of the Mental Status: What Is It?

The mental status represents an attempt to *objectively* describe the behaviors, thoughts, feelings, and perceptions of the patient *throughout the course of the interview itself*. Although it primarily focuses upon how the patient looked during the interview, when recording the mental status, recent psychiatric symptoms not present during the interview but uncovered as recently being experienced by the patient are also recorded. These observations are usually typed as a separate section in the patient's electronic health record (EHR). The general topics covered by the mental status are categorized as follows: (1) appearance and behavior, (2) speech characteristics and thought process, (3) thought content, (4) perception, (5) mood and affect, (6) sensorium, cognitive ability, and insight.[2] Clinicians may vary on the exact categories that are used, and some clinicians collect all of these observations into a single narrative paragraph (although I find this somewhat confusing). In any case, the clinician attempts to convey the state of the patient during the course of the interview.

When documenting the mental status, checklists are often commonly used as well and can quickly alert the reader of the EHR to the presence of psychopathology. A cautionary note: checklists alone are *never* adequate for a mental status. A checklist without the accompanying descriptive mental status paints a woefully weak clinical picture of the patient. It also invites a malpractice suit, for a good lawyer will quickly pounce on the clinician's appearance of being both disinterested and negligent in taking the time to critically hunt for evidence of psychopathology, as evidenced by a lack of a descriptive component to the mental status.

There exist two broad aspects to the mental status. First, there is the type of questioning that is required to be done in any standard initial assessment when undertaking a review and exploration of the patient's psychiatric symptoms. We are familiar with these types of questions from the previous chapters of this book. Interviewers use such sensitive questioning to explore various diagnostic categories, from mood disorders to anxiety disorders, as well as uncovering troubling pathologic processes such as psychosis and suicidal thought that can occur across many disorders. These questions are not done in an artificial "section" of the interview. As we have seen earlier, this review of psychiatric symptoms is woven gracefully throughout the body of the interview.

Thus, most of the mental status is not done in a specific section of the interview. Nor, if the interviewer skillfully structures the interview following the principles of facilics, will a patient be aware that a mental status is being performed. A good mental status is artfully hidden within the natural flow of an initial interview, and consists both of questions focused upon uncovering psychiatric symptoms and our observations of the patient's appearance and behaviors as we ask those questions.

On the other hand, there does exist a second, more formal part to the mental status. In this part, the interviewer tests the patient's cognitive functioning. Here one will see the interviewer devoting a specific section of the interview to questions on orientation, concentration, memory, and intellectual functioning. One can easily recognize when an interviewer is performing a formal cognitive mental status exam, for they will be using specific "cognitive tests" such as digit spans, three-object recall, and constructions. This aspect of the mental status – formal cognitive testing – is more optional in nature and will be expanded depending upon the diagnostic suspicions and age of the patient (suspected delirium, dementia, etc.). Later in our chapter, we will discuss and observe a complete cognitive mental status being performed, known as the Folstein Mini-Mental State Examination.

At this point, I believe it will be useful to turn our attention to our first video module. In it I will further clarify the various aspects of the mental status including the interface between the performance of the mental status and its placement and documentation in the EHR. I'll also demonstrate several practical techniques for gracefully weaving aspects of the mental status throughout the interview.

VIDEO MODULE 16.1

Title: Principles and Components of the Mental Status

Contents: Contains didactic material delineating those aspects of the mental status that are related to a psychiatric review of symptoms, ongoing observations during the interview, and immediate cognitive functioning. Clarifies the relationship of these interviewing processes to their documentation under the six standard headings of a mental status in an EHR: (1) appearance and behavior, (2) speech characteristics and thought process, (3) thought content, (4) perception, (5) mood and affect, and (6) sensorium, cognitive functioning, and insight. Also contains video demonstrations of how to use natural gates to gracefully perform a psychiatric review of symptoms throughout the body of the interview.

Documenting the Mental Status

It is difficult to discuss the performance of the mental status without carefully considering the process of documenting it in the EHR (or in some instances a written record). The recorded document (whether typed or written) frequently reflects the clinician's activities during the interview itself. For example, if the clinician has a difficult time moving into a relatively pure vantage point of observing the patient, then the mental status frequently reflects this inability with omissions, premature assessment opinions, or misplaced bits of the history of the present illness that "explain the patient's psychopathology." In this light, a disorganized or confusing clinical document is usually a reflection of an equally disorganized interview. Thus, one of the most effective ways to explore how to do the mental status is to explore how it is documented, which will be the focus of this chapter.

Subjective opinions, diagnostic formulations, and other conceptual perspectives do not belong in the mental status. The mental status should represent an earnest attempt to describe *objectively* what is being encountered during the actual clinical interview. It therefore represents a unique and highly valuable aspect of the psychiatric record, because it serves as an area in which a clinician can read about the appearance, behaviors, and level of symptomatology of the patient, as recorded by a fellow mental health professional at a given point in time. The clinician can then compare the patient's current presentation with the past in an effort to determine evidence of improvement or decline. The use of the mental status in this more disciplined fashion trains clinicians to effectively utilize the vantage point of looking at the patient with as clear an eye as is possible, exactly as Sir William Osler counseled in our opening epigram.

The mental status complements other aspects of the EHR and is relatively distinct from them. By way of example, the History of the Present Illness (HPI) describes the pertinent historical aspects of the patient's behavior, the patient's concerns, and the patient's symptomatology up until the interview itself. The HPI is primarily culled from the patient's own words, but the clinician frequently also pulls from the patient's family, previous clinicians, written documents, and other sources of information. The mental status *only includes information gathered from the patient,* in the same sense that a physical examination only includes the immediate blood pressure reading of the patient, not the history of blood pressure readings taken by previous clinicians.

In a similar vein, the Narrative Summary and Clinical Formulation, a different section of the EHR appearing towards the end of the document, allows the clinician to piece together the patient's history and immediate presentation into a cohesive whole, utilizing the added perspective of the clinician's opinions and knowledge base. It is in the Narrative Summary and Clinical Formulation that the clinician shares his or her DSM-5 diagnostic impressions, conceptions of the etiology of the patient's problems, and possible treatment interventions within the patient's matrix.

The History of the Present Illness and the mental status should be as objective a relating of the facts associated with the patient's presentation as possible. They do not include the clinician's impressions of what those facts may mean. Thus, in the HPI and mental status, a clinician will document the patient's symptoms, but they will not proffer their DSM-5 diagnostic impressions. A diagnosis is a subjective formulation of what the facts mean. Hence, diagnostic impressions and treatment recommendations belong in the part of the EHR designated Narrative Summary and Clinical Formulation. All of this material – related to how to document the initial assessment – is nicely described, simplified, and illustrated with examples in Appendix III.

On a practical level, one of the reasons why it is important to emphasize these distinctions in this chapter is the fact that clinicians frequently waste an inordinate amount of time repeating themselves in the EHR. If a good description of the patient's delusions appears in the HPI, then the mental status need only refer to this material rather than repeat it, because the focus should be the current thought content of the patient as illustrated below:

Thought Content

The patient has a history of an extensive delusional system regarding communist infiltration (see HPI). In the interview itself he continues to believe that his place of work is teeming with communists. He even believed that the psychiatric nurse he had just met was also a communist. Upon asking whether his mind might be playing tricks on him, he reported, "I'm not crazy. I know for a fact that the communist invasion has begun, will you help me?" He currently denies the belief of an alien invasion from Jupiter, which he had believed earlier this year, as reported in the HPI.

Note that the clinician does not go into detail about the specifics of the delusional system, because those details had already been related in the HPI. Moreover, the clinician does not discuss his assessment of the patient's distance from his delusion with a statement such as, "This patient clearly remains very delusional and psychotic," for such an appraisal is most effectively made in the Narrative Summary and Clinical Formulation, where the clinician provides his or her clinical opinions. Instead, the clinician carefully records the exact words of the patient, which demonstrate the patient's adamant belief in his delusional system. The focus is once again where it belongs in the mental status, on the actual behaviors and thoughts of the patient during the interview itself.

To become an accurate observer, the clinician must learn how to look, in a relative sense, without the contamination of previous beliefs and theoretical biases. This objective stance is one of the prerequisites of a sound mental status and of the vantage point of looking at the patient. To convey one's observations accurately, it becomes critical for one to utilize a common language. There is no room for a sloppy use of terminology, because such a practice can clearly confuse other clinicians, potentially biasing them towards faulty observations themselves.

Upon graduation from a psychiatric residency or graduate school in nursing, counseling, clinical psychology, or social work, all mental health professionals will be expected to be able to perform and document a sound mental status. The organization and terms used in the mental status are quite specific and accurately defined. To a trainee, the terms are not necessarily self-evident. But by the time of graduation the mental health professional must feel at home with the terms, be able to utilize them proficiently to describe underlying and subtle psychopathology, and be able to *rapidly* translate their observations into a sound clinical record. This chapter attempts to provide the tools with which to accomplish these goals, whether one finds oneself working in a community mental health center, an inpatient psychiatric unit, a specialized clinic, a high school or college counseling center, or an emergency department.

Consequently, we shall now examine each of the six components of the mental status as it might appear in a standard EHR. An effort will be made to summarize commonly utilized descriptive terms, clarify confusing terms, point out common mistakes, and provide an example of a well-documented mental status as a model for the reader as he or she begins clinical rotations. As the clinician becomes adept at documenting the mental status, he or she will also be developing improved interviewing skills using the vantage point of looking at the patient with a highly skilled focus and increased awareness.

Components of the Mental Status

1. Appearance and Behavior

In this section the clinician attempts to accurately describe the patient's outward behavior and presentation. One place to start is with a description of the patient's clothes and self-care. As Wallace suggests, it is probably best to avoid interpretations when describing the patient's clothing and presentation. Instead, the clinician records the exact data that ultimately leads to the opinions written in the subsequent Narrative Summary and

Clinical Formulation. In this regard, the clinician should describe the patient's apparel as opposed to relying solely on subjective terms such as "stylish," because not everyone would agree upon the meaning of the word "stylish."[3]

Striking characteristics, whether decorative in nature (as in tattoos) or unwanted (such as scars and deformities), should be noted, as well as any tendencies for the patient to look older or younger than his or her chronological age. Eye contact is usually mentioned. Any peculiar mannerisms are noted, such as twitches or the patient's apparent responses to hallucinations, which may be evident through tracking movements of the eyes or a shaking of the head as if shutting out an unwanted voice.

The clinician should note the patient's motor behavior; common descriptive terms include restless, agitated, subdued, shaking, tremulous, rigid, pacing, and withdrawn. Displacement activities, such as picking at a cup or chain smoking, are frequently mentioned. An important and frequently forgotten characteristic is the patient's apparent attitude toward the interviewer. With these ideas in mind, let us first take a look at a relatively poor description.

CLINICIAN A

The patient appeared disheveled. Her behavior was somewhat odd and her eye contact didn't seem right. She appeared restless and her clothing seemed inappropriate.

Although this selection gives some idea of the patient's appearance, one does not come away with a feeling for what it would be like to meet this patient. Generalities are used instead of specifics. Let us look at a description of the same patient that captures her presence more precisely.

CLINICIAN B

The patient presents in tattered clothes, all of which appear filthy. Her nails are laden with dirt, and she literally has her soiled wig on backwards. She is wearing two wrist watches on her left wrist and tightly grasps a third watch in her right hand, which she will not open to shake hands. Her arms and knees moved restlessly throughout the interview, and she stood up to pace on a few occasions. She did not give any evidence of active response to hallucinations. She smelled badly but did not smell of alcohol. At times she seemed mildly uncooperative.

This passage clearly presents a more vivid picture of her behavior. The reader now has an idea of what her odd behaviors consist of. The clinician has included pertinent negatives, indicating that she shows no immediate evidence of hallucinating as might be seen in a delirium. In this example, one can almost intuit some of the thinking processes of the clinician with regard to the development of a differential diagnosis. This is a hallmark of a well-organized mental status. Each section adds a new series of pieces to the puzzle, suggesting certain diagnoses and making others less likely. For instance, this patient's agitation may be suggestive of a manic picture.

2. Speech Characteristics and Thought Process

The clinician can address various aspects of the patient's speech, including the speech rate, volume, and tone of voice, and structure of the speech. Before proceeding, let me clarify some commonly misunderstood and misused terms.

You will occasionally see the generic term "thought disorder" used in a document. Beware of it. It is often used inappropriately. Technically, the term "thought disorder" is incomplete, and hence misleading, for it contains two different types of pathologic disorders: (1) Problems with the formation of thought (derailment, severely tangential thought, disjointed illogical thought). This psychopathologic sign is more appropriately called a "*formal* thought disorder," for it refers to problems with the *formation* of the patient's thoughts. Because it deals with thought process and will be displayed in the patient's speech, it is appropriately addressed in this section of the mental status. (2) Problems with the content of the patient's thought, what we typically mean by a delusion. This type of thought disorder is more appropriately called a "*content* thought disorder," for there are problems with the content of the patients thinking. The term "content thought disorder" is seldom used in medical records (most clinicians simply prefer using the term delusion). Having nothing to do with the patient's *process* of thinking or resultant speech patterns, problems with delusions are *not* appropriately addressed in this section of the mental status.

I also mention this distinction to alert the reader to a common error seen in medical records. Many clinicians are under the misconception that the term "formal thought disorder" is *synonymous* with the term "psychotic." As a result, they mislabel *any* patient who is psychotic as having a formal thought disorder. But a patient could be strikingly psychotic (grossly delusional, actively hallucinating, and wildly agitated) but *not* have problems in how they are forming their thought; hence, such a patient would not have a *formal* thought disorder.

There exists so much confusion regarding the terms "thought disorder," "formal thought disorder," and "content thought disorder" that I suggest you do not use them, although you will certainly see them in clinical records, especially older records. Instead, in this section of the mental status devoted to speech characteristics and thought process, I think you will find the following terms useful and capable of describing your patient's problems succinctly and accurately:

- *Rate of speech:* The rate of speech refers to what one would expect – how fast or slow the patient's speech appears. Slowed speech could be seen in depressed states as well as somnolent deliria. Increased speech rate is frequently seen in manic states, agitated psychoses, and drug-related euphorias.
- *Pressured speech*: This is not the same as rapid speech (although they generally occur together). In pressured speech the normal pauses seen with speech disappear. It may possibly best be described as a "speech *sans* punctuation." It is very hard to get a word in edgewise with a patient who has pressured speech and equally hard to interrupt them. Note that a patient's speech could have a normal rate but still be pressured (occasionally seen with hypomania or with patient's displaying a histrionic style).

Sometimes pressured speech is only mildly pressured, whereas, at other times, the patient's speech may virtually gush forth in an endless stream. Pressured speech is commonly seen in mania, agitated psychotic states, or during extreme anxiety or anger.

- *Tangential thought:* The patient's thoughts tend to wander off the subject as the patient proceeds to take tangents off his or her own statements. There tends to be some connection between the preceding thought and the subsequent statement. An example of fairly striking tangential thought would be as follows, "I really have not felt very good recently. My mood is shot, sort of like it was back in Kansas. Oh boy, those were bad days back in Kansas. I'd just come up from the Army and I was really homesick. Nothing can really beat home if you know what I mean. I vividly remember my mother's hot cherry tarts. Boy, they were good. Home cooking just can't be beat." In tangential thought the patient's wanderings go off-course and never return to the original topic. In contrast, in "circumstantial thought," which is identical in nature to tangential thought, the patient's thoughts wander off but eventually the patient returns to the original topic.

- *Derailment/loosening of associations:* The DSM-5 uses the term derailment. Derailment is also called loosening of associations in the clinical literature. With derailment, the patient's thoughts at times appear unconnected. Of course, to the patient, there may be obvious connections, but a normal listener would have trouble seeing them. In mild forms, derailment may represent severe anxiety or evidence of a schizotypal character structure. In moderate or severe degrees, unless the loosening is a product of malingering, it is an indicator of psychosis. An example of a moderate to severe degree of derailment would be like this: "I haven't felt good recently. My mood is shot, fluid like a waterfall that's black, back home I felt much better, cherry tarts and Mom's hot breath keeps you going and rolling along life's highways." If derailment becomes extremely severe, so as to become essentially incoherent, it is sometimes referred to as a "word salad." Derailment (loosening of associations) is a classic example of a formal thought disorder.

- *Flight of ideas:* In my opinion, this is a relatively weak term, because it essentially represents combinations of the above terms, which is why most trainees find it confusing. For flight of ideas to occur, the patient must demonstrate tangential thought or a loosening of associations in conjunction with a significantly pressured speech and usually speeded up speech. Generally, there are connections between the thoughts but, at times, a true loosening of associations is seen. A frequently, but not always, seen characteristic of flight of ideas is the tendency for the patient's speech to be triggered by distracting stimuli or to demonstrate plays on words. When present, these features represent more distinguishing hallmarks of a flight of ideas. Flight of ideas is commonly seen in mania but certainly can appear in any severely agitated or psychotic state.

- *Thought blocking:* The patient stops in mid-sentence and never returns to the original idea. These patients appear as if something had abruptly interrupted their train of thought and, indeed, usually something has, such as a hallucination or an influx of confusing ideation. Thought blocking is very frequently a sign of psychosis. It is *not* the same as exhibiting long periods of silence before answering questions. Some dynamic theorists believe it can also be seen in neurotic conditions, when a repressed impulse is threatening to break into consciousness.

- *Illogical thought:* The patient displays illogical conclusions. This is different from a delusion, which represents a false belief but often has logical reasoning behind it. An example of a mildly illogical thought follows: "My brother has spent a lot of time with his income taxes so he must be extremely wealthy. And everyone knows this as a fact because I see a lot of people deferring to him." These conclusions may be true, but they do not necessarily logically follow. Of course, in a more severe form, the illogical pattern may be quite striking as with, "I went to Mass every Sunday, so my boss should have given me a raise. That bum didn't even recognize my religious commitment." Patients presenting with severely illogical thought are sometimes viewed as having a formal thought disorder, for their thoughts can be so illogical as to appear to be unrelated.

Let us take a look again at the woman we have already begun to describe. The first example, once again, could use some improvement:

CLINICIAN A

Patient positive for loosening of associations and tangential thought. Otherwise grossly within normal limits.

This clinician has made no reference to the degree of severity of the patient's loosening of associations. Specifically, does this patient have a mild loosening of associations or does she verge upon a word salad? Moreover, the clinician makes no reference to her speech rate and volume, characteristics that are frequently abnormal in manic patients and patients with an agitated psychosis. The following brief description supplies a significantly richer database, providing further diagnostic information and a means of noting improvement or deterioration for future clinicians treating the patient who need to know how the patient presented:

CLINICIAN B

The patient demonstrates a moderate pressure to her speech accompanied at times by loud outbursts. Even her baseline speech is slightly louder than normal. Her speech is moderately tangential, with rare instances of a mild loosening of associations. Without thought blocking or illogical thought.

Slowly one is beginning to develop a clearer picture of the degree of this patient's psychopathology. More evidence is mounting that there may be both a manic-like disturbance and a psychotic process. In any case, coupled with her strikingly disheveled appearance, the clinician may be increasingly suspicious that the patient is having trouble managing herself. All of this information may suggest the need for hospitalization and it would support such a decision if a malpractice suit ever challenged this clinical decision in the future.

3. Thought Content

This section refers primarily to five broad phenomena: (1) ruminations, (2) obsessions, (3) compulsions, (4) delusions (the "content thought disorder" referred to above), and (5) the presence of suicidal or homicidal ideation.

Ruminations

These are frequently seen in a variety of anxiety states and are particularly common in depressed patients. Significantly depressed patients will tend to be preoccupied with worries and feelings of guilt, constantly turning the thoughts over in their minds. The thinking process itself does not appear strange to these patients, and they do not generally try to stop it. Instead, they are too caught up in the process to do much other than talk about their problems. In contrast, obsessions have a different flavor to them, although they may overlap with ruminations at times.

Obsessions

An obsession is a recurrent idea, thought, fantasy, or image that intrusively enters the mind of the patient and is hard to stop thinking about. A patient may relate that it is hard "to shake" the thought or image or "get away from it." Obsessions can create an immensely intense anxiety, in which patients feel that they are bad for having them or that something horrific will occur if one does not do something about them. Unlike the case with ruminations, patients generally find these obsessive thought processes to be both odd and painful. They frequently have tried various techniques to interrupt the process.

Common themes for obsessions include thoughts of committing violence, homosexual or heterosexual fears, issues of right and wrong, and worries that one has been contaminated by germs, dirt, filth, or poisons. Sometimes the obsessions also consist of fears that one has done something bad that harmed another person (such as a fear that one has left a stove on that may result in a fire or that one has hit somebody with his or her car when, in reality, the patient merely hit a speed bump). If one takes the time to listen carefully to the patient, bearing the above phenomenological issues in mind, the clinician can usually differentiate between ruminations and obsessions.

As we shall see below, in order to relieve the intense anxiety caused by the obsession, the patient will frequently feel a need to either do a specific action (e.g. wash one's hands if there is an obsession about germs) or perform a mental act (e.g. repeat a phrase over and over such as "I've turned the stove off" in response to an obsessive thought that the house is going to burn down because the stove was left on) to relieve the anxiety. These compensatory actions or mental acts are called compulsions.

Compulsions

Compulsions are strong urges to perform a specific behavior or mental act, which the patient often recognizes as silly, odd, abnormal, or unnecessary. Nevertheless, it is very difficult for the patient to resist a compulsion. As noted above, they often arise as a method of relieving the intense anxiety caused by an unsettling obsession. Common compulsive behaviors include repeated hand washing, checking to see if one has left something unlocked or turned on, returning to see if one has hit somebody with a car, and cleaning something like a plate or counter top repeatedly.

Compulsive mental acts include such things as repeatedly counting, repeatedly saying a phrase or prayer, or answering a question over and over again in one's mind. For instance, a patient may suddenly have the intrusive obsession that he or she offended someone earlier in the day. To relieve this anxiety, the patient will feel compelled to re-imagine the earlier encounter over and over, each time saying to themselves, "See, I didn't say anything bad." In a similar vein, the patient may develop a need to ask another person a question in order to be reassured about a disturbing obsession. For instance, a patient may ask a spouse, "I'm not ugly am I?" just to hear the spouse say, "No, you look fine." This is known as a reassurance compulsion. Compulsions are often, but not always, triggered by obsessions (one washes one's hands because of fears of contamination).

Completing the compulsive behavior or mental act may give the patient a feeling of relief; but, unfortunately, as soon as the obsession returns, the patient feels compelled to repeat the relieving behavior or mental act. The patient may repeat this process many times in a row until it "feels right." Some patients could repeat such thoughts and behaviors hundreds of times, being pre-occupied by them for hours, to the point of being disabled by the process. If one interrupts the patient while this process is occurring, the patient will frequently feel a need to start the whole process again.

Obsessions and compulsions are seen in obsessive–compulsive disorder (OCD), an extremely painful and disruptive condition that is surprisingly common and amenable to treatment. As noted in an earlier chapter, patients are so embarrassed by these symptoms that it is rare for them to share these symptoms with a therapist (sometimes even after years of therapy). Consequently, it is critical in the initial assessment to ask every patient about obsessions and compulsions.

Delusions

Delusions represent strongly held beliefs that are not correct or not held to be true by the vast majority of people in the patient's culture, as described in detail in Chapter 11 on psychotic process.

Thought Concerning Dangerousness to Self and Others

This is a complex area that warrants our detailed exploration in Chapters 17 and 18. Suffice it to say that – since all patients should be asked about current dangerousness – issues including suicide, non-lethal self-damaging behaviors (such as the self-cutting seen in borderline process), self-mutilation (as seen in some psychotic processes), and violence towards others, this should always be addressed in the mental status of the EHR.

In general, the clinician should make some statement regarding the presence of suicidal wishes, plans, and degree of intent to follow the plans in an immediate sense. If a plan is mentioned, the clinician should state to what degree any action has been taken on it. It should also be noted whether any violent or homicidal ideation is present and to what degree, in the same fashion as with suicidal ideation. The same material should be addressed regarding non-lethal self-damaging behaviors and self-mutilation if psychotic process is present.

Let us return to our patient with two sample excerpts concerning thought content:

CLINICIAN A

The patient is psychotic and can't take care of herself. She seems delusional.

This excerpt is just simply sloppy. The first statement has no place in the mental status, because it is the beginning of the clinician's clinical assessment. The description of the delusion is threadbare and unrevealing. The clinician has also omitted the questioning concerning lethality. Assuming that the clinician asked but forgot to record this information, the clinician may sorely regret this omission if this patient were to kill herself and the clinician was taken to court. A more useful description is given below.

CLINICIAN B

The patient appears convinced that if the watch is removed from her right hand, the world will come to an end. She proceeds to relate that consequently she has not bathed for 3 weeks. She also feels that an army of rats is following her and is intending to enter her intestines to destroy "my vital essence." She denies current suicidal ideation or plans. She denies violent or homicidal ideation. Also denies any thoughts of self-mutilation. Without ruminations, obsessions, or compulsions.

Now we have clear-cut evidence of someone who is clearly psychotic with concrete delusions. Because there is psychotic process present, the clinician has also indicated that evidence of self-mutilatory process was explored and none was reported. The next question is whether hallucinations play a role in her psychotic process.

4. Perception

This section refers to the presence or absence of hallucinations or illusions, which were described in detail in Chapter 11. Hallucinations can be auditory, visual, tactile, olfactory, or dealing with taste. It is of value to note that there sometimes exists a close relationship between delusions and hallucinations. It is not uncommon for the presence of hallucinations to eventually trigger the development of delusional thinking, but the two should not be confused.

Let us assume that a patient is being hounded by a voice screaming, "You are possessed. You are a worthless demon." If the patient refuses to believe in the reality of an actual entity producing the voice, then one would say that the patient is hearing voices but is not delusional. If, on the other hand, the patient eventually begins to believe in the existence of an entity whose voice the patient is hearing and feels that this entity is planning her death, then the patient is said to have developed a delusion as well as to be experiencing auditory hallucinations.

Hallucinations, no matter which sensory channel in origin, arise without any specific trigger from the environment. For instance, a person experiencing a *visual hallucination* will see something in open space. Such a patient may be looking down an empty hallway and suddenly see a demon pacing back and forth. Illusions, which can also occur in any sensory modality, always are triggered by some real sensory input. A person experiencing a *visual illusion* will distort something that is actually being seen. For instance, a person experiencing a visual illusion might be looking at their dog and suddenly the dogs face will begin to change contorting into the head of a werewolf. Both hallucinations and illusions can be horrifying in nature.

We can now turn to our two clinicians:

CLINICIAN A

Without abnormal perceptions.

The question arises as to whether it is appropriate in the mental status to use phrases such as, "grossly within normal limits" or "without abnormality." Generally speaking, the mental status is improved by the use of more precise and specific descriptions, but sometimes clinical situations require flexibility. For example, if the clinician is working under extreme time constraints, then such global statements may be appropriate, but in most situations it is preferable to state specifically the main entities that were ruled out, because this essentially relays to the reader that the clinician actually looked for these specific processes. Stated differently, with these global phrases, the reader does not know whether they are accurate or the end result of a sloppy examination. If one has performed a careful examination, it seems best to let the reader know this fact.

Another problem with the phrasing used by Clinician A is the fact that he has stated that the patient does not, in actuality, have hallucinations; but perhaps this patient is simply withholding information because she fears that the voices will indicate she is "crazy" or that she will be committed involuntarily if she admits to hearing them. Numerous reasons exist for a patient to not share the presence of hallucinations or illusions with a clinician, including the fact that the voices may have told the patient not to speak to the clinician. Thus, it may be more accurate to state that the patient denied having hallucinations rather than stating categorically that the patient is without them. With these ideas in mind, a slightly more sophisticated report would be as follows:

CLINICIAN B

The patient denied visual, auditory, and tactile hallucinations and any other perceptual abnormality such as illusions.

---

5. Mood and Affect

Mood is a symptom *reported by the patient* as to how the patient has been feeling recently in general and tends to be relatively persistent. Affect is a physical indicator *directly observed in the interview by the clinician* as to the immediate feelings of the patient. It is demonstrated by the patient's facial expressions and other nonverbal clues during the interview itself and frequently is of a transient nature. Mood is a self-reported symptom; affect is a physical sign that can be observed.

If a patient refuses to talk or refuses to describe his or her mood, then the clinician can say essentially nothing about mood in the mental status itself, except that the patient refused to comment on mood. Later, in his or her Clinical Formulation, the clinician will have ample space to describe his or her impressions of what the patient's mood had been. In contrast to mood, in which the clinician is dependent upon the patient's self-report, the clinician can always say something about the patient's affect.

Thus it is conceivable that a patient who is quite depressed could deny his or her depression, while still appearing sad, even crying, during the interview. Such a situation would be reported as follows, "The patient demonstrated a sad affect throughout most of the interview, including several short episodes of crying. However, when questioned as to her mood she reported, 'I'm feeling just fine, really I am.'"

Later, in the Narrative Summary and Clinical Formulation, the clinician would note that the patient's reported mood was inconsistent with both the HPI and the mental status, perhaps suggesting the presence of active mechanisms of denial or repression. In this situation, some clinicians are tempted to ignore what the patient states, persisting in relaying *in the mental status* that the patient's mood is depressed. But this prevents the reader from seeing the patient's denial mechanisms. It is much better to let the story speak for itself, while providing one's final assessment in the proper section of the written report. Let us now return to our patient:

CLINICIAN A

The patient's mood is fine and her affect is appropriate but angry at times.

This statement is somewhat confusing. In which sense is her affect appropriate? Is it appropriately fearful for a person who believes that rats are invading her intestines, or does the clinician mean that her affect is appropriate for a person without a delusional system? The clinician should always first state what the patient's affect is and then comment upon its appropriateness.

The following are clinically accepted terms that you will find useful in describing your patient's affect: normal (broad) affect with full range of expression; restricted affect (some decrease in facial animation); blunted affect (fairly striking decrease in facial animation); a flat affect (essentially no sign of spontaneous facial expression); buoyant affect; angry affect; suspicious affect; frightened affect; flirtatious affect; silly affect; threatening affect; labile affect; and edgy affect. The following description gives a much clearer feeling for this patient's presentation:

CLINICIAN B

When asked about her mood, the patient angrily retorted, "My mood is just fine, thank you!" Throughout much of the interview she presented a guarded and mildly hostile affect, frequently clipping off her answers tersely. When talking about the nurse in the waiting area she became particularly suspicious and seemed genuinely frightened. Without tearfulness or a lability of affect.

6. Sensorium, Cognitive Functioning, and Insight

In this section, the clinician attempts to convey a sense of the patient's basic level of functioning with regard to the level of consciousness, intellectual functioning, memory, insight, and motivation. It is always important to note whether a patient presents with a normal level of consciousness, using phrases such as "the patient appeared alert with a stable level of consciousness," or "the patient's consciousness fluctuated rapidly from somnolence to agitation." As we saw in our chapters on mood disorders and psychosis, the presence of a fluctuating level of consciousness is particularly disturbing, mandating that the clinician determine whether or not the patient is experiencing a delirium, for deliria can result in permanent brain damage or death.

As discussed in Video Module 16.1, it should be noted that the data for this section may evolve from two processes: the informal cognitive examination and the formal cognitive examination. The informal cognitive examination is artfully performed throughout the interview in a non-invasive fashion. The clinician essentially "eyeballs" the patient's orientation, concentration, and memory by noting the way in which the patient responds to questions.

If the clinician chooses to perform a more formal cognitive examination, it can range from a brief survey of orientation, digit spans, and short-term memory to a much more comprehensive examination, perhaps lasting 20 minutes or longer. We will shortly be looking at and viewing the performance of several commonly utilized questions and tasks used to test cognitive functioning.

Let us examine an EHR that could use some polishing, by Clinician A:

CLINICIAN A

The patient seemed alert. She was oriented. Memory seemed fine and cognitive functioning was grossly within normal limits.

Once again, this clinician's report remains vague. Most important, the reader has no idea exactly how much cognitive testing was performed. No mention has been made of the patient's insight or motivation, either. The following excerpt provides a clearer picture:

CLINICIAN B

The patient appeared alert with a stable level of consciousness throughout the interview. Indeed, at times, she seemed hyper-alert and overly aware of her environment. She was oriented to person, place, and time. She could repeat six digits forwards and four backwards. She accurately recalled three objects after 5 minutes. Other formal cognitive testing was not performed. Her insight was very poor, as was her judgment. She does not want help at this time and flatly refuses the use of any medication.

Clinician B has created a significantly more useful description of our patient's mental functioning than Clinician A. The presence of a hyper-alert quality to the patient was completely missed in the first description. This hyper-alert state suggests the need to be aware of a possible delirium, but the likelihood that a delirium is present has been decreased by the fact that the patient is well oriented and can perform digit spans capably. It is further decreased by her ability to recall three objects after 5 minutes, all of which information was nicely documented by Clinician B. This shifts the reader's attention of this EHR towards the consideration of other types of states that can cause hyper-alert conditions such as manic states, psychotic states, drug-induced states, and situational stress.

In addition, Clinician B has introduced for us the use of several formal cognitive tests, such as the use of digit spans and three-word recall. It is an opportune time to delineate effective ways for performing a more comprehensive cognitive exam. Such testing can help to uncover evidence of both dementia and delirium. Cognitive tests, which have been developing for over 100 years, can be given singly or in groups as was recorded in the preceding document by Clinician B. They are sometimes further grouped together into a battery of tests to be given in a standardized fashion.

One such exam is called the Folstein Mini-Mental State Examination (MMSE), which can help to spot both dementias and deliria.[4,5] The MMSE is easy to use and usually only takes about 10 to 20 minutes to administer. The MMSE covers a broad group of cognitive functions. Areas included are: orientation, initial memory registration, attention and calculation, short-term recall, language recognition, and the ability to follow commands. These areas are tested with a variety of questions and tasks that are ultimately scored up to a 30-point maximum. Numerous references, including the original article cited above, are readily available for readers wanting to learn more details regarding the MMSE. The MMSE has been in use since 1972, which has resulted in an excellent empirical validation of its contents. It should be noted that, at the time of this writing, payment appears to be required for the use of the Folstein MMSE form (www4.parinc.com).

On the other hand, other excellent standardized batteries are available, without cost, that can help clinicians to spot dementias and deliria. One such battery is the Montreal Cognitive Assessment (MoCA; www.mocatest.org),[6] which is easily done in a short amount of time and is available in a variety of languages. Some people (of which I am one) feel that the MoCA is more efficient at uncovering delirium than the Folstein.

Indeed, if our patient from above had appeared mildly disorientated, or had done poorly on her digit spans and/or three-word recall test, we would have been more suspicious of the possible presence of delirium, which could be life threatening as described in Chapter 11. With such a presentation, we could have utilized some of the individualized tests from the MoCA, or, if we had the standardized MoCA with us (it is only a single sheet of paper, moreover, it can be pulled up quickly on the web), we could have applied the entire test. I highly recommend becoming familiar with the MoCA.

In addition, the Confusion Assessment Method (CAM) has been specifically developed to spot delirium, and many feel it is one of the best tests for this specific task. In Chapter 11, when discussing methods for spotting delirium, I described the CAM (see page 489).[7] The interested reader will also find a nice review of the many tests specifically developed for spotting and tracking the progress of deliria in a paper by Grover and Kate.[8]

In Video Module 16.2 I demonstrate four tests (all of which have similar variants in the MoCA) that I have found to be particularly useful for spotting subtle deliria: digit spans (repeating digits forwards and/or backwards), the vigilance test (having the patient tap on a table every time he or she hears a specific letter – implanted in a string of random letters), drawing a clock, and drawing a cube. I demonstrate them as I have adapted them for my independent use. If used as part of the MoCA, you would do them exactly as indicated on the form as it has been standardized. I described these tests in some detail earlier (see pages 488–489), and I suggest reviewing them before watching Video Module 16.2, below.

These four tests require a good deal of sustained attention and concentration from patients to perform accurately. Consequently, because of the common presence of distractibility, deficits in attention, and problems with fluctuations in the level of consciousness in delirium, delirious patients will often show deficits in such testing. Naturally, such patients will often have problems with orientation, which should also be routinely tested if delirium is suspected. As noted earlier (see page 489), delirial patients also often have problems in handwriting (dysgraphia).

Towards the goal of enhancing our abilities to uncover cognitive deficits – in addition to demonstrating the four specific tests mentioned above – our next video module describes a variety of specific person-centered nuances related to formal cognitive testing.

VIDEO MODULE 16.2

Title: The Formal Cognitive Mental Status Examination: The Art of Sensitively Uncovering Cognitive Deficits

Contents: Contains both didactics and annotated interview excerpts of four cognitive tests including the digit-span examination, the vigilance test, drawing a clock, and drawing a cube.

At this point we are almost at the end of our discussion of the mental status. A simple exercise can demonstrate the power of a well-documented mental status: Simply go back and read, in a consecutive fashion, the excerpts written by Clinician A. One is left with a rather bland and nebulous picture of the woman in question. Afterwards, read the model excerpts, in succession, by Clinician B. A strikingly more vivid picture of the woman appears. She suddenly seems more human, and the reader can easily picture her warily pacing the room. This, then, is the goal of the mental status: to ultimately provide a fellow clinician with a reliable image of the patient's actual presentation over the course of the interview.

It should be openly acknowledged that, in actual practice, the documented mental status may need to be significantly briefer. However, the principles outlined above remain valid, and can help to ensure that an accurate, albeit briefer, mental status does not degenerate into an inept mental status. For more tips and strategies on detailing the electronic health record or written document, please see Appendix III, which also includes quality assurance guidelines and a sample assessment.

If the reader is interested in learning more about the mental status, several excellent resources are available. Dave Robinson's text provides a practical, no-nonsense approach for advancing one's skills in everyday practice.[9] Perhaps the most sophisticated exploration of the mental status can be found in the outstanding book by Trzepacz and Baker, which is also rich in detail and examples of clinical application.[10] If one wants to learn more about the complexities of the mental status when used to uncover hidden neurologic disorders, a skill of immense importance when neurologic diseases such as tumors present with psychiatric symptoms, one cannot go wrong with Strub and Black's classic text *The Mental Status in Neurology, 2nd Edition*, which is not only filled with practical interviewing techniques but has a gentle compassion woven throughout its pages.[11] Finally, if the student is particularly interested in an advanced knowledge of the formal cognitive mental status and/or specializes in care of the elderly, Hodge's text is on the mark.[12]

In conclusion, the impact status and the mental status create in the clinician a sharpening of the mind's eye. With time, these observational skills become more and more keenly honed, allowing the clinician to quickly and gracefully learn from observing the patient, to successfully utilize the vantage point of looking at the patient. The slightest welling of the eyes becomes an opening into the pain of the patient; a subtle loosening of associations, a hint that psychotic process is nearby; a downward glance during a suicide assessment, an alert that dangerous intent is being hidden. Without these observational skills, the clinician is at risk of being swallowed up by the patient's world as opposed to learning from it. With them, the clinician has the ability to transform the mental status from an exercise in *seeing much* to a skill for *seeing wisely*.

REFERENCES

1. Osler W. *Aequanimitas: with other addresses to medical students, nurses and practitioners of medicine*. Birmingham, AL: The Classics of Medicine Library, Division of Gryphon Editions, Inc.; 1987. p. 111, 332.
2. Mezzich JE, Dow JT, Rich CL, et al. Developing an efficient clinical information system for a comprehensive psychiatric institute. II: initial evaluation form. *Behav Res Meth Instr* 1981;16(4):464–78.
3. Wallace E. *Dynamic psychiatry in theory and practice*. Philadelphia, PA: Lea & Febiger; 1983. p. 157.
4. Roffman JL, Silverman BC, Stern TA. Diagnostic rating scales and laboratory tests. In: Stern TA, Fricchione GL, Cassem NH, et al., editors. *Massachusetts General Hospital handbook of general hospital psychiatry*. 6th ed. Philadelphia, PA: Saunders/Elsevier; 2010. p. 61–71.
5. Folstein MF, Folstein SE, McHugh PR. "Mini-mental state": a practical method for grading the cognitive state of patients for clinicians. *J Psychiatr Res* 1975;12:189–98.
6. Nasreddine ZS, Phillips NA, Bédirian V, et al. The Montreal Cognitive Assessment, MoCA: a brief screening tool for mild cognitive impairment. *J Am Geriatr Soc* 2005;53(4):695–9.
7. Inouye SK. *The Confusion Assessment Method (CAM) Training Manual and Coding Guide*. Boston, MA: Hospital Elder Life Program; 2003 Available at: <http://www.hospitalelderlifeprogram.org/uploads/disclaimers/Long_CAM_Training_Manual_10-9-14.pdf>; [accessed September 2015].
8. Grover S, Kate N. Assessment scales for delirium: a review. *World J Psychiatry* 2012;2(4):58–70.
9. Robinson DJ. *The mental status exam explained*. 2nd ed. Port Huron, MI: Rapid Cycler Press; 2002.
10. Trzepacz P, Baker RW. *The psychiatric mental status examination*. Oxford, UK: Oxford University Press; 1993.
11. Strub R, Black F. *The mental status examination in neurology*. 4th ed. Philadelphia, PA: F. A. Davis Company; 2000.
12. Hodges JR. *Cognitive assessment for clinicians*. Oxford, UK: Oxford University Press; 2007.

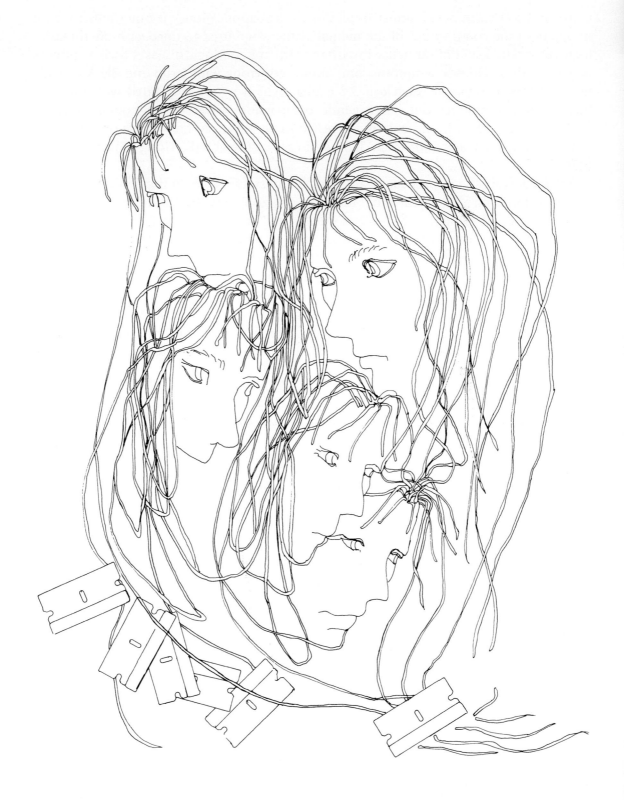

CHAPTER 17

Exploring Suicidal Ideation: The Delicate Art of Suicide Assessment

Dying
Is an art, like everything else.
I do it exceptionally well.

I do it so it feels like hell.
I do it so it feels real.
I guess you could say I've a call.

Sylvia Plath
Lady Lazarus

INTRODUCTION

These words written by Sylvia Plath invoke the coolness of death. They are even more unsettling when one realizes that their author would eventually go on to kill herself, her words acting not only as art but also as prophecy. Her death added one more digit to the annual suicide statistics in 1963. According to the Centers for Disease Control and Prevention (CDC), in 2014 there were 42,773 documented suicides in the United States. From 1999 through 2014, the age-adjusted rate in the United States has increased by 24%, with the 2014 rate being 13.00 deaths per 100,000. In the United States, roughly one person dies by suicide every 12 minutes.[1]

Moreover, these figures probably represent conservative estimates, because they exclude dubious accidents, such as one-driver automobile fatalities, which may actually represent masked suicides. In any case, suicide is the tenth leading cause of death in the United States, and, after unintentional injuries, the most common cause of death in 15 to 24 year olds.[2]

Indeed, suicide is ubiquitous. It honors no boundaries. For clinicians, exploring suicidal ideation and intent is a daily task. Whether our patient is young or old, rich or poor, a quiet recluse or an infamous Hollywood icon, suicide is often a player – a final arbiter that, if heeded, ends the play. Many of us have been touched by suicides among our patients, friends, family members, and colleagues. Contemplation of suicide may even be a part of our own past or future history.

Suicide assessment is a task that requires a gentle sensitivity and a tenacious persistence. All of the interviewing skills previously discussed are put to their most rigorous test. As we shall soon see, many of the validity techniques from Chapter 5 serve as the foundation stones for uncovering suicidal ideation and intent. If ever there were a moment of critical importance in interviewing, it is the moment when one listens for the harbingers of death. This arena is not a place for haphazard approaches or reliance solely upon intuitive skills.

To better understand how to effectively perform a suicide assessment, it is important to respect the complexity of the task, for a suicide assessment is an integrated process that unfolds in real time as the interview itself proceeds. Much as differential diagnosis consists of two processes: (1) the interviewing process of data gathering, and (2) the cognitive process of formulating the diagnoses from the data *as it is being gathered*, a suicide assessment consists of both a data-gathering process and a cognitive/intuitive process of arriving at a formulation of risk from the data that is being gathered. It is actually a bit more complicated, for there exist two distinct data-gathering components. As I have delineated in previous writings,[3-5] a suicide assessment is a three-part task that demands three distinct skill sets:

1. Uncovering information related to risk factors, warning signs, and protective factors that are associated with suicide (a data-gathering process)
2. Eliciting the patient's suicidal ideation, planning, behaviors, desire, and intent (a data-gathering process)
3. Arriving at a clinical formulation of risk based on these two databases (a cognitive and intuitive process)

In order to become more adept at suicide assessment, we will examine all three of these areas in this chapter. In Section I, we will examine risk factors, warning signs, and protective factors. In Section II, we will explore a flexible interviewing strategy, the Chronological Assessment of Suicide Events – the CASE Approach – designed to help patients more openly share the truth about their suicidal ideation and intent. In both sections we will address the implications of these databases on the formulation of risk.

SECTION 1: RISK FACTORS, WARNING SIGNS, AND PROTECTIVE FACTORS: THEIR ROLE IN THE CLINICAL FORMULATION OF RISK

Important Distinctions and Critical Limitations

Risk Factors Versus Risk Predictors (Warning Signs)

It is important to understand the distinction between "risk factors" and "risk predictors." A risk factor is a characteristic of a large sample of people who have died by suicide that appears to be statistically more common than would be expected. In contrast, risk predictors are characteristics of a specific living person that may indicate an increased likelihood of a potential suicide attempt by that unique individual. In contemporary clinical literature, the term "warning signs" has come into vogue as a replacement for the term "risk predictor."

Risk factors often include demographics (such as age or sex), living circumstances (such as the presence of a severe stressor or the lack of a significant other), historical associations (a family member has committed suicide or the patient has a previous history of attempting suicide), and clinical condition (such as the presence of acute alcohol intoxication or psychosis). Risk factors sometimes overlap with warning signs, as is the case with the presence of alcohol intoxication and the presence of psychosis.

It has always been hoped that risk factors and warning signs, if studied collectively in a specific patient, would be able to accurately predict the risk of an imminent suicide attempt. Such is not the case. Not a single piece of research has shown that the presence of any collection of risk factors and warning signs can accurately predict the imminent dangerousness of a patient. Interestingly, as we shall discuss later, there is some empirical evidence that the uncovering of valid information related to the patient's suicidal ideation, planning, behaviors, and intent (the second data-gathering task in a sound suicide assessment) does appear to have some degree of predictive capability.[6]

This does not mean that risk factors cannot help us to save a life. It simply means that using risk factors as a predictive algorithm is not of much use. Ultimately, people kill themselves not because they fit a statistical profile of risk factors and warning signs. They kill themselves because they have decided to do so. When a middle-aged man whose business has collapsed pulls the trigger of a gun or a college student who has failed a semester takes a fatal step off a bridge, it is caused by phenomenological rather than statistical events. Statistical analysis does not cause suicidal behavior, it helps us to retrospectively understand it. Human pain, coupled with human decision, causes it.

An example can help to illustrate the limitations of using statistical algorithms to predict suicide risk. Let us rate a patient's dangerousness using the SAD PERSONS Scale, a ten-point risk factor scale that we will examine later in this chapter. The presence of each factor is allotted a point value of one. The closer one approaches to ten points, the more dangerous the person is supposed to be. But is this true?

Let us look at a middle-aged woman who has the following characteristics: she is not particularly depressed, has never attempted suicide, does not drink alcohol or use drugs, has a loving nuclear family (including two healthy parents and three loving brothers living nearby), has a wonderful spouse, has no organized suicide plan, and has no chronic illnesses. She lacks nine of the ten risk factors on the SAD PERSONS Scale. The very highest she could score is one point out of ten (if she has the last risk factor). Using this scale, the clinician would rate the patient's immediate risk as quite low.

However, the last risk factor on the scale is the presence of psychotic process. Our hypothetical patient is unfortunately in the throes of a postpartum psychosis. She is convinced that demons have entered her daughter and are torturing her relentlessly. The voice of the main demon, which she believes is Satan himself, is hounding her minute by minute. He harangues her, "You must pay for your sins. Kill yourself *now* or we will torture your daughter and burn her flesh forever in the fires of Hell." The woman turns to the clinician, eyes wide with fear, begging frantically, "Do something. You've got to stop them. I can't let them do this to her. You've got to stop them."

Rather dramatically, our scale has failed us as a predictive instrument. The patient, despite a very low risk rating on the SAD PERSONS Scale, is potentially at very high risk. She is most likely best served by acute hospitalization.

If risk factors are not necessarily reliable risk predictors, one might wonder why we study them at all. The answer lies in the utility of risk factors to alert the clinician not to the fact that the patient is definitely at higher risk but that there is a good reason to suspect that the patient may be at higher risk. Such a realization suggests that the situation may require a particular tenacity in the clinician's approach, even, as we shall see, possible changes in interviewing technique – in order to uncover suicidal intent.

It may even signal one of the most dangerous of situations – a patient who has truly decided to kill himself or herself and is intent on hiding this information. With such a patient, a high number of risk factors (and/or a high number of warning signs) may suggest the wisdom of contacting a corroborative source such as a spouse. Such a corroborative source may provide a picture of the patient's suicidal intent that is markedly different from the patient's self-report.

I remember one patient who was adamantly denying suicidal ideation in our emergency department, whose high risk factors suggested the need to contact his wife. Her comment was telling, "Thank God he's down there. I don't care what he's saying, he's done nothing but talk about suicide for a month and I saw him with his pistol out last week." In short, the elicitation of numerous risk factors may trigger both analytic and intuitive suspicions that all is not as it appears to be.

The search for risk factors and warning signs provides other benefits as well; sometimes, it suggests lines of questioning related to the presence of a type of psychopathology. For instance, uncovering the presence of psychotic process may indicate the need for specific lines of questioning, such as inquiries about the presence of command hallucinations, which proved to be so telling with the hypothetical middle-aged woman described above. Consistent elicitation and formulation of risk factors serve yet one more practical function: conditioning the clinician to consider suicide risk with every patient. Such a clinical habit can only prove to be beneficial over time. It will prompt careful suicidal formulation even when the clinician is feeling pressured, weary or harried, or is simply having an "off day."

Static Versus Dynamic Risk Factors

Our last example leads into another distinction that is of value before we begin our study of risk factors/warning signs and their implications in the assessment of dangerousness. Risk factors (as well as warning signs) can be viewed as either being "static" or "dynamic" in nature.

Static risk factors are those characteristics of the patient that cannot be changed. Thus risk factors such as the following cannot be altered: age and sex of the patient, history of previous attempts, presence or absence of spouse or partner, situational stresses that cannot be changed (death of a child in a car accident). In contrast, dynamic risk factors have the potential to be altered. Such factors include the presence of substance abuse, psychotic process, specific situational stresses that can be changed (e.g., current unemployment), and the presence of depression and other psychiatric disorders. Some dynamic factors may include other wings of the patient's matrix where inroads can be made as with changes in the patient's family dynamics or a revitalization of the patient's spirituality.

In recent years, there has been an increased interest among suicidologists in dynamic risk factors and dynamic warning signs, for they represent signposts towards matrix treatment planning. Each dynamic risk factor represents a possible point for collaborative treatment planning with the patient as well as possible interventions on other wings of the patient's matrix from familial (family psychoeducation and/or therapy) to environmental (procuring housing or food stamps).

Protective Factors

Before exploring those factors that may contribute to suicidal risk, it is useful to examine those factors that may diminish it, factors that reflect wellness as opposed to stress, conflict, and psychopathology. Protective factors are characteristics, attributes, or situations that prospectively may reduce the likelihood that a person will attempt or complete a suicide. Western Michigan University has conceptualized protective factors as originating from two foci – "personal protective factors" and "external or environmental protective factors."[7] They culled their useful list from several sources including the Center for Disease Control and Prevention (CDC)[8] and the Suicide Prevention Resource Center.[9]

We will begin by looking at the personal protective factors. These factors originate from the various wings of the human matrix (from the biological and psychological wings to the patient's framework for meaning):

1. Attitudes, values, and norms prohibiting suicide, e.g., strong beliefs about the meaning and value of life
2. Social skills, e.g., decision making, problem solving, and anger management
3. Good health and access to mental and physical health care
4. A healthy fear of risky behaviors and pain
5. Hope for the future – optimism
6. Sobriety
7. Medical compliance and a sense of the importance of health and wellness
8. Impulse control
9. Strong sense of self-worth or self-esteem
10. Sense of personal control or determination
11. Access to a variety of clinical interventions and support for seeking help
12. Coping skills
13. Resiliency
14. Reasons for living
15. Being married or a parent

David Rudd has noted several other valuable personal protective factors including: wanting to maintain a pregnancy, children being present in the home, fear of social disapproval, and fear of suicide and death itself. Rudd postulates that the latter fear is a particularly good sign, for it indicates that the patient has not yet habituated to death.[10]

These personal protective factors are complemented by various external or environmental protective factors such as:

1. Strong relationships, particularly with family members
2. Opportunities to participate in and contribute to school or community projects and activities
3. A reasonably safe and stable environment
4. Restricted access to lethal means
5. Responsibilities and duties to others
6. Pets

In the next section, as we explore the use of risk factors and warning signs in the clinical formulation of risk, we will keep in mind that an astute interviewer will look for protective factors as well. They play an important role as potential mitigating elements when conceptualizing foreseeable risk.

Uncovering and Weighing Risk Factors and Warning Signs: The State of the Art

Definitions and distinctions in hand, we are now ready to launch our inquiry into risk factor analysis. With the following two case illustrations, we will attempt to accomplish the following goals:

1. Introduce the commonly cited risk factors and warning signs associated with suicide (as well as potential protective factors)
2. Demonstrate specific questions for effectively eliciting these factors
3. Illustrate the use of specialized interview strategies indicated by the presence of specific risk factors (such as questions to ask psychotic patients)
4. Briefly introduce the formulation of acute versus chronic risk, partially based on the presence or absence of specific risk and protective factors

Clinical Illustrations

Clinical Illustration #1: Michael

Michael is a 21-year-old male who comes to the emergency department at 1:00 A.M. accompanied by a male friend. Michael's shaggy hair hangs to his large shoulders, which cap a body obviously shaped by the rigors of a weight-lifting room. Michael reports feeling "odd" for months and has frequent ideas of reference. He also displays a loosening of associations sporadically. He relates, "It all comes down to the way the clouds kiss the moon." Other than this sentence, he demonstrates no illogical thoughts, tangential thought, or thought blocking, and he denies hallucinations. His speech has a gentle quality to it, with a peculiarly long latency before responses, as if he is preoccupied with a disturbing decision. His affect is guarded with periods of unusual intensity.

He denies feeling depressed and reports few neurovegetative symptoms of depression. He claims to have felt "upset" since he witnessed the brutal slaying of a friend by a motorcycle gang member. As he warms to the interviewer, he admits to recent abuse of alcohol, speed, lysergic acid diethylamide (LSD), and marijuana. When asked about whether he wants to kill himself, he replies testily, "I've no intention of killing myself (pause), ... that's what I'm fighting for." He refuses to elaborate. At the end of the interview, he refuses admission.

At this point, the clinician is faced with a formidable disposition problem. Does the suicide risk of this patient warrant hospitalization, or can he be treated as an outpatient? A second consideration is the fact that even if admission is warranted, the patient is refusing such treatment. There appear to be inadequate grounds for involuntary commitment. Can the interviewer discover adequate grounds, if necessary? With these issues in mind, we can begin an examination of risk factors.

In the first place, Michael's sex and age are statistically consistent with an increased suicide risk. With regard to sex, men more frequently successfully die by suicide roughly three to four times more frequently than women. On the other hand, women attempt suicide roughly three to four times more frequently than do men, although there is wide variation depending upon factors such as age and culture.[11] Perhaps this increased "suicide efficiency" in men relates to the choice of the means of suicide. Men more frequently choose violent methods (e.g., guns and hanging), which provide a more certain means of death, although more and more women are choosing guns as their method of suicide.

With regard to age, in general, suicide risk is greater for both sexes with increasing age. In women, the suicide rate increases until mid-life, after which it tends to reach a plateau. In White men, the suicide rate increases with older age, the highest rate being in White men over 70 years of age. Disturbingly, especially with males, there has been a sharp increase in the suicide rate since 2006 for the age group of 45–64.[12] In both men and women, the curve is complicated by a bimodal tendency, with a second peak occurring in late adolescence and young adulthood,[13] a point of special significance with regard to Michael.

Suicide represents the second highest cause of death in 15 to 24 year olds, accounting for nearly 5100 deaths in the United States in 2014.[14] It has been estimated that a staggering half a million adolescents and young adults perform suicidal behaviors each year.[15] The Youth Risk Behavior Survey (YRBS) is conducted annually by the CDC. The 2009 survey showed the disturbing statistic that 13.8% of high school students had seriously considered suicide in the previous 12 months; 10.9% had formulated a plan; and 6.3% proceeded with the plan. Of those attempting suicide, 12.9% required medical attention.[16] Moreover, a clinician should always keep in mind that, even though young children rarely kill themselves, some still do. This fact is driven home by the knowledge that 302 children aged 5 to 14 years killed themselves in 1996.[17]

Ramifications of race and culture are complex and nuanced, representing factors far beyond the limitations of our chapter because of the tremendous diversity in the world. Although in the United States the White population is generally at a higher risk, it is important to realize that there has been a disconcerting rise in Black suicides, especially among young adult urban males.[18] There is also a disturbingly high rate of suicide in

Native Americans, although this rate can vary significantly from tribe to tribe, with Apache having much higher rates than the Navajo and Pueblo.[19] For the interested reader, good reviews that do justice to the complexities of racial, ethnic, and cultural demographics on suicide are available.[20,21]

In the United States, a major subculture that has seen a distinctive increase in suicides is the military – both in soldiers returning from fronts such as Iraq and Afghanistan and in aging veterans. More than 1900 service members died from 2001 to 2009 by suicide. This represents an increase over the decade of approximately 50%, with the highest rates being in the Army and Marines. Bates and colleagues have written an excellent review of suicide assessment and management in the military.[22]

However, there is more to worry about with Michael than the implications of his sex and age, both of which are static risk factors, because the interviewer left the encounter feeling that Michael might be psychotic. The presence of psychosis, with or without depression, should alert an initial interviewer when evaluating suicide potential. Michael's age is a common time for the initial emergence of schizophrenia and psychotic mania. College counselors must be adept at spotting early psychotic symptoms and exploring the psychotic processes that can lead towards suicide and violence towards others.

Psychosis should be considered a major suicide warning sign, because disruption in rational thought often removes the final obstacle to self-destruction. In particular, three disturbing processes that could possibly push a patient towards violence to self or others should be carefully evaluated when the clinician is suspicious of the presence of psychosis; these are: (1) command hallucinations, (2) feelings of alien control, and (3) religious preoccupation. In Chapter 12 we discussed in detail effective interviewing approaches for uncovering command hallucinations (see pages 528–532). Let us now turn our attention to the other two processes in psychosis that increase the risk of violence.

Alien control is the feeling that one is being controlled by an outside agent. It is probably most often related to belief in demon possession, but other forms of "alien entity" may be suspected by the patient, including actual interplanetary aliens (a fear sparked by an upsurge in the cultural belief in alien abduction); the fear may be of being personally invaded or externally controlled by them. At other times the delusion is tied into other paranoid concerns, such as a neighbor having implanted a device inside the patient that is controlling the patient or driving the patient towards violence to self or others.

In our high-tech and wired culture, patients may believe that they are being controlled by radio waves, satellites, characters from a television screen, entities or messages being communicated by the web, a computer, or a smart phone. A psychotic patient who is actually being taunted or flamed via e-mail, social media, chat room, or texting may feel that their antagonist has the ability to make them act on commands to harm themselves or others. Of course, a psychotic patient could also have delusions that such is the case when there are no real-life antagonists or antagonistic messages being received.

If a patient has already described delusional material in the interview, the clinician can often gracefully tie an inquiry regarding alien control directly into the delusional material, as with: "Jim are you worried that the demon may have possessed you?" or "Do you think that your neighbor is trying to take you over or control your thoughts somehow?" If the answer is yes, one can further explore for alien control with questions such as, "Are you concerned the demon is trying to get you to do something such as harm yourself, kill yourself, hurt others, or anything that you wouldn't normally want to do?" It is not uncommon for alien control to be associated with dangerous command hallucinations such as commands to kill oneself or self-mutilate as with enucleating one's eyes.

In a patient that is clearly psychotic but has not described paranoid material, a clinician can raise the topic of alien control relatively unobtrusively with questions such as the following (introduced with a shame attenuation):

"I'm wondering, with all this stress, have you been having any sensations that seem odd or a little scary such as the feeling that something is trying to take you over or possess you in some way?"

It is important to remember that feelings of alien control may represent a particularly dangerous psychotic process if the "other agent" presses the patient to commit suicide or homicide (or both). It is not unknown for a patient to fight off such potentially lethal urges on a minute-by-minute basis. Thus any patient who presents in an initial interview with psychotic process should be asked about alien control at some point in the interview.

The third significant psychotic concern arises when the patient exhibits a specific type of excessive religious preoccupation. This type of rumination centers on ideas that God wants the patient to perform certain acts in order to prove the patient's love for God. These acts may include suicide, homicide, or self-mutilation. Such ideas may also be associated with command hallucinations. This time, however, the commands originate from an entity as ultimately persuasive as God. Patients may believe that their faith is being tested and may perhaps compare themselves with Abraham, who was commanded by God to sacrifice his own son, Isaac. This "Abraham syndrome" can prove fatal. At other times, patients may feel that Satan is pushing them toward violence.

In a related fashion, the patient may be preoccupied with specific verses from the Bible that suggest violent action. Such a biblical injunction may be interpreted from Matthew 5:29, in which lustful wanderings of the eye are handled in a rather absolute fashion:

> So if your right eye is an occasion of sin to thee, pluck it out and cast it from thee; for it is better for thee that one of thy members should perish than that thy whole body should be thrown into hell. And if thy right hand is an occasion of sin to thee, cut it off and cast it from thee; for it is better for thee that one of thy members should be lost than that thy whole body should go to hell.[23]

Psychotic process can prod the patient to act on such phrases. I vividly remember a patient who had viewed his acts of masturbation as an "occasion of sin." He subsequently tried to cut his hand off at the wrist with a steak knife, his Bible open to this exact verse. Bizarre methods of self-mutilation such as autocastration and the removal of the tongue may result when verses such as this one are twisted by psychotic thought.[24]

Preoccupation with this Bible verse presents a rather unique problem. Generally speaking, clinicians should not shy away from asking directly about dangerousness to self or others, as will be stressed repeatedly throughout this chapter. But here we have a caveat, for it seems ill advised to directly ask an actively hyper-religious psychotic patient about this Bible verse. To do so, risks that the psychotic process, at a later date, may distort the clinician's inquiry into some type of psychotic message. The psychotic process could convince the patient that the interviewer was functioning as an agent of God, communicating God's wish that the patient cut off his hand or enucleate his eye. Such post-interview psychotic twisting can prove to be dangerous indeed. How does one get around this dilemma, for clearly it is important to try to determine if a hyper-religious psychotic patient is preoccupied with this Bible verse?

In such a situation, after doing my utmost to secure the best possible engagement with the hyper-religious patient, I have found it useful to ask, "Are there parts of the Bible that seem particularly important to you?" I then follow this question with a second question, "Are there parts of the Bible where you feel God or something else is directing you to do something specific, perhaps even to harm yourself?" I believe that these two questions in tandem may often prompt a patient who is preoccupied with the Bible verse above to share his or her preoccupation with the clinician.

Before leaving the topic of psychotic process and its relation to suicide, an important and easily overlooked consideration should be mentioned. Patients with schizophrenia more frequently attempt suicide, not due to active psychotic processes, but due to devastating demoralization and depression resulting from years of pain, frustration, and low self-esteem caused by the disease process itself.[25-27] As mentioned in Chapter 12 on psychosis, schizophrenia rapes the soul of the patient, robbing an individual of the chance to pursue the dreams that motivate all of us. The core pains of losing a sense of internal control and, subsequently, of losing meaning in life can prove unbearable, even for the most courageous of people.

As people suffering from schizophrenia often perceive themselves to be hopelessly damaged, their reasons for living are gradually extinguished. It has been postulated that patients with the following characteristics may be most at risk: young age, chronic relapses, good educational background, high performance expectations, painful awareness of the illness, fears of further mental deterioration, suicidal ideation or threats, and hopelessness.[28]

Michael illustrates yet another important factor in the determination of lethality. He is a heavy drug abuser. The presence of chronic alcohol abuse or other drug abuse should be viewed as another risk factor, because these agents may decrease impulse control or precipitate psychotic process. However, alcohol is not only a problem with regard to poor impulse control; it also appears to cause long-term problems with suicidal ideation. It has been shown that people with chronic depression directly caused by alcohol abuse are at a significantly higher risk of making a serious suicide attempt.[29]

The acutely intoxicated patient presents a particular problem, because the intoxication predisposes the patient toward a suicide attempt in two ways. First, impulse control may be significantly lowered. Second, because of cognitive impairment, the patient may inadvertently commit suicide in a variety of fashions, such as forgetting that a large number of pills were taken earlier that evening and subsequently ingesting "just a few more." Such miscalculations can result in a fatal overdose. Because of these factors, even chronic emergency room visitors who present with serious suicidal ideation while acutely intoxicated should be observed until they sober up. Frequently, as the alcohol wears off, the suicidal ideation disappears and may not even be remembered.

These points also highlight the fact that significant organic impairment of the sensorium can increase risk. Fluctuating levels of consciousness or impaired concentration warrant careful attention during the mental status examination.

At this juncture, Michael presents a disturbing clinical dilemma. Too many gaps exist in the knowledge base to enable the clinician to make a sound decision. In addition, the presence of significant risk factors (recent severe stressor, recent isolation from support systems, and heavy use of drugs and alcohol), especially the suspected presence of psychotic process, suggests the usefulness of corroborative interviewing despite his denial of suicidal ideation. An interview with Michael's friend unearthed the following material.

Michael had not been himself since the murder of his friend who was, indeed, brutally murdered. Recently, Michael had seemed more distant than usual and was using a "load of uppers." He had been discharged about 3 weeks ago from a psychiatric hospital. Unfortunately, Michael was at odds with his family; he was currently living by himself in a dingy apartment and was subsisting on food stamps. The friend knew of no previous suicide attempts.

But there was another piece of information from Michael's friend that proved troubling in nature. It surfaced as follows:

Clin.:   Any other things about Michael that might be of importance?

Friend: I don't think so – except, well it's probably not that important.

Clin.:   What were you going to say?

Friend: Well, you know, he's just more wound up all the time. Sometimes he looks positively wired.

Clin.:   What's he do that makes you say that?

Friend: Oh, he paces and he looks sort of, I don't know, frightened. It's really sort of weird. I guess it's just that he's so damn intense about everything. I keep telling him to chill, but he doesn't.

The element of concern in this new information is the presence of intense anxiety in Michael. As we shall soon see, research by Jan Fawcett and others has suggested that increased anxiety, especially if acute and intense, may play a role in impulsive suicide attempts.[30] On inpatient units, there is evidence that patients with high levels of anxiety and agitation are more likely to kill themselves. This knowledge provides some support to the value of time-limited use of antianxiety agents at effective doses, when such patients "hit the unit." Keep in mind that almost 5 to 6% of suicides in the United States occur in psychiatric and medical inpatient units,[31] with about 4.7% occurring on psychiatric units (hanging being the leading method of suicide).[32] Michael's anxiety could be related to a variety of factors, including psychotic anxiety, concurrent panic attacks, or his use of speed. No matter what the cause, there is reason for concern.

When asked whether he had seen Michael with any type of potential weapon, his friend remarked, "I hadn't really thought about it, but he does carry a hunting knife he got after he left the hospital. But he's had hunting knives before." Michael lost his girl-friend about a month after the murder. When asked if he could stay with Michael until he had an outpatient appointment (hunting for a potential protective factor), the friend quietly replied, "No way, I just can't do it. Maybe his mom or something could do it."

In the first place, the above scenario illustrates the important principle of interviewing appropriate friends or family members, because they may provide invaluable information. In an emergency room situation, it is often critical to talk with significant others before making a decision regarding a patient's safety. Don't forget that if there are serious concerns about safety, these concerns outweigh confidentiality. It is sometimes necessary to contact relatives against a person's will. These contacts should be made, if at all possible, after consulting with a supervisor or colleague, and the reason for the decision to break confidentiality should be clearly stated in the chart, as should the role of the consultation.

In general, corroborative sources should be asked if they have witnessed anything that suggests possible suicide intent on the part of the patient. After a general inquiry, specific questions such as the following may be useful:

a. "Has he made any comments about being 'better off dead?'"
b. "Has he joked about killing himself?"
c. "Have there been any statements about 'things being better soon?'"
d. "Does he have any potential weapons in the house, such as guns or knives?"
e. "Has he ever tried to hurt himself before, even in small ways such as taking a few pills too many?"
f. "Has he appeared depressed or tearful?"
g. "Is he spending more time alone than usual?"

With this type of questioning, other than determining lethality, one is also searching for information that would fulfill involuntary commitment criteria. If using New Hampshire criteria (criteria differ from one state to another), one checks to see if the patient has participated in behavior that is a clear danger to himself or to others. The criteria are also met if the patient has expressed a desire to harm himself/herself or others while taking some steps to fulfill this desire (e.g., purchasing a weapon). In the case of Michael, his friend knew of no such behavior, except for the purchase of the hunting knife, although it was unclear as to whether the knife was bought for innocuous or dangerous purposes. It is noteworthy that teenage males tend to use firearms and hanging as the methods of choice, whereas females lean towards less lethal methods such as overdosing and carbon monoxide poisoning.[33] Any household with an adolescent at risk should get rid of any guns. This may be one of the single best measures for preventing the suicide of an adolescent or adult.

The corroborative interview also provides a chance to better determine stressors (key triggers for suicide) and social supports (key protective factors). With regard to stress, the clinician should search for situations such as unemployment and financial collapse, domestic violence, family disruption, rejection by a significant other, abrupt changes in career responsibilities, serious medical illness, death of spouse or child, or a catastrophic stress (e.g., witnessing a murder in Michael's case). Recent research by Wang and colleagues suggests that financial stress and assaultive violence may represent the two most powerfully correlated life stressors with attempted suicide.[34] Indeed, financial stress was more highly correlated with attempted suicide than any psychiatric disorder except major depressive episode. Their work also supported the common sense view that multiple major stressors in the past year are correlated with significantly higher risk.

Concerning support systems, a lack of friends, family, or societal supports, such as church organizations, has often been reported as a risk factor. In particular, one should be looking for evidence of recent losses, such as Michael's estrangement from his girlfriend and his family. These represent not only acute losses, but also the elimination of potentially powerful protective factors.

In their practical primer on the assessment and treatment of suicidal patients, Fremouw, de Perczel, and Ellis point out that one of the more striking statistical correlations with suicide remains the increased risk associated with the absence of a spouse. The highest risk is with people who are separated, followed in descending level of risk, by people who are divorced, widowed, or single. People who have never been married are twice as likely to commit suicide as people currently happily married. Divorced and widowed people have even higher rates.[35]

The innovative "interpersonal theory of suicide" developed by Thomas Joiner and colleagues has shed even more light on the delicate interplay between the psychological, interpersonal, familial, and cultural wings of the matrix with regard to suicidal potential.[36,37] Joiner and colleagues believe that one of the most dangerous forms of suicidal desire is caused by the simultaneous presence of two sensations related to interpersonal experience: (1) a thwarted sense of belongingness, and (2) a perception that one is a burden to others.

According to Joiner, from a psychological standpoint, the juxtaposition of these two interpersonal sensations becomes significantly more dangerous when the feelings are so extreme that a third component is added to the mixture – the inward drive to follow through with his or her suicidal ideation. In short, the patient has become more psychologically capable of proceeding with the act of suicide. As Joiner points out, suicide is difficult to complete. To do so, a person must overcome a variety of psychological hurdles, including fear of death, fear of pain, and fear of physical complications if one survives the suicide (trauma, permanent brain impairment or coma, etc.). In addition, humans are wired biologically to survive at all costs. This innate drive to prolong life is immensely powerful.

Joiner and colleagues believe that one of the factors that helps patients to mobilize the drive to follow through with suicidal action is the degree with which they are familiar with death, hence, more comfortable with it. By being exposed to death frequently one may become desensitized to a fear of death – in much the same fashion that exposure to heights can help a person overcome a fear of heights. This phenomenon of desensitization may help to explain why people with certain occupations such as police, paramedics, military personnel, and medical/nursing staff may be more prone to attempt suicide. It also helps to explain why people with chronic illnesses where death is always in the background, including psychiatric illnesses with a high potential for death (such as electrolyte imbalance in anorexia nervosa), are more likely to proceed with a suicide attempt, for they have become familiar with the possibility of death on a daily basis. It also provides some theoretical understanding of why people who have attempted suicide are more likely to die by a suicide, for "practice makes perfect" in the sense of creating familiarity with the process and, hence, less fear of proceeding with it. The clinician should try to determine the degree with which the patient has mobilized his or her psychological will and capability to proceed with the act as per the above factors.

In my opinion, Joiner's factors become even more pregnant with danger when accompanied by a hopelessness that these interpersonal failings cannot be improved. One can see how the above sensations can also coalesce to create a concurrent damaging matrix effect on the wing dealing with the patient's framework for meaning, for the unfortunate entwining of these factors can convince the patient that his or her life has no meaning. Without a reason to be, indeed, having concluded that others will be better off if one is dead, it is easy to understand how a patient can be pulled towards the relief promised by a handgun.

Joiner and colleagues suggest that thwarted belongingness can be assessed with questions such as the following[38]:

1. "Do you feel connected to other people?"
2. "Do you live alone?"
3. "Do you have someone you can call when you are feeling badly?"

They use a normalization to assess perceived burdensomeness, as with "Sometimes people think, 'The people in my life would be better off if I was gone.' Do you think that?"

Although not available for Michael, in many instances, immediate family members and loved ones are available supports, serving as potentially powerful protective factors. Their availability can be particularly useful when sending a patient home who is safe for discharge but who is clearly experiencing intermittent suicidal thoughts. Until the next appointment, the family can play a crucial role in monitoring for any increase in suicidal thought or intent. To do so, they must be comfortable asking the patient about suicidal thoughts.

In such cases, I generally find it is valuable to have a discussion with the patient and the family together, talking openly about suicidal concerns and the design of a collaborative safety plan. Such a procedure helps to communicate to both the patient and family that it is safe and appropriate to discuss suicidal ideation frankly. In fact, the patient's ideation may prove more deadly if it is not discussed.

There is an art to helping families communicate effectively when a patient is being discharged into the care of family members, a potentially frightening situation for those involved. When alone with the patient I ask, "Would you be comfortable with your mom or dad asking you whether you were having any suicidal thoughts?" If the patient answers "yes," I have found the following question to be particularly useful:

"How would you like them to ask you about that later tonight and in the next couple of days? I mean exactly what words would you like them to use?"

This inquiry conveys control to the patient in a key arena, at a time when many patients are feeling that others are taking control of them. Sometimes patients simply respond, "They should just ask me if I'm having thoughts of killing myself." Other patients may say something like, "Well, they could say 'Are you having any tough thoughts?'" Whatever the patient feels most comfortable with (as long as it is clear to all involved that this is a question about suicide) can then be presented as the preferred method for asking about suicidal thought. I then press the patient as to whether he or she really can agree to truthfully answer this question, as well as whether he or she is prepared to share with the parents what the thoughts are in detail.

If the patient agrees, I meet again separately with the parents (spouse, roommate, or whomever is going to be staying with the patient). I ask if they feel comfortable asking the patient about suicidal thoughts. If they answer "yes," then I share with them how the patient has requested this inquiry be done. I have the family member ask me the question in a role-play style, to make sure they are comfortable saying the words. (It is one thing to agree to say the words, it is another thing altogether to actually say them – practice is invaluable.)

I then meet with the patient and the family to consolidate the plan with all present. At this point, I ask the parents to practice by asking the patient in front of me. Finally, I ask the patient how this felt and ensure that all in the room are comfortable with their means of communication about this critical topic. I have found that such collaborative approaches can significantly increase the likelihood that the patient will relay dangerous suicidal ideation if it should arise in the near future. As we have seen so often in this book, when it comes to interviewing – technique counts.

With regard to the factors discussed earlier, including long-term supports, immediate supports, and recent stressors, Michael gives cause for much concern. The risk is further heightened by the relatively recent discharge of Michael from a psychiatric hospital (which could provide "no information at this time because the medical records department are closed"). In particular, the first month following a patient's discharge represents a particularly high-risk period.[39] Michael has no known suicide history. With regard to previous attempts, corroborative informants often provide information that is withheld by the patient. Previous attempts are clearly associated with increased risk. At a minimum, 30 to 40% of suicide completers have had one or more prior attempts. Put into perspective, whereas roughly only 12 per 100,000 people in the United States die by suicide per year, 15,000 out of 100,000 (i.e., 15 per 100) people with prior attempts will ultimately go on to die by suicide over the course of their lives.[40]

In this regard, prior attempts and the availability of the current method of choice remain major risk factors. As we shall see later, this combination amplifies the level of concern if the current method and the current interpersonal/situational stressors are similar to dangerous attempts from the past.

Concerning Michael's clinical disposition, the interviewer investigated one more pertinent external protective factor – the mental health system itself. The charge nurse, when queried, related that the outpatient department was flooded with people requiring appointments and was backlogged for several weeks. She thought that it was highly unlikely that Michael could be seen the next day. Thus, because of a lack of immediate social support and a relative lack of professional support, the clinician felt very uneasy about outpatient triage. However, despite many statistical risk factors, it is unclear how lethal a risk Michael presents. It must be remembered that he denied suicidal intent, albeit in a somewhat quizzical fashion. Furthermore, at present, there are insufficient grounds to commit Michael.

At this point, the interviewer made a wise, but often under-used, decision to interview the patient again. This time the clinician would make an even more concerted effort to bring psychotic ideation to the surface, while listening persistently for adequate grounds to commit Michael, if indeed he appeared more imminently suicidal. In this illustration, we will see the clinician deftly using Robinson's "greasing the wheels of psychosis," a technique we described in Chapter 11 (pages 474–475). The following dialogue evolved after about 10 minutes:

Pt.: I don't think there's anything that could have been done. Peace is what is needed. Peaceful mankind … but it all seems so weird and I try to stop them.

Clin.: To stop who? (greasing the wheels)

Pt.: Bad people … bad people who push me and make me do things, make me watch things.

Clin.: Have you ever felt like someone or something was really trying to take you over? (checking for alien control)

Pt.: Oh … they take me over, or try to, but I don't let them.

Clin.: Who are you talking about? (greasing the wheels)

Pt.: Something inside me, something about my heart, scratching at my heart, my muscle.

Clin.: It sounds very frightening.

Pt.: Very frightening, but I won't do it.

Clin.: What do they want you to do? (greasing the wheels)

Pt.: To cut it out, to cut the scratching out of my heart, to bring peace to mankind, to wipe off the pain. But I won't do it unless I see the sign. The clouds will kiss the moon, you'll see.

Clin.: What do they want you to use to cut yourself?

Pt.: My knife.

Clin.: Have they ever made you hold the knife in your hands? (further elaboration of alien control)

Pt.: Oh yes … one night, I think it was last night, they put it in my hand. I told them I didn't want to, but they made me hold it with the point pressing on my chest, just waiting.

Clin.: And what did they want you to do?

Pt.: To thrust it deep inside my heart, to let my scratching out, to let my God in, to thrust steel truth into God.

The interviewer has succeeded. He has been granted access to the patient's inner world, which proves to be grossly psychotic, as was initially suspected. By probing along the lines of alien control, the interviewer has skillfully uncovered both suicidal ideation and action. In the earlier interview, Michael had denied suicidal ideation probably because he felt that an alien force wanted him to die, not his own will. In his mind this was murder, not suicide. Clearly, Michael warrants hospitalization, and adequate grounds for commitment are now available if necessary. It should be noted that the interviewer had gently guided Michael towards a concrete description of his suicidal actions in the hope that grounds for commitment would emerge. Many times a patient will not grant such information unless he or she is sensitively guided towards it.

Perhaps a review of some basic principles illustrated by Michael may be of value here:

1. A relatively small but significant number of people who attempt suicide are actively psychotic.
2. Any evidence of psychosis warrants a thorough evaluation of lethality.
3. Three particularly dangerous areas of psychotic process are command hallucinations, feelings of alien control, and hyper-religiosity. These areas should be actively probed by the interviewer if they are not elicited spontaneously.
4. Recent evidence suggests that many suicides in schizophrenia occur in response to depressive episodes while the patient is relatively non-psychotic.
5. Demographic material such as age, sex, and marital status may indicate risk factors for suicide.
6. Recent losses and poor social support systems also represent risk factors for suicide.
7. Financial devastation and physical assault (keep in mind domestic violence and violence within prisons) represent two of the most powerful stressors related to suicide attempts.
8. The combination of feeling thwarted in ones attempts to belong to a group coupled with a sense of being a burden to others may represent one of the most potent of emotional milieus conducive to suicide, especially if the patient feels that there is no hope these situations can be ameliorated.
9. When patients feel more familiar and comfortable with the idea of death, they may have increased their psychological capability of following through on suicidal action.
10. Alcohol, drugs, or any physiologic insult to the central nervous system may increase the likelihood of suicide or homicide.
11. When evaluating systems of immediate outpatient support, one should carefully consider whether the mental health system itself is prepared to offer adequate support.
12. Interviews with corroborative informants may yield valuable information.

At this point, it may be best to move on to our second patient, who presents some new areas of concern when considering lethality.

Clinical Illustration #2: Mrs. Kelly

Mrs. Kelly, a 50-year-old married mother of three, has arrived for an outpatient initial assessment, accompanied by her eldest daughter. Mrs. Kelly appears frail, walking as if each step presented a personal challenge. There remains a glint in her eye, but it is a weary one. Her hands are grossly deformed by the ravages of rheumatoid arthritis. She reports feeling very depressed, and her speech is punctuated by heavy sighs. She complains of many neurovegetative symptoms of depression. They have persisted for more than 6 months, "although I've not felt normal since the arthritis began over 7 years ago." She continues tearfully, "I'm not the same woman my husband married." She manages to smile as she wryly adds, "You know, if my memory serves me right, I used to move a little faster."

When asked about suicide, she admits to having thought of it occasionally but denies any intention of pursuing it. She has no organized plan. She relates an increasing sense of hopelessness, adding, "I think I'm starting to lose my fight. I think my husband would be better off with me dead, at least he says so." She is without evidence of psychosis and does remarkably well when tested for cognitive dysfunction.

Her daughter relates that her mother used to be a real fighter. At one time she was "the belle of the ball." With the onset of the arthritis, she had been forced into a strikingly more sedate lifestyle. Her illness has greatly affected her husband, who always wants to be active socially. They bicker constantly. Her daughter has seen no evidence of suicidal behavior in her mother but is frightened of what her mother will do when she becomes bedridden.

Mrs. Kelly's case certainly raises different concerns than those encountered with Michael. In the first place, she appears to be significantly depressed. As expected, the presence of a depression represents one of the most significant of suicide risk factors. It is important to keep in mind the possibility of atypical depression. Indeed, various somatoform disorders, such as the psychogenic pain syndrome, may be accompanied by depression. With such an atypical presentation, an interviewer can be lulled into a feeling of false security concerning suicide potential.

The presence of a severe psychiatric disorder, such as a major depression, is probably the single strongest statistical correlate with suicide risk. Sometimes clinicians ask me, "What is one of your best tips for predicting suicide potential?" and one of my favorite responses is simply, "Do a good diagnostic assessment." Reviews of completed suicides have shown that up to 90% of all suicides, including both adolescents and adults, occur in people suffering with a psychiatric disturbance.[41] Affective disorders lead the pack. They are followed by substance abuse, anxiety disorders, schizophrenia, and people coping with a severe personality disorder such as borderline personality disorder.[42]

There is also increasing evidence that people who experience frequent panic attacks are at a higher risk. If the panic attacks occur in conjunction with a severe depression, then a "red flag" should go up. In a study of almost 1000 patients with a mood disorder, Fawcett found that depressed patients who experienced panic attacks demonstrated three times the suicide rate of other patients, accounting for nearly two thirds of the suicides in the first year of the study.[43,44] More recent research has supported the idea that patients with mood disorders who co-morbidly present with severe psychic anxiety have a higher rate of suicide.[45] Anxiety disorders in general clearly play a role in suicide, as reflected in a major survey by Nepon and colleagues that found that over 70% of individuals with a lifetime history of a suicide attempt had an anxiety disorder.[46,47]

With regard to physical illness, Mrs. Kelly highlights the fact that severe illnesses are often associated with increased suicide risk. The clinician should pay particular attention to illnesses that result in markedly decreased mobility, disfigurement, and chronic pain. Mrs. Kelly's rheumatoid arthritis unfortunately creates all three of these burdens. The interviewer should also note the impact of illnesses in which the patient perceives a horrifying demise. Illnesses such as Huntington's chorea, multiple sclerosis, severe diabetes, and severe chronic obstructive pulmonary disease may present more suffering than many of us can bear to accept and that some individuals would choose to accept. The interaction of medical illnesses with the patient's underlying personality structure also warrants attention. In some instances, people locked into damaging structures such as narcissistic, histrionic, or borderline personalities may have enormous difficulty dealing with disease processes that people lucky enough to have more mature coping skills can handle better.

Leonard has described three personality types that may be predisposed to suicide when stressed.[48] The first type is a controlling personality; these patients tend to constantly manipulate their environment. They are often hard-driven and feel a need to be "on top of things." They frequently pilot their way into roles of power and authority. When such people are suddenly struck by the loss of control caused by a crippling illness, they may attempt to escape through death. Mrs. Kelly certainly may possess some of these dynamics, because she had always been an "on the go" person. Her daughter's fear of what will happen when her mother becomes bedridden represents a well-founded concern.

A second personality type is exemplified by a dependent-dissatisfied approach to life, a common element of people suffering with borderline personality disorders and people with "passive-aggressive" structures. Such people often leave a long line of exasperated caretakers in their wake. When the last source of aid finally closes the door, these people are suddenly left without any means of emotional support. Suicide may loom as the only viable option. Finally, a third predisposing characterological type involves people who have evolved a truly symbiotic relationship with a significant other. These people are at high risk if their sustaining support dies or abandons them.

All of these examples emphasize one of the most important hallmarks of suicide, which we have already seen elaborated by Joiner's work. Suicide is an interpersonal phenomenon. As such, an evaluation of suicide potential not only involves consideration of the identified patient, but it also requires an evaluation of the interpersonal systems surrounding that patient. At times, this evaluation proceeds through the use of corroborative interviews. At other times, the interviewer must depend on information provided solely by the patient. In either case, a careful consideration of the interpersonal and familial wings of the matrix is always warranted.

Using a simplistic but practical approach, the interviewer should attempt to determine whether the patient is returning to a supportive or hostile environment. If the patient's family or friends provide a caring milieu, this bodes well for the patient. However, even in this situation, a paradoxical problem can arise if the patient begins to feel guilty "about being a burden to everyone." As Joiner has suggested, comments such as Mrs. Kelly's, "I think my husband will be better off with me dead," should prick up the ears of the interviewer. Following this line of reasoning, after suicide has been broached as a topic, questions such as the following can be revealing:

a. "If you would kill yourself, how do you think that would affect your family?"
b. "What do you think your spouse would feel if you killed yourself?"
c. "What are your thoughts about your responsibilities for your family and children if you kill yourself?"[49]

Such questioning may lead directly to evidence of an interpersonal maelstrom or into an exploration of the framework for meaning that will keep the patient alive, such as the need to care for a child or grandchildren. On the darker side, as the evaluation proceeds, the interviewer makes inquiries to check whether a supposed support system (individual) in reality wishes, at some level, that the patient were dead. A death wish may be unconscious or conscious, innocuous or sinister. The clinician's recognition of such death wishes is not a moral judgment passed upon a potential support system, but rather an objective attempt to see the potentially lethal ramifications arising from such situations. A premature dismissal of such factors may represent a dangerous naiveté on the part of the interviewer. Certainly, in the case of Mrs. Kelly, one wonders to what degree the marital alliance has been severely strained. At some level, does Mr. Kelly "want out?"

An unconscious or conscious death wish may show itself by a lax attitude of the family towards appropriate precautions against suicide. The clinician may discover that the safety suggestions of previous mental health professionals, such as removing a firearm, have not been followed by the family.

The most striking example of this type of dangerous process that I have encountered was a man who presented to our emergency room with his 15-year-old son who had been depressed for months. Tragically, this man had lost his eldest son to suicide. This older son had killed himself with a hunting rifle given to him on his fifteenth birthday by his father. In the interview with the current patient, his father blandly told me that despite his son's depression, he had opted to give him a hunting rifle on his fifteenth birthday several weeks earlier!

Likewise, there may be resistance to hospitalizing a seriously lethal patient; however, the motivation behind this may be rather different. From the perspective of psychological defense mechanisms, family members may see a falsely rosy picture because of denial or repression.

More disturbingly, clinicians will undoubtedly encounter, at some point in their practice, a death wish laced with true malice. Perhaps it will be a spouse who has long been denied a divorce or a battered significant other unable to retaliate. These family members, rightly or wrongly, may consciously wish the patient dead. It is not known how many times people have waited a few hours before calling for help when they have happened upon a "sleeping" family member surrounded by empty pill bottles.

I remember one patient that I hospitalized from the emergency room whose spouse yelled at her in the emergency room, "take the damn pills, in fact I'll stuff them down your throat, and trust me I won't call a soul." The uncovering of such vicious interaction should serve as a warning to a clinician. It may influence a clinician to hospitalize a patient who might otherwise have been safely discharged to a more supportive environment.

Another aspect of the hostile interpersonal environment may be a scenario in which a patient is angry with family members. With revenge in mind, a patient may kill himself or herself, hoping to "show them they'll be sorry when I'm gone." Questions such as, "What have you pictured your funeral being like?" may provide revealing insights into the patient's motive for suicide. It is not at all unusual to receive answers such as, "They will all be really hurt, realizing at last what they've done to me." In a similar vein, some authors have viewed suicide as the result of a murderous impulse turned inward, a symbolic murder with an ironic satisfaction.[50]

Reasoning of the types described earlier emphasizes the importance of determining whether the patient is developing powerful interpersonal excuses for suicide. The more rational the suicide appears to the patient, the more concerned the interviewer should become. It becomes particularly ominous when the excuse has a humanistic flavor to it, as with "It's the only way I can really help my family." Such thinking may be the first note in a death toll.

Leaving the interpersonal realm and returning to Mrs. Kelly, several indicators suggest a lowered suicide risk. In the first place, she denies immediate hopelessness. Aaron Beck's work with the cognitive aspects of suicide has suggested that the presence of hopelessness may be an ominous sign. In fact, hopelessness may be an even better indicator of lethality than the severity of depressive mood.[51] Flipped towards a positive statement, in my opinion, hope may be the single most powerful antidote to suicide.

Viewed from a logical perspective, suicide usually represents a last resort that is taken when no other alternatives are apparent to the patient. *A trigger is pulled, a step off a bridge is taken, when a person is looking into the future and sees no possible way that his or her pain will ever end.* Moreover, a sense of helplessness is often coupled to this state of despair. Patients generally kill themselves for one major reason, to escape what appears to them to be inescapable pain.

Further questioning also revealed that regarding the spiritual wing of her matrix Mrs. Kelly was not only raised a Catholic but also that she strongly practiced her faith and believed that suicide was a mortal sin punishable by eternal damnation. At this intensity, religion is probably acting as a major protective factor that diminishes suicide risk. Other patients may have different frameworks for meaning, such as caring for their children or fulfilling other important societal roles. In any case, the clinician should seek out evidence of such powerful deterrents.

A peculiar and unsettling twist can enter the picture with regard to children. Some patients may decide that their children would be worse off after the patient's suicide. For instance, the patient's spouse may have alcoholism with an active history of abusing the children both physically and sexually. In these cases, the patient may contemplate taking the lives of the children before killing himself or herself. Although this happens rarely, one only needs to read the newspapers in order to learn about such tragedies. If suspected, validity techniques, such as normalization, may be useful when moving unobtrusively into this extremely sensitive area.

> **Pt.:** My husband will never change. He likes to hurt us. We have no future, and I now realize that suicide is my only option.
>
> **Clin.:** You mentioned "we." What do you think is going to happen to your children after you kill yourself?
>
> **Pt.:** (long pause) I don't really know.
>
> **Clin.:** Sometimes parents consider taking the lives of their children (normalization), has that thought ever crossed your mind?
>
> **Pt.:** Yes, it has … it's a terrible thought, but it has.
>
> **Clin.:** What have you thought of doing?

Another positive note in Mrs. Kelly's presentation is the lack of a recent, abrupt change in clinical condition in either direction. The sudden onset of severe sleeplessness, agitation, or marked dysphoria may indicate that the patient is rapidly approaching a pain level that he or she cannot tolerate. On the other hand, one hears of the often-quoted clinical observation that an unexpected improvement in clinical condition may be masking a sinister outcome. The patient's peace may be secondary to the patient's decision to commit suicide. Suddenly, the patient perceives an end to the suffering. The most upsetting decision of the patient's life is over.

A problem concerning "improvement" surfaces from the fact that sometimes depressed patients appear more likely to attempt suicide when they begin to improve. Suicide is less common while they are in the troughs of their depression. This curious finding is probably related to the fact that, as they initially improve, they regain initiative and energy, even though their dysphoric mood may remain severely intense. The clinician should keep this in mind when encountering a patient who has recently started taking an antidepressant. This phenomenon should not be confused with the more frequent and concerning side effect – discussed in Chapter 9 – of suicidal ideation and dysphoric manic symptoms being released by the use of antidepressants.

Finally, further interviewing revealed that Mrs. Kelly has no immediate models for suicide; neither friends nor family members have ever attempted suicide. If one discovers a legacy of suicide in a family tree, this should arouse concern on the part of the interviewer.

In addition to modeling, a positive family history of suicide represents a significant risk factor for several reasons: (1) some illnesses that predispose to suicide such as major depression, bipolar disorder, and schizophrenia possess a genetic predisposition (there is growing evidence of a genetic component to some personality disorders such as borderline personality disorder as well), (2) suicidal ideation may itself have a genetic and epigenetic predisposition,[52,53] and (3) a patient may psychologically identify with a relative and/or namesake who died by suicide, thus feeling, "Everyone has always said that I am just like my Aunt Sally and I am. And I intend to kill myself when I'm 30, just like she did. At least she finally got some relief."

At this point, a summary of issues illustrated by Mrs. Kelly may clarify some principles.

1. The presence of disease may increase suicide risk, especially if it leads to immobility, disfigurement, or severe pain.
2. The interviewer should search for evidence of feelings of hopelessness or helplessness.
3. A hostile interpersonal environment may substantially increase the risk of suicide.
4. A strong framework for meaning, such as a deeply held religious conviction, may decrease risk. It should be sought for by the clinician.
5. Sudden changes in clinical condition, either positive or negative, may indicate an increased risk.
6. Rational excuses for committing suicide may indicate increased intention.
7. The presence of a positive family history of suicide should be actively looked into by the clinician.
8. Suicide assessment should always include a search for major psychiatric disorders such as major depression, bipolar disorder, schizophrenia, anxiety disorders such as obsessive–compulsive disorder and panic disorder, alcohol and drug abuse, and severe personality disorders such as borderline personality disorder.
9. Pay particular attention when intense anxiety is a co-morbid feature of any psychiatric disorder.

Risk Factors and Warning Signs: Summary and Effective Utilization

Useful Mnemonics

Through the examination of the two case studies, the risk factors and warning signs most often cited in the literature have been surveyed. When pressured by time constraints, clinical demands, and the other usual pressures of being a mental health professional, it is sometimes difficult to remember all these issues. To facilitate their recall, the following two acronyms have been developed.

The first acronym, the SAD PERSONS Scale (Table 17.1), was developed by Patterson, Dohn, Bird, and Patterson and was the first widely used acronym in the field.[54] It serves as a useful checklist of pertinent risk factors, many of which are static risk factors. There is no predictive value in assigning numbers to it. The second acronym, the NO HOPE Acronym (see Table 17.1), first described in the second edition of this book, attempts to add further depth to the evaluation of suicide potential with a greater emphasis upon dynamic risk factors.

The acronym NO HOPE, itself, emphasizes the need to inquire about feelings of hopelessness as per Beck's research.

Table 17.1 Useful Acronyms in Suicide Assessment

SAD PERSONS SCALE	NO HOPE ACRONYM
• **S**ex	• **N**o framework for meaning
• **A**ge	• **O**vert change in clinical condition
• **D**epression	
	• **H**ostile interpersonal environment
• **P**revious attempt	• **O**ut of hospital recently
• **E**thanol abuse	• **P**redisposing personality factors
• **R**ational thinking loss	• **E**xcuses for dying are present and strongly believed
• **S**ocial supports lacking	
• **O**rganized plan	
• **N**o spouse	
• **S**ickness	

Loose Ends and a New Mnemonic

A new mnemonic was devised under the auspices of the American Association of Suicidology in 2006.[55] It was an attempt to focus solely upon dynamic risk factors, (emphasizing those dynamic factors that are best supported by research literature as representing warning signs of imminent risk). The three-word mnemonic is as follows:

IS PATH WARM
  Ideation (suicidal)
  Substance abuse

  Purposelessness
  Anger
  Trapped
  Hopelessness

  Withdrawing
  Anxiety
  Recklessness
  Mood change

Most of the factors in this mnemonic have already been nicely covered in the previous two acronyms, but it provides several nuances. One of its best features is the insight it provides into some of the phenomenology experienced by people about to kill themselves. It delineates a subtle distinction between the cognitive *belief* of hopelessness and the emotional *sensation* of "feeling trapped." A patient might arrive at the cognitive conclusion that there is no hope for relief from his or her psychological pain, but it may be the persistent, unrelenting, and very real sensation that he or she is trapped that ultimately urges the person to pull a trigger or jump from a bridge. In essence, the need to get away from this highly dysphoric internal sensation may be the phenomenological driving agent resulting in the suicide attempt.

I also like the phenomenological refinement of the feeling of "purposelessness" as a major component of the broader risk factor of loss of meaning. It highlights a distinctive feeling state that one should be on the lookout for when interviewing a potentially suicidal patient. It ties in nicely with Joiner's emphasis upon imminently suicidal patients perceiving that they are a burden to others.

Differentiating Between Concerns of Chronic Suicide Risk Versus More Immediate Risk

Perhaps one of the most important indicators that Mrs. Kelly is probably not at high risk in the near future is the fact that she convincingly denies current suicidal intent and has no organized plan to harm herself. This point illustrates the usefulness of making a distinction between chronic suicide potential and more immediate suicide potential. If a patient presents with a variety of risk factors present over a significant period of time, then the patient may well represent a chronic risk for suicide. Such is the case with Mrs. Kelly, who presents with the following risk factors: presence of a major psychiatric disorder (depression), increasing age, debilitating illness, increasing sense of hopelessness, a strained marital alliance that may actually represent a hostile environment, and the slow evolution of a rational excuse for suicide.

However, the presence of numerous risk factors does not necessarily indicate a more immediate risk of suicide, as evidenced by Mrs. Kelly, who most likely could be safely triaged to an outpatient therapist despite her substantial list of risk factors (although she would probably benefit from hospitalization).

More important, the absence of most risk factors does not necessarily indicate the lack of a serious risk if certain critical risk factors or warning signs are present. We saw this earlier in this chapter with the patient who had minimal risk factors but was experiencing a postpartum psychotic episode with command hallucinations to kill herself to stop Satan from torturing her baby. Thus, it is important to determine what factors suggest that a patient is at a reasonably foreseeable risk of suicide in the immediate and near future, perhaps suggesting the wisdom of hospitalization.

The Tetrad of Lethality: Four Common Indicators That Hospitalization May Be Required

It is important to remember that clinicians cannot truly predict risk in the sense of being able to state categorically that a suicide attempt will occur and when. As Simon has wisely pointed out, even terms such as "imminent risk" can be misleading, for they imply better predictive capabilities than are reasonable.[56] Instead, as clinicians we have within our capabilities (and responsibilities both clinically and medico-legally) the ability to estimate whether there is a reasonably foreseeable increased risk of suicide in a specific patient.

Arguably, the issue of foreseeability is at its most intense focus when a clinician is working with a patient whose presenting risk is suggesting that hospitalization may be indicated (occasionally involuntarily). This decision as to whether to recommend (or sometimes require) hospitalization versus outpatient care is a tough one. You will most frequently encounter it in emergency rooms and inpatient units (is it safe to discharge the patient or allow the patient to go on a pass home?) but it can occur in any clinical setting from an outpatient mental health clinic to a college counseling center or a private practice office. Consequently, we will focus, as we conclude this section, on this complex decision point.

In my opinion, the four most dangerous situations suggesting the need for hospitalization, which form a lethal tetrad, include: (1) an immediately recent serious suicide attempt, (2) the presence of acutely disturbing psychotic processes suggestive of lethality, (3) the relaying of serious suicidal intent by the patient in the interview (or recent behaviors outside the interview indicating serious intent), and (4) a patient who flatly denies suicidal ideation because they strongly intend to proceed with suicide and do not want to be stopped. The presence of any one of these situations can warn the clinician that the patient may be at a foreseeably higher risk for a suicide attempt in the near future. With respect to triage, in my opinion, the clinician should strongly consider hospitalization for the patient, even if opposed by the patient.

By way of illustration, Michael and Mrs. Kelly appear to represent two ends of this continuum. Mrs. Kelly lacks all the elements of the tetrad of lethality. Specifically, she has no recent history of a serious suicide attempt; she has no evidence of psychosis; and she gives no feeling from the interview of current suicidal ideation. Thus, despite the fact that she has numerous risk factors, she is probably not in immediate danger. On the other hand, Michael presented with three of the four elements of the tetrad and thus was worrisome indeed.

These two presentations highlight the point that there is no mechanical formula that one can use for determining suicidal potential. Instead, clinicians utilize an expertise in which they carefully weigh various risk factors, historical elements, and pieces of information gleaned from the interview. Perhaps a summary of these factors and their interplay would be helpful at this time.

As we look back at the first element of the tetrad of lethality, the presence of a presenting serious attempt, certain points may help to determine the significance of the attempt. First, the clinician should ascertain the potential dangerousness of the method used. For example, taking a few extra aspirin is a great deal less disconcerting than shooting oneself or ingesting lye. Moreover, the threat of an overdosage by a physician, who understands the use of medications, may be more worrisome than the same threat in a non-medical person.

Second, the clinician should determine whether the patient appeared to really want to die or not. Looked at differently, did the patient leave much room for rescue? The interviewer should search for factors such as the following: Did the patient choose a "death spot" where the patient could easily be discovered? Did the patient choose a spot where help was nearby? Did the patient leave any hints of suicidal intention that could have brought help, such as an easily accessible suicide note? Did the patient contact someone after the suicide attempt?[57] The absence of these elements may indicate that the patient was frighteningly serious.

Concerning the second element of the tetrad of lethality – ominous psychotic process – we have already discussed in detail the ramifications of dangerous command hallucinations and how to explore them in Chapter 12 (see pages 528–532) as well as the other dangerous psychotic processes earlier in this chapter. There is no need to reiterate them here.

However, the third element of the tetrad – the relaying of serious suicidal intent by the patient in the interview – which is primarily dependent upon the clinician's interviewing skills, in my opinion, represents the single most important indication of suicide potential. Indeed, recent research offers some support for this contention.

The pioneering work of Kelly Posner in the development of the Columbia Suicide Severity Rating Scale[58] has provided research that has demonstrated some modest, yet promising predictive capabilities. The Columbia Suicide Severity Rating Scale is a semi-structured interviewing format that focuses less on classic risk factors (although the clinician is still urged to consider them in the final formulation of risk when using the tool). Instead, it focuses upon the elicitation of the patient's suicidal ideation, planning, actions, and intent. Posner believes that it is this emphasis that gives the tool its predictive capabilities.

And here we are led to our fourth element of the tetrad of lethality, the patient who denies suicidal ideation because they truly intend to die and are flat-out lying to the interviewer. Never forget this possibility. It is arguably the most dangerous of all possibilities. It is easily missed.

The presence of an inordinately high number of risk factors, a single particularly intense risk factor, or the concurrent lack of protective factors may be the initial alerting phenomenon to the interviewer. Often (but not always), there is an accompanying terseness or annoyance to the patient's responses regarding suicidal thoughts.

If one is suspicious that a patient is lying or minimizing suicidal intent, every reasonable effort should be made to uncover, from other sources, evidence of the patient's high lethality. Corroborative sources are of immense importance here, as is past psychiatric history and past presentations regarding suicide attempts. If one is suspicious that a patient is withholding serious intent, in many instances it is wise to consult with another clinician. Sometimes, if possible, it is useful to have a second clinician interview the patient with the hope that the patient may be more open in sharing his or her real intent.

Once the clinician has decided that the patient is safe for outpatient care, it remains important to consider the relative intensity of the patient's risk, for this intensity will determine many aspects of follow-up, such as the frequency of sessions with the therapist, the establishment of familial and community supports, and communications with referrals, to ensure that the agreed-upon follow-up proceeded as planned. An analysis of risk factors, warning signs, and protective factors can provide aids to this decision making and the concurrent collaborative treatment planning. For the interested reader, a variety of excellent material has been written regarding the cognitive and intuitive subtleties of risk formulation.[59-65]

We can now turn our attention to the second of the clinical tasks required in a sound suicide assessment – the interviewing techniques used to uncover the patient's suicidal ideation, desire, planning, actions, and intent. It is here that we may have the greatest chance to save a life.

SECTION 2: THE ELICITATION OF SUICIDAL IDEATION, PLANNING, BEHAVIORS, AND INTENT

The uncovering of suicidal ideation and intent is a complex arabesque that unfolds as a dyadic phenomenon, impacted by the psychological states, biases, and personalities of both the interviewer and the interviewee. It is not an exaggeration to say that the resolution of this arabesque is a life and death matter. In this section, we will approach this task via four gateways: (1) elements impacting upon the assessment process such as a patient's hesitancy to share suicidal thought, countertransference, and clinical myths, (2) the importance of eliciting a comprehensive database related to suicidal ideation and the impediments to doing so, (3) setting the stage for the elicitation of suicidal ideation, and (4) an exploration of the practical application of the Chronological Assessment of Suicide Events (the CASE Approach) as a sensitive and flexible method for exploring suicidal ideation, planning, behaviors, and intent.

It should also be noted that phenomenological characteristics associated with self-damaging non-lethal behaviors such as self-cutting, self-burning, and head banging, as seen in disorders such as borderline personality disorder, were delineated in Chapter 14 (see pages 584 and 607). This chapter will focus solely upon the elicitation and exploration of suicidal thoughts and behaviors related to lethality, as opposed to non-lethal self-harm. As noted earlier, the phenomenology of self-damaging non-lethal behaviors is strikingly different than the phenomenology of lethal thoughts and behaviors, and the two should not be confused with one another.

1. Before the Interview Begins: Secrets, Countertransference, and Problematic Myths

There exists little doubt that as mental health professionals we will all be interviewing a patient at some point in our careers who has decided to kill himself or herself. As we talk, the patient will have already accepted an invitation to die. The question becomes whether the patient will decide to share his or her secret with us.

In such a situation, the interviewer – if viewed as a measuring instrument – should be set at the highest level of sensitivity. The clinician essentially should try to elicit even the smallest of suicidal thoughts, because such ideations may have important implications for disposition and treatment. Moreover, once the patient has felt comfortable sharing his or her superficial suicidal thoughts, the door may widen for the sharing of deeper and more dangerous suicidal secrets.

In the following pages, an attempt is made to offer various principles that may significantly increase the likelihood that suicidal ideation will be shared. As usual, each interviewer must ultimately develop an individually tailored style, but these suggestions may serve as useful stimulants for thought. We begin by simply admitting that suicide is a taboo topic. It is normal for a patient to be hesitant to share their suicidal thoughts, especially with a total stranger, who holds the power to involuntarily hospitalize them. Who wouldn't be careful in such a situation?

Several points immediately come to mind concerning lethality questioning and its sensitive nature. They can be summarized as follows:

1. The least hesitancy in a patient's response may suggest that the patient has had such thoughts, even if he or she proceeds to deny them.
2. Answers such as "No, not really," often indicate that there has been concrete suicidal ideation. The interviewer can often break the resistance with a concerned tone of voice and a question such as, "What kind of thoughts have you had?"
3. The interviewer should look carefully for any body language clues that the patient is being deceptive or feels anxious.
4. To increase clinician awareness of such nonverbal clues, note taking should be avoided during the elicitation of suicidal ideation.
5. The clinician should be aware of and avoid giving any nonverbal clues of their discomfort with the topic of suicide, such as might be shown by increased interviewer displacement activities or looking away from the patient.
6. *The clinician's nonverbals and eye contact should be used to maximize engagement, creating as conversational a feel to the interview during the elicitation of suicidal ideation as possible, for engagement should be maximized to enhance uncovering the truth regarding suicidal intent from the patient.*

This is an opportune time to address the potential limitations of semi-structured interviews (such as the Columbia Suicide Severity Rating Scale) when eliciting suicidal ideation and intent. Semi-structured interviews generally *require that the clinician must periodically look away from the patient* to be prompted – by a paper or a computer screen – as to what questions to ask and/or to subsequently document the answers to these questions. In my opinion, *the resulting inability to attend fully to the nonverbal leakage of deceit (as well as limitations in using one's own nonverbal behaviors to more powerfully engage the patient)* limits the use of semi-structured interviews in some suicide assessment situations. Such situations include interviewing a poorly engaged or angry patient, working with an intensely suicidal patient who intends to withhold his or her true suicidal intent, or any patient where deceit is an issue. In a similar light, these tools can further hinder engagement – which is of extreme importance in uncovering the truth while eliciting suicidal ideation and intent – by disrupting the naturalistic conversational flow of the interview as the interviewer keeps breaking it off to be prompted on what to ask next.

Sometimes psychopathological states may also suggest that the use of a semi-structured interview may be unwise. Such is the case when encountering an actively paranoid and/

or agitated patient. Paranoid patients are prone to project malicious intentions behind note taking or the act of a clinician reading questions from a computer screen or piece of paper (such as developing delusional beliefs that the interviewer is falsifying the patient's history, preparing commitment papers, or receiving messages from an outside source with malicious intent towards the patient). The use of note taking, prompting, or typing in such situations is, in my opinion, not only potentially disengaging, it is potentially dangerous with regard to triggering a potential assault. Considering the above limitations to the use of semi-structured interviews, I do *not* feel they should be used in emergency rooms or by crisis clinicians in face-to-face interviews.

This is also an opportune time to look at a common myth concerning the search for suicidal ideation. Simply stated, the myth reads: "I might give patients the idea to kill themselves, if I raise the topic."

In the first place, to my knowledge, there is not a single case example of such a process unfolding. In the second place, the idea of suicide is not a cultural secret. A patient would have to be unusually backward to have never heard of suicide before encountering the clinician. And thirdly, and probably most important, suicide is extremely hard to do. It will take a lot more than a single interviewer's discussion of the topic to lead someone to make the decision.

To the contrary, as discussed earlier, the clinician's frank discussion allows the patient to share a heavy burden, made much heavier by the isolation imposed by taboo-induced silence. Moreover, the demonstration that suicidal ideation can be openly discussed conveys that help may be only a spoken word away. Suddenly, suicidal ideation is no longer a sin to be hidden, but rather a problem to be solved.

It should be added that later in the interview, it might be worthwhile to repeat the inquiry. Sometimes hesitancies to share may vary with time. If the interviewer is not satisfied with the first inquiry, a second one may yield some surprises.

The clinician must also ensure that his or her own anxiety over suicidal issues is not conveyed to the patient. Such anxiety may be misinterpreted as an indication of moral disapproval. If, indeed, the patient picks up evidence of moral condemnation through tone of voice or body language, the patient may shut up like a frightened child before an unforgiving parent. With this in mind, it becomes important for the interviewer to be keenly aware of countertransference issues. An awareness of such issues may surface by asking questions of oneself such as:

a. What are my beliefs about suicide?
b. Do I feel that suicide is sinful or unnatural?
c. Do I feel that people who commit suicide are weak?
d. Do I ever picture myself as capable of taking my own life?
e. Have I known anyone in my family or friends who killed themselves? How does this fact affect the way that I approach the issue in my interviews?

The answers to such questions may help the interviewer to spot any characteristics of their own interviewing style (avoiding the topic, diminishing the exploration of the topic, changes in tone of voice or eye contact) that may inadvertently lead a patient to withhold suicidal thought and intent.

It also seems pertinent to raise a countertransference issue that many interviewers do not like to admit, but one that I think is present in most of us. Namely, if we uncover serious suicidal ideation, we are potentially creating a mess for ourselves. For instance, if suicidal plans emerge, we may need to significantly prolong our assessment when we are already strapped for time. Family members may need to be involved. We may have to deal with an irate patient or equally irate family member if we need to proceed with involuntary commitment. And, finally, we may have to spend a day in court if commitment occurs. The bottom line is: if we do our job well, we may have to pay a not-so-insignificant price. These realistic concerns can emerge as countertransference in the guise of processes such as failing to inquire about suicide, waiting until the end of the interview to ask about it, poorly setting the stage, hurrying the assessment, and asking questions in a manner that decreases the sensitivity of the questions themselves.

With regard to the last concern, it is important to avoid using negative statements of inquiry as described in Chapter 3 (see page 83) as illustrated below:

> **Pt.:**   Sometimes things are simply too much. My husband can't stop yelling, the dog is barking, kids screaming, too much, just too much.
>
> **Clin.:**   You've *not* thought of killing yourself? (statement of negative inquiry)
>
> **Pt.:**   Why no, I haven't thought of that really.

Such a negative leading question may suggest to the patient that the interviewer does not morally approve of suicide and may be judgmental if told of suicidal ideation. In reality, it may merely represent the hassled interviewer's unconscious prayer that nothing serious comes up. Unfortunately, to the interviewee, it clearly indicates that this interviewer wants "no" for an answer. As a general rule, interviewees try to please interviewers. Validity clearly becomes an issue here. I watched such an interaction in which the patient denied suicidal ideation to an initial interviewer. A second interviewer re-approached the same patient at the end of the first clinician's interview. This time, the second interviewer avoided the statement of negative inquiry. He subsequently discovered that the patient had overdosed on aspirin about 5 days earlier.

Concerning the issue of patient hesitancy, a second general principle comes to mind that can be simply stated: Do not accept the first "no." I am consistently amazed at how many people flatly deny suicidal ideation when first asked, despite the presence of such ideation. The clinician should seldom, if ever, leave the topic after a single denial. As we are about to see, there exist many reasons for a patient to be hesitant to share suicidal thought and intent.

2. The Importance of Uncovering Suicidal Ideation and Why It Is Hard to Do So

Roadblocks to Sharing Suicidal Ideation

The first rule of life is to reveal nothing, to be exceptionally cautious in what you say, in whatever company you may find yourself.

Elizabeth Aston, *The Darcy Connection*[66]

Many patients who find themselves in the company of mental health professionals unfortunately may adopt the above dictum, especially when they are asked about suicide. It is the interviewer's task to transform this potentially dangerous hesitancy.

On a positive note, some patients who are seriously suicidal may actually share their real intent, secondary to their own ambivalence and/or the effective interviewing skills of the clinician. Such information subsequently serves to sculpt safe triage and treatment planning, whether offered in an outpatient clinic, college campus counseling center, emergency department (ED), inpatient unit, or over the telephone with a crisis counselor.

This information may also be useful in a prospective sense if accurately documented; a thorough record of suicidal ideation and action provides subsequent clinicians with a baseline of the patient's suicidal activity at a specific point. This reference point can be used by future clinicians – such as crisis intervention clinicians or inpatient staff contemplating a pass for a patient – to determine whether the patient's current suicidal ideation is increasing or decreasing.

But not all dangerous patients relay suicidal ideation to clinicians.[67] One could argue that many dangerous patients – those who truly want to die and see no hope for relief from their suffering – would have little incentive to do so. Even if their ambivalence about attempting suicide leads them to voluntarily call a crisis line or go to an ED, they may be quite cautious about revealing the full truth, for a large part of them still wants to die. Such patients may be predisposed to share only some of their suicidal ideation or action taken on a particular plan, while hiding their real intent or even their method of choice (such as a gun tucked away at home).

Many reasons exist why patients, with various ranges of intent, may be hesitant to openly share, including the following:

- The impulsive patient may lack extensive suicidal ideation before his attempt. (This is one reason it may be necessary to hospitalize a patient who denies suicidal ideation.)
- The patient has had marked suicidal ideation and is serious about completing the act, but is purposely not relaying suicidal ideation or is withholding the method of choice because he does not want to be thwarted. (Another reason to hospitalize a patient who may be denying or minimizing suicidal ideation.)
- The patient feels that suicide is a sign of weakness and is ashamed to acknowledge it.
- The patient feels that suicide is immoral or a sin.
- The patient feels that discussion of suicide is, literally, taboo.
- The patient is worried that the clinician will perceive him as crazy.
- The patient fears that he will be locked up if suicidal ideation is shared or, if during a crisis call, that the police will appear at his door.
- The patient fears that others (parents, spouse, other family members, friends, school administrators, potential employers) will find out about his suicidal thoughts through a break in confidentiality, perhaps fearing that the information may be maliciously posted in a chat room or on Facebook, or even used as a texted taunt.

- The patient does not believe that anyone can help.
- The patient has alexithymia (a condition in which people have trouble describing emotional pain or material).[68]

It is sometimes easy to believe that if we ask directly about suicide, the patient will answer directly – and truthfully. From the above considerations, it is apparent that this is not necessarily the case. The real suicidal intent of a patient can be more accurately conceptualized by the following "Equation of Suicidal Intent"[69-71]:

Real Suicidal Intent = Stated Intent + Reflected Intent + Withheld Intent

Thus, a patient's actual intent may equal his stated intent, reflected intent, and withheld intent, any one of these three or any combination of the three. The more intensely a patient wants to proceed with suicide, the more likely he or she is to withhold his or her true intent. In addition, the more taboo a topic is (e.g., incest and suicide), the more one would expect a patient to withhold information. In such instances, both conscious and unconscious processes may underlie the withholding of vital information.

From a psychodynamic perspective, a curious paradox can arise. If a patient believes that suicide is a sign of weakness or of sin, unconscious defense mechanisms (such as denial, repression, rationalization, and intellectualization) may create the *conscious* belief that the patient's intent is much less than it actually is. When asked directly about his or her suicidal intent, such a patient may provide a gross underestimate of his or her potential lethality, even though the patient is genuinely trying to answer the question honestly.

From a phenomenological perspective, it is not surprising that some seriously suicidal patients relay their actual intent in stages during the interview. Whether evaluating such patients in an ED or on a crisis line, it is not uncommon for them to share some information, read how the clinician responds, then share some more information, re-evaluate "where this session is going," and so on.

Indeed, patients with serious suicidal intent who are trying to decide how much to reveal, may share information about a mild overdose while consciously withholding their main method of choice (such as a gun) – for they are aware that once they share this information there is a risk that the gun will be removed – until they arrive at a decision during the interview that they do not want to die, at which point they may feel safe enough to share the full truth with the clinician.

Reflected Intent: One of the Master Keys to Unlocking Real Intent

Reflected intent is the quality and quantity of the patient's suicidal thoughts, desires, plans, and extent of action taken to complete the plans, which reflects how much the patient truly wants to commit suicide. The extent, thoroughness, and time spent by the patient on suicidal planning may be a better reflection of the seriousness of the intent and the proximity of the desire to act on that intent, than is the actual stated intent.

Such reflections of intent may prove to be life-saving pieces of the suicide assessment puzzle. The work of Thomas Joiner[72,73] has provided insight into the importance of acquired capability for suicide (e.g., strength of the psychological drive to complete the suicide, intensive planning, multiple past attempts, availability of method of choice), as a reflection of the seriousness of intent and the potential for action.

A wealth of research and theory from an unexpected source – motivational theory – can help us better understand the importance of reflected intent. We will be exploring motivational theory and motivational interviewing in detail in Chapter 22 in Part IV on advanced interviewing techniques. At this juncture, suffice it to say that these theories and interviewing approaches provide a foundation for better understanding why people do things and how to help them to be motivated to do things of benefit to their wellness. Prochaska's and DiClemente's[74,75] transtheoretical stages of change – precontemplation, contemplation, preparation, action, and maintenance – helped to lay the foundation from which Miller and Rollnick's influential work on motivational interviewing eventually arose.[76,77] When it comes to motivation to do something that is hard to do but good for one (e.g., counseling), the extent of the patient's goal-directed thinking and his subsequent actions might be much better indicators of intent to proceed than his stated intent. In short, the old adage "actions speak louder than words" appears to be on the mark in predicting recovery behavior.

For instance, a patient in alcohol counseling may make all sorts of positive proclamations to the counselor about his intent to begin attending Alcoholics Anonymous (AA). Nevertheless, it is the amount of time he spends thinking about the need for change (reading the AA literature), arranging methods to make this change (finding out where the local AA meetings are), and the actions taken for change (tracking down someone to drive him to the meetings) that, according to Prochaska's theory, may better reflect the intent to change than the patient's verbal report.

Motivational theories are usually related to initiating difficult-to-do actions for positive change. But they may be equally applicable to initiating a difficult-to-do action that is negative, such as suicide (Joiner has pointed out that suicide can be quite a difficult act with which to proceed[78]). Once again, the amount of time spent thinking, planning, and practicing a suicide attempt may speak louder about imminent risk than the patient's immediate words about his intent.

Pitfalls of an Incomplete Elicitation of Suicidal Ideation

Premature Crisis Resolution

Arguably, the single most important task in a suicide assessment, whether in a face-to-face interview or over the phone, is to estimate the immediate risk of suicide and to triage safely with appropriate follow-up. Much of this determination of risk is contingent on an accurate estimate of the patient's suicidal intent. However, significant errors can be made, whether a clinician is functioning in an outpatient clinic, college counseling center, a private practice setting, in an emergency department, or while manning a crisis line.

Picture a patient who mentions suicidal thought and openly admits to a plan (e.g., overdosing on several aspirin weeks ago) yet is withholding much of his intent (as well as his method of choice) because of a strong desire to die. The clinician explores the ideation related to overdosing and then prematurely (before carefully eliciting other suicidal ideation and planning that may better reflect the patient's true intent and method of choice) begins crisis transformation. Being a skilled clinician, during the course of the interview, the crisis is effectively resolved. The patient reports feeling much better. Indeed, temporarily the patient feels much better and no longer feels suicidal, telling the interviewer, "You really helped me tonight. I feel so much better." Recognizing that the patient responded nicely to therapeutic intervention, during the closing phase of the interview the clinician makes a recommendation for follow-up, "Sometime in the near future, I urge you to seek out a therapist. I think you will do really well in therapy."

Because the clinician did not do a thorough assessment of reflected intent before beginning crisis intervention (prematurely assuming that the method first supplied by the patient – overdosing – was the patient's method of choice), the clinician is unaware that the patient has been thinking about shooting himself for weeks, has gotten his gun out on several occasions (loaded it once), and was in need of a much more careful follow-up, including prompting the patient's mother to remove the gun. Unfortunately, 3 days after the "successful" crisis intervention, the patient's girlfriend unexpectedly leaves him, he begins drinking, and his suicidal intent returns with a vengeance and the sound of a gunshot.

Lost Data for the Receiving Clinician

A clinician who helps a patient to open up about suicidal ideation and who uses effective interviewing techniques, such as the CASE Approach, may have an unusually good opportunity to obtain an accurate picture of both stated and reflected intent during the initial interview. The patient may be affectively charged at the time of presentation and such emotional turmoil may make the patient's unconscious and conscious defenses less active so that it is easier for the truth to emerge.

It is of great value for a triage clinician, such as a school counselor, primary care clinician, or crisis line counselor, to gather as much information as possible at this time, because during the trip to the ED a surprising number of patients undergo a miraculous "transportation cure." In short, by the time the reach the ED or the therapist's office the next day, they clam up. It is important for professional gatekeepers to gather as much information as possible regarding reflected intent, because the receiving mental health professional, whether in an emergency room later that night or in a community mental health center 2 days later, may be dependent upon this relayed information for making a formulation of risk.

The Power of a Thorough Elicitation of Suicidal Ideation, Behavior, and Intent to Save a Life

The Issue of Credibility

Especially in situations in which the patient is not known to the interviewer, such as may occur in emergency rooms and during consultation and liaison assessments following a suicide attempt, a determination of the credibility of the patient's self-report is of vital importance. In such situations, one can compare the validity of what is being reported to what has been documented in the past. Although previous charts are not always available (electronic records may diminish this problem), when they are, information documented on reflected intent may be invaluable in assessing the reliability of the patient's current self-reporting.

A marked discrepancy between what the patient reports about past suicidal ideation and what is actually documented may be the best indicator that the patient is (or is not) telling the truth. Such a contradiction may guide the clinician to seek corroborative sources of information and/or to discuss the discrepancies with the patient. It also emphasizes the need to re-evaluate the patient's immediate safety.

Reaching for Life

Regarding future safety, the act of eliciting a thorough database on suicidal ideation and actions may be of value not only in the content of the database obtained, but in the therapeutic fashion in which this information is garnered. Clinicians who have been trained to use an engaging strategy for eliciting suicidal ideation, such as the CASE Approach, may often create a positive interpersonal experience during the initial assessment. Such a patient may remember the sense of safety and comfort he felt openly talking with this clinician who neither over-reacted nor under-reacted to the patient's description of his suicidal thought. If, in the future, the same patient becomes dangerously suicidal – and is debating whether to call for help or proceed with the attempt – the patient may decide to reach for the phone rather than a gun.

3. Setting the Platform for the Suicide Inquiry

It is clear from the above discussion why it is important to elicit a valid and comprehensive database regarding suicidal ideation, planning, and behaviors, all of which may provide the clearest reflection of the patient's real intent. Now we can begin our exploration of how to do so effectively, a process that begins by setting the platform for the inquiry.

Suicide remains one of the most taboo of all subjects and people can have significant feelings of shame and guilt about having ideas of killing themselves. Consequently, it becomes critical that clinicians time their inquiry in such a way as to maximize the likelihood of uncovering the intimate thoughts of the patient regarding their suicidal intent in a sensitive fashion. Many a clinician has "lost the truth" through the poor timing of the inquiry, sometimes resulting in the permanent loss of engagement as well.

Perhaps the single most common timing problem is asking about suicide too early in the interview. This is sometimes caused by the interviewer's "need to know" or the desire to "get the tough questions out of the way." Such premature inquiry regarding such a critically sensitive topic can be off-putting, disengaging, and artificial sounding; it may lead to a significant breakdown in the alliance with a potentially dangerous loss of valid information and of willingness to collaborate with subsequent recommendations for safety and follow-up.

The "Elicitation of Suicidal Ideation Triad"

The optimum time for raising the topic of suicide can be conceptualized as the intersection of three factors: (1) the presence of sound engagement, (2) the presence of intense emotional/affective discharge in the patient, and (3) the patient hints at the topic (a factor that is not always present). Let's look at each of these in more detail.

Step 1 of the Elicitation Triad: Enhancing Engagement With a Potentially Suicidal Patient

Because people are much more likely to share sensitive material with someone with whom they feel comfortable talking, if the interviewer chooses to be the first to raise the subject of suicide, it is generally best to wait to do so until engagement is maximized. Such patience can significantly enhance the likelihood that the patient will share openly. Naturally, such maximization of engagement takes time, frequently occurring fairly deep into the interview, after the patient has had the chance to interface in an engaging fashion with the clinician on a variety of other topics such as the presenting crisis, stressors, painful symptoms, etc.

Sometimes in phone interventions, the inquiry occurs even later than with face-to-face interventions, because communication of factors such as empathy, as the noted social scientist Edward T. Hall commented (see Chapter 8), are often primarily conveyed by nonverbal cues and cultural rhythms rather than the words we speak. The lack of many nonverbal communicators puts telephone clinicians at a distinct disadvantage in creating rapid alliances compared to face-to-face interviewers (a single warm smile may communicate more empathy than a dozen empathic statements over a phone).

Step 2 of the Elicitation Triad: Helping the Potentially Suicidal Patient to Share Highly Charged Emotional States

To better prepare the patient to openly share suicidal ideation, the interviewer attempts to create an atmosphere in which the patient feels optimally safe and unguarded. If one reflects upon it, the most conducive atmosphere is probably a rather unusual state. In this state, the patient should feel maximally safe with the interviewer while being intensively involved, psychologically, with the painful emotion that is pulling the patient towards suicide. I have found that the presence of intense emotional involvement usually tends to lower both unconscious and conscious defenses, thus increasing the likelihood that suicidal ideation will be shared.

More specifically with regard to timing, it is useful to raise the topic of suicidal ideation during a point in the conversation in which the patient is experiencing and expressing significant emotional pain. At such moments of intense affective discharge, the defense mechanisms and prohibitions regarding stigmatization are often overwhelmed by the pain, once again resulting in a more open sharing of the extent of suicidal ideation and intent. Patients will often spontaneously enter these areas of intense involvement; but at other times, the interviewer must skillfully create gateways that lead them there.

Three Gateways to Suicidal Ideation

There appear to be three primary affectively charged gateways that lead people toward sharing their thoughts of suicide. These gates are: (1) depression, anxiety, and hopelessness, (2) a sense of turmoil, anger, or confusion over a situational/interpersonal stress, and (3) psychotic process (less common but critical when present). Generally speaking, it pays the interviewer to refrain from asking about suicidal ideation until the patient is obviously emotionally involved in one of these three areas. The clinician does not pop the question to the patient; the clinician leads up to it.

If the interviewer suspects that the patient has been depressed, then the interviewer may wait to inquire about suicide until the patient gives evidence of being involved in intense depressive affect by tone of voice, depressive sighing, and/or tearfulness. In some cases, the interviewer may need to gently lead the patient into these areas, because the patient may be using denial or other mechanisms to avoid such painful affect.

This principle of guiding the patient towards emotional involvement also applies to the second gate, in which the patient contemplates suicide secondary to some specific situational/interpersonal turmoil. Sensitively setting the stage by allowing the patient to ventilate their immediate stressors – whether a divorce, financial catastrophe, death of a loved one, or medical illness – also provides the interviewer with the time needed to better establish an enhanced degree of blending with the patient. This time devoted to engagement is time well spent, for it will further increase the likelihood of eliciting valid information about the patient's suicidal intent. Generally, this evolving process reaches a peak somewhere in the middle of the interview.

With regard to psychotic gateways, we can return to the first clinical presentation we used in this chapter: Michael, the psychotic young man who cryptically commented, "It all comes down to the way the clouds kiss the moon." As you will recall, Michael, at first, essentially denied suicidal ideation, refusing to elaborate on the subject. Perhaps the stage for sharing had not been adequately set.

In contrast, in the clinician's second interview with Michael, the clinician sensitively entered the gateway provided by Michael's psychotic process. As the interviewing dyad entered the world of Michael's psychotic anguish, Michael's affective involvement became more intense, leading to an increased desire to relieve his pain by sharing his burdens with a compassionate listener. Obviously, for this process to be effective, the interviewer must have previously decreased the patient's initial paranoia. Consequently, at this delicate point when secrets are shared, the interviewer will be perceived as an ally worthy of such trust.

With regard to psychosis, such well-timed focusing upon affectively charged content may naturally lead the patient into a mildly dissociated state, in which conscious and unconscious defenses are diminished, with direct questions often yielding surprisingly direct answers. Processes mentioned earlier, such as command hallucinations, alien control, and hyper-religiosity, may be described more openly by the patient at these times. In essence, the interviewer has created a powerful gateway through which to enter the realm of suicidal ideation.

Before leaving the creation of gateways for allowing patients to share highly charged material, two other technical points should be mentioned. First, if one gate fails, then the interviewer can try a different gate. For instance, the interviewer may hit denial of suicidal intent when flowing with depressive ideation in a man with a psychotic depression. If approached by the gate of psychosis, this same man may admit to suicidal ideation.

Second, some interviewers may initially approach suicidality with a mildly ambiguous question that invites the interviewee to discuss suicidal ideation without spelling it out.

Such questions as, "Have you ever thought of a way of ending your pain?" or "Have you ever wished that you could go to sleep and never wake up?" can be effective indirect gateways to suicidal thought. *If the patient does not follow this type of lead, the clinician must always ask directly about suicide* as described earlier. This technique may be of value in patients who appear exceptionally anxious about being interviewed, thus providing a back door through which the patient may feel more comfortable about entering a discussion of suicide, as follows:

Pt.:	Nothing seems to matter much anymore and everything seems wrong.
Clin.:	How do you mean?
Pt.:	I can't sleep, I can't eat, and every minute seems worse than the one before. I'm not kidding when I say I feel miserable.
Clin.:	Have you ever thought of a way of ending your pain?
Pt.:	Yes, yes I have … I thought of blowing my brains out (nervous laughter), but that's a little messy.
Clin.:	Sounds scary.
Pt.:	Yes it is.
Clin.:	Do you have a gun in the house?
Pt.:	Yes I do … beside my bed.

As we shall soon see, such indirect methods of raising the topic of suicide are often not necessary, for there exist a variety of effective and sensitive direct methods that leave no possibility for miscommunication about what is being asked.

Step 3 of the Elicitation Triad: The Patient Hints at Suicide or Raises the Topic Spontaneously

Although not always present, a third indicator of an excellent time to raise the topic is if the patient not only is engaged and affectively charged but also hints at the possibility of suicide with comments such as, "I'm not even sure whether it is worth going on," or "Maybe my kids would be better off without me." Obviously, the timing of raising the topic of suicide is unique to each patient and should never be approached in a cookbook fashion at a pre-designated time of the interview.

Sometimes an interviewee will hint at suicidal ideation late in the scouting phase or early in the body of the interview. Such hints suggest that the stage may already be set and that the patient is ready to share. If spontaneous gates appear, they should generally be pursued by the interviewer, as follows:

Pt.:	My life is very different for me now. Over the past several years it seems to have gone empty.
Clin.:	How do you mean?
Pt.:	After the divorce I was on automatic pilot, but eventually it all sunk in, it all seemed horribly empty, not worth continuing, much as it seems now. But I have managed and have had some brighter days.

> **Clin.:** When you say, it seemed not worth continuing, did you have any thoughts of killing yourself?
>
> **Pt.:** Yes … and I still do.
>
> **Clin.:** What kinds of things have you thought of doing?
>
> **Pt.:** I thought of taking pills and I did that once …

If the clinician does not pick up on such nuances by referring to them directly, the conversation can quickly move to new topics. If this movement occurs, the clinician may have missed the most opportune spot for inquiry. By bringing up such thoughts, the metacommunication of the patient seems to be a simple one, "Ask me about suicide." When given such an open gate, it seems unwise to walk by it. By not following up, the interviewer may discover that later on, due to an unexpected problem with engagement, the interviewee will no longer feel comfortable about sharing. The suicidal ideation will remain unspoken; a most deadly situation.

On the other hand, if a patient *unknown to the interviewer* immediately opens an interview or a crisis call with a statement about suicide, I have found it wise to acknowledge the statement and my concerns about it, but postpone a more active exploration of suicidal ideation and planning until a later moment in the interview (at which point I will have had the chance to shore up the engagement to maximize the likelihood of uncovering the truth). A statement such as the following can be used:

"I'm really glad that you called, Mr. Jackson. This was the right number to call. I'd like to help you with your suicidal thoughts. Perhaps we could start with you telling me a little bit about what you've been going through and what kinds of stresses have led you to have thoughts of killing yourself."

As the interviewer proceeds to sensitively explore the patient's stresses and pain, the engagement process often greatly accelerates, reaching a point where the patient is more likely to truthfully share the details of his or her suicidal thoughts and plans. When engagement has been optimized, the interviewer can sensitively raise the topic using a referred gate as follows, "Earlier you had mentioned that you were having thoughts of killing yourself. What kinds of thoughts have you been having?"

At this point in our discussion, it is time to look at the actual exploration of the patient's suicidal ideation, the exploration of which is both a delicate and complex art.

4. Eliciting Suicidal Ideation, Planning, and Intent Using the Chronological Assessment of Suicide Events (CASE Approach)

Background, Rationale, and Limitations

When one reviews the enormous body of literature on suicide assessment, one is first struck by the great number of studies, scales, papers, and books. The second striking finding is the relative lack of writing about the practical aspects of "how to do the interview." The vast majority of the writings focus on such topics as risk factors, warning signs, and the clinical judgment process itself, which are all very important. However, one critically important subject is often given short shrift.

Few resources, other than some of the excellent research on semi-structured interviews and patient self-reporting of suicidal intent, focus upon the second aspect of data gathering – arguably the most important one – how does one go about effectively uncovering the patient's unique suicidal ideation, planning, actions, and intent? More specifically, was the necessary material gathered and was it gathered in a way that maximized both engagement and validity? During a suicide assessment, one can ask for all the "right data," but if it is invalid data, one might as well not be asking. In the last analysis, the cornerstone of all suicide assessments is the degree to which the clinician's interview style leads to the highest level of truthfulness from the patient. In other words, to what degree does this person, contemplating death by his or her own hands, let us into his or her secret world? The stakes are high.

As with the earlier writings and presentations on the CASE Approach,[79-92] which was first introduced in the second edition of this book and subsequently described in a variety of clinical settings ranging from college counseling centers and substance abuse clinics to the military and correctional facilities, primary care clinics, emergency rooms, and general mental health centers, the rest of this section will address this relative void in the literature on the art of eliciting suicidal ideation. I have become convinced over the years that errors in clinical risk assessment frequently do not arise from poor clinical reasoning. They often arise from sound clinical reasoning that, unfortunately, was based upon a poor clinical database.

In my opinion, the two biggest errors in eliciting suicidal ideation tend to be errors of omission (involving critical data related to the patient's suicidal ideation, planning, actions, and intent) and errors in which the interviewer's style of questioning or engagement resulted in the patient providing misleading information regarding these very same highly sensitive areas.

The reason interviewers make these mistakes, and I make them too, is quite easy to see. Complicated suicide assessments have a way of occurring at complicated times. They often happen in the middle of an extremely hectic clinic day or in the chaotic environment of a packed emergency room. In these days of managed care, time pressures, and waiting lists, clinicians often find themselves in the unenviable position of feeling that there is not enough time to do anything well. However, a suicide assessment must always be done well. A mistake can result in an unnecessary death and a terrible tragedy. It can also result in a lawsuit, which is much less important, but very disturbing in its own right.

Thus in many suicide assessment scenarios, we find a harried clinician, performing an extremely pressured task, in an unforgiving atmosphere. No wonder mistakes are made. Under such difficult clinical conditions, it is very easy to see and understand why we may make mistakes such as unintentionally forgetting to ask for important data. The truth is that we always will make such mistakes, because we are only human. However, the question is, "Are there techniques and strategies that can greatly diminish the likelihood of such mistakes?" I think that there are.

I believe that the trick lies in developing a flexible but consistent approach to exploring suicidal ideation and in practicing this approach until it becomes second nature, much like a martial artist practices a series of attack and defense movements, called *katas*, over and over again until they become so natural that they are "instinctive." At this point, the movements have become gateways to intuition and, more important, they will be there when the martial artist most needs them: when the martial artist is tired, distressed, feeling beaten or, possibly, even fighting for his or her life. That is exactly what we want as clinicians – a set of graceful and reliable interviewing techniques that will reliably be there when we most need them, no matter how tired we are or how hectic the crisis situation.

Designed specifically to address the above concerns, the CASE Approach is a flexible, practical, and easily learned interviewing strategy for eliciting suicidal ideation, planning, behavior, desire, and intent. It is not presented as the right way to elicit suicidal ideation or as a standard of care, but as a reasonable way that can help clinicians develop their own way. From an understanding of the CASE Approach, clinicians can directly adopt what they like, reject what they do not like, and add new ideas.

Specific interviewing techniques and strategies from the CASE Approach can be used and/or adapted to any suicide assessment protocol the clinician deems useful, from a totally personalized protocol to more formal protocols like the Collaborative Assessment and Management of Suicidality (CAMS) of Jobes.[93] It can be used to help generate a valid database that can be subsequently entered into the predictive engines of semi-structured interviews such as the Columbia Suicide Severity Rating Scale[94] at moments when the interpersonal process of semi-structured interviewing may not be effective or indicated.

The goal of the CASE Approach is to provide clinicians with a practical framework for exploring and better understanding how they uncover suicidal ideation, no matter what suicide assessment protocol or style of clinical formulation they ultimately want to use. In such a fashion, the clinician can develop an individualized approach with which they personally feel comfortable and competent.

Note that the CASE Approach complements, not replaces, the two other critical components of a sound suicide assessment protocol delineated earlier in this chapter (the interviewing process of gathering risk factors and the cognitive/intuitive process of subsequently formulating risk). The CASE Approach is not a method of gathering information about the risk factors and warning signs; *that information must be gathered in other regions of the same interview,* either before one employs the CASE Approach or afterwards (or some before and some afterwards). It is also not a cognitive algorithm for determining a clinical formulation of risk. Indeed, the CASE Approach says nothing about the process of clinical formulation.

The CASE Approach *solely* addresses the complex interviewing task of uncovering the patient's suicidal ideation, planning, behaviors, and intent in such a fashion that the very best and most accurate information on this highly sensitive material can be delineated. The resulting phenomenological picture of the patient's suicidal ideation, planning, and actual intent can then be used in conjunction with the risk factors, warning signs, and protective factors to begin the cognitive/intuitive process of determining clinical risk.

The Question of Validity: Its Central Role in the CASE Approach

Validity is the cornerstone of suicide assessment. Nothing more directly determines the effectiveness of the interviewer in gathering information that may forewarn of dangerousness. If the patient does not invite the clinician into the intimate details of his or her suicidal planning, the best clinician in the world, armed with the best risk factor analysis available, will be limited in his or her ability to determine whether the patient is at acute, high risk.

Two elements are critical for enhancing validity, both of which we have already emphasized in previous chapters: (1) the therapeutic alliance should be as robust as possible, and (2) the interviewer can intentionally and flexibly utilize specific validity techniques such as those delineated in Chapter 5.

With regard to the former element, unless the interviewer has actively and effectively engaged the patient in the interview process preceding the elicitation of suicidal ideation – and during it – it is unlikely that the use of validity techniques will be particularly effective or that the truth will be uncovered. *Thus, empathic connection and compassion are the two foundation stones of any successful elicitation of suicidal ideation and intent.* Towards this end, all of the engagement techniques discussed previously in our book are pivotal aspects of a successful exploration of suicidal thought and planning.

Here the innovative work of David Jobes and the CAMS, referenced above, is well worth emphasizing. The CAMS is an integrated approach to providing sound collaborative suicide assessment and intervention during ongoing therapy. Indeed, its sophistication and power of engagement move the CAMS from pure assessment into the realm of therapy itself, and I urge you to familiarize yourself with its techniques. Born from a cognitive therapeutic perspective, the CAMS uses a set of structured assessment tools and a well systematized approach to provide ongoing monitoring of suicidal intent, while simultaneously providing an avenue for communicating positive re-enforcement for effective control of suicidal thought. Jobes has designed the CAMS so that clinicians can flexibly use bits of the approach or utilize it with full implementation as seems to best suit the needs of the patient.

For us, the most telling principle of the CAMS, as fits our chapter here, is the concept of collaborative interviewing. Both the CAMS and the CASE Approach are collaborative interviewing strategies. As Jobes emphasizes, patients will relay the truth – and be more open to sharing the depth of their suicidal angst and the proximity of their intention to act on that angst – in direct proportion to the degree that they feel the interviewer is listening with a compassionate ear and without judgment. In this sense, we want to communicate to our patient that we are working as a collaborative team to explore their suicidal thoughts, including reasons to live and reasons to die, in an effort to find hope and relief.

Having ensured the engagement process and communicated a collaborative, non-judgmental attitude towards the patient's feelings and perspectives, we are then better able to employ the second, extremely valuable element for enhancing validity – the intentional use of validity techniques and interviewing strategies as delineated in the CASE Approach.

At this point, it may be beneficial to review the seven validity techniques utilized in the CASE Approach. The first step is to raise the topic of suicide in a sensitive fashion while maintaining engagement.

Two Validity Techniques for Sensitively Raising the Topic of Suicide

Normalization

A valuable interviewing principle to employ before raising sensitive or taboo topics is to metacommunicate to the patient that it is safe to discuss the topic. Two different interviewing techniques come to mind that employ this principle effectively.

As you will recall from Chapter 5 (see pages 159–161) normalization, first introduced in the second edition of this book, is the simple, yet effective, technique in which the clinician begins a question by suggesting that he or she has heard the behavior in question from other patients, metacommunicating that the patient is far from alone in having experienced this feeling or behavior. Normalizations often, but not always, begin with words such as, "Sometimes people who have ..." Outside of the topic of suicide, a typical normalization may sound like this: "Sometimes when people get really angry they say things they later regret, has that ever happened to you?" One can see how normalizations can foster a safe environment for patients to share delicate information.

With regard to raising the topic of suicide, I have found the following normalization to be quite effective:

"Sometimes when people are in a tremendous amount of pain, they find themselves having thoughts of killing themselves. Have you been having any thoughts like that?"

or

"Sometimes when people are going through very difficult times like you are, they find themselves having thoughts of killing themselves. Have you been having any thoughts like that?"

Clinicians can use numerous variations of normalization to raise the topic of suicide depending upon specific situational stresses that may be prompting suicidal ideation, as with:

"Sometimes when people lose a spouse they loved as much as you loved Anna, they have thoughts of killing themselves, have you been having any thoughts like that?"

Rudd suggests that the following normalization can be used as a lead-in to raising the topic of suicide: "It's not unusual for someone that is depressed to feel hopeless and have thoughts about death or dying."[95] From this lead-in, one can follow with, "Have you been having any thoughts about killing yourself?"

Other common phrases used to begin normalizations include:

a. "It is not uncommon for people who ..."
b. "Many of my patients have told me that when they are ..."
c. "Patients often tell me that when they are as depressed they ..."

Shame Attenuation

With shame attenuation (see pages 160–164 for in-depth discussion), also introduced in the second edition of this book, the patient's *own pain* is used as the gateway to sensitive topics such as suicide (note that in the following question there is no mention of any other people, as would be seen when using a normalization). Thus the interviewer is indicating that it is safe to discuss the taboo topic by metacommunicating that, "I get it, I get how much pain you are in, and I understand why you might be having the thoughts or feelings that you are having." This metacommunication is simply communicated in practice with questions such as the following:

"With everything you're going through, have you been having any thoughts of killing yourself?"

or

"With all of your pain, have you been having any thoughts of killing yourself?"

You will note that these two shame attenuations have a subtle difference between them. This difference may have implications on when to use each. I have found the first shame attenuation (which emphasizes the patient's current situational stresses) to be particularly useful with patients who – earlier in the interview – have related a series of stresses as being the main trigger for seeking help. In contrast, when interviewing a patient who has been suffering from a major psychiatric disorder such as schizophrenia, bipolar disorder, or post-traumatic stress disorder for years, I find that these patients frequently powerfully identify with the word "pain" and have, indeed, contemplated suicide not so much as a response to current stressors but as a release from the chronic pain caused by these disorders.

Shame attenuations are very simple and somewhat less wordy than most normalizations. This technique can be used for raising the topic of suicide (and many other sensitive topics) with just about any patient in a wide range of circumstances.

A Note on Word Choice: "Killing Yourself" Versus "Committing Suicide"

You will notice that in the examples of both normalization and shame attenuation I used the words "killing yourself." If a clinician feels more comfortable substituting words such as "thinking of suicide" or "taking your life" when using normalization or shame attenuation, they should feel free to do so, for they are equally direct. All of these phrases are good at avoiding the confusion that can arise when clinicians raise the topic of suicide with more nebulous words such as, "have you thought of hurting yourself?" that a patient may interpret as an inquiry into non-lethal methods of self-harm (such as self-cutting or burning oneself).

My own preference is to use the words "killing yourself," for I feel that when the idea of suicide enters the mind of a person for the very first time, it probably doesn't enter with relatively sophisticated phrases such as "Maybe I should take my own life," or "Maybe I should commit suicide." I think it is more likely that most people matter-of-factly say to themselves things like, "Maybe I should just kill myself."

In addition, there is another reason that I don't recommend using the word "commit." I believe that in many cultures the word "commit" carries a pejorative connotation, as with "committing a crime," "committing a sin," or "committing adultery." Consequently, I like to phrase the question with the same words that I think the patient is more likely to have used – for it may resonate more empathically in that fashion – as well as avoiding the potential stigmatization associated with words such as "commit."

If the patient denies any suicidal ideation, I often inquire a second time, softening the second inquiry by asking for even subtle suicidal ideation, "Have you had any fleeting thoughts of killing yourself, even for a moment or two?" Sometimes the answer is surprising, and it may prompt hesitant patients to begin sharing the depth of their pain and the extent of their ideation.

Five Validity Techniques Used to Explore the Extent of Suicidal Ideation

Behavioral Incident

A patient may provide distorted information for any number of reasons, including anxiety, embarrassment, protecting family secrets, cultural norms, unconscious defense mechanisms, or conscious attempts at deception. These distortions are more likely to appear if the interviewer asks a patient for opinions rather than behavioral descriptions of events.

As we discussed in Chapter 5 (see pages 165–170), behavioral incidents, originally delineated by Gerald Pascal, are questions that build a picture of specific events. They may be questions that ask for specific facts, behavioral details, or thoughts (called fact-finding behavioral incidents), such as, "How many pills did you take?", "Did you put the razor blade up to your wrist?", or "How many pill bottles did you actually store up?" Alternatively, they may be questions that simply ask the patient what happened sequentially (called sequencing behavioral incidents), such as, "What did you do right after you took the pills?" As we shall soon see, by using a series of behavioral incidents, the interviewer can sometimes help a patient enhance validity by re-creating, step by step, the unfolding of a potentially taboo topic such as a suicide attempt.

As Pascal states, it is generally best for clinicians to make their own clinical judgments on the basis of the details of the story itself, rather than relying on patients to provide "objective opinions" on matters that have strong subjective implications.

Gentle Assumption

Gentle assumption (see pages 170–171) – originally defined by Pomeroy and colleagues for use in eliciting a valid sex history – is used when a clinician suspects that a patient may be hesitant to discuss a taboo behavior. With gentle assumption, the clinician assumes that the potentially embarrassing or incriminating behavior is occurring and frames his or her question accordingly, in a gentle tone of voice. Questions about sexual history, such as, "What do you experience when you masturbate?" or "How frequently do you find yourself masturbating?" have been found to be much more likely to yield valid answers than, "Do you masturbate?" If the clinician is concerned that the patient may be potentially disconcerted by the assumptive nature of the question, it can be further softened by adding the phrase "if at all" (e.g., "How often do you find yourself masturbating, if at all?"). If engagement has gone well and a gentle, non-accusatory tone of voice is used, patients are rarely bothered by gentle assumptions.

In eliciting suicidal ideation, gentle assumption is used at a specific juncture. After the patient's first method of suicide has been thoroughly explored by the clinician, gentle assumption is used to search for other methods of suicide (keeping in mind that a dangerous patient may not have mentioned his or her "method of choice" when first asked about suicide). In this regard, I have found the simplest of the gentle assumptions to be quite useful, as with:

"What other ways have you thought of killing yourself?"

Denial of the Specific

After a patient responds with words such as "no other ways" or "none" to a gentle assumption, it is surprising how many other methods will be uncovered if the patient is asked a series of questions about specific entities. As we discussed in Chapter 5 (see pages 171–173), this technique appears to jog the memory, and it also appears to be harder to falsely deny a specific question as opposed to a more generic question such as a gentle assumption. Examples of denial of the specific concerning drug use would be: "Have you ever tried crystal meth?", "Have you ever smoked crack?", and "Have you ever dropped acid, even once?"

With regard to suicide, even after gentle assumptions have been used, some patients (especially patients who strongly want to die) may still have withheld their methods of choice for fear they may be removed from their possession. Sometimes, if engagement has been carefully nurtured, they may share the method of choice following the clinician's sensitive use of a denial of the specific. The following are prototypes of denial of the specific with suicide:

"Have you been having any thoughts of shooting yourself?"

"Have you been having any thoughts of overdosing?"

"Have you been having any thoughts of hanging yourself?"

"Have you been having any thoughts of jumping off a bridge or one of the buildings on campus?"

Clinical caveat: It is important to frame each denial of the specific as a separate question, pausing between each inquiry and waiting for the patient's denial or admission before asking the next question. The clinician should avoid combining the inquiries into a single question, such as, "Have you been having any thoughts of shooting yourself, overdosing, or hanging yourself?" A series of items combined in this way is called a "cannon question."

Such cannon questions frequently lead to invalid information because patients only hear parts of them or choose to respond to only one item in the string – often the last item. In addition, when used correctly – one at a time, waiting for the patient's response before using the next denial of the specific – a savvy clinician is looking for nonverbal signs of deceit. If a cannon question is used, the patient only needs to lie once. But if a series of denials of the specific is utilized, the patient may have to lie repeatedly. Each lie provides the clinician with a chance to spot the nonverbal indicators that truth is hiding. *Also note, when used to uncover suicidal ideation, denials of the specific are only utilized if the clinician suspects that the patient is withholding a suicidal plan.* The resulting, previously withheld, plan might even turn out to be the patient's method of choice.

Catch-All Question

The catch-all question (see page 173) allows an interviewer to unobtrusively see "if something has been missed" by literally asking if such is the case. It is useful in many situations involving sensitive material, including those areas that may generate suicidal thought:

1. "We've talked about a lot of different things that you've been concerned about your son doing at school; do you have any other concerns that we haven't had a chance to talk about yet?"
2. "Are there any other bad experiences you had in Iraq, perhaps even with fellow soldiers, that we haven't talked about yet?" (may uncover sexual assault)

Concerning suicidal ideation itself, the catch-all question can be worded as follows:

"We've been talking about a lot of different ways you've been thinking about killing yourself; are there any ways you've thought about, that we haven't talked about yet?"

The answers are sometimes surprising.

Symptom Amplification

As you will recall from Chapter 5 (see pages 173–174), this technique is based on the observation that patients often minimize the frequency or amount of their disturbing behaviors, such as the amount they drink or gamble. Symptom amplification bypasses this minimizing mechanism: It sets the upper limits of the quantity in the question at such a high level that the clinician is still aware that there is a significant problem even when the patient downplays the amount. For instance, when a clinician asks a patient who abuses hard liquor, "How much can you hold in a single night … a pint, a fifth?" and a minimizing patient responds, "Oh no, not a fifth, I don't know, maybe a pint pretty easily," the clinician is still alerted that there is a problem despite the patient's minimizations.

The beauty of the technique lies in the fact that it avoids the creation of a confrontational atmosphere, even though the patient is minimizing behavior. *To be viewed as symptom amplification, the interviewer must always suggest an ascending series of numbers that begin at a high number and go even higher.* It is also worth repeating that symptom amplification is used in an effort to determine an actual quantity and it is *only* used if the clinician suspects that the patient is about to minimize.

With regard to uncovering suicidal ideation, we will find this technique to be invaluable in uncovering how much time a patient is preoccupied with suicidal thoughts and urges. Symptom amplifications with regard to suicidal thought can be phrased in a variety of ways, always fashioning the words to the unique cultural and intellectual characteristics of the patient. I find the following phrasing useful with patients who have been lucky enough to receive a higher education:

"On your very worst days, how much time do you spend thinking about killing yourself: 70% of your waking hours, 80% of your waking hours, 90%?"

On the other hand, this phrasing may be problematic with patients who have done poorly or dropped out of middle or high school, for such patients may not be accustomed to using percentages. Instead, the symptom amplification can be made more effective by switching to something more concrete, as with a reference to hours:

"On your very worst days, how much time do you spend thinking about killing yourself: 10 hours a day, 14 hours a day, 18 hours a day?"

As we have seen repeatedly in this book, flexibility is the name of the game, sculpting questions to suit the unique qualities, perspectives, and cultural characteristics of the patient.

The Macrostructure of the CASE Approach: Avoiding Errors of Omission

As I mentioned earlier, besides recovering invalid data (a problem the validity techniques attempt to address), the other major problem for front-line clinicians when uncovering suicidal ideation is making errors of omission. Two questions are of immediate relevance: (1) Why do interviewers frequently miss important data while eliciting suicidal ideation, and (2) Is there a way to decrease errors of omission?

To find our answers to these questions, we only need return to our understanding of facilics, as described in Chapter 4. You will recall that according to facilic principles, clinicians tend to make more errors of omission as the amount and range of required data increases. Errors of omission decrease if the clinician can split a large amount of data into smaller, well-defined regions. With such well-defined and limited data regions, the interviewer can more easily recognize when a patient has wandered from the subject. The clinician is also more apt to easily track whether the desired inquiry has been completed and does not feel as overwhelmed by the interview process.

Earlier in this book, we saw how facilic principles can provide a powerful framework for sensitively structuring the entire initial assessment. We will now see how facilic principles can help the clinician to creatively and flexibly structure specific data regions within that interview, a process that can dramatically decrease errors of omission while enhancing engagement. Once again, the goal is to create a conversational feeling in the patient as one is exploring suicidal thought, as opposed to an artificial sensation that one is "being interviewed."

Facilic principles are applied to the elicitation of suicidal ideation by organizing the sprawling set of clinically relevant questions into four smaller and more manageable regions. The regions represent four contiguous timeframes from the distant past to the present, hence the name "chronological." In each region, the clinician investigates the suicidal ideation and actions present during that specific timeframe. Generally, each region is explored thoroughly before moving to the next; the clinician consciously chooses not to move with a patient's tangential wandering unless there is a very good reason to do so. In the description below, the term "suicide events" can include any of the following: death wishes, suicidal feelings and thoughts, planning, behaviors, desire, and intent.

Although mentioned earlier, I believe it is important to emphasize the following point. Before using the CASE Approach in the interview (and while using it), it is critical that the interviewer has been maximizing the therapeutic alliance with the techniques and strategies delineated in Part I of this book. Engagement. Engagement. Engagement. These are the three most important factors at play in a suicide assessment.

In the CASE Approach, the interviewer sequentially explores the following four chronological regions in this order (Figure 17.1):

1. Presenting suicide events (often falling within the past 48 hours or several weeks)
2. Recent suicide events (over the preceding 2 months)
3. Past suicide events (from 2 months ago back in time)
4. Immediate suicide events (suicidal feelings, ideation, and intent that arise *during the interview itself*)

The sequencing of the regions was specifically designed to maximize both engagement and the validity of the obtained data. For many patients, once the topic of suicide has been raised, it seems natural to talk about the presenting ideation or attempt, if one exists, first. Following this exploration, it is easy for the interviewer to make a natural progression into recent ideation followed by past suicide events.

When performed sensitively by the interviewer, explorations of the three timeframes that occurred before the interview generally improve both engagement and trust as the patient realizes that it is safe to talk about suicidal ideation. Once trust has been maximized, it is hoped that this positive alliance will increase the likelihood of the patient sharing valid information. It is then an opportune time to explore suicidal ideation and intentions that are being experienced by the patient *during the interview itself* (the region of immediate suicide events), a critically important area of a suicide assessment.

For instance, a patient about to go on a pass from an inpatient unit may be planning to commit suicide. During the interviews directly preceding the pass, such a patient may be having suicidal thoughts such as, "Don't give it away. Just look fine. Get home. Get the gun. Just get home. Get the gun." Here, the most subtle nuances of facial expression or hesitancy of speech may indicate that a dangerous suicide plan is being withheld.

The Microstructure of the CASE Approach: Exploring the Four Specific Timeframes

Step 1: The Exploration of Presenting Suicide Events

Whether the patient spontaneously raises the topic of suicide, or the topic is sensitively uncovered with techniques such as normalization or shame attenuation, the subsequent ideations, plans, and actions revealed by the patient are called "presenting events," in the sense that this is the suicidal ideation that the patient *presents* when the topic of suicide is broached. Such presenting suicide events are those ideas, plans or actions that have occurred in the past several days or perhaps couple of weeks. If a patient presents

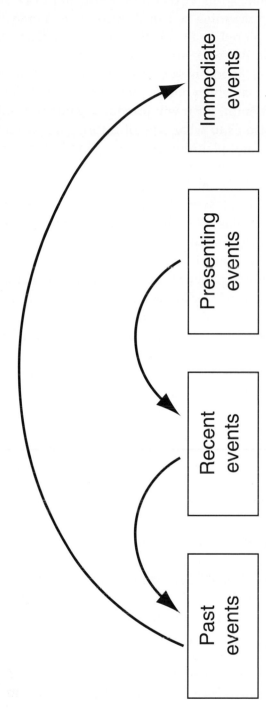

Figure 17.1 Chronological Assessment of Suicide Events (CASE Approach).

with such current suicidal behavior or with pressing suicidal ideation, it becomes critical to understand their severity. Depending upon the severity of the ideation or attempt, the patient may require hospitalization, crisis intervention and/or close follow-up.

Note that the patient's presenting suicide "events" may merely be plans or ideation, but these too must be explored in detail, for they may reflect the seriousness of the patient's intent to proceed. But what specific information would give the clinician the most accurate picture of the seriousness of presenting suicidal ideation or of an actual suicide attempt? Let us look at which puzzle pieces could be of value in determining the seriousness of an actual attempt, for it will provide a guide not only to the exploration of an attempt itself, but also as to what type of information would be useful to garner regarding suicidal ideation and planning without action having been already taken:

- How did the patient try to attempt suicide? (What method was used?)
- How serious was the action taken with this method? (If the patient overdosed, what pills and how many were taken? If the patient cut himself, where was the cut, and did it require stitches and, if so, how many?)
- How serious were the patient's intentions? (Did the patient tell anyone about the attempt afterwards? Did the patient hint to anyone beforehand, either in direct conversation or indirectly through social media like Facebook, a chat room, or by texting? Did the patient make the attempt in an isolated area or in a place where he was likely to be found? Did the patient write a suicide note, give away prized possessions, or say goodbye to significant others in the days preceding the event? How many pills were left in the bottle? [Note that patients with serious intent may go to great lengths to take as many pills as they can keep down, whereas a patient who has left many pills in the bottle may be reflecting less intent to die.] Another useful question is, "How many pills did you think it would take to kill yourself?")
- How does the patient feel about the fact that the attempt was not completed? (A very good question here is, "What are some of your thoughts about the fact that you are still alive now?")
- Was the attempt well planned or an impulsive act? Did the patient research suicide on the web or in books?
- Did alcohol or drugs play a role in the attempt?
- Were interpersonal factors a major role in the attempt? These factors might include sensations of failure, feelings of being ostracized or unwanted, or the notion of being a burden, and that the world would be better off without the patient. Alternatively, there may be anger towards others (as in a suicide attempt undertaken to make others feel pain or guilt, often a spouse, parent, other family member, friend, or employer).
- Did a specific stressor or set of stressors prompt the attempt?
- At the time of the attempt, how hopeless did the patient feel?
- Why did the attempt fail? (How was the patient found and how did the patient get help?)

Answers to such questions can provide invaluable information regarding how serious the attempt was, reflecting the patient's true intent to die, no matter what the patient's stated intent might be. Moreover, all the statistical risk factors in the world will not tell us if a specific patient intended death during an attempt, but the answers to the above questions may give us a better hint. As we addressed earlier in the chapter – excluding patients who accidentally kill themselves during manipulative gestures – people kill themselves because they have decided to do so. Suicide is not only an emotional act of the heart, it is also a cognitive decision of the mind. The above information can provide us with more direct access into the shadowy recesses of this decision-making process.

If no actual attempt has been made, then it is the reflected intent – the extent of suicidal desire, ideation, planning, and procurement of means – that the clinician will use in the clinical formulation of risk to determine the triage (inpatient versus outpatient) and rapidity of follow-up if outpatient care is recommended. Information uncovered in other parts of the interview regarding risk factors, protective factors, and warning signs is coupled with the above information to make these triage decisions.

The Concept of Creating a Verbal Video

At first glance, especially for a clinician in training, the above list of questions may appear intimidating to remember. Fortunately, one of the validity techniques discussed earlier – Pascal's behavioral incident – can provide the clinician with a simpler and more logical approach than memorization. The reader will recall that behavioral incidents are used when the clinician asks for a specific piece of data (e.g., "Did you put the gun up to your head?") or asks the patient to continue a description of what happened sequentially (e.g., "Tell me what you did next").

In the CASE Approach, during the exploration of the presenting events, the interviewer asks the patient to describe the suicide attempt or ideation itself from beginning to end. During this description, the clinician gently, but persistently, uses a series of behavioral incidents to guide the patient in the creation of a so-called "verbal video" of the attempt, step by step. In essence, as the patient describes the attempt, the clinician should be able to see the attempt unfolding in his or her mind as if watching a streaming video. Readers familiar with cognitive–behavioral therapy (CBT) and dialectical behavioral therapy (DBT) will recognize this strategy as one of the cornerstone assessment tools – often called a behavioral (chain) analysis.

If the patient begins to skip over an important piece of the "video" (I like to refer to such omissions as "Nixon Gaps"), the clinician gently stops the patient and "rewinds the video" by asking the patient to return to where the gap began. The clinician then uses a string of behavioral incidents from that point forward to fill in the gap, until the clinician feels confident that the missing information has been provided.

Let us see the power of this simple interviewing strategy at work. We will join an interview at a point in which the patient, whom we shall call Indira, has just mentioned that she had thought of overdosing:

Clin.:   Indira, with everything you've been going through, have you been having any thoughts of killing yourself? (shame attenuation)

Pt.:   (pauses) Oh, yeah, they come and go.

Clin.: And what have you thought of doing? (fact-finding behavioral incident)

Pt.: Taking a bunch of pills.

Clin.: Did you ever get any pills out while you actually were thinking of overdosing? (fact-finding behavioral incident)

Pt.: Yeah, yeah. Just recently.

Clin.: When was that? (fact-finding behavioral incident)

Pt.: Oh, that was, let's see, that was just about 4 days ago. I'd just come back from work. It was already dark out. I'd been having one of my "rough days."

Clin.: And where were you, Indira, when you actually got the pills out? (fact-finding behavioral incident)

Pt.: I was in the upstairs bathroom (pauses), that's where I keep the pills.

Clin.: Sounds like a rough time. Help me to understand better what exactly happened. So you were in the bathroom, you had the pills out, what happened next? (sequencing behavioral incident)

Pt.: I took a bunch of Benadryl. I sometimes use them to knock myself out at night. I've always been hesitant to use actual sleeping pills because I'm worried I might get hooked on them.

Clin.: And how many pills did you actually take? (fact-finding behavioral incident)

Pt.: Not a lot.

Clin.: Roughly how many? (Clinician wisely uses a behavioral incident to determine what Indira actually means by "not a lot")

Pt.: Oh, I'd say only about five or six.

Clin.: Were there any left in the bottle? (fact-finding behavioral incident)

Pt.: Oh yeah, it was basically full of pills. I'd bought a new bottle at the pharmacy a couple of months before.

Clin.: Had you bought the pills with the idea of using them to kill yourself? (fact-finding behavioral incident)

Pt.: Oh my gosh no! I wasn't even having suicidal thoughts back then.

Clin.: Indira, on that night, did you take any other type of medication or street drug? (fact-finding behavioral incident)

Pt.: Nope, that was it.

Clin.: What happened next? (sequencing behavioral incident)

Pt.: I ended up in the emergency room.

And here we have our first Nixon Gap. Having skillfully used a series of behavioral incidents to create a verbal video, the clinician has a clear rendering of what had happened during the actual overdose. But the clinician has absolutely no idea how Indira got to the emergency room. The clinician will now follow our interviewing principle for transforming Nixon Gaps. She will re-wind the video.

Clin.: Indira, right after you took the Benadryl, what did you do next? (sequencing behavioral incident)

Pt.: Oh, I called my sister.

Clin.: And what did you say to her? (sequencing behavioral incident)

Pt.: (pauses, looks a bit sheepish) I told her I did something stupid, that I took some pills I shouldn't have taken and would she mind taking me down to the emergency room.

> Clin.: And what happened next? (sequencing behavioral incident)
>
> Pt.: Like the good sister she is, she took me right down to the emergency room. (pauses) … Thank the gods.

The interviewer, by re-winding the video in response to a missing sequential bit of data, has uncovered a vital piece of the puzzle. It is a piece of the puzzle that might otherwise have been missed in the hectic pace of a busy emergency room with five patients backed up waiting to be seen. And it is a piece of the puzzle that reflects less intent to die from Indira, a piece of the puzzle that might help to prevent an unnecessary hospitalization. The quickness with which Indira called her sister, the small number of pills ingested, and the large number of pills left untouched all point towards a lower level of intended lethality. From this excerpt, we can see how the simple strategy of creating a verbal video and re-winding it – if pieces are missing – provides a valuable method for gathering important elements of reflected intent that can be subsequently used in the clinical formulation of risk.

More Tips on Making a Verbal Video With Behavioral Incidents

This sequential use of behavioral incidents not only increases the clinician's understanding of the extent of the patient's intent and actions, it also decreases any unwarranted assumptions by the clinician that may distort the database. Creating such a verbal video, the clinician will frequently cover all of the material described above in a naturally unfolding conversational mode, without much need for memorization of what questions to ask when.

The serial use of behavioral incidents can be particularly powerful at uncovering the extent of action taken by the patient regarding a specific suicide plan, an area in which patients frequently minimize. Generally, once the verbal video is kick-started, the clinician will rely fairly heavily on sequencing behavioral incidents (such as "What happened next?" and "What did you do then?"). In response to these sequencing behavioral incidents many patients will provide you with the facts that are most useful for indicating their dangerousness and seriousness of intent (facts I like to call "lethal points").

If the patient gets stuck, starts to wander, or starts to omit important lethal points necessary for determining dangerousness, you can use an occasional (or even a series) of fact-finding behavioral incidents to ensure that the important information is forthcoming. For example, the types of fact-finding behavioral incidents that can help you to secure "lethal points" may look something like this in a patient who actually took some actions with a gun:

"Do you have a gun at home?"

"Have you ever gotten the gun out while you were having thoughts of killing yourself?"

"When did you do this?"

"Where were you sitting when you had the gun out?"

"Did you load the gun?"

"Did you put the gun up to your body or head?"

"Did you take the safety off or load the chamber?"

"How long did you hold the gun there?"

"What thoughts were going through your mind then?"

"What stopped you from pulling the trigger?"

"What did you do with the gun?"

"Where is the gun now?"

By utilizing the easily remembered strategy of creating a verbal video, clinicians can feel more confident that they are obtaining a valid picture of how close the patient actually came to committing suicide. The resulting scenario may prove to be radically different – and more suggestive of danger – from what would have been assumed if the interviewer had merely asked, "Did you come close to actually using the gun?" to which case an embarrassed or cagey patient may quickly reply, "Oh no, not really." Once again, we see an example of reflected intent being potentially more accurate than the patient's stated intent.

Also note in the above sequence the use of questions such as, "When did you do this?" and "Where were you sitting when you had the gun out?" These types of questions, also borrowed from CBT, are known as "anchor questions," for they anchor the patient into a specific memory as opposed to a collection of nebulous feelings. Such a refined focus will often bring forth more valid information as the episode becomes both more real and more vivid to the patient.

Indeed, I have found it to be useful over the years to "kick-start" my verbal videos with the flexible use of the following four steps. When a patient spontaneously raises a new method of killing himself – or proffers a new one when asked – the following steps create a graceful lead-in to the creation of a verbal video:

1. Ask the patient if he or she has ever gotten the method out while thinking about killing themselves – a technique called "the method-in-hand question"
2. Ask when the last time was
3. Ask where the patient was at the time
4. Invite the patient to walk you through what happened by summarizing the situation and literally inviting the patient to help you understand better – a statement called a "summarizing invitation"

Summarizing invitations often are loosely worded as follows: "It sounds like last night was a very difficult time. It will help me to understand exactly what you experienced if you can sort of walk me through what happened step by step. Two nights ago, you were on the 5th Street bridge, you'd picked out a spot, what did you do next?"

Following this four-step kick-start, the interviewer then proceeds to make the verbal video using a series of sequencing and fact-finding behavioral incidents. The metaphor of making a verbal video has been popular with trainees, as well as front-line staff, for the clinical task seems clear and is easily remembered even at 3 A.M. in a busy emergency department.

Uncovering the Patient's Apparent and Not-so-Apparent Motivations for Suicide

There exists another beneficial but rather peculiar "side effect" of using behavioral incidents to find out how far a person has taken actions towards suicide. Not infrequently, while patients are describing their actions, they spontaneously discuss some of the advantages and disadvantages about killing themselves. This listing often provides important clues with regard to which "way they are leaning." As with all aspects of the CASE Approach, the creation of a verbal video is not a rigidly applied "cookbook strategy." It is used as a flexible guideline that clinicians adapt as necessary to the unique needs of the suicide assessment.

By way of illustration, sometimes at such moments, it is an ideal time for the interviewer to lead the dialogue into a deeper exploration as to what the patient hopes to achieve by his or her own death. In his wonderfully insightful and very practical book, *Suicide Risk: The Formulation of Clinical Judgment*, John T. Maltsberger points out the diversity of goals – in addition to the almost universal goal of wanting release from unrelenting pain – in which patients can view their own death by suicide, some of which can be driven by anger or psychotic process[96]:

1. Suicide is a gateway leading into a dreamless sleep (nothingness).
2. It will effect reunion with someone or something that has been lost.
3. It will be a way of escaping from a persecutory enemy, interior or exterior (psychotic process).
4. It will destroy an enemy who seems to have taken up a place in the patient's body or some other part of himself (psychotic process).
5. It will provide a passage into another, better world.
6. It will provide an opportunity to get revenge on someone else by abandoning him or by destroying his favorite possession (the patient's body), and one can then watch him suffer from beyond the grave.

The clinician can ask questions that explore regions such as the above, and the answers can provide insight into the drives motivating the individual patient towards death, perhaps providing further insight into the imminent risk of a suicide attempt. These beliefs can serve as surprisingly powerful, and sometimes odd, motivators for suicide, especially in people who see no other ways of resolving their current pain or who find existence, as we know it, to be a bleak proposition.

This was highlighted in the mass suicide of 39 people in a rich suburb of San Diego in 1997. The idea that suicide could provide a method of passage to a better world was the driving force behind the members of the Heaven's Gate cult. The cult members believed that their death would carry them to a better world aboard an alien spacecraft, which just happened to be tagging a ride inside the tail of the Hale-Bopp Comet.

Clinical Illustration of Step 1: Exploring the Region of Presenting Suicide Events

Frank Thompson is a good soul. He is also a tired soul. He commented to the charge nurse, "I've had a good life, I don't know, maybe it's just time to pass on." Frank has been a farmer in the rolling hills of Western Pennsylvania for over 5 decades. His dad was a farmer. His grandfathers were both farmers. He was married to a wonderful woman, Sally, for 50 years. She died 2 years ago from brain cancer. Frank is plagued by diabetes and moderately severe heart and lung disease, having sucked on far too many cigarettes for far too many years. Since Sally's death he has developed a mild drinking problem.

Frank has five children, 21 grandchildren, and a pack of great grandkids to boot. His children are supportive, but only one lives nearby – Nick. It is Nick who has brought his dad in to the ED. Nick received a call from his dad earlier in the morning that he wasn't doing well. Nick got off work early and was caught off-guard by the depressive look of his father. Later during the night, while the two of them were sitting on the front porch, his dad shared a secret that prompted Nick to get in the car and bring him down to the ED immediately. Apparently his dad had taken a handful of aspirin and some antibiotics 2 days ago.

We are picking up this re-constructed interview about 20 minutes in, when the clinician is about to enter the region of presenting events using the CASE Approach. We will see elements of the four-step kick-start used flexibly as fit the needs of this particular patient. This reflects the important principle, noted earlier, that no elements of the CASE Approach are undertaken in a rigid "cookbook" manner. All elements are available to you to use flexibly as will most benefit the exploration of your patient's pain and suicidal ideation:

Pt.: It's been a long haul over the past 2 years. Sometimes too long a haul, if you know what I mean. I'm way too old for all this crap.

Clin.: And it's got to be hard to do it alone. (empathic statement)

Pt.: You bet! With Sally gone it's all so very different.

Clin.: I'm sure the pain of her loss is beyond words. With that amount of pain on board Mr. Thompson, have you had any thoughts of killing yourself? (shame attenuation used to gently raise the topic of suicide)

Pt.: I suppose my son may have already said something to you ... I took some pills ... I know it was dumb, but nothing came of it anyway.

Clin.: When was that? (behavioral incident, anchoring as to time)

Pt.: Couple of nights ago. But like I said nothing came of it. I'm not sure I need any help. I'm not going to do anything stupid, you don't have to worry about that. (Note that the clinician is not going to take the patients "stated intent" as necessarily an accurate picture of his real intent. Instead, the clinician is going to uncover Mr. Thompson's reflected intent by weaving a verbal video using behavioral incidents.)

Clin.: You know what Mr. Thompson ... that may be true, but I just want to get a better feeling for what you've been going through so we can make a wise decision together. Where were you when you took the pills? (behavioral incident serving as an anchor point to place)

Pt.: In the kitchen. I was sitting in a little kitchen nook where Sally and I used to eat lunch. I always loved that little place.

Clin.: (gently smiling) Yeah, I bet it brings back warm memories of Sally. (empathic statement)

Pt.: (smiling back) Yeah, it does.

Clin.: Maybe you could sort of walk me through what happened that night, Mr. Thompson. So you were at the kitchen nook where you and Sally used to sit, you took some pills, what kind of pills did you take? (summarizing invitation to the verbal video)

Pt.: Some aspirin, some penicillin.

Clin.: How much did you take of each one? (behavioral incident)

Pt.: About a handful of each. (Note that there can be quite a difference in what a patient means by a "handful." It is a perfect time to clarify with a behavioral incident.)

Clin.: When you say a handful, how many of each do you mean? (behavioral incident)

Pt.: About ten of each.

Clin.: Any other pills?

Pt.: (pause) … I also took about five digoxin I'm on; more than I'm supposed to, I know that. (This is a fact that the son was unaware of and had not been shared with the charge nurse by Mr. Thompson.)

Clin.: Did you have any pills left? (behavioral incident)

Pt.: Not a lot, I don't keep many pills in the house and my prescriptions have basically run out.

Clin.: Did you look for any other pills? (behavioral incident)

Pt.: (pause) … Not really pills (pause) … I did go through the drawer wondering if there was any rat poison around, but I realized that was stupid, too. (pause) … Trust me, suicide is not the answer, God did not put us on this earth to kill ourselves. (Unexpected information is coming to the surface. Clearly the son has not been told everything. The searching for the rat poison reflects more suicidal intent than might be expected from phrases like, "God did not put us on this earth to kill ourselves.")

Clin.: I'm glad you feel that way. And maybe we can help some too. At least I hope so.

Pt.: Maybe.

Clin.: You know, right after you took the pills, what was the next thing you did? (sequencing behavioral incident)

Pt.: Went to bed, just to sort of to see what would happen? I was just so tired of it all.

Clin.: How did you feel about the fact that you woke up okay?

Pt.: I don't know. Sort of didn't care. It's just the way it is.

Clin.: Had you been drinking at all, even a little bit? (behavioral incident)

Pt.: Nope. I'm trying to lay off the stuff. It just gets me more depressed. Don't get me wrong, I'm still drinking, but not over the past couple of days. (Notice that the clinician does not pursue a complete drug and alcohol history here; this will be carefully delineated as a risk factor in a different section of the interview – the drug and alcohol history – or may have already been done earlier in the interview.)

Clin.: I know from your son that you called him the next day. Had you tried any other ways of killing yourself before you called him? (behavioral incident)

Pt.: Nope. I just thought I needed a rest of some sort, and I wanted to talk it over with Nick.

> Clin.:   Good. How about over the past 2 months, have you had any other thoughts of overdosing? (behavioral incident, the clinician is gracefully moving into the region of recent suicide events with a bridging question)

Step 2: The Exploration of Recent Suicide Events

The region of recent events may very well represent – from the perspective of motivational theory – the single richest arena for uncovering reflected intent. It is here that a skilled interviewer may uncover suicidal ideation and planning that provides a more accurate indication of the patient's real intent than what the patient states. Here is where a talented clinician can save the life of a patient who strongly wants to die and *consciously* minimizes his real intent for fear of what will happen (possible hospitalization, involuntary commitment, or removal of the method of choice). It is also the arena in which a more accurate picture of the patient's intent may emerge with a patient whose *unconscious* defense mechanisms may be minimizing their conscious awareness of the intensity of their real suicidal intent.

Vague forays such as, "How much have you been thinking about suicide?" and "Have you thought about any other ways?" – if left at that – are invitations for miscommunication and under-reporting of suicidal ideation with truly dangerous patients. With the CASE Approach, this region is explored by determining exactly what types of plans for suicide the patient has had and how far the patient has acted on these plans. Such concrete behavioral information can provide a more direct measure of lethality. The best way to approach this process is through the following three steps: (1) find out what plans have been contemplated, (2) determine how far the patient took actions on these plans, and (3) determine how much of the patient's time is spent on these plans and accompanying ruminations about suicide.

This database looks somewhat formidable in scope, although it is obviously of great potential value. Keep in mind that we are trying to gather the most valid and comprehensive database that will allow us to make our best educated guess about the patient's lethality – because it is always a guess. However, we want to make this guess from the best view of "where the patient is at" that we can possibly garner. The material uncovered in our exploration of recent events is a mother lode of reflected intent simply waiting to be mined by a skilled interviewer. *Most importantly, it is the region in which a patient with extremely high suicidal intent might be hiding his or her true method of choice (which was intentionally withheld during the exploration of the presenting events).*

Fortunately, as was the case with our exploration of the region of the presenting event, we already have the tools necessary to do the task engagingly and with a minimum of time. Once again the behavioral incident (and the creation of verbal videos) will be of great use, but this time it will be combined with the other validity techniques described earlier: gentle assumption, denial of the specific, the catch-all question, and symptom amplification. Let's see how it is done.

The task is rather straightforward. We will delineate the list of methods and the extent of action taken upon them by weaving these validity techniques into easily remembered strategies. I will describe a single approach, but the reader should feel free to design new approaches in a flexible fashion as the needs arise. Once again, there is no cookbook

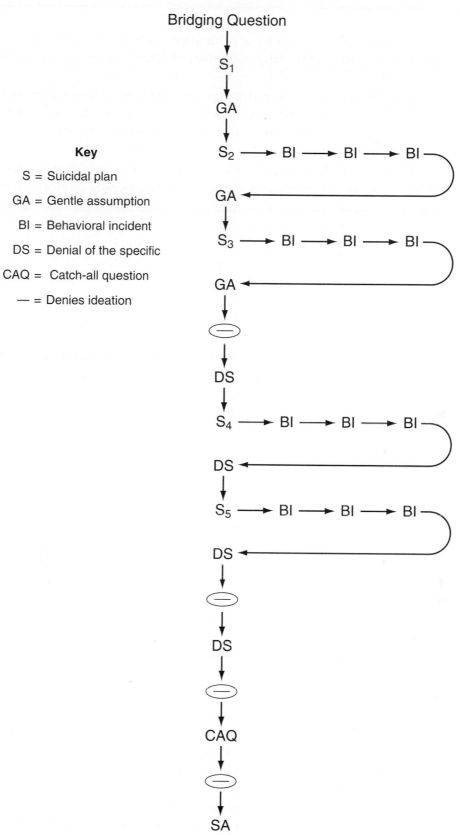

Figure 17.2 Exploring region of recent events.

approach that is correct, but the following principles can make the exploration of recent ideation and actions surprisingly easy and natural. First, let us make a note about timeframe.

Sometimes when the clinician raises the topic of suicide with techniques like normalization or shame attenuation, the patient's reported events do not lie within the previous 48 hours or several weeks (*in essence there is no presenting event*); in which case, the clinician immediately begins exploring the region of recent events.

On the other hand, if the patient reports a true presenting event, after the verbal video is created of that method, the clinician will need to use a bridging question to transition into the region of recent suicide events (Figure 17.2). Often this transition is initiated by smoothly eliciting any thoughts in the past 2 months related to the same plan that the patient discussed in the presenting events (as was done in the interview with Mr. Thompson). Thus if a patient had described thoughts of shooting himself in the exploration of presenting events, the clinician would, after finishing the verbal video, create a bridge into the timeframe of recent events as follows, "Over the past 2 months, have you had any other thoughts of shooting yourself?"

Once any markedly intense recent thoughts or actions regarding the same method, if present, have been explored with a verbal video within the timeframe of recent events (previous 2 months), a gentle assumption is used to look for a different suicide method within the timeframe of recent events (previous 2 months). As mentioned earlier, my favorite gentle assumption is the simplest one, "What other ways have you thought of killing yourself?"

If a second method is uncovered, sequential behavioral incidents are used to create another verbal video reflecting the extent of action taken. The interviewer continues this use of gentle assumptions, with follow-up verbal videos as indicated with each newly uncovered method, until the patient denies any other methods when asked, "What other ways have you thought of killing yourself?"

Once the use of a gentle assumption yields a blanket denial of other methods, *if (and only if)* the clinician feels that the patient may be withholding other methods of suicide, the clinician uses a short series of denials of the specific. The interviewer must use his or her clinical judgment to decide whether or not the use of denials of the specific is indicated. None would be warranted if the patient had low risk factors, high protective factors, and had convincingly reported minimal or no suicidal ideation to that point in the interview.

However, if the clinician's intuition is suggesting that the patient may be withholding critical suicidal ideation, especially if the clinician suspects that the patient is withholding his or her method of choice, then denials of the specific can be employed. Denials of the specific can be surprisingly effective at uncovering a previously withheld suicide method and plan. The interviewer doesn't drive this technique into the ground with an exhaustive series of methods, but simply asks for any unmentioned methods that are common to the patient's culture and which the clinician is suspicious that this specific patient might be withholding.

By way of example, if the patient has talked about overdosing, guns, and driving a car off the road, the clinician might employ any one or a number of the following denials of the specific, pausing after each for an answer:

"Have you been having any thoughts about cutting or stabbing yourself?"

"Have you been having any thoughts about hanging yourself?"

"Have you been having any thoughts about jumping off a bridge or other high place?"

"Have you been having any thoughts about carbon monoxide?"

As before, if a new method is revealed, the clinician uncovers the extent of action taken by creating a verbal video with the use of a series of behavioral incidents. It is here – with the selective and well-timed use of denials of the specific – that a highly dangerous patient that has been purposefully withholding his or her method of choice, may suddenly share it, perhaps prompted by a wedge of healthy ambivalence. The number of denials of the specific asked is usually small, sometimes only one. You will determine the number by how the patient is answering and your intuitive feel for whether or not a method is being withheld.

Following the use of denials of the specific, the clinician generally utilizes the catch-all question ("We've been talking about a lot of different ways you've been thinking about killing yourself; is there a way you've thought about, that we haven't talked about?"). The catch-all question's value lies in the fact that some hesitant, yet ambivalent, patients with dangerous intent may have continued to hide their actual method of choice when responding to denials of the specific. This is particularly true when the patient's method of choice is an *unusual* method not covered by the clinician's denials of the specific (many odd methods are now openly discussed on the web). If there is enough ambivalence, the patient at this point may share his or her method of choice.

In other instances, some patients may inadvertently pause after being asked the catch-all question, revealing, through nonverbal leakage, that other plans may have been considered. A simple comment, said gently, can be surprisingly powerful at such moments as with, "Mr. Thompson, it looks like you may have thought of some other ways. I know it can be hard to talk about suicide, but I really want to help you. Try to share with me your thoughts even if they were fleeting in nature." The resulting information is sometimes life saving.

The catch-all question is useful in two other ways. Sometimes, a clinician, when using a list of denials of the specific, inadvertently forgets to mention the culturally common method that the patient happens to be intending to use. In such cases, the method may be relayed in response to the catch-all question. The catch-all question can also prompt the patient to share that he or she has done a web search on suicide, offering further glimpses of the patient's reflected intent.

I believe that whether indirectly tapped by the catch-all question or by direct questioning, at some point clinicians should explore the extent that the patient has been online, hunting for information on suicide. Unfortunately, numerous sites exist that provide advice and encouragement on suicide. A patient may even find a chat room in which participants are urging the patient to proceed with suicide. In our wired age, time spent googling and searching for information on suicide has become an important indicator of reflected intent.

After establishing the list of methods considered by the patient and the extent of action taken on each method, the interviewer hones in on the frequency, duration, and intensity of the suicidal ideation with a symptom amplification such as: "On your very worst days, how much time do you spend thinking about killing yourself … 10 hours a day, 14 hours a day, 18 hours a day?"

The above strategy is easy to learn and simple to remember. It also flows imperceptibly, frequently increasing engagement, as the patient is pleasantly surprised at how easy it is to talk to the clinician about issues that had been carried as secret burdens of shame. It also becomes apparent to the patient that the interviewer is quite comfortable talking about suicide and has clearly discussed it with many others. This represents yet another shame-reducing metacommunication.

Clinical Illustration of Step 2: Exploring the Region of Recent Events

There is no better way to illustrate the power of this strategy than to see it at work with Mr. Thompson. The clinician has uncovered information suggesting that Mr. Thompson's real intent may be greater than his initially stated intent would suggest. Moreover, his list of risk factors is high and his support systems, other than his nearest son, Nick, have been markedly weakened by the loss of his wife. The fact that he is wrestling with the notion that it is "wrong" to kill oneself, may be creating both ambivalence (good) and a skewed self-admission – secondary to unconscious defense mechanisms – as to the depth of his suicidal desire and intent (bad).

Notice that the clinician is quite explicit with the timeframe, stating the exact duration as opposed to using a vague term such as "recently." This specificity is important because it helps the patient remain focused on the timeframe of interest while decreasing time-wasting sidetracks.

> **Pt.:** Nope. I just thought I needed a rest of some sort, and I wanted to talk it over with Nick.
>
> **Clin.:** Good. How about over the past 2 months, have you had any other thoughts of overdosing? (behavioral incident, the clinician is gracefully moving into the region of recent suicide events with a classic bridging question)
>
> **Pt.:** A few times but I never got no pills out or nothing.
>
> **Clin.:** What other ways have you thought about killing yourself? (gentle assumption)
>
> **Pt.:** Oh not much … I suppose I thought about hangin' myself, but that is not a good way to die. You know, it doesn't always work, at least that's what I been told.
>
> **Clin.:** Have you ever gotten a rope out or something else to use to hang yourself? (behavioral incident, method-in-hand question)
>
> **Pt.:** No sir, I haven't.
>
> **Clin.:** What other ways have you thought about killing yourself? (gentle assumption)
>
> **Pt.:** Well, I have gone out to the barn to see if we still had some of that pesticide I used a couple of years ago.
>
> **Clin.:** And? (variant of a sequencing behavioral incident)
>
> **Pt.:** Oh we did. And … and I was thinking about taking some and then burning the barn down with me inside it.

Clin.: Hmmm.

Pt.: Yeah, (pause) … sort of Hollywood-ish (smiles), but it's no good, way too apt to not work out right.

Clin.: Did you ever go out there and actually pick up the pesticide with the actual intention of using it? (behavioral incident, method-in-hand question)

Pt.: Hell no! I ain't no bug, it's no way to go. (smiles sheepishly again)

Clin.: How often did you actually go out to the barn thinking about that? (behavioral incident, note that despite the patient's strong disavowal of the method, the interviewer's question and the patient's response will provide further reflection of potentially serious intent)

Pt.: Maybe four or five times, I don't really remember exactly.

Clin.: What other ways have you thought of killing yourself? (gentle assumption)

Pt.: That's about it. Nothing else really.

The CASE Approach is doing exactly what it is supposed to be doing – getting those puzzle pieces out on the table that might better reflect the severity of Mr. Thompson's suicidal intent. The resulting information is a bit surprising. The use of the gentle assumptions has resulted in a method (pesticides and burning down the barn) that quite frankly the clinician would not have thought to ask about. Gentle assumptions allow patients to provide such individualized plans that may never have come to the clinician's awareness otherwise. The number of times Mr. Thompson went to the barn is also disturbing. Despite his ability to still retain a sense of humor, the depth of his angst is becoming more and more apparent.

Note that Mr. Thompson has now denied any other methods when presented with the gentle assumption, "What other ways have you thought about killing yourself?" The clinician is about to use a short string of denials of the specific. His persistence is prompted by the presence of high risk factors, the clear depth of Mr. Thompson's anguish, and by the fact that during the exploration of presenting events, and thus far in the exploration of recent events, details are being uncovered that Mr. Thompson had not shared earlier. The clinician is not entirely certain that the Mr. Thompson's method of choice has yet been shared. In addition, there was one other fact that seemed odd to the clinician:

Clin.: What about carbon monoxide, you know with a car or tractor? (denial of the specific)

Pt.: My old barn is so drafty, you couldn't do that if you tried. (smiles weakly)

Clin.: Have you thought of jumping off a building or bridge? (denial of the specific)

Pt.: Nope.

Clin.: You know Mr. Thompson, most farmers I know like to hunt or at least have a gun around to protect their livestock; and sometimes when they are in a lot of pain like you've been having, they think of shooting themselves. I'm wondering if that has crossed your mind? (denial of the specific introduced with a normalization)

Pt.: (long pause, looks away ever so slightly) I suppose.

Clin.: Did you ever picture a place where you might shoot yourself? (behavioral incident, a variation of anchoring to place in the four-step kick-start of a verbal video)

Pt.: There is a place down by Willow Creek that was the favorite place that Sally and I used to go. (pause) … It's just lovely, even in the winter it's lovely. (sigh) And I've often thought that if I had to go, that's where I would do it.

Clin.: Did you ever go there with a gun, thinking you might kill yourself? (behavioral incident, method-in-hand question)

Pt.: Yeah, (pause) … yeah, I've done that.

Clin.: Did you load the gun? (behavioral incident)

Pt.: Yeah.

Clin.: What did you do next? (sequencing behavioral incident)

Pt.: Put it in my mouth. I read somewhere that's how you should do it. (pause) … Someone told me once they knew a guy who did that but didn't point it upwards so the darn thing shot right out the back of his neck (slight chuckle) hard to believe (shakes his head).

Clin.: Sounds like you were pretty close though.

Pt.: Yeah. Yeah. I guess I was.

Clin.: Was the safety off? (behavioral incident)

Pt.: Yeah. (looks down)

Clin.: (said very gently) You really miss her don't you?

Pt.: (patient bursts into tears) Oh God, I miss her. She made my world. She was my world.

Clin.: What made you put the gun down, Mr. Thompson? (behavioral incident)

Pt.: I don't really know. Maybe I thought I should be around for all my grandkids, but I just don't know anymore.

Clin.: Mr. Thompson, roughly when was this? (behavioral incident)

Pt.: About 2 weeks ago.

Clin.: Right around then, when things were really tough, how much time were you spending thinking about killing yourself, 10 hours a day, 14 hours a day, 18 hours a day? (symptom amplification)

Pt.: (lifts head up and looks the clinician right in the eye) The truth is – I couldn't get it out of my mind.

This interviewer is earning his pay. He may also be saving Mr. Thompson's life. Mr. Thompson's intent to kill himself is much higher than his originally stated intent conveyed. In addition, it was only through the skilled use of a denial of the specific that the patient's true method of choice emerged. With this added information reflecting the potential seriousness of Mr. Thompson's suicidal intent, hospitalization appears to be more appropriate, and there is now an opportunity to have the gun or guns removed from the farmhouse as well.

From the perspective of interviewing technique, notice that once the use of a gun was uncovered, the clinician deftly used a series of behavioral incidents to create a verbal video of what actually happened. Fact-finding behavioral incidents such as, "Did you load the gun?" and sequencing behavioral incidents such as, "What did you do next?" provided concrete information regarding the seriousness of Mr. Thompson's intent.

Also note that the string of behavioral incidents led the patient to remember and describe his inner world at the time of the gun incident. This is a rather common phenomenon. Although the behavioral incident was designed to improve the validity of hard behavioral data, as patients begin to re-imagine their experiences, they are often drawn into their internal cognitions and emotions at the time. This often provides a window into the soul of the patient. Within the patient's soul, we may find strong reasons to live. As Jobes and Mann[97] have pointed out, an understanding of a patient's reasons for living is an important aspect of suicide assessment that has traditionally not been given the attention in the literature that it warrants. On the other hand, as with Mr. Thompson, the clinician may find a shattered soul where there seems to be only good reasons to die, as reflected by his telling comment, "She was my world."

Note that the interviewer saw no reason to utilize the catch-all question, for the interviewer felt comfortable that Mr. Thompson had finally shared his method of choice and was not thinking of using another unusual suicide method. This conscious decision making once again highlights that the CASE Approach is not a rigidly pre-determined method of exploring suicidal ideation.

For instance, the extensiveness of the questioning during the region of recent events is dependent on the interviewer's ever-evolving "read" on the dangerousness of the patient. If a patient has low risk factors, high protective factors, denies any thoughts of suicide during the exploration of presenting events, and reports only one fleeting thought of shooting himself (no gun at home) during the early exploration of the recent events, a clinician most likely would not use denials of the specific, the catch-all question, or symptom amplification. It would not make sense to do so, and might even appear odd to the patient.

Step 3: The Exploration of Past Suicide Events

Clinicians sometimes spend too much time on this area. Patients with complicated psychiatric histories (e.g., some people with a borderline personality disorder) may have lengthy past histories of suicidal material. One could spend an hour solely reviewing this material. It would be an hour poorly spent.

Within the time constraints of busy practices and managed care, initial assessments by mental health professionals usually must be completed within a "50-minute hour" or less, with much less time available in an emergency department. When exploring the region of past suicide events, I have found it to be useful to simplify the task by operationalizing it.

In this regard, I only seek information about past suicidal behaviors (no longer looking for episodes of isolated suicidal thought). *In addition, in this region of the CASE Approach, the clinician only seeks information that could potentially change the immediate clinical triage and follow-up for the patient.* I have found the following questions to be of value in this regard, and the interviewer limits his or her inquiry into the region of past events to these germane topics:

- If past suicide attempts are revealed, what is the most serious past suicide attempt? (Is the current ideation focused on the same method? "Practice" can be deadly in this arena.)

- Are the current triggers and the patient's current psychopathological state similar now as to when the most serious attempts were made? (Does the patient view the current stressors and options in the same light as during the most dangerous past attempt? A patient may be prone to suicide following specific stressors such as the break-up of relationships or during specific psychopathological states, such as episodes of acute intoxication, intense anxiety, depression, mania, or psychosis.)
- Specific psychological states may also trigger suicidal action, as with the confluence of the sensation that one does not belong to a social group coupled with the feeling of being a burden to others, as Joiner has delineated. Consequently, it can be useful to take a quick assessment of the patient's internal phenomenology at the time of a serious past attempt to see if it resonates with current phenomenology.
- What is the approximate number of past gestures and attempts? (Large numbers here can alert the clinician to suicide attempts made as a means of communication and/ or receiving comfort, perhaps making one less concerned, or may alert the clinician that the patient has truly exhausted all hope, making one more concerned. In either case, it is important to know.
- When was the most recent attempt outside of the 2 months explored in the region of recent events? (There could have been a significant attempt within the last 6 months that may signal the need for more immediate concern.)

Clinical Illustration of Step 3: Exploring the Region of Past Events

Let us return to our interview with Mr. Thompson and see what it uncovers. The interviewer has already decided that Mr. Thompson is best served by hospitalization, but wisely realizes that it is valuable to continue exploring the extent of Mr. Thompson's suicidal history. It is possible that puzzle pieces will be uncovered that may be useful to future clinicians in determining potential safety, including those clinicians who will be making the tough decision as to when Mr. Thompson will be safe for discharge from the inpatient unit.

In my opinion, once a patient feels safe enough to share openly about suicidal ideation, it is important to uncover as much accurate information as possible, for the patient may clam up, sometimes entirely, with the next clinician. In this sense, future clinicians who must make complex triage decisions may be entirely dependent upon the information we have garnered from the patient. This is particularly important if you are referring a patient to an emergency department for possible admission from an outpatient setting such as a school counseling center or a mental health clinic. As mentioned earlier, many a patient, during the process of getting to the emergency room, will undergo a remarkable "transportation healing." In short, the patient becomes unwilling to share openly with the emergency room clinicians for fear of hospitalization.

    Pt.:   (lifts head up and looks the clinician right in the eye) The truth is – I couldn't get it out of my mind.

    Clin.:   With a loss like the loss of Sally, who wouldn't be in great pain, Mr. Thompson (strategic empathic statement of high valence). I wish we could bring her back for you, but we can't, but maybe we can help with the pain.

Pt.:   I sure hope so, because I can't go on like this.

Clin.: We'll do our best. (pauses) … One thing I want to understand better and may help me to help you better is to understand if you have ever had pain so great in the past that suicide passed through your mind? (clinician is making the chronological transition to past suicide events using a behavioral incident)

Pt.:   (sighs) Not really.

Clin.: When you say "not really," I have a feeling there is a little something there.

Pt.:   Well, many, many years ago (faintly smiles, making eye contact), when I was young and restless, before Sally, a girlfriend broke up with me.

Clin.: And?

Pt.:   Well, like I said, I was a young guy then and didn't think things through, but I got my dad's gun out.

Clin.: Did you load it?

Pt.:   He kept it loaded.

Clin.: What did you do with it? (sequencing behavioral incident)

Pt.:   Nothin'. Put the damn thing away. Even then I knew that was not the answer.

Clin.: Sounds like you made the right decision. (empathic statement)

Pt.:   Yeah. Yeah. I guess I did.

Clin.: One thing for sure is, you never would have met Sally if you had followed through back then.

Pt.:   Well, that's for sure. (pauses) … I wouldn't want to have missed that. No, I wouldn't want to have missed that. I suppose you never really do know what the future holds.

Clin.: No we don't. (said gently) Have you had any other attempts? (behavioral incident)

Pt.:   No way. I've never given it another thought until recently.

Clin.: How about even fleeting thoughts like when you and Sally lost your house in the depression? (behavioral incident)

Pt.:   Never, just never crossed my mind.

There is not a lot here of concern. Nevertheless, a few useful puzzle pieces have come onto the table. The gun history as a teenager is so long ago that it probably pales in significance. But it does give weight to the idea that guns will probably be the most likely method of choice with Mr. Thompson, even in the future, a point that will be of importance down the pike during long-term follow-up.

The dialogue demonstrates an even more interesting teaching point. Although the CASE Approach is an assessment strategy, interviewers are free to flexibly insert moments of counseling. Moreover, it is imperative that empathy be enhanced throughout the use of the CASE Approach. This interviewer gets an "A" in both regards.

The bridging comments into the region of past events were nicely empathic as evidenced by, "With a loss like the loss of Sally, who wouldn't be in great pain, Mr. Thompson. I wish we could bring her back for you, but we can't, but maybe we can help with the pain."

In addition, the interviewer's reflection, "One thing for sure is, you never would have met Sally if you had followed through back then" gently opened the door towards a potentially protective cognition (good things can happen in the future even though bad things are happening now). The clinician was wise to let Mr. Thompson walk through the door himself (to arrive at his own insight independently), which he did as reflected by his words, "Well, that's for sure. (pauses) … I wouldn't want to have missed that. No, I wouldn't want to have missed that. *I suppose you never really do know what the future holds.*" Note that the interviewer does not pursue therapeutic lines at this point, for that will be better addressed by a therapist on the unit, but the interviewer has delicately planted a seed of hope.

Step 4: The Exploration of Immediate Suicide Events

In this region, the interviewer focuses upon any new suicidal ideation, desire, and intent that the patient may be *experiencing during the interview itself.* The interviewer also makes inquiries as to whether the patient thinks he or she is likely to have further thoughts of suicide after leaving the office, ED, or inpatient unit, or gets off the phone following a crisis call. The region of immediate events can also include appropriate safety planning, although many clinicians, including myself, tend to address safety planning later in the interview. For me, I find that safety planning often fits more naturalistically in the closing phase of the interview itself, where it can be gracefully integrated into the collaborative treatment planning. The focus of the exploration of immediate events is thus on the present and future (easily remembered as the region of Now/Next). The ultimate goal is to gather information that can help the clinician to further delineate the patient's immediate suicidal intent.

Exploring immediate desire (the intensity of the patient's pain and desire to die) and the patient's intent (the degree with which the patient has decided to actually proceed with suicide) is clarified by discerning the relationship between the two, for they are not identical despite being intimately related. A patient could have intense pain with a strong desire to die yet have no intent, as reflected by, "I could never do that to my children." Conversely, over time, a patient's pain could become so intense, that it over-rides his or her defenses that had prevented the transformation of pain into the decision for action, resulting in a patient who impulsively acts.

A sound starting place is the question, "Right now, are you having any thoughts about wanting to kill yourself?" From this inquiry, a question such as the following can be utilized to further explore the patient's desire to die:

"On a scale from 0 to 10, how would you describe how bad the pain is for you in your divorce right now ranging from a 0 'It's sort of tough, but I can handle it okay' to a 10 'If it doesn't let up, I don't know if I can go on.' Where would you place yourself on that scale?"

Questions such as the two below can help delineate whether the patient's desire for relief has been transformed into an intent to act:

"I realize that you can't know for sure, but what is your best guess as to how likely it is that you will try to kill yourself during the next week, from highly unlikely to very likely?"

"What keeps you from killing yourself?"

It is important to explore the patient's current level of hopelessness and to assess whether the patient is making productive plans for the future or is amenable to preparing concrete plans for dealing with current problems and stresses. Questions such as, "How does the future look to you?", "Do you feel hopeful about the future?", and "What things would make you feel more or less hopeful about the future?" are useful entrance points for this exploration. If not addressed in an earlier timeframe, an exploration of reasons for living can be nicely introduced here with, "What things in your life make you want to go on living?"

Developing a safety plan – whether done here or later during the closing phase of the interview – is frequently facilitated by asking questions such as "What would you do later tonight or tomorrow if you began to have suicidal thoughts again?" From the patient's answer, one can sometimes better surmise how serious the patient is about ensuring his safety. Such a question also provides a chance for the joint brainstorming of plans to handle the re-emergence of suicidal ideation. Sound safety planning often includes a series of steps that the patient will take to transform and/or control suicidal ideation if it should arise. Such planning could begin with something as simple as taking a warm shower or listening to soothing music and end with calling a crisis line or contacting a cab to return to the hospital if out on a pass.

Now is a good time to address the complex issue of whether "safety contracting" as opposed to "safety planning" may be of use with any specific patient. In my opinion, each patient is unique in this regard. Safety *contracting* has become somewhat of a controversial topic. To understand its practical use, it is important to remember that, in addition to metacommunicating care and concern on the part of the interviewer, there are two main reasons or applications for safety contracting: (1) as a method of deterrence and (2) as a sensitive means of suicide assessment.

These applications are radically different, and their pros and cons are equally dissimilar. The intensity of the debate, in my opinion, is generated because most of what is "debated" in the literature deals primarily with its application as a deterrent (its role as an assessment tool being relatively ignored in the literature). Indeed, in my opinion, if safety contracting is examined solely as a means of deterrence, then it has many significant limitations when compared to safety planning.

For instance, safety contracting may frequently be counterproductive in patients dealing with borderline or passive-aggressive pathology. With such patients it is sometimes best to avoid the whole issue of safety contracting, because it may embroil the dyad in ineffective debates with statements such as, "I don't know what to tell you. I guess I'm safe, but on the other hand, I can't make any guarantees. Do you know anybody who can?"

If one uses safety contracting as a deterrent, it is critical to use it cautiously. As Miller and colleagues have pointed out, it guarantees nothing and may yield a false sense of security.[98,99] Moreover, it should never be done before a sound suicide assessment has been completed. Generally speaking, I believe that safety contracting *as a deterrent* is viewed by most suicidologists as generally inferior to sound safety planning.

The power of the patient's superego and the power of the therapeutic alliance may play significant roles in whether safety contracting – employed as a deterrent – may have use with a specific patient in relatively rare circumstances. I am convinced that in some patients it may play a role in deterrence, as with a patient in a long-standing therapeutic alliance, with minimal characterological pathology, and a powerful superego. I have had several seasoned therapists tell me after workshops that they have had patients clearly state that the safety contract functioned as a deterrent. One patient relayed on a Monday after a particularly bad weekend that, "The only reason I am alive today is our contract, for I couldn't do that to you. I couldn't break my word to you." Nevertheless, in my opinion, safety contracting has limited use as a deterrent, and, for the most part, I prefer safety planning as a tool for deterrence.

But deterrence is not the only reason – and in my opinion, is not the main reason – to use safety contracting. It may be more useful – albeit in relatively infrequent situations – as an exquisitely sensitive assessment tool. In its capacity as an assessment tool, it is selectively used and, in my opinion, should only be used in the *absence* of passive-aggressive or borderline personality pathology. It is selectively utilized in the relatively rare instances, in which a clinician is leaning towards non-hospitalization after completing a suicide assessment, but is bothered by his or her intuition that the patient is more dangerous than the patient has stated. Sometimes the interviewer may analytically feel that something does "not add up here."

In such cases, the clinician may ask a patient, "Sean (use patient's first name if used throughout the interview), can you promise me that you will not act on any suicidal thoughts before you would call me, or one of my staff, 24/7, any hour of the day or night? And can you really promise me that?" Such a statement is said with a sincere and earnest tone and while looking the patient directly in the eyes. The intimacy of the interaction creates a gentle but real "interpersonal push" on the patient to be truthful. Such an "interpersonal push" may prompt nonverbal leakage of hidden ambivalence or dangerous suicidal intent.

When used in this highly selective fashion, as the interviewer asks whether the patient can promise to contact the clinician or appropriate staff before acting on any suicidal ideation, the interviewer scans the patient's face, body, and tone of voice for any signs of hesitancy, deceit, or ambivalence. Here is the proverbial moment of truth. Nonverbal leakage of suicidal desire or intent at this juncture can be, potentially, the only indicator of the patient's true immediate risk.

Using the interpersonal process of safety contracting as an assessment tool, the clinician may completely change his mind about releasing a patient based on a hesitancy to contract, avoidance of eye contact, or other signs of deceit or ambivalence displayed while reluctantly agreeing to a safety contract.

I vividly remember one patient, who adamantly did not want to be admitted to the hospital, that I was about to discharge from my ED, but whom I felt intuitively something was askew, despite a careful suicide assessment. I decided to employ safety contracting *as an assessment tool*. When I asked whether he could promise to call us before ever acting on any suicidal ideation, he hesitated and briefly glanced down. When I pointed out that it looked hard for him to make the contract, he welled up and said, "I just want to die."

I commented, "You know, I think we should just bring you into the hospital," at which point he looked at me and said with a pained foreboding, "You probably should." It was a chilling moment. I believe he was planning to kill himself that night. He subsequently agreed to be admitted.

The interviewer who notices such nonverbal clues of ambivalence can simply ask, "It looks as though this contract is hard for you to agree to. What's going on in your mind?" The answers can be benign or alarming (as above) and the resulting piece of the puzzle – which could only be provided by the process of safety contracting – may lead to a change in disposition. This use of safety contracting *as an assessment tool*, based on non-verbal leakage of suicidal intent, unlike safety contracting as a deterrent (which probably has limited use in an ED), may be particularly useful in an ED.

As one would expect logically, safety *planning*, in my opinion, is much less useful *as an assessment tool* than safety contracting. Unlike safety contracting, which has a powerful interpersonal push that triggers the nonverbal leakage alerting clinicians to the presence of patient ambivalence or serious suicidal intent, safety planning is an ultra-collaborative process when done well. The elimination of the interpersonal push with safety planning markedly decreases its ability to effectively prompt nonverbal leakage of suicidal intent. Thus the use of safety contracting and safety planning is complicated. CASE-trained clinicians neither generically condemn nor condone the use of either, but attempt to make a wise decision based on the specific needs of the patient and the clinical task at hand (deterrence or assessment).

For a practical review of how to effectively use safety contracting, the reader is referred to "Safety Contracting: Pros, Cons, and Documentation Issues," from the appendix in my book, *The Practical Art of Suicide Assessment: A Guide for Mental Health Professionals and Substance Abuse Counselors*,[100] where one will also find references to numerous articles on the subject. Remember that safety contracting is no guarantee of safety whatsoever.

Finally, it cannot be re-emphasized enough that if, following the interview, the clinician has continuing concerns about the safety of the patient or the validity of the patient's self-report, corroborative sources may need to be contacted.

Clinical Illustration of Step 4: Exploring the Region of Immediate Events

To better see this line of questioning in action, let us wrap up by returning to Mr. Thompson.

> **Pt.:** Never, just never crossed my mind.
>
> **Clin.:** You know, how about right now. We've been talking for quite some time and I'm wondering how you are feeling about killing yourself right now?
>
> **Pt.:** I'm not really sure. (pauses) … I just don't know. I actually feel a little bit better after talking with you, but I just don't know.
>
> **Clin.:** Do you see much hope for the future? (behavioral incident)
>
> **Pt.:** Not a lot. Maybe a little.
>
> **Clin.:** I'm wondering, Mr. Thompson, if you walked out of here tonight, what would be stopping you from killing yourself, say a couple of days from now, or a week or two down the road?

Pt.: You really want to know?

Clin.: I really want to know.

Pt.: Probably nothing (sighs) … probably nothing, although I bet you guys are going to get rid of my guns.

Within the region of immediate events, there is no need to proceed with Mr. Thompson, for his answers in response to the CASE Approach have suggested a level of dangerousness indicating the need for hospitalization. Note that there is no reason for the clinician to utilize safety contracting as either a deterrent (for the clinician has already decided that inpatient hospitalization is indicated) nor as an assessment tool (for the simple reason that there is nothing left to assess, the patient's potential for lethality is striking).

Indeed, the clinician has completed the CASE Approach. In this example, as the interviewer was uncovering the patient's suicidal ideation, planning, and behaviors, the clinician was simultaneously beginning to generate a cognitive/intuitive formulation of risk. Coupling the data from the CASE Approach with an understanding of Mr. Thompson's risk factors garnered earlier in the interview (elderly, ill, major interpersonal loss, feeling isolated, and potentially feeling that he may be a burden) and lack of protective factors (other than his one son there is minimal family support, little sense of hope, resilience or purpose) the clinician can proceed to finalize a formulation of risk.

With the help of the CASE Approach, the interviewer has uncovered a remarkably rich view of the internal world of Mr. Thompson's suicidal thoughts, plans, actions, and behaviors. Most importantly, with adept interviewing in the region of recent events, the interviewer has uncovered his method of choice, which was unknown to others until that moment, and a method of choice that Mr. Thompson had purposely withheld earlier in the interview.

As we wrap up our introduction to the CASE Approach, it is an ideal time to turn to our integrated video material. The CASE Approach is a sophisticated interviewing strategy with many steps, all of which can potentially help us to save a life. In the following series of video modules, you will find material designed to help simplify, clarify, and consolidate the material we have been exploring. I will also demonstrate the CASE Approach as I adapt it for use with patients who vary in their degrees of dangerousness.

By the time you have completed viewing the video modules, I believe you will have significantly enhanced your understanding of the CASE Approach. With both the use of role-playing, and from your future clinical experience, you will undoubtedly find your skill set improving. I believe you will also find a reassuring increase in your confidence to uncover dangerous suicidal intent. Someday, I believe these enhanced skills will help you to save a life.

VIDEO MODULE 17.1

Title: The Delicate Art of Uncovering Suicidal Ideation and Intent – Part 1: Core Principles and Theory

Contents: Consolidates and expands the reader's understanding of the challenges and nuances of uncovering suicidal intent with particularly dangerous patients. *The video module adds material not covered in the text itself.*

Important note to the reader: *After viewing Video Module 17.1 the reader should proceed directly to Video Module 17.2 for the second component of a three-part series on effectively using the CASE Approach.*

VIDEO MODULE 17.2

Title: The Delicate Art of Uncovering Suicidal Ideation and Intent – Part 2: From Theory to Practice (Annotated Video Clips)

Contents: Contains both expanded didactics and various annotated interview excerpts demonstrating the use of the CASE Approach in its entirety.

Important note to the reader: *After viewing Video Module 17.2 the reader should proceed directly to Video Module 17.3 for the third component of a three-part series on effectively using the CASE Approach.*

VIDEO MODULE 17.3

Title: The Delicate Art of Uncovering Suicidal Ideation and Intent – Part 3: Flexibly Utilizing the CASE Approach with Patients of High Lethality (Annotated Video Clips)

Contents: Contains both expanded didactics and various annotated interview excerpts demonstrating the use of the CASE Approach with patients demonstrating varying degrees of high lethality. Explores how to flexibly adapt the CASE Approach with such patients and the impact on the clinical formulation of risk determined from the patient's responses.

Important note to the reader: *After viewing Video Module 17.3 you can return directly to the text below for the conclusion of Chapter 17 or you may view Video Modules 17.4, 17.5, and 17.6, which are OPTIONAL modules that can be used to consolidate your understanding of the material from Video Modules 17.1, 17.2, and 17.3.*

VIDEO MODULE 17.4

Title: CASE Approach Illustrated: Complete Interview with Amy #1 without Didactics and without Labels for Interviewing Techniques

Contents: The interview excerpts from Video Module 17.2 (showing the interview with patient Amy #1) appear here as they naturally occurred (without any didactic material inserted), providing a chance to better experience the actual flow of the interview. The labeling of the specific interview techniques as they appeared at the bottom of the video in Video Module 17.2 has also been removed. Thus this module can be used by the reader (individually) or by faculty (within the classroom) to function as a springboard for discussion, consolidate understanding, or as an opportunity to test one's ability to correctly identify the individual validity techniques as they appear sequentially during the use of the CASE Approach.

VIDEO MODULE 17.5

Title: CASE Approach Illustrated: Complete Interview with Amy #1 without Didactics but *with* Labels for Interviewing Techniques

Contents: *This module is identical to Video Module 17.4 except for the return of the labels for the individual validity techniques.* Each validity technique is tagged with a label as it is demonstrated. This format provides an ideal method to once again consolidate an understanding of the validity techniques utilized in the CASE Approach as well as a chance "to check the answers" if one used Video Module 17.4 as an opportunity to test one's abilities to identify the individual validity techniques as they appear sequentially during the use of the CASE Approach.

VIDEO MODULE 17.6

Title: CASE Approach Illustrated: Complete Interviews with Amy #2 and with Amy #3 without Didactics and *without* Labels for Interviewing Techniques

Contents: The interview excerpts from Video Module 17.3 (showing the interviews with patients Amy #2 and Amy #3) appear here as they naturally occurred (without any didactic material inserted) providing a chance to better experience the actual flow of the interviews. The labeling of the specific interview techniques as they appeared at the bottom of the video in Video Module 17.3 has also been removed. Thus this module can be used by the reader (individually) or by faculty (within the classroom) to function as a springboard for discussion, consolidate understanding, or as an opportunity to test one's ability to correctly identify the individual validity techniques as they appear sequentially during the use of the CASE Approach.

CONCLUDING COMMENTS

In Section 2 of this chapter, we have learned how to use the CASE Approach to sensitively and deeply enter the patient's world of suicidal preoccupation. The resulting information regarding methods of suicide contemplated, the determination of a method of choice, the actions taken towards procuring the method and practicing it, as well as the severity of the patient's angst and desire to relieve that angst, all provide reflections of the patient's true suicidal intent.

As described in Section 1 of this chapter, our information regarding the patient's intent is used to complement a careful review – performed during the same interview as the CASE Approach – of the patient's risk factors, warning signs, and protective factors. Having completed these two data gathering steps (e.g., uncovering the pieces of the puzzle) the clinician is ready to put the puzzle together with the third step of a sound suicide assessment – the clinical formulation of risk. In our formulation of risk, we use both our cognitive and intuitive skills to arrive at a determination of the patient's foreseeable likelihood of acting upon his or her suicidal thoughts.

During this assessment process, something else has also been accomplished – something very important, because the interviewer has helped the patient to share painful information, which, in many instances, the patient has shouldered alone for too long. At a different level, perhaps the thoughtfulness and thoroughness of the questioning, as illustrated with the CASE Approach, have conveyed that a fellow human cares. To the patient, such caring may represent the first realization of hope. Such was the case with Mr. Thompson.

REFERENCES

1. Center for Disease Control and Prevention (CDC). *Data for 2014 from CDC website. WISQARS Leading Causes of Death Reports.* Available at: <http://www.cdc.gov/injury/wisqars/leading_causes_death.html>; [accessed May 2016].
2. Center for Disease Control (CDC). *Data for 2014 from CDC website.* [accessed May 2016].
3. Shea SC. The interpersonal art of suicide assessment: interviewing techniques for uncovering suicidal intent, ideation and actions. In: Simon RI, Hales RE, editors. *The American psychiatric publishing textbook of suicide assessment and management.* 2nd ed. Washington, DC: American Psychiatric Publishing; 2012. p. 29–56.
4. Shea SC. *The practical art of suicide assessment: a guide for mental health professionals and substance abuse counselors.* Newbury, NH: Mental Health Presses; 2011 [re-issue of a book first published by John Wiley & Sons, Inc.; 2004].
5. Shea SC. The delicate art of eliciting suicidal ideation. *Psychiatr Ann* 2004;**34**:385–400.
6. Posner K, Brown GK, Stanley B, et al. The Columbia-Suicide Severity Rating Scale: initial validity and internal consistency findings from three multisite studies with adolescents and adults. *Am J Psychiatry* 2011;**168**:1266–77.
7. *Western Michigan University Suicide Prevention Program.* Available at: <http://www.wmich.edu/suicideprevention/basics/protective>; [accessed May 2016].
8. Centers for Disease Control and Prevention (CDC) Website. *Suicide: Risk and Protective Factors.* Available at: <www.cdc.gov/ViolencePrevention/suicide/riskprotectivefactors.html>; [accessed May 2016].
9. Suicide and Prevention Resource Center (SPRC) Website. *Understanding Risk and Protective Factors for Suicide.* Available at: <http://www.sprc.org/sites/sprc.org/files/library/RiskProtectiveFactorsPrimer.pdf>; [accessed May 2016].
10. Rudd MD. The clinical risk interview. In: Simon RI, Hales RE, editors. *The American psychiatric publishing textbook of suicide assessment and management.* 2nd ed. Washington, DC: American Psychiatric Publishing; 2012. p. 57–73.
11. Maris RW, Berman AL, Silverman MM. Suicide, gender, and sexuality. In: *Comprehensive textbook of suicidology.* New York, NY: The Guilford Press; 2000. p. 145–69.
12. American Foundation for Suicide Prevention. <https://afsp.org/about-suicide/suicide-statistics/>; [accessed April 2016].
13. Center for Disease Control (CDC). *Data for 2014 from CDC website.* [accessed May 2016].

14. Center for Disease Control (CDC). *Data for 2014 from CDC website.* [accessed May 2016].
15. Husain SA. Current perspectives on the role of psychosocial factors in adolescent suicide. *Psychiatr Ann* 1990;**20**:122–7.
16. Ash P. Children, adolescents, and college students. In: Simon RI, Hales RE, editors. *The American psychiatric publishing textbook of suicide assessment and management.* 2nd ed. DC: American Psychiatric Publishing; 2012. p. 349–66.
17. Nisbet PA. Age and lifespan. In: Maris RW, Berman AL, Silverman MM, editors. *Comprehensive textbook of suicidology.* New York, NY: The Guilford Press; 2000. p. 127–44.
18. Maris RW, Berman AL, Silverman MM. Racial, ethnic, and cultural aspects of suicide. In: *Comprehensive textbook of suicidology.* New York, NY: The Guilford Press; 2000. p. 170–92.
19. Wendler S, Matthews D, Morelli PT. Cultural competence in suicide risk assessment. In: Simon RI, Hales RE, editors. *The American psychiatric publishing textbook of suicide assessment and management.* 2nd ed. Washington, DC: American Psychiatric Publishing; 2012. p. 75–88.
20. Wendler S, Matthews D, Morelli PT. 2012. p. 75–88.
21. Maris RW, Berman AL, Silverman MM. 2000. p. 145–69.
22. Bates MJ, Bradley JC, Bahraini N, Goldenberg MN. Clinical management of suicide risk with military and veteran personnel. In: Simon RI, Hales RE, editors. *The American psychiatric publishing textbook of suicide assessment and management.* 2nd ed. Washington, DC: American Psychiatric Publishing; 2012. p. 405–52.
23. *The holy bible, revised standard version.* New York, NY: Thomas Nelson, Inc.; 1971.
24. Lion JR, Conn LM. Self-mutilation: pathology and treatment. *Psychiatr Ann* 1982;**12**:782–7.
25. Drake RE, Gates C, Cotton PG, Whitaker A. Suicide among schizophrenics: who is at risk? *J Nerv Ment Dis* 1984;**172**:613–17.
26. Roy A. Depression, attempted suicide, and suicide in patients with chronic schizophrenia. *Psychiatr Clin North Am* 1986;**9**:193–206.
27. Amador XF, Friedman JH, Kasapis C, et al. Suicidal behavior in schizophrenia and its relationship to awareness of illness. *Am J Psychiatry* 1996;**153**:1185–8.
28. Drake RE, et al. 1984, p. 617.
29. Elliott AJ, Pages KP, Russo J, et al. A profile of medically serious suicide attempts. *J Clin Psychiatry* 1996;**57**:567–71.
30. Fawcett J. Depressive disorders. In: Simon RI, Hales RE, editors. *The American psychiatric publishing textbook of suicide assessment and management.* 2nd ed. Washington, DC: American Psychiatric Publishing; 2012. p. 109–22.
31. Busch KA, Clark DC, Fawcett J, Kravitz HM. Clinical features of inpatient suicide. *Psychiatr Ann* 1993;**23**: 256–62.
32. Xiong GL, Barnhorst A, Hilty D. Inpatient psychiatric treatment. In: Simon RI, Hales RE, editors. *The American psychiatric publishing textbook of suicide assessment and management.* 2nd ed. Washington, DC: American Psychiatric Publishing; 2012. p. 109–22.
33. Ash P. 2012. p. 350.
34. Wang Y, Sareen J, Afifi TO. Recent stressful life events and suicide attempts. *Psychiatr Ann* 2012;**42**(3):101–8.
35. Fremouw WJ, de Perczel M, Ellis TE. *Suicide risk: assessment and response guidelines.* New York, NY: Pergamon Press; 1990.
36. Joiner T. *Why people die by suicide.* Cambridge, MA: Harvard University Press; 2005.
37. Van Orden KA, Witte TK, Cukrowicz KC, et al. The interpersonal theory of suicide. *Psychol Rev* 2010;**117**(2):575–600.
38. Joiner TE, Van Orden KA, Witte TK, Rudd MD. *The Interpersonal theory of suicide: guidance for working with suicidal clients.* Washington, DC: American Psychological Association; 2009. p. 57.
39. Tanney BL. Psychiatric diagnoses and suicidal acts. In: Maris RW, Berman AL, Silverman MM, editors. *Comprehensive textbook of suicidology.* New York, NY: The Guilford Press; 2000. p. 311–41.
40. Maris RW, Berman AL, Silverman MM. Suicide attempts and methods. In: *Comprehensive textbook of suicidology.* New York, NY: The Guilford Press; 2000. p. 284–308.
41. Tanney BL. 2000. p. 319–20.
42. Tanney BL. 2000. p. 320.
43. Fawcett J, Scheftner WA, Fogg L, et al. Time-related predictors of suicide in major affective disorder. *Am J Psychiatry* 1990;**147**:1189–94.
44. Fawcett J, Clark DC, Busch KA. Assessing and treating the patient at risk for suicide. *Psych Annals* 1993;**23**:245–55.
45. Fawcett J. 2012. p. 109–12.
46. Nepon J, Belik SL, Bolton J, Sareen J. The relationship between anxiety disorders and suicide attempts: findings from the National Epidemiological Survey on Alcohol and Related Conditions. *Depress Anxiety* 2010;**27**:791–8.
47. Antar LN, Hollander E. Anxiety disorders. In: Simon RI, Hales RE, editors. *The American psychiatric publishing textbook of suicide assessment and management.* 2nd ed. Washington, DC: American Psychiatric Publishing; 2012. p. 123–41.
48. Fawcett J. Saving the suicidal patient – the state of the art. In: Ayd F, editor. *Mood disorders: the world's major public health problem.* Baltimore, MD: Ayd Medical Communication; 1978.

49. Fremouw WJ, et al. 1990. p. 44.
50. Everstine DS, Everstine L. *People in crisis: strategic therapeutic interventions*. New York, NY: Brunner/Mazel; 1983.
51. Beck A. Hopelessness and suicidal behavior. *J Am Med Assoc* 1975;**234**:1146–9.
52. Maris RW, Berman AL, Silverman MM. The biology of suicide. In: *Comprehensive textbook of suicidology*. New York, NY: The Guilford Press; 2000. p. 377–81.
53. Checknita BA, Benoit L, Turecki G. An epigenetic view of suicide and early life adversity. *Psych Annals* 2012;**42**(3):89–94.
54. Patterson WM, Dohn HH, Bird J, Patterson G. Evaluation of suicidal patients: the SAD PERSONS scale. *Psychosomatics* 1983;**24**:343–9.
55. Rudd MD, Berman AL, Joiner TE Jr, et al. Warning signs for suicide: theory, research, and clinical applications. *Suicide Life Threat Behav* 2006;**36**(3):255–62.
56. Simon RI. Imminent suicide: the illusion of short-term prediction. *Suicide Life Threat Behav* 2006;**36**(3):296–301.
57. Weisman AD, Worden JM. Risk-rescue rating in suicide assessment. *Arch Gen Psychiatry* 1972;**26**:553–60.
58. Posner K, Brown GK, Stanley B, et al. 2011. p. 1266–127.
59. Shea SC. Putting it all together: safe and effective decision making. In: *The practical art of suicide assessment: a guide for mental health professionals and substance abuse counselors*. Newbury, NH: Mental Health Presses; 2011.
60. Simon RI. Suicide risk assessment. In: Simon RI, Hales RE, editors. *The American psychiatric publishing textbook of suicide assessment and management*. 2nd ed. Washington, DC: American Psychiatric Publishing; 2012. p. 3–28.
61. Rudd MD. *The assessment and management of suicidality (practitioner's resource)*. Sarasota, FL: The Professional Resource Exchange; 2006.
62. Rudd MD. The clinical risk interview. In: Simon RI, Hales RE, editors. *The American psychiatric publishing textbook of suicide assessment and management*. 2nd ed. Washington, DC: American Psychiatric Publishing; 2012. p. 57–73.
63. Joiner TE, Van Orden KA, Witte TK, Rudd MD. Risk assessment. In: *The interpersonal theory of suicide: guidance for working with suicidal clients*. Washington, DC: American Psychological Association; 2009. p. 53–82.
64. Jobes DA. *Managing suicidal risk: a collaborative approach*. 2nd ed. New York, NY: Guilford Press; 2016.
65. Chiles JA, Strosahl KD. *Clinical manual for the assessment and treatment of suicidal patients*. Washington, DC: American Psychiatric Publishing; 2004.
66. Aston E. *The Darcy connection: a novel*. Austin, TX: Touchstone Publishing; 2008.
67. Hall RCW, Platt DE, Hall RCW. Suicide risk assessment: a review of risk factors for suicide in 100 patients who made severe suicide attempts: Evaluation of suicide risk in a time of managed care. *Psychosomatics* 1999;**40**(1):18–27.
68. Mays D. Structured assessment methods may improve suicide prevention. *Psychiatr Ann* 2004;**34**(5):371.
69. Shea SC. Suicide assessment: part 1: uncovering suicidal intent, a sophisticated art. *Psychiatr Times* 2009;**26**(12):17–19. Available at: <www.PsychiatricTimes.com>; [accessed May 2016].
70. Reed MH, Shea SC. Suicide assessment in college students: innovations in uncovering suicidal ideation and intent. In: Lamis DA, Lester D, editors. *Understanding and preventing college student suicide*. Springfield, IL: Charles C. Thomas, Ltd.; 2011.
71. Shea SC. 2012. p. 31.
72. Joiner TE Jr. *Why people die by suicide*. Cambridge, MA: Harvard University Press; 2005.
73. Joiner TE Jr, Van Orden KA, Witte TK, Rudd MD. *The interpersonal theory of suicide: guidance for working with suicidal clients*. Washington, DC: American Psychological Association; 2009.
74. Prochaska J, Norcross J, DiClemente C. *Changing for good*. New York, NY: William Morrow and Co; 1992.
75. Prochaska J, DiClemente C. *The transtheoretical approach: crossing traditional boundaries of therapy*. Homewood, IL: Dow Jones-Irwin; 1984.
76. Miller W, Rollnick S. *Motivational interviewing: preparing people to change*. 2nd ed. New York, NY: The Guilford Press; 2002.
77. Rollnick S, Miller WR, Butler CC. *Motivational interviewing in health care: helping patients change behavior (applications of motivational interviewing)*. New York, NY: The Guilford Press; 2007.
78. Joiner TE Jr, Van Orden KA, Witte TK, et al. 2009. p. 53–63.
79. Knoll J. Correctional suicide risk assessment & prevention. *Correctional Mental Health Report: Practice, Administration, Law* 2009;**10**(5):65–80.
80. Reed MH, Shea SC. Suicide assessment in college students: innovations in uncovering suicidal ideation and intent. In: Lamis DA, Lester D, editors. *Understanding and preventing college student suicide*. Springfield, IL: Charles C. Thomas, Ltd.; 2011.
81. Shea SC. The chronological assessment of suicide events: a practical interviewing strategy for eliciting suicidal ideation. *J Clin Psychiatry* 1998;**59**(Suppl. 20):58–72.
82. Shea SC *Tips for uncovering suicidal ideation in the primary care setting. Part of the 4-part CD-ROM series Hidden diagnosis: uncovering anxiety and depressive disorders (version 2.0)*. GlaxoSmithKline, 1999.
83. Shea SC. Practical tips for eliciting suicidal ideation for the substance abuse professional. *Counselor, the Magazine for Addiction Professionals* 2001;**2**:14–24.

84. Shea SC. The Chronological Assessment of Suicide Events (the CASE Approach): an introduction for the front-line clinician. *NewsLink (Newsletter of the American Association of Suicidology)* 2002;29:12–13.
85. Shea SC. The delicate art of eliciting suicidal ideation. *Psychiatr Ann* 2004;34:385–400.
86. Shea SC. Suicide assessment: part 1: uncovering suicidal intent, a sophisticated art. *Psychiatr Times* 2009;26(12):17–19. Available at: <www.PsychiatricTimes.com>; [accessed May 2016].
87. Shea SC: *Suicide assessment: part 2: uncovering suicidal intent, using the Chronological Assessment of Suicidal Events (CASE approach)*. Available at: <www.PsychiatricTimes.com>; [accessed May 2016].
88. Shea SC *Innovations in Uncovering Suicidal Ideation With Vets and Soldiers: The Chronological Assessment of Suicide Events (CASE Approach)*. Presented at: the Department of Defense/Veterans Administration Annual Suicide Prevention Conference, San Antonio, TX, 2009.
89. Shea SC. *The practical art of suicide assessment: a guide for mental health professionals and substance abuse counselors.* Newbury, NH: Mental Health Presses; 2011 [originally published John Wiley & Sons, Inc., 2002].
90. Shea SC *Innovations in Eliciting Suicidal Ideation: The Chronological Assessment of Suicide Events (CASE Approach)*. Presented at: the Annual Meetings of the American Association of Suicidology 1999–2013.
91. Shea SC, Barney C. Macrotraining: a how-to primer for using serial role-playing to train complex clinical interviewing tasks such as suicide assessment. *Psychiatr Clin North Am* 2007;30:e1–29.
92. Shea SC. The interpersonal art of suicide assessment: interviewing techniques for uncovering suicidal intent, ideation and actions. In: Simon RI, Hales RE, editors. *The American psychiatric publishing textbook of suicide assessment and management.* 2nd ed. Washington, DC: American Psychiatric Publishing; 2012. p. 29–56.
93. Jobes DA. *Managing suicidal risk: a collaborative approach.* New York, NY: Guilford Press; 2006.
94. Posner K, Brown GK, Stanley B, et al. 2011. p. 1266–77.
95. Rudd MD. 2012. p. 61.
96. Maltsberger JT. *Suicide risk: the formulation of clinical judgment.* New York, NY: New York University Press; 1986.
97. Jobes DA, Mann RE. Reasons for living versus reasons for dying: examining the internal debate of suicide. *Suicide Life Threat Behav* 1999;29:97–104.
98. Miller MC. Suicide-prevention contracts: advantages, disadvantages, and an alternative approach. In: Jacobs DG, editor. *The Harvard Medical School guide to suicide assessment and intervention.* San Francisco, CA: Jossey-Bass; 1999.
99. Miller MC, Jacobs DG, Gutheil TG. Talisman or taboo? The controversy of the suicide prevention contract. *Harv Rev Psychiatry* 1998;6:78–87.
100. Shea SC. 2011. p. 287–303.

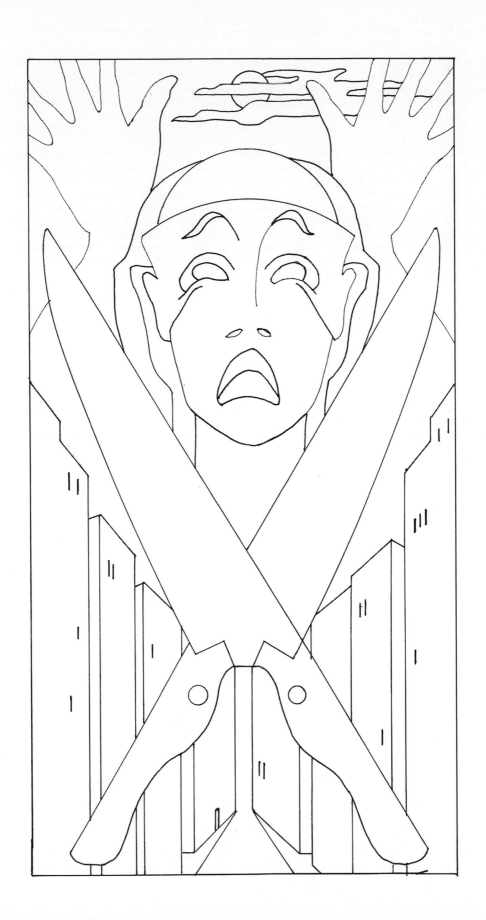

CHAPTER 18

Exploring Violent and Homicidal Ideation: From Domestic Violence to Mass Murder

Domestic violence causes far more pain than the visible marks of bruises and scars.

Dianne Feinstein[1]
United States Senator

INTRODUCTION

Background

We live in a violent society. Violence permeates our imaginations, from the images produced by Hollywood for the big screen to the smaller images created by television moguls that stream across our televisions, tablets, and smart phones. Even more disturbingly, our newscasts, newspapers, and news-related webzines are brimming with violent imagery. They provide hard evidence that violence is all too real – not just a product of our imaginations. We need only remind ourselves that the most likely place for a person to be assaulted is within the walls of his or her own home to see the ubiquitous nature of violence in our culture.

Domestic violence – whether it be intimate partner violence (IPV), older adult abuse, or child abuse – is an everyday reality that recognizes no geographical, ethnic, racial, or socioeconomic boundaries. Recent prevalence data show that 23.6% of women in the United States report experiences of threatened, attempted, or completed physical or sexual assault during their lifetime from an intimate partner.[2] Snider reports the staggering statistic that an estimated 2.2% to 12% of all women who are treated in an emergency department present with injuries related to IPV.[3-8] It is also sobering to realize that among 15- to 34-year-olds, homicide was the third leading cause of death in the United States in 2014. Equally disturbing, or perhaps even more so, is the fact that 364 children between the ages of 1 and 4 were murdered in the same timeframe.[9]

As mental health clinicians, we encounter issues regarding violence on a daily basis, including not only the various forms of domestic violence mentioned thus far, but violence stemming from a variety of situations and environments including gang violence, home invasion, sexual violence, racial/ethnic hate crimes, general criminal violence, workplace violence, psychotic-induced violence, torture, war, terroristic violence, and miscellaneous others. As part of our ongoing work we often find ourselves trying to help the victims of violence to regain a sense of safety and integrity.

This chapter focuses on the daunting, and sometimes nerve-racking, task of spotting the individual who is about to commit violence. As with previous chapters in this book, the goal is to provide practical background theory amplified by specific interviewing strategies and techniques that can make this endeavor both more easily approached and more successful in its outcome. The focus is upon techniques that may help one to spot an individual who is more likely to commit violence in the near future (1–2 weeks from the interview date). I use the word "may" because we have yet to find methods that have been empirically proven to be effective in this task. Such a lack of evidence does not suggest that we should simply throw up our hands saying, "one cannot accurately predict imminent violence." To the contrary, it suggests that we should do our very best to use whatever interviewing techniques seem to make the most sense and appear to be the most logical as we await the development of a better empirical and phenomenological evidence base.

This chapter is designed to be a primer on interviewing techniques for uncovering potential violent behaviors and intent in our patients. The goal is to provide readers with a sound foundation for approaching this task in a sensitive and effective fashion for immediate use in their clinical practices. In addition, as a primer, it is designed to refer the interested reader to more advanced resources for further study. In this regard, many excellent textbooks on the risk assessment regarding violence are available. Three of my favorites are *Violence Assessment and Management* by Simon and Tardiff,[10] *Clinician's Guide to Violence Risk Assessment* by Mills, Kroner, and Morgan,[11] and Meloy and Hoffman's *International Handbook of Threat Assessment.*[12]

Characterizing Violence: Three Practical Domains for Clinicians

One of the first issues of interest is the finding that violence can be inflicted by very different types of people in many different types of settings. Reid Meloy describes two of these distinctive categories – affective violence and predatory violence.[13] In the first category, affective violence, we find individuals who, because of intense anger and emotion, impulsively act out violently, often in response to interpersonal stress and frequently under the influence of alcohol and drugs. This is often the arena of IPV, child and older adult abuse, and violence undertaken at the job, in our schools, or on the streets. This type of violence probably arises from a very different "headspace" than Meloy's second categorization. With predatory violence, the killer or perpetrator has often thought out the violence beforehand, frequently derives pleasure from the violent act itself, and feels little, if any, remorse. This is the domain of many rapists, sadistic perpetrators of children, and individuals with sociopathic personality structures.

Although there are undoubtedly significant biologic underpinnings to the above styles of violence, I think it is useful to include a third category of violent behavior – "biologically induced violence." This term specifically describes those individuals whose violence is directly caused by brain pathophysiology or structural pathology. The first sub-category, pathophysiology, includes individuals who are suffering from biochemical abnormalities such as schizophrenia, mania (especially dysphoric mania), or acute ingestion of drugs such as lysergic acid diethylamide (LSD), phencyclidine (PCP), or "bath salts." The second sub-category, structural damage, includes people suffering from diseases such as brain tumors, partial complex seizures, intracranial infections, brain trauma, multiple sclerosis, and Alzheimer's disease. Violent behavior sometimes erupts from combinations of the above three categories (affective, predatory, and/or biologically induced) as well.

By reminding ourselves of these three "domains of violence," we can sometimes increase our suspicion of when to search for violent ideation, ensuring that we are searching frequently enough. With regard to this latter point, clinicians, owing to various factors including schools of training, countertransference, and lack of familiarity, can sometimes have "blind spots." For instance, an example of a blind spot can occur for clinicians who do not frequently work with people with psychotic processes. In such a situation, it can be easy to miss the subtle indications of active psychosis, and, consequently, the clinician may not undertake the type of questioning that such psychotic process suggests (see pages 464–466, 528–532, and 690–692).

Another blind spot can occur when it becomes necessary to explore for evidence of the psychological, physical, or sexual sadism sometimes seen in predators. Such explorations can be unnerving and, consequently, are sometimes avoided by clinicians. It should be noted, however, that there are times when such avoidance, if consciously chosen, is not only appropriate but also wise. For instance, if a female interviewer unexpectedly uncovers a sexual sadist whose victims are female, the details of this patient's violent history may, in some cases, be better taken by a male clinician, and vice versa for a male interviewer if men are the patient's victims.

Regarding the much more everyday problem of domestic violence – although most of our patients are not perpetrators – in essence, almost every patient who is seen is a potential perpetrator of domestic violence (from IPV to the abuse of children or older adults). Indeed, some of our patients are involved in other types of violence from gang violence to physical bullying in schools (the term "bullying" being a bad euphemism for psychological abuse and/or physical assault). One simply cannot know unless one asks. And to ferret out the truth, one must ask using effective questions. Of course, even then, one may not be receiving accurate information. Moreover, in my opinion, trainees in psychiatric residencies and graduate programs are often inadequately trained to uncover violence from domestic violence to predatory violence including rape, pedophilia, and mass murder. This chapter attempts to fill some of the gaps in this training.

The logical question arises – are there methods for increasing our ability to look for violent ideation, behaviors, and intent? I believe that there are. Fortunately, we have already developed the foundation, because, as Tardiff emphasizes in his excellent pocket guide, *Assessment and Management of Violent Patients*,[14] a sound homicide assessment has much in common with a sound suicide assessment. The techniques that we found so valuable in the Chronological Assessment of Suicide Events (the CASE Approach) in the previous chapter are directly adaptable to the elicitation of violent ideation and intent. This is one of the main reasons that this chapter is much shorter than that on suicide assessment: Our main tool has already been described. When the techniques and strategies for uncovering suicidal ideation are adapted and revised to uncover potentially violent and/or homicidal ideation, the strategy is called the Chronological Assessment of Dangerous Events (the CADE Approach).

The Organization of the Chapter and the Role of Structured Risk Assessments

Before delineating the risk factors for violence and the intricacies of the CADE Approach, I would like to better delineate what the chapter is (and what it is not), as well as suggesting some further useful resources for topics that are clinically quite important but go beyond the scope of the chapter. First, although we will touch upon how to take the puzzle pieces uncovered during an interview and put them together into a clinical formulation of risk, being a book on clinical interviewing, our main focus will be upon how to most effectively uncover the puzzle pieces themselves. The emphasis is upon helping clinicians who must make the difficult decision as to whether a particular patient has an increased likelihood of violence either upon immediately leaving the interview or during the next few days to 2 weeks.

In the second place, a variety of structured approaches to risk assessment (the Historical Clinical Risk Management-20 [HCR-20], the Classification of Violence Risk [COVR], and the Violence Risk Appraisal Guide [VRAG]),[15] as well as various psychological testing measures (Hare's Psychopathy Checklist Revised [PCL-R], Novaco Anger Scale, etc.),[16] have been developed over the past several decades. The structured interviews, such as the HCR-20, focus upon the gathering of statistical risk factors, both static and dynamic. This emphasis upon statistical prediction is generally referred to as an "actuarial approach" in the literature, in contrast to a clinical approach. It is important to realize that these structured instruments have not been shown to have predictive capabilities in the assessment of immediate (within 24 to 48 hours post interview) and imminent (up to 2 weeks post interview) violence risk, which are the relative timeframes of interest to us in this chapter.

Consequently, I personally do not recommend the routine use of such structured interviews in the initial assessment for everyday clinicians (related to their length of time in administration, lack of evidence of predictive capability in immediate and imminent risk prediction, the need to take one's eyes off the patient intermittently with the possible missing of nonverbal clues of deceit, and the disruption of a naturalistic flow of conversation with possible disengagement and consequent loss of validity).

On the other hand, although it remains unclear whether they might play a role in predicting violence in the next several days after seeing a patient, they have been shown to be of definite value in helping to better predict violence over the course of several months. For instance, the COVR, an innovative piece of risk assessment software, has been validated for predictive use over the subsequent 20 weeks after its completion. Thus, if a clinician is going to be seeing a patient in an ongoing fashion, or is being asked to provide a relative prediction of violence in the next 6 months – as a forensic consultant might be asked – these innovative tools appear to be valuable, with research suggesting that they may be more accurate at predicting violence than many clinicians when used for assessing violent behavior over these longer timeframes. I certainly recommend becoming familiar with them, but they will not be the focus of this chapter.

It should be mentioned that, in general, there remains a great deal of debate about a clinician's abilities to predict violence, including immediate (within 24 to 48 hours post interview), imminent (up to 2 weeks post interview), short-term (up to 6 months post interview), and long-term (greater than 6 months post interview). It is beyond the scope of this chapter to explore this debate, but the interested reader will find plenty of valuable information in both recent and classic works, such as the MacArthur Study, and contributions from pioneering writers such as Monohan, Lidz, Applebaum and others.[17-24]

As was the case with suicide, we will begin with a review of statistical risk factors, bolstered by the knowledge that has been provided by the promising research on the HCR-20. As we saw in the evaluation of immediate and imminent suicide potential, statistical risk factors can serve as significant aids in assessment, for they can alert us to specific venues worth exploring (dangerous psychotic process, current substance abuse, intense interpersonal anger, etc.), as well as making us suspicious of deceit from the patient (as evidenced by the appearance of a large number of risk factors in a patient who dismissively denies any violent ideation).

To accomplish the tasks of this primer, it is divided into three parts. In Part 1, Risk Factors for Violence, we will explore the many risk factors that research has demonstrated may help with the assessment of violent risk. In Part 2, Clinical Formulation of Risk – The Tetrad of Lethality, we will explore four clinical situations that may suggest that our interviewee may be predisposed to a violent act in the very near future. Finally, in Part 3, The Art of Eliciting Violent and Homicidal Ideation, we will move to the main focus of this chapter – interviewing techniques for uncovering violent ideation, planning, behaviors, and intent.

PART 1: RISK FACTORS FOR VIOLENCE

Past Violence

The single most robust statistical indicator of violence is a history of previous violence.[25,26] If you want to be a "betting man," here is the place to put your money. As Tardiff notes, a general tendency for marked problems with impulse control may also be part of the picture. In this regard, it is also important to ask about destruction of property, criminal record, reckless driving, reckless spending, sexual acting out, and suicide attempts.[27]

Sex, Age, and Environment

Young men have the highest rate of violent behavior. Growing up in an impoverished area – where violence may be more frequent and peer pressure towards violent behavior may be strong – carries a higher risk of violent behavior. It is also noteworthy that growing up in a family in which one was abused or where one watched other family members being abused may also be associated with an increased risk of violence.[28,29]

Presence of Psychiatric Disorders

The most significant diagnosis here is the presence of alcoholism and street drug use. Other common correlates with violence are antisocial personality disorder; borderline personality disorder; and psychiatric disorders secondary to a general medical condition, including conditions such as intellectual disabilities and dementia, as well as disorders where psychotic or manic process may emerge. It should be kept in mind that most people with psychotic process, most of the time, are very safe. It is an unfortunate and detrimental myth among the lay public that people with schizophrenia, by definition, are dangerous. On the other hand, as we found to be the case regarding suicide risk, during the exacerbation of specific types of psychotic process (e.g., paranoid delusions, command hallucinations) such patients are definitely at a higher risk of violence. We will talk more about the clinical implications of this fact shortly.

With regard to antisocial personality disorder, be on the lookout for a subset of this personality disorder referred to as psychopathy in the literature. It should be noted that most people with antisocial personality disorders are not psychopathic. This psychopathic group is a relatively small subset of this personality disorder, but a significantly more dangerous one. In psychopathy, the patient lacks almost all superego function and tends to exhibit marked enjoyment of violence towards others including animals. Psychopathy is the realm of Meloy's predatory violence, where one encounters serial rapists, serial murderers, and people prone to torturing others.

Violence is also seen with intermittent explosive disorder, which has a 2.7% 1-year prevalence rate.[30] Be careful though, for some clinicians inappropriately apply this diagnosis. It can only be used when there is no other psychiatric disorder present that could explain the violence such as schizophrenia, schizoaffective disorder, bipolar disorder, post-traumatic stress disorder, disruptive mood dysregulation disorder, etc. In this light, it is not an appropriate diagnosis in domestic violence if alcohol use, drug use, or antisocial personality disorder is present.[31]

Other Factors Suggested by the HCR-20

We can round out our exploration of potential risk factors for violence by referring to the revised version of the HCR-20. In this instrument, risk factors are elicited in three domains: (1) "historical" items, (2) "clinical" items, and (3) "risk management" items.[32] Historical factors not already described above include: young age at first violent incident, relationship instability, employment problems, early maladjustment, and prior supervision failure (as with probation officers). Regarding clinical risk factors, the items in the HCR-20 that we haven't already discussed above include: lack of insight and negative attitudes. The last five items of the HCR-20 are related to risk management and include: the violent plan lacks feasibility, exposure to destabilizers, lack of interpersonal support, noncompliance with remediation attempts in the past, and current stress.

Some of this material will be naturalistically uncovered when taking the social history (relationship problems, employment problem, and lack of interpersonal supports); others will emerge as the interviewer explores the past treatment history (prior supervision failure, noncompliance issues); and some will become apparent as the history of the present stressors and disorders unfolds (lack of insight, negative attitudes, and current stressors).

The potential predictive power of a history of past violence, as well as the appearance of violence (and marked maladjustment) in childhood, highlight the importance of exploring past violent behaviors with patients suspected of near future violence. Questions for performing such explorations will be delineated in our discussion of the CADE.

PART 2: CLINICAL FORMULATION OF RISK – THE TETRAD OF LETHALITY

As was the case with suicide assessment, a clinician's final clinical formulation of risk is not made solely based on statistical risk factors. These risk factors are carefully weighed in addition to information about the patient's immediate presentation. Moreover, as with suicide assessment, the clinical formulation of risk is not limited to an analytic weighing of risk factors, protective factors, and expressed violent ideation, planning, and intent. It also includes the clinician's intuitive insights garnered during the interview.

In my opinion, four aspects of the patient's immediate presentation can alert the clinician to the potential for immediate, imminent, or short-term violence. This tetrad of lethality is as follows: (1) the patient is presenting subsequent to a recent serious act of violence (often brought in by police), (2) the presence of a type of psychotic process that may precipitate violence, (3) indication from the interview itself that the patient intends to engage in violence, and (4) the patient is lying and significant corroborative evidence exists that violence is more likely in the immediate, imminent, or short-term timeframe. The reader probably recognizes that this homicidal tetrad looks very similar to the tetrad of lethality for suicide.

1. Patients Presenting With a Recent Violent Episode

With regard to the first element – a history of presenting recent violence – generally, the more severe the violent act and the greater the degree to which the patient remains hostile and angry, the more the clinician should feel concerned. But it is here that an understanding of some of the differences that Meloy points out between violent individuals of an affective style versus a predatory style may help the clinician to predict violence. For instance, if the patient has a history of an affective style of violence, then the continuing presence of a simmering anger during the interview should alert the clinician that hospitalization may be necessary for the purposes of a "cool down." On the other hand, an unwary clinician can be lulled into a false sense of safety by the apparent calm demeanor of a predator, even right after or before performing an act of violence. Never forget that in the presence of a predator it is important to "look through" the person's presenting affect, because it is almost always a mask.

Another important aspect of history concerns the issue of whether the potential victim has been an object of the patient's violence before, as is often the case in domestic violence. If so, this fact should alert the clinician, because the risk of violence may increase in a "powder keg" environment such as one in which the former victim is present. Keep in mind that most homicides occur between people well known to each other.

A powder keg environment may also develop when the potentially homicidal patient is placed around other people who have poor impulse control. In short, anger may beget anger, and violence may breed violence. Furthermore, the presence of alcohol use or drug use, in either the patient or in the patient's companions, may increase the risk of violence as well. It is important for the interviewer to actively hunt for evidence of such powder keg environments. As with suicide, corroborative interviews may be revealing in this regard.

2. Patients Presenting With Dangerous Psychotic Process

As mental health professionals, we do our best to de-stigmatize serious mental illnesses, including those that involve psychotic process. Part of this de-stigmatization process is to challenge the popular myth that all patients with disorders such as schizophrenia and bipolar disorder are, by the nature of their diseases, particularly dangerous. On the other hand, in our efforts to de-stigmatize these illnesses, as we found to be the case in suicide, it is sometimes easy to forget that the presence of specific types of psychotic process do make some patients more dangerous at certain times. And when these processes are active, people are in potential danger.

In an informative article, Lake points out the paradoxical fact that it is the psychotic patients themselves who are often at highest risk of harm.[33] Psychotic process, such as command hallucinations, may lead them to self-mutilate or attempt suicide. Another avenue to danger for these patients can come from police, who may have been called because of the patient's disruptive behavior. For instance, some psychotic patients attempt "suicide by cop"; at other times, poorly trained police may use unnecessary lethal force.

Moreover, mental health professionals are at a significantly higher risk. For instance, the annual rate for nonfatal violence in all occupations in the United States from 1993 to 1999 was 12.6 per 1000 workers according to the Department of Justice National Crime Victimization Study. During the same period, the rate for psychiatrists was 62.2 per 1000 workers and 69 per 1000 for custodial mental health workers.[34]

Of the roughly 10 million people in the United States who are suffering from a severe mental illnesses such as schizophrenia, schizoaffective disorder, bipolar disorder, and other psychotic processes, it has been estimated that about 14% will commit a violent act in any given year.[35] Keeping in mind that nearly 40 to 50% of the patients with a severe mental illness are untreated, these statistics are not overly surprising. Ironically, the stigmatization of these people has probably contributed to the striking lack of resources that our society chooses to offer them, a fact that increases the likelihood that the patients will act out violently, thus continuing their stigmatization in a vicious circle.

In any case, it is important to remember that, statistically speaking, people suffering with a serious mental disorder, such as those involving psychotic process, are about five times more likely to be violent than a person without such a disorder. (To put this in perspective though, people with alcohol or substance use disorders are about 10 to 16 times more likely to be violent than a person without a mental disorder.[36]) This does not mean that a specific patient with a serious mental illness, such as schizophrenia or bipolar disorder, is five times more dangerous. *They usually are not more dangerous than the population without a mental disorder, unless that specific patient is experiencing, at that specific time, the types of dangerous psychotic processes described below (or marked manic symptoms).*

If we become adept at utilizing the types of interviewing techniques discussed below (and those presented in earlier chapters) hopefully we will be better able to prevent psychotic violence. This mission not only protects potential victims but also protects our patients, whose violent actions are generally beyond their control, caused by a biological maelstrom in their brains. Many of these patients, once their psychotic process moves into remission, must live with a horrifying guilt for the rest of their lives. Some choose not to do so (suicide). One need only talk with a patient who has committed infanticide during a postpartum psychotic episode to understand the immense pain of these patients and the tragedy of their afflictions. This section tries to avert such tragedies.

Command Hallucinations, Alien Control, and Hyper-Religiosity

Concerning psychotic violence, the same three processes as seen with a suicide assessment are of concern. Once again, if psychotic process is spotted, the interviewer should actively pursue evidence of: (1) command hallucinations, (2) alien control, and (3) hyper-religiosity. *In Chapters 11, 12, and 17 practical interviewing strategies and techniques for exploring these three areas of psychotic dangerousness were delineated in detail* (see pages 464–466, 528–532, and 690–692). If you have not read these sections, I urge you to do so, for the clinician's ability to utilize effective interviewing techniques in this area can literally be life saving.

Regarding your exploration of psychotic hyper-religiosity, remember to pay particular attention to "missions from God to rid the earth of some evil." Such an intense preoccupation with right and wrong may be signaling underlying homicidal ideation. The search for specifics may be rewarding, as follows in this reconstructed dialogue:

Pt.: The world is filled with scum. Derelicts and bums. I hate them all. God wants them gone.

Clin.: How do you mean?

Pt.: God has his ways.

Clin.: Has he given you any ideas of how to get rid of them?

Pt.: Yes he has. He wants me to cut their eyes out. And I might do just that.

Clin.: Have you thought of anyone in particular that you might hurt?

Pt.: Sam … what a scumbag. I've thought of him.

Clin.: What have you thought of doing to him?

As we saw earlier, command hallucinations, alien control, and psychotic hyper-religiosity are risk factors common to both suicidal and violent behaviors. But with regard to violence assessment, there is one more risk factor of immense importance.

Uncovering Paranoid Process

In talking about psychotic-induced violence, another important avenue to pursue is the presence of paranoia. Although paranoia can be seen relatively frequently in schizophrenia and schizoaffective disorder, it is also commonly seen in bipolar disorder as well as during psychotic major depressive episodes. In particular, the anger seen in dysphoric manias (see pages 368–374) often demonstrates a paranoid quality to it, ranging from hostile wariness to frank paranoid delusional process.

In this regard, patients experiencing psychotic dysphoric manias may be more prone to violence, whether violence to individuals (family, colleagues, clinicians, or strangers) or, much more rarely, to episodes of mass murder (school shootings, mall shootings, etc.). Some authors feel that the type of violence seen in psychotic rampage murders is more likely to be caused by dysphoric manias than by schizophrenia.[37] No matter what the etiology of the violent ideation triggered by paranoid process, the interviewer should search for evidence that the patient so believes in the delusional material that methods of acting upon it have been pursued, as the following prototypic dialogue illustrates:

> **Pt.:** The neighbors know everything, I can't keep their eyes out of my brain.
>
> **Clin.:** What are they planning on doing to you?
>
> **Pt.:** They're going to cut off my feet but I'm not going to let them.
>
> **Clin.:** What have you thought about doing to protect yourself?
>
> **Pt.:** I'm going to scissor them.
>
> **Clin.:** How do you mean?
>
> **Pt.:** I'll stick a pair of scissors in their spines.
>
> **Clin.:** Have you armed yourself with scissors or some other weapon at home?
>
> **Pt.:** Yes I have. Last night I patrolled my house with a pair of scissors and a knife.

This degree of acting on the premise that the delusion is a real threat should strongly suggest hospitalization. Any neighbor of this man may be in serious danger for merely accidentally crossing his path. But the point is, it is not enough to find out if a paranoid delusion is present. The clinician needs to find out what the patient intends to do about it. *A variety of interviewing techniques for determining the dangerousness of paranoid ideation were described in detail earlier in this book* (see pages 464–470) *and are well worth familiarizing yourself with, if you have not already done so.*

Complexities of Spotting Individuals Contemplating Mass Murder and Other Paranoid-Induced Violence

Before leaving the exploration of paranoid process, let us briefly turn our attention to mass murderers. Although mass murders are sometimes caused by nonpsychotic individuals, it is important to realize that a significant percentage are caused by patients suffering with psychotic process. The likelihood of interviewing a potential mass murderer is not high, but it is a possibility. Nearly half of psychotic perpetrators of mass murder received mental health care prior to their rampages.[38] They also have a tendency to give warnings about their intended violence through personal revelation directly (comments to friends, family, fellow students) or indirectly (via websites, social media, etc.).

Examples of mass murder being triggered by psychotic process include Seung-Hui Cho, who killed 32 students at Virginia Tech in 2007 (gave warning); James E. Holmes, who killed 12 people in a movie theater in Aurora, Colorado in 2012 (gave some warning); and Jared Loughner, who killed six people, as well as seriously injuring United States Representative Gabrielle Giffords, on January 8, 2011 (gave many warnings over several years). Thus we can see that no matter where we work, from a college counseling center to a community mental health center, emergency department, or inpatient unit, we may be interviewing a person whose psychotic process and dangerousness may be discoverable with appropriate training.

According to Lake, people prone to psychotic-induced mass murder tend to share the following characteristics: They usually act alone and often in daylight hours. Curiously, they seldom try to get away; consequently, many are killed at the scene of the crime by police. Their plans are usually well thought out. They may recognize that their actions are illegal, but they believe that the act must be done for the greater good (their delusions or voices tell them that great harm will occur to many others, or themselves, if they do not kill the intended people, etc.). In this regard, they may feel they are killing Satan, protecting children from demons, preventing a global holocaust, or preventing sinister plans for mass torture or genocide. In this sense, they have little or no distance from their delusional thinking, i.e. they are absolutely convinced that their delusional material is true. Interestingly, despite the fact that alcohol and drugs are common in violent acts, these patients tend to be free of alcohol and/or street drugs at the time of the murders.[39]

Knoll and Meloy have proposed that psychotically triggered mass murderers often possess a common phenomenology to their paranoid process as it unfolds towards implementation.[40] I feel that the cognitive progression described by Knoll and Meloy is actually also commonly seen in acts of paranoid-related violence towards individuals. Thus, in my opinion, a better understanding of Knoll and Meloy's concepts can be of value when exploring paranoid process with any patient. I will present each step of their fourfold model and follow each step with some examples of questions that may help to uncover the reflected dangerousness of each step.

In the first step, the person must perceive that there exists a present danger. Whether this perception evolves from intense feelings of inadequacy (perhaps even a projection of self-hate) or simply is triggered by external acts of abuse from other people, the patient becomes convinced that they (or others) are at risk of serious harm or death. As we saw earlier in the book – when describing dysphoric mania – this process often crystallizes into an ongoing dark mood characterized by resentment, fear, anger, and righteous condemnation of others (either specific people who have rejected or hurt them or the world at large, as with hate towards a political system, misogyny, government, or "the in-class"). The following types of questions may be of use in exploring this phenomenology:

1. "Tell me a little bit more about the people you think are trying to hurt you?"
2. "What are some of the specific things these people do to hurt you or others?"

3. "Do these people have any sense of remorse or guilt for what they have done?"
4. "Do they make fun of you, taunt you, or reject you?"
5. "How set are they upon hurting you or killing you?"

In the second step, the person experiencing paranoia will move inside themselves to contemplate the likelihood that there are non-violent and/or legal ways of preventing their persecutors from hurting them. If they decide that there is no way to stop them, violence becomes the only viable force for protection. Ironically, at this point, violence is seen as defensive, necessary, and good. As any of us would, if we felt that someone was going to kill us and there was no possible way of stopping them from doing so, we would do what we needed to do to protect ourselves, our families, or other innocent people who were threatened. Thus the decision to act violently is neither illogical nor immoral from the patient's psychotic worldview. The following questions are of use in exploring this step:

1. "Have you tried anything to reason or compromise with these people?"
2. "Are there avenues for you to ensure your safety (safety of your child, etc.) such as going to the police, moving away, talking with the principal, etc.?"
3. "On a scale from 0 to 10, with 0 being 'these people will not actually try to kill me' to 10 being 'I am absolutely sure that they will try to kill me,' what number represents your risk from them? Do you understand what I mean by the question?"
4. "How soon do you think you need to act to protect yourself?"

In the third step of the cognitive progression described by Knoll and Meloy, the patient has decided that there is no avenue for safety or means of retribution for wrongdoing by others than violence towards them. In this step, the patient frequently begins to both fantasize and picture the act of violence and its impact on his or her persecutors:

1. "What have you pictured doing to protect yourself?" (or to "right this wrong," "seek vengeance," "provide just punishment," if more applicable to the patient's story)
2. "Do you spend time having any fantasies about hurting them or making them pay for what they have done?"
3. "How would you go about punishing or killing them?"
4. "Are there movie scenes or gaming sequences that please you, that you picture yourself doing to these people?"
5. "Would you make them pay for their crimes?"
6. "Do you have fantasies of torturing the person?"
7. "What do you picture saying to them as you are about to kill them?"
8. "How much time do you spend picturing or fantasizing doing what you are thinking about doing, 50% of your day, 70%, 90%?" (symptom amplification)

In the fourth step, the patient moves from fantasy towards implementation. In short, the patient begins to make a resolution to proceed with his or her act of proactive protection and/or vengeance/retribution against society or a specific group in society. In essence, this step is explored using the CADE, but here is a preview of some useful questions:

1. "How would you kill this person/s?" (use name of potential target if known)
2. "What other ways have you thought or killing them?" (gentle assumption)
3. "Have you gone on the web to find methods for killing these people?"
4. "Have you gotten the weapon/s you need?"
5. "Have you practiced using it/them?"
6. "Do you have a plan for actually doing it?"
7. "Have you picked a date?"

In this last section, one can use Resnick's "confrontation with a paranoid persecutor" (see page 465) and the techniques of David Robinson (see page 465) to better delineate the likelihood of imminent future violence.

If you encounter a patient who has developed a marked paranoid delusional system, with any hints of violence, I would urge you to consult with a fellow clinician to discuss various potential strategies for proceeding and to actively make sure of your own safety. It is important that you proceed in the safest manner with this patient in future sessions; also consider warning potential victims, if deemed necessary under the Tarasoff principles. The Tarasoff decision is a legal ruling in the United States that requires clinicians to contact potential victims – whom the clinician feels may be at danger – even if it requires breaking confidentiality. You will find excellent material regarding the Tarasoff's decision in any of the three general textbooks on violence assessment mentioned earlier in the chapter (see page 764).

As a final note regarding rampage mass murder, Knoll and Meloy's model was designed to provide insight into mass murders related to psychotic process, and I have adapted it for use with psychotic violence aimed at a specific individual (a scenario that an everyday clinician is much more likely to encounter during his or her career). To some degree, the model is also useful for exploring violent ideation in a nonpsychotic individual with whom one is worried about the potential for mass murder.

Instead of focusing upon the concept of paranoid process as in Knoll and Meloy's model, consider the four steps as being part of an evolving bitterness, contempt, and hatred for a specific group, such as people who have verbally or physically abused a student (euphemistically called bullying) or are viewed as being unworthy of their financial or societal status. Sometimes the potential perpetrator feels that he or she has been unfairly rejected by a specific group of people (as might be demonstrated by a misogynistic hatred for women by a loner male who feels consistently romantically rejected). In short, nonpsychotic mass murderers frequently act out of a profound belief that they have been wronged by specific elements of society. The four steps of the Knoll/Meloy model can be adapted as follows: (1) the potential perpetrator will feel that the wrongdoing will continue, (2) the perpetrator will feel there is no way to right the wrong and/or justly punish the wrongdoers other than violence, (3) the perpetrator will begin to fantasize violence towards the wrongdoers, and, finally, (4) the perpetrator will make a resolve to act out the violence (moving towards planning, procuring the means for the violence, and implementation).

3. Indication From the Interview That the Patient Intends to Engage in Violence

As illustrated with the last set of questions, patients may describe their violent/homicidal ideation, planning, and intent during the interview itself. As with suicide assessment, this particular set of puzzle pieces can be invaluable in assessing a reasonably foreseeable increase in the potential risk of violence in the near future. This "set of risk factors" warrants its own elaboration. The validity techniques and interviewing strategies that allow one to explore this area more effectively are so important that we will devote the entire last part of this chapter to their description and illustration. But what if the patient lies despite the use of these techniques?

4. The Patient Is Lying and Collaborative Evidence Suggests Intended Violence

Ironically, the first thing to remember about the information elicited from the patient, with regard to violent intent, is not to rely upon it. Family members and friends may be far superior sources of information. The police, previous and current therapists, and crisis clinicians may also hold critical pieces of information.

A Few Caveats Regarding Domestic Violence

Perpetrators of domestic violence, whether IPV, older adult abuse, or child abuse, frequently minimize or deny it altogether. Oftentimes the victims of the violence can give a better history and hence allow for a more accurate picture as to whether or not they are in danger of more violence in the immediate or imminent future. We are focusing upon methods for interviewing the perpetrators of violence in this chapter, but a few caveats are in order here regarding interviews with the victims as a means of gathering information for violence risk assessment with the perpetrator.

You may find yourself in a situation, such as in an emergency room or inpatient unit, where the perpetrator and the victim present simultaneously. Although you may uncover significantly more valid information from the victim, the situation requires caution and foresight before proceeding.

Domestic violence, from child abuse to sexual IPV, is primarily driven by the perpetrator's need for power and control over his or her partner, elder parent, sibling, disabled family member, or child. Keep in mind that a clinical interview in which a perpetrator shares his or her thoughts and/or behaviors can feel threatening to the perpetrator. *Before proceeding with such an interview, clinicians should bear in mind that the assessment itself may increase the risk of new violence to the adult or child victims.* Consultation may be indicated before (as well as after) proceeding with an interview of the perpetrator. Moreover, in my opinion, a frank discussion of safety issues with the collaborative generation of a safety plan is often best done with the victim of the violence before proceeding to interview the perpetrator.

Other guiding principles include: Do not ask the alleged batterer about the violence in front of the alleged victim. And avoid telling the perpetrator information provided earlier by the victim regarding the perpetrators violent behavior. Instead, try to use corroborating information from police, neighbors, courts, medical personnel, etc. A variety of other considerations are important that go beyond the focus of this chapter. The above tips, as well as coverage of many other considerations and practical questions are available on the web from the Oregon Department of Human Services (DHS).[41] This resource provides excellent questions for use with the victims of domestic violence as well as the perpetrator. I strongly recommend it. Another rich resource for practical questions to ask the victims of domestic violence has been created by Anne Ganley and Susan Schechter, which I also heartily recommend.[42]

Returning to our focus – information from victims that may increase the accuracy of our prediction of more imminent or short-term violence – a valuable study by Snider and colleagues provides several excellent questions. The questions grew out of the pressures encountered in emergency department work to quickly and safely uncover the risk of future domestic violence. A group of 20 questions were studied with regard to their predictive capabilities. Five of the questions proved to be of particular value. These questions relate to interviews of female victims of IPV. I think you will find them to be of use[43]:

1. "Has the physical violence increased in frequency or severity over the past 6 months?"
2. "Has he (the abuser) ever used a weapon or threatened you with a weapon?"
3. "Do you believe he is capable of killing you?"
4. "Have you ever been beaten by him while you were pregnant?"
5. "Is he violently and constantly jealous of you?"

In addition to collaborative sources, whether exploring the potential for domestic violence or any other kind of violence, one should not forget the immense value of previous medical records, a resource that should become progressively more accessible as the use of electronic health records (EHRs) evolves. In the EHR one can look for arrests, violent episodes, involuntary commitments, and a history of restraining orders. Court records can also be of value. In addition, any material a patient has made public via the web, including social media, can potentially be of use if one suspects a patient is considering violent behavior. Mass murderers frequently leave a trail on social media.

The issue of the EHR raises another important point. As Applebaum and Roth point out,[44] one of the major reasons why receiving hospitals reverse involuntary commitments at the door is because important information elicited from the patient, family, or police is not adequately recorded by the interviewer or the information is not passed on to the receiving center. It is often best not only to include these written documents but also to call the receiving institution and speak directly about your concerns with the clinician who will be assessing the patient. EHRs will hopefully enhance inter-hospital communication as both the EHR systems improve and issues related to confidentiality are more explicitly delineated.

PART 3: THE ART OF ELICITING VIOLENT AND HOMICIDAL IDEATION

With regard to the strategy for eliciting violent ideation, the flexible use of the same strategies as used with the CASE Approach can be very revealing. First, as with suicide assessment, the clinician carefully "sets the stage." Second, the clinician proceeds to explore presenting, recent, past, and immediate violent events (both ideation and behaviors) in that order.

Once again, the major goal consists of determining whether a concrete violent plan has been reached and whether any actions have been taken on it, as well as obtaining any other information that represents "reflected intent." The interviewer also looks for information suggesting that the patient is about to impulsively act out violent ideation. *A point to keep in mind is that if the interviewer suspects that the patient truly intends to harm a specific person, the clinician has the legal responsibility to warn that potential victim, as mandated by the Tarasoff decision.*

Setting the Stage

One aspect to consider when setting the stage for asking about violent ideation and intent is the wide variety of gates available. Homicide has more than the three gates that are useful when dealing with suicidal ideation. Some of these homicidal gates include: (1) psychosis, (2) interpersonal conflict, (3) need for money and other practical concerns, (4) revenge, (5) jealousy, (6) political concerns, (7) gang membership and organized crime, (8) terroristic violence, and (9) violence for pleasure and pathologic sexual desires. Naturally, any of these gates could be used to enter an exploration of dangerousness.

Regarding IPV, one way of setting the stage is to get the patient to describe in detail his or her worst argument with the significant other. Let us look at a clinician interviewing a suspected male perpetrator of IPV. Once the patient has depicted the intensity of the angry encounter in question, the interviewer might ask, "When you and your wife/partner are arguing like that, has she/he ever sort of lost her/his control and hit you or attacked you?" After the patient responds to this inquiry, one is much more likely to get a valid response to the follow-up, "How about you, during arguments like that? How frequently have you struck your wife/partner or grabbed her/him, if at all?"

By first asking about the other person's potential violence, it helps the patient, whom you actually suspect of violence, to feel equally heard and hence safer with you. This sense of safety can directly lead to a more valid self-reporting of the patient's own violent behavior. Notice also the clinician's use of the validity technique of gentle assumption with the phrase, "... how frequently have you struck your wife/partner or grabbed her/ him, if at all?" as opposed to a phrase such as, "... have you ever struck your wife/partner or grabbed her/him?" Of course, IPV is sometimes a two-way affair, and this approach can also uncover this process.

Ganley and Schnechter have delineated a series of questions that sensitively allows one to raise the topic of domestic violence. It provides the clinician with a gentle manner with which to explore the extent of violence with a victim. Yet it also elegantly employs the above strategy of first asking the patient – even if you are suspicious the patient might be the perpetrator of the IPV – if he or she has been a victim of IPV from his or her partner. Note that they begin this exploration through the use of a "normalization" and follow through with a heavy employment of fact-finding behavioral incidents[45]:

a. "All families disagree and have conflicts. I am interested in how your family resolves conflict. I am interested in how you and your partner communicate when upset."
b. "What happens when you or your partner disagree and your partner wants to get his/her way?"
c. "Have you ever been hurt or injured in an argument? Has your partner ever used physical force against you or anyone else or broken or destroyed property during an argument? Have you ever felt threatened or intimidated by your partner? How?"
d. "If your partner uses physical force against a person or property, tell me about one time that happened? Tell me about the worst or most violent episode? What was the most recent episode? Are you afraid of being harmed or injured?"
e. "Have you ever used physical force against your partner? If so, tell me about the worst episode. What was the most recent episode? Is your partner afraid of you?"

Even if there is little suspicion of violence in the initial interview, as Tardiff suggests, it should be routinely screened for with questions such as those above or even simple bridging questions such as, "Have you ever lost your temper?"[46] Once the topic of violence is raised, if violent thought or violent behavior is uncovered, one is ready to carefully explore the extent of the violence, searching for both stated intent and reflected intent. As with suicide assessment, the term "reflected intent" refers to feelings, thoughts, planning behaviors, and actions that suggest the possibility of impending violent behavior. Keep in mind that such thoughts and actions may better reflect the patient's real intent than what the patient states when directly asked questions such as, "Do you feel you will act on your violent thoughts?"

Chronological Assessment of Dangerous Events (the CADE Approach)

Please note that in order to understand the following section, the reader must first have read the information in the previous chapter on the Chronological Assessment of Suicide Events (the CASE Approach; see pages 722–757). To not do so, a reader risks being confused or, worse, misinterpreting the use of some of the following techniques.

Presenting Event

If the patient is brought in following a violent episode, the same principles that are used in exploring a presenting suicide attempt can be of use. Whether the patient is a perpetrator of domestic violence or some other type of violence, the clinician should guide the patient into a creation of a metaphorical "verbal video" through the use of a series of behavioral incidents. (Note that throughout Part 3, I am sometimes using a male-to-female act of violence as an example; women are often perpetrators of domestic violence as well.) Walk the perpetrator through the act of violence step by step. If he or she skips over an area, "rewind the video" and ask the patient to once again walk you through the incident: "Go back for a minute, Jim, to when you slapped your son, what happened next?" Be sure to clarify the actual acts of violence. If the patient says he hit his wife, ask him, "Did you use your fist, an open-hand, or any type of weapon?"

It is also important to understand the patient's motivation for the violence and how pre-planned, as opposed to impulsive, it may have been. It is very useful to explore the patient's feelings about the act of violence with simple and direct questions such as, "How do you feel about having hit your child?" and "How do you feel about your child now?" It is also important to find out what happened after the violence and how the patient ended up in front of you.

While delineating the verbal video, the severity of the violence should be carefully elicited using behavioral incidents to avoid the minimization so often seen by abusive or violent individuals. In this light, patient-opinion questions such as, "Did you hurt him/her badly?" are replaced with, "Did you leave any bruises?", "Did she/he need to go to an emergency room?", "Did she/he receive any stitches?" (ask how many), "Did she/he have any broken bones?", "Were X-rays taken?" All of these questions can help cut through minimization and denial. In this regard, the validity technique of symptom amplification may also be useful, such as with, "How many times did you actually strike Mary, 10 times, 20 times, 30?"

It is also useful to ask directly, "At any point, did you threaten to kill Jimmy (name of victim)?" I believe it is also useful to ask questions such as, "During your anger, were you ever afraid that you were out of control, because when people get this angry they often feel out of control at some point?" and "At any point, did the urge to kill your son cross your mind, even for an instant?" It is critical that these questions not be asked in a critical or judgmental fashion, but with a matter-of-fact genuine interest in what happened. After exploring this region thoroughly, the clinician smoothly moves into the region of recent violent activity.

Exploration of Recent Violent Events

This is an extremely important region in the violence assessment, and it covers the past 2 months. As stated earlier, a history of violence is a powerful predictor of future violence. A history of recent violent behavior may be an even more compelling predictor. This is especially true if the person of the intended violence has recently been assaulted by the patient, as is often the case in domestic violence, including IPV, child abuse, and the abuse of older adults.

The same consistent and persistent strategy used during the exploration of recent suicidal ideation and plans in the CASE Approach is also of use here. The emphasis is on uncovering the extent of actual planning and action that has been taken toward harming the potential victim in the past 2 months. This exploration is designed to uncover the methods of violence, the timing of the proposed or completed assault, the place of the assault, and whether or not accomplices were/are to be involved.

Naturally, as with the CASE Approach, there is no guarantee that our questioning will result in truthful answers, but these questions are designed to maximize the likelihood that it will. Some patients may be irritated or angered by such questioning, in which case the interviewer should back off and attend to engagement. At a minimum, although no more material about recent violent ideation may be garnered in that specific interview, the patient's response may suggest that violent ideation has been present.

As with suicide, once the concrete methods and circumstances are elicited, the clinician makes an effort to determine the frequency and intensity of the patient's violent thoughts. Questions such as the following may be of use: "How many times in the past 5 to 8 weeks have you been thinking about hurting Debbie, daily, couple times a day, more often?" (a variation of a symptom amplification) and "How close do you think you have come to actually hitting her?"

As we have started to see, when the clinician applies the CADE Approach to the assessment of recent violence, a heavy reliance is made upon the same validity techniques that were used in suicide assessment, including the behavioral incident, gentle assumption, denial of the specific, the catch-all question, and symptom amplification. Such interviewing can be quite difficult because of the emotional charge attached to it, especially if the clinician is in the presence of a particularly violent patient or a sexual predator. It is not an arena for the squeamish. Clinicians need to practice these techniques. Role-playing and group discussion of these approaches can be very useful.

As stated earlier, in an initial interview there exist situations in which a clinician, in my opinion, should give significant consideration to deferring such questioning to another clinician. For instance, if a female interviewer unexpectedly uncovers a sexual sadist whose victims are female, the details of this patient's violent history and recent thoughts concerning a potential act of violence are often best taken by a male clinician, and vice versa for a male interviewer if men are the patient's victims. If one feels uneasy during an interview, it is always okay to gently excuse oneself from the interview and consult with a colleague and/or supervisor about how to proceed. In fact, it is advisable to do so. If one is concerned about clinician safety, if available, safety officers should be contacted before anyone proceeds with the patient's assessment.

It is critical that the clinician explore the region of recent violent events with a matter-of-fact tone of voice and quiet confidence. When asked in a calm, straightforward manner, such questions sometimes result in surprisingly straightforward answers, particularly with a patient who has some guilt over his or her behaviors. Let's watch a demonstration of these techniques. Let us picture a patient who presents to the clinic secondary to depression. He has a pleasant affect and is dressed casually in shorts and a T-shirt. His age is 27, although he looks younger. A relatively recent stressor has been a break-up with his girlfriend, which was initiated entirely by her. The patient attributes much of his pain to this break-up. To the clinician's surprise, the patient relates some stalking behavior.

As the interview proceeds, keep your eye on the clinician's clever maneuvering as he attempts to make sure that enough information has been related about the intended victim, in order that she could be alerted by the police if Tarasoff's decision needs to be invoked:

Clin.: Timothy, when you say you've been following Judy around, what exactly do you mean? (behavioral incident)

Pt.: I … I … I sort of keep track of her, you know, where she's been, stuff like that.

Clin.: Is that easy to do, I mean does she live near you now? (behavioral incident)

Pt.: Yeah, she's still in the city. It ain't that hard.

Clin.: Do you follow her to work? (behavioral incident)

Pt.: Sometimes, but more like when she comes home.

Clin.: Now where does she work and how far is it from there to her home? I want to understand what it is really like for you, when you are following her. (behavioral incident)

Pt.: She's working at Clement's Pharmacy. She takes the subway home. It don't take her long. [Got it! If the patient's ex-girlfriend needs to be warned, there is now adequate information to find out who she is, in the necessity of a Tarasoff's warning. In this case, there is no indication that such a warning is needed yet. Later, after the violence assessment is done, the clinician will ask for the girlfriend's last name. But to do so now may "spook" the patient into withholding information, creating a potentially dangerous situation.]

Clin.: Now when you say that you follow her at home, what exactly do you mean? (behavioral incident)

Pt.: I wait to see if she's coming or going, see if she's with anyone.

Clin.: Do you ever look in her windows or use binoculars to look through the windows? (behavioral incident)

Pt.: Thought of it, but I've never done it.

Clin.: Do you ever take pictures of her or video her with your cell phone? (behavioral incident)

Pt.: No, I'm only interested in following her, you know, seeing her in the flesh.

Clin.: How many nights during the past month have you followed her, 10, 15, 20 times? (symptom amplification)

Pt.: I don't think that often. Maybe six, seven times.

Clin.: Are you thinking about hurting her when you follow her? (behavioral incident)

Pt.: No, I'd never hurt her.

Clin.: What are some of the reasons you think you follow her? (behavioral incident)

Pt.: I don't really know, I guess I miss her.

Clin.: Sounds like you really do. (pause) You know, what you're doing is called stalking. It's actually illegal. Do you feel like you need to stop?

Pt.: Sort of. I guess so.

Clin.: Maybe we could help you to stop (pause). Would you like that?

Pt.: Yeah.

Clin.: We'll take a look at that later. You know, earlier, you had told me that you had a sexual relationship with …

Pt.: Well, we didn't really have sex, I mean, we kissed a lot, but she wouldn't have sex with me.

Clin.: Okay, even so, sometimes after a break-up, people still have sexual thoughts about the other person (normalization); has that been true for you?

Pt.: Yeah.

Clin.: What type of sexual fantasies do you have about her? (gentle assumption)

Pt.: I just sort of think about having sex with her, you know, that kind of stuff.

Clin.: Do you masturbate to these fantasies sometimes? (behavioral incident)

Pt.: Oh yeah, I like to masturbate.

Clin.: When you masturbate to her, do you ever have fantasies of forcing sex on her? (behavioral incident)

Pt.: Sort of.

Clin.: What do you picture doing? (behavioral incident)

Pt.: I … I … I just sort of make her have sex with me.

Clin.: In your fantasies, do you ever use a weapon to do that?

Pt.: (looks uncomfortable) Sometimes I picture having a knife with me.

Clin.: I know this is very difficult material to talk about, Timothy, but you're doing a great job of explaining. I ask these questions so that I know what you're really feeling and if there is something you want help with, then I can help better. Getting back to the knife, do you ever picture cutting her with it? (behavioral incident)

Pt.: I have. (pauses) Not often though, I mean that. I'd never do it. I don't think it's right.

Clin.: I can see the idea of doing it upsets you. Maybe you'd like to get rid of some of these thoughts. When you have the fantasies about her, where do you cut her? (Behavioral incident – this is an attempt to more clearly delineate the degree of lethality of the fantasy material.)

Pt.: Oh man I don't want to talk about this. I really don't picture it very often. I would never do it. (The clinician decides to "back off" a bit so as not to lose the engagement with the patient.)

Clin.: When you follow her, do you ever carry a knife or any other weapons? (behavioral incident)

Pt.: Hell no. I'm not going to do anything to her. I'm just sort of mad at her, that's all. I've never hurt anybody in my life.

Clin.: Good. That's good to hear. Well, Timothy, how about other women? What have your relationships been like over the years?

Pt.: Well there haven't been many. I get mad about that too.

Clin.: What kind of fantasies about forcing sex have you had about other women, if any? (gentle assumption)

Pt.: Not a lot. But I have them, every once in awhile.

Clin.: Timothy, have you ever followed another woman, even for a short distance, ever? (behavioral incident)

Pt.: Never.

Clin.: Have you ever raped anybody, you know, forced sex on them? (behavioral incident)

Pt.: No. (pause) … Sometimes I worry about that though.

Clin.: How do you mean? (behavioral incident)

Pt.: Oh, you know, having these thoughts I've been talking about. I know they're not right. (patient looks uncomfortable)

Clin.: Are you okay talking about this stuff? I know it's hard to do.

Pt.: (sighs) Yeah, sort of. I almost feel better. I've never told anybody this stuff.

Clin.: I'm glad you can talk about it. Maybe we can get you some help to stop the thoughts. You mentioned that you know this is bad. I'm wondering what other kinds of sexual thoughts you may have had that you feel sort of bad about having? (gentle assumption) Now might be a good time to talk about them.

Pt.: Nothing, really.

Clin.: Do you buy porn magazines or look at porn on the web? (behavioral incident)

Pt.: Oh yeah. I masturbate to the pictures.

Clin.: Sometimes those magazines and websites have pictures that excite some people and turn off other people (variant of normalization). Do your magazines ever have pictures of children in them? (behavioral incident)

Pt.: Some of them.

Clin.: Do you look at them? (behavioral incident)

Pt.: Sort of, but they don't turn me on.

Clin.: Have you ever masturbated to them? (behavioral incident)

Pt.: (sheepish affect) A couple of times, but I really didn't get off on it that much.

The interview continues. This clinician is uncovering very important material, and there appears to be growing evidence that we may be in the presence of a predator or "predator in the making." Timothy's anger towards women is disturbing and certainly fits the profile of someone capable of rape. Obviously, pedophilia will need to be explored in much greater detail in future therapy.

The probability that Timothy has committed some type of sexual aggression is high, although he is currently denying it. The clinician is doing a good job of engaging Timothy, while gaining entrance to his very private and dark world. As the clinician wraps up this survey of potential sexually related crimes, he might opt to use a catch-all question to see if anything has been missed such as, "Timothy, you've done a great job of sharing very difficult material and we have talked about a lot of different things today; is there anything you've been doing that you're concerned might not be right, or is perhaps sexually unusual, because I could let you know exactly whether it is or isn't? That might be a relief to you."

I have provided a fairly extensive illustration here, because I find that training on uncovering violence, including sexual violence, is frequently under-emphasized in training programs across disciplines. This is somewhat surprising, because such interviewing must be done, at least occasionally, in most settings, from private practices to managed care clinics, college counseling centers, and community mental health centers. Obviously, it is a more frequent exercise in emergency rooms and inpatient units. Any person with a history of violence of any kind should be screened for sexual violence, and there exists a disturbingly high frequency of incest, rape, and pedophilia in general, often in people who have no other history of violence. Moreover, partner rape is a disturbingly common aspect of IPV.

While exploring the region of recent violence in a person who is currently committing domestic violence, keep in mind the power of symptom amplification for obtaining a more accurate picture of the frequency of the violence, which is usually minimized without this technique. For example, as mentioned earlier, a question such as, "How many times do you think you've hit her?" can become much more effective by adding "… 20 times, 40 times, maybe more?" This technique is also useful in disrupting minimization, while eliciting the frequency of acts of violence in the more distant past, which is our next topic of discussion.

Elicitation of Past Violent Events

As with the use of the CASE Approach for suicidal ideation, because of time constraints the clinician must be careful not to overdo this section in the initial assessment. On the other hand, this section warrants some explorations that are not necessarily used in suicide assessment because of the high correlation of future violence with a history of past violence. It is also during the review of past violence that the astute clinician may find some of the best evidence that he or she is in the presence of a predator, as opposed to a patient whose violence is triggered by affective charge or brain pathophysiology/structural damage.

Key elements for review include: (1) What is the worst act of violence? (2) Approximately how many acts of violence have occurred? (3) When was the most recent act of violence? (4) Has violence been done to anyone in the past against whom there is current violent ideation or fantasy? (5) Has a weapon been used in the past and, if so, is it being considered for use presently? (6) Is there an arrest history, jail history, and/or history of restraining orders related to violence?

With regard to uncovering the worst act of violence in the past, as was utilized in the presenting and recent history, the clinician can use a series of behavioral incidents to create a verbal video. As you walk the patient through the incident, be sure to elicit specific details, for they can illustrate the severity of the violence better than a patient's opinion such as, "Yeah, I hurt him pretty bad." Particularly severe violence should alert you to the potential dangerousness of the patient, and one can follow up in the next section of the CADE Approach to see if a similar act of violence is being currently thought about as the interview itself is unfolding.

Some questions about past acts of violence may help uncover predatory violence. Specifically, one is interested in seeing if the patient has much of a superego, which may show itself by the degree of guilt and shame the patient feels about past violence. In this regard, Meloy suggests exploring the patient's thoughts and feelings before, during, and after previous violent acts.[47] This gives a potential window into superego constraints and also whether or not violent thoughts "trouble" versus "arouse" the individual, the latter finding being more disturbing.

Two other useful questions along these lines are: "Is there anything you have done that has made you feel guilty?" and "If the price were right, is there anything you would not do?"[48] The presence of sociopathy and predatory process sometimes blossom with such questioning.

Predators and people with sociopathy are not beyond experiencing pride in what they do. Consequently, they can sometimes fall into admitting self-incriminating dangerous ideation through the use of an induction to bragging (see pages 164–165) as with, "Mick you seem very clever to me, you clearly know how to cover your tracks unusually well. If you could figure out how to rape one of the students at that college without getting caught, you know, a completely foolproof way, do you think you'd do it?" If he answers yes, the clinician simply follows up with, "What have you thought of doing?"

After exploring this region thoroughly, it is time for the clinician to bridge into an exploration of immediate violent ideation and intent.

Elicitation of Immediate Violent or Homicidal Ideation

As with suicidal ideation, the clinician asks about immediate violent ideation with a calm and non-judgmental tone of voice. Once again, this is no time to mince words, and, if an intended victim has been mentioned, the clinician should ask directly about his or her safety with questions such as, "Timothy, right now, are you planning on hurting or killing Judy?" Other useful questions include, "How well do you feel in control of your desires to attack Judy?", "After you leave here, do you think your thoughts about hurting Judy will return?", and "If you get any violent thoughts, what are you going to do about them?" Another important issue is whether or not the patient is intending to seek out the person with whom he or she is currently angry. One can feel slightly more comfortable if the patient says, "No, I need to stay away from her. I realize that," and means it. In contrast, comments such as, "I gotta at least talk to her. She's got to understand. I know she will," are far from reassuring.

Generally speaking, safety contracts, *utilized as assessment tools*, are, in my opinion, significantly less effective in this arena compared with their use as a suicide assessment tool. They may serve a purpose, as a means of assessment, with certain patients who you feel are truly upset by their violence. In contrast, with sociopaths and predators I feel they are of no use, for these patients have essentially no sense of guilt.

With regard to their use *as a deterrent* to violent behavior, safety contracts are even less effective than when used in suicide assessment. My personal opinion is that they are essentially worthless for this purpose. Obviously, with predators or sociopaths they are useless, for these patients are professional liars. Even with perpetrators of affective violence, they have no deterrent value, in my opinion. Keep in mind that many patients with affectively triggered violence, once they are in an angry exchange with the object of violence, all bets are off again, no matter what would have been genuinely intended in a safety contract.

With predators and people with antisocial structure, in most instances I believe the very act of safety contracting can often make one look naive and almost silly. Respect for the clinician can drop, as the predator silently thinks, "What a stooge." It is often much better to address the lack of trust with comments like, "Jim, I think both you and I know that from your history, I'd be very foolish to trust you – and I don't. That doesn't mean I don't want to help you, but it just means you've got to earn my trust, and vice versa. I would like to hear from you, as best you can, how dangerous you think you are right now." This type of candor may catch the predator off-guard and sometimes engages him or her in the sense that you are at least seen as a more worthy opponent.

In contrast to the suicide assessment, another thing that is different during the exploration of immediate violent ideation is the simple fact that the patient may assault you, not only while exploring this region but also at any time in the interview. The role of the patient's immediate mental status in predicting such an assault or the likelihood of imminent violence if released, is very important. Always be careful. Most assaults upon clinicians can be avoided, and the key is to think about safety at all times and to quit the interview if safety becomes an issue. If it crosses your mind that perhaps you are in danger, you should probably leave the room. Your intuition may be warning you of imminent assault.

Although clinicians have not shown outstanding accuracy at predicting short-term (weeks to months) violence, there is evidence that immediate violence can often be predicted. Solid predictors pretty well follow common sense and include items such as irritability, boisterousness, physical threats, verbal threats, attacks on material objects, and confusion.[49]

This last point emphasizes the need during an initial interview, especially in emergency departments, always to consider whether or not the person in front of you may become violent due to a biological cause. Keep alert for evidence of alcohol intoxication or street drug abuse, including alcohol on the breath, unsteady gait, slurred speech, dyscoordination, nystagmus, pupillary signs, and confusion. Such things as tremors, incontinence, abnormal eye movements, poor hygiene, cushingoid facies, and exophthalmos could all indicate an organic cause for violence.[50] Naturally, all violent patients in an emergency department require physical examination, testing of vital signs, and laboratory tests as medically indicated.

On a final note, regarding the use of the CADE in incest, once you have utilized the CADE Approach in relation to the principle child suspected of being abused by the perpetrator, it is important to find out if other children in the family have been molested. Gentle assumption can be particularly effective here as with, "Which of your other children have you had thoughts of having sex, even fleeting thoughts of doing so?" If the patient denies any such thoughts, I would consider using a denial of the specific regarding each child in the family, as with, "How about, Jackie, have you ever had any thoughts whatsoever about her?" These patients are so apt to lie and minimize their thoughts and actions, that denials of the specific can sometimes yield surprises, especially because you might spot nonverbal evidence of deceit as you inquire separately about each child.

CONCLUSION

If the above strategies have been skillfully employed, a rich database will often have been achieved, and the clinician will have essentially ended the assessment of violent ideation across all four chronological regions. Using this information plus the statistical risk factors gained from other regions of the interview and corroborative sources, the clinician can make his or her best clinical estimation of immediate or imminent violence. In the last analysis, a major limiting factor for the interviewer, as with suicidal ideation, remains the interviewer's own skill, tenacity, sensitivity, and intuition.

On a macro level, violence will probably be a lasting characteristic of human nature. As individual clinicians, we are limited in what we can accomplish in its elimination. But on a micro level, if we can utilize the techniques explored in this chapter to spot and prevent only one act of violence – whether domestic in nature, gang related, or psychotic-induced – we will have done a very good thing. If we use these tools over the course of our careers to prevent multiple acts of violence, we will have done a great thing. Our efforts will prevent not only the bruises and scars caused by violent actions, but the horrors and pains that lie in their wake, to which Dianne Feinstein so elegantly alluded in our opening epigram. We can shut the doors of our offices at the end of a day content to know that our efforts will have made the world a better place.

TRANSITIONAL DIRECTIONS TO PART IV: ADVANCED INTERVIEWING AND SPECIALIZED TOPICS

Please proceed to the ebook for Part IV of the text, where the following five bonus chapters and all appendices appear (directions for access to the ebook appear on the inside of the front cover of the book):

Chapter 19: Transforming Anger, Confrontation, and Other Points of Disengagement

Chapter 20: Culturally Adaptive Interviewing: The Challenging Art of Exploring Culture, Worldview, and Spirituality

Chapter 21: Vantage Points: Bridges to Psychotherapy

Chapter 22: Motivational Interviewing (MI): A Foundation Stone in Collaborative Interviewing

Chapter 23: Medication Interest Model (MIM): Moving from Mere "Adherence" to Genuine Interest and Effective Use

REFERENCES

1. Feinstein D. <http://www.pinterest.com/explore/domestic-violence-quotes/> [accessed March 2015].
2. Black M, Breiding M. Adverse health conditions and health risk behaviors associated with intimate partner violence – United States, 2005. *MMWR Morb Mortal Wkly Rep* 2005;**57**:113–17.
3. Snider C, Webster D, O'Sullivan CS, Campbell J. Intimate partner violence: development of a brief risk assessment for the emergency department. *Acad Emerg Med* 2009;**16**(11):1208–16.
4. Morrison LJ, Allan R, Grunfeld A. Improving the emergency department detection rate of domestic violence using direct questioning. *J Emerg Med* 2000;**19**:117–24.
5. Abbott J, Johnson R, Koziol-McLain J, Lowenstein SR. Domestic violence against women: incidence and prevalence in an emergency department. *JAMA* 1995;**273**:1763–7.
6. Hofner MC, Python NV, Martin E, et al. Prevalence of victims of violence admitted to an emergency department. *J Emerg Med* 2005;**22**:481–5.
7. Feldhaus KM, Koziol-McLain J, Amsbury HL, et al. Accuracy of 3 brief screening questions for detecting partner violence in the emergency room. *JAMA* 1997;**277**:1357–61.
8. Dearwater SR, Coben JH, Campbell JC, et al. Prevalence of intimate partner abuse in women treated at community hospital emergency departments. *JAMA* 1998;**280**:433–8.
9. Center for Disease Control and Prevention (CDC). *Data for 2014 from CDC website. WISQARS Leading Causes of Death Reports*. Available at <http://www.cdc.gov/injury/wisqars/leading_causes_death.html> [accessed May 2016].
10. Simon RI, Tardiff K, editors. *Textbook of violence assessment and management*. Washington DC: American Psychiatric Publishing, Inc.; 2008.
11. Mills JF, Kroner DG, Morgan RD. *Clinician's guide to violence risk assessment*. New York, NY: The Guilford Press; 2010.
12. Meloy R, Hoffman J. *International handbook of threat assessment*. New York, NY: Oxford University Press; 2013.
13. Meloy JR. The prediction of violence in outpatient psychotherapy. *Am J Psychother* 1987;**41**(1):38–45.

14. Tardiff K. *Assessment and management of violent patients*. Washington, DC: American Psychiatric Press; 1996. p. 127–35.
15. Monahan J. Structured risk assessment of violence. In: Simon RI, Tardiff K, editors. *Textbook of violence assessment and management*. Washington DC: American Psychiatric Publishing, Inc.; 2008. p. 17–34.
16. Rosenfeld B, Pivovarova E. Psychological testing in violence risk assessment. In: Simon RI, Tardiff K, editors. *Textbook of violence assessment and management*. Washington DC: American Psychiatric Publishing, Inc.; 2008. p. 59–74.
17. Monahan J, Steadman H, Silver E, et al. *Rethinking risk assessment: the macarthur study of mental disorder and violence*. New York, NY: Oxford University Press; 2001.
18. Monohan J, Appelbaum P. Reducing violence risk: diagnostically based clues from the MacArthur Violence Risk Assessment Study. In: Hodgins S, editor. *Effective prevention of crime and violence among the mentally ill*. Dordecht, the Netherlands: Kluwer Academic Publishers; 2000. p. 19–34.
19. Aegisdottir S, White MJ, Spengler PM, et al. The meta-analysis of clinical judgment project: fifty-six years of accumulated research on clinical versus statistical prediction. *Couns Psychol* 2006;**34**:341–82.
20. Lidz CW, Mulvey EP, Gardner W. The accuracy of predictions of violence to others. *JAMA* 1993;**269**:1007–11.
21. Lidz CW, Mulvey EP, Apperson LJ, et al. Sources of disagreement among clinicians' assessments of dangerousness in a psychiatric emergency room. *Int J Law Psychiatry* 1992;**15**:237–50.
22. Gardner G, Lidz CW, Mulvey EP, Shaw EC. Clinical versus actuarial predictions of violence in patients with mental illness. *J Consult Clin Psychol* 1996;**64**:602–9.
23. Mossman D. Assessing predictions of violence: being accurate about accuracy. *J Consult Clin Psychol* 1994;**62**:783–92.
24. Appelbaum PS, Roth LH. Assessing the NCSC guidelines for involuntary civil commitment from the clinician's point of view. *Hosp Community Psychiatry* 1988;**39**:406–10.
25. Blomhoff S, Seim S, Friis S. Can prediction of violence among psychiatric inpatients be improved? *Hosp Community Psychiatry* 1990;**41**:771–5.
26. McNeil DE, Binder RL, Greenfield TK. Predictors of violence in civilly committed acute psychiatric patients. *Am J Psychiatry* 1988;**145**:965–70.
27. Tardiff K. 1996. p. 130.
28. Tardiff K. 1996. p. 131.
29. Blomhoff S, et al.. 1990. p. 771–5.
30. *Diagnostic and statistical manual of mental disorders*. fifth ed, DSM-5. Washington DC: American Psychiatric Publishing; 2013. p. 467.
31. DSM-5. 2013. p. 466–7.
32. Webster C, Douglas K, Eaves D, Hart SD. *HCR-20: Assessing risk for violence (version 2)*. Vancouver, BC, Canada: Simon Fraser University; 1997.
33. Lake CR. Psychotic rampage murderers, part I: psychotic versus non-psychotic and a role for psychiatry in prevention. *Psychiatr Ann* 2014a;**44**(5):216–25.
34. Lake CR. 2014a. p. 219.
35. Lake CR. 2014a. p. 216.
36. Lake CR. 2014a. p. 218.
37. Lake CR. Psychotic rampage murderers: part II   psychotic mania, not schizophrenia. *Psychiatr Ann* 2014b;**44**(5):226–35.
38. Lake CR. 2014a. p. 223.
39. Lake CR. 2014a. p. 216–17.
40. Knoll J, Meloy R. Mass murder and the violent paranoid spectrum. *Psychiatr Ann* 2014;**44**(5):236–43.
41. Oregon DIIS. *Quick Reference Guide: Working with Domestic Violence, an excerpt from Child Welfare Practices for Cases with Domestic Violence*, 2011. <www.dhs.state.or.us/policy/childwelfare/manual_1/i-ab4att6.pdf> [accessed March 2015].
42. Washington State Administrative Office of the Courts. *DV Manual for Judges, 2006, B Appendices*. Adapted from Domestic Violence: A National Curriculum for Child Protective Services, 1996, written by Ganley AL, Schecter S. Available at <http://wscadv.org/resources/assessment-of-risk-posed-to-children-by-domestic-violence/> [accessed November 2015].
43. Snider C. 2009. p. 1212.
44. Appelbaum PS, Roth LH. 1988. p. 408.
45. Washington State Administrative Office of the Courts. *DV Manual for Judges*, 2006, Appendix B-7, Handout 4-4.
46. Tardiff K. 1996. p. 129.
47. Meloy JR. 1987. p. 41.
48. Hare RD. *The Hare PCL-R, interview and information schedule*. North Tonawanda, NY: Multi-Health Systems; 1990, 1991. p. 10.
49. Linaker OM, Busch-Iverson H. Predictors of imminent violence in psychiatric patients. *Acta Psychiatr Scand* 1995;**92**:250–4.
50. Reid WH. Clinical evaluation of the violent patient. *Psychiatr Clin North Am* 1988;**11**:527–37.

Part V

Specialized Topics and Advanced Interviewing

To the Reader

Part IV of the text appears in our e-book as 5 bonus chapters accompanied by the Appendices and Glossary (directions for access to the ebook appear on the inside of the front cover of the book)

Chapters

Appendices and Glossary

Group A: Articles for Clinicians and Trainees

- Havens L. Approaching the mind in clinical interviewing: the techniques of soundings and counterprojection. *Psychiatr Clin North Am* 2007;**30**(2):145–56.

- Murray-Swank A, Dixon LB, Stewart B. Practical interview strategies for building an alliance with the families of patients who have severe mental illness. *Psychiatr Clin North Am* 2007;**30**(2):167–80.

- Josephson AM, Peteet JR. Talking with patients about spirituality and worldview: practical interviewing techniques and strategies. *Psychiatr Clin North Am* 2007;**30**(2):181–97.

Group B: Articles for Faculty and Interviewing Mentors

- Shea SC, Green R, Barney C, et al. Designing clinical interviewing training courses for psychiatric residents: a practical primer for interviewing mentors. *Psychiatr Clin North Am* 2007;**30**(2):283–314.

- Shea SC, Barney C. Facilic supervision and schematics: the art of training psychiatric residents and other mental health professionals how to structure clinical interviews sensitively. *Psychiatr Clin North Am* 2007;**30**(2):e51–96.

- Shea SC, Barney C. Macrotraining: a "how-to" primer for using serial role-playing to train complex clinical interviewing tasks such as suicide assessment. *Psychiatr Clin North Am* 2007;**30**(2):e1–29.

- Shea SC, Barney C. Teaching clinical interviewing skills using role-playing: conveying empathy to performing a suicide assessment – a primer for individual role-playing and scripted group role-playing. *Psychiatr Clin North Am* 2015;**38**(1):147–83.

Glossary of Interview Supervision Terms

Index

Page numbers followed by *"f"* indicate figures, *"t"* indicate tables, *"b"* indicate boxes, and *"e"* indicate online content.